Compliments of

 Bristol-Myers Squibb Company

HOSPITAL
AND
INSTITUTIONAL
SALES GROUP

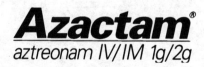

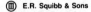

The Handbook of Surgical Intensive Care

Practices of the Surgical Residents at the Duke University Medical Center

Third Edition

H. KIM LYERLY, M.D.
Assistant Professor of Surgery and Pathology
Duke University Medical Center
Durham, North Carolina

J. WILLIAM GAYNOR, M.D.
Chief Resident
General and Cardiothoracic Surgery
Duke University Medical Center
Durham, North Carolina

M Mosby
Year Book

St. Louis   Baltimore   Boston   Chicago   London   Philadelphia   Sydney   Toronto

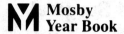

Mosby Year Book

Dedicated to Publishing Excellence

Sponsoring Editor: Nancy E. Chorpenning
Associate Managing Editor, Manuscript Services: Deborah Thorp
Production Coordinator: Nancy C. Baker
Proofroom Manager: Barbara Kelly

4   5   6   7   8   9   0 CL/MA 96   95   94   93

NOTICE
Every effort has been made to ensure that the drug dosage schedules herein are
accurate and in accord with the standards accepted at the time of publication.
However, as new research and experience broaden our knowledge, changes in
treatment and drug therapy occur. Therefore, the reader is advised to check the
product information sheet included in the package of each drug he plans to administer
to be certain that changes have not been made in the recommended dose or in the
contraindications. This is of particular importance in regard to new or infrequently
used drugs.

Library of Congress Cataloging-in-Publication Data

The Handbook of surgical intensive care : practices of the surgical
  residents at the Duke University Medical Center / [edited by] H. Kim
Lyerly, J. William Gaynor.—3rd ed.
     p.   cm.
  Includes bibliographical references and index.
  ISBN 0-08-151254-6
  1. Surgical intensive care—Handbooks, manuals, etc.   I. Lyerly,
H. Kim.   II. Gaynor, J. William.
  [DNLM] 1. Critical Care—handbooks.   2. Postoperative care—
-handbooks.   3. Preoperative care—handbooks.   WO 39 H23571
RDB1.5.H36   1991
617'.919—dc20
                                                         91-33631
                                                            CIP

This edition is dedicated to David C. Sabiston, Jr., M.D., professor, teacher, and role model. As chairman of the Department of Surgery, his unique contributions, generosity and tireless efforts on behalf of the residents in surgery, past and present, at the Duke University Medical Center are acknowledged with gratitude and high esteem.

CONTRIBUTORS

All contributors are from the Duke University Medical Center, Durham, North Carolina.

Terence J. Boyle, B.Sc., FRCSI
International Research Fellow, General and Cardiothoracic Surgery

Gene D. Branum, M.D.
Senior Assistant Resident, General and Cardiothoracic Surgery

William C. Brown, M.D.
Chief Resident, Plastic, Reconstructive and Maxillofacial Surgery

Louis A. Brunsting, M.D.
Teaching Scholar in Cardiothoracic Surgery, General and Cardiothoracic Surgery

Thomas D. Christopher, M.D.
Teaching Scholar in Cardiothoracic Surgery, General and Cardiothoracic Surgery

Nancy J. Crowley, M.D.
Senior Assistant Resident, General and Cardiothoracic Surgery

Samuel M. Currin, M.D.
Chief Resident, Urology

Robin G. Cummings, M.D.
Chief Resident, General and Cardiothoracic Surgery

Thomas A. D'Amico, M.D.
Research Fellow, General and Cardiothoracic Surgery

Andrew M. Davidoff, M.D.
Research Fellow, General and Cardiothoracic Surgery

R. Duane Davis, Jr., M.D.
Senior Assistant Resident, General and Cardiothoracic Surgery

Joseph R. Elbeery, M.D.
Senior Assistant Resident, General and Cardiothoracic Surgery

Gregory P. Fontana, M.D.
Senior Assistant Resident, General and Cardiothoracic Surgery

Herbert E. Fuchs, M.D.
Chief Resident, Neurosurgery

Stanley A. Gall, Jr., M.D.
Research Fellow, General and Cardiothoracic Surgery

J. William Gaynor, M.D.
Chief Resident, General and Cardiothoracic Surgery

Robert C. Harland, M.D.
Senior Assistant Resident, General and Cardiothoracic Surgery

Jeffrey S. Heinle, M.D.
Senior Assistant Resident, General and Cardiothoracic Surgery

Scott H. Johnson, M.D.
Senior Assistant Resident, General and Cardiothoracic Surgery

J. Scott Kabas, M.D.
Senior Assistant Resident, General and Cardiothoracic Surgery

Allan D. Kirk, M.D.
Research Fellow, General and Cardiothoracic Surgery

H. Kim Lyerly, M.D.
Assistant Professor, Surgery and Pathology

George M. Maier, M.D.
Teaching Scholar in Cardiothoracic Surgery, General and Cardiothoracic Surgery

James R. Mault, M.D.
Research Fellow, General and Cardiothoracic Surgery

Charles E. Murphy, M.D.
Teaching Scholar in Cardiothoracic Surgery, General and Cardiothoracic Surgery

Mark D. Plunkett, M.D.
Senior Assistant Resident, General and Cardiothoracic Surgery

Scott K. Pruitt, M.D.
Research Fellow, General and Cardiothoracic Surgery

Cemil M. Purut, M.D.
Research Fellow, General and Cardiothoracic Surgery

Robert L. Quigley, M.D.
Chief Resident, General and Cardiothoracic Surgery

Lewis B. Schwartz, M.D.
Research Fellow, General and Cardiothoracic Surgery

Mark W. Sebastian, M.D.
Research Fellow, General and Cardiothoracic Surgery

Phillip P. Shadduck, M.D.
Senior Assistant Resident, General and Cardiothoracic Surgery

Michael A. Skinner, M.D.
Chief Resident, General and Cardiothoracic Surgery

Craig L. Slingluff, Jr., M.D.
Chief Resident, General and Cardiothoracic Surgery

Dean C. Taylor, M.D.
Chief Resident, Orthopaedic Surgery

Mark Tedder, M.D.
Research Fellow, General and Cardiothoracic Surgery

Douglas S. Tyler, M.D.
Senior Assistant Resident, General and Cardiothoracic Surgery

Charles D. Veronee, M.D.
Cardiac Fellow, Anesthesiology

Christopher R. Watters, M.D.
Chief Resident, General and Cardiothoracic Surgery

Ronald J. Weigel, M.D., Ph.D.
Senior Assistant Resident, General and Cardiothoracic Surgery

FOREWORD

It is astonishing how rapidly the fame of the second edition of the *Handbook of Surgical Intensive Care: Practices of the Surgery Residents at the Duke University Medical Center* edited by H. Kim Lyerly, has spread throughout the United States, Canada, South America, and Europe. Further convincing evidence of this spectacular record is the fact that this *Handbook* is currently being translated into both Spanish and German, which will greatly enhance its impact worldwide. In the *foreword* to the last edition, it was emphasized that the success of the *Handbook* was predictable in view of the remarkable capabilities of the editor, who prepared a work with emphasis on every detail. With this approach, the management of many clinical problems that arise in surgical intensive care units was carefully presented. Dr. Lyerly's keen commitment to the last edition has established this *Handbook* as the finest in the field.

In this third edition, Dr. J. William Gaynor, Chief Resident in Surgery and a member of the Cardiothoracic Surgical Residency Program, was chosen as the co-editor. His achievements provide much evidence that he is also an extraordinary young academic surgeon who is thoroughly committed to the principle that hard work is the key to success. Drs. Gaynor and Lyerly have extensively revised this edition with a number of new contributors and a thorough update of every chapter.

With the increasing complexity of patients in *surgical intensive care units,* it is essential to remain abreast of the most recent contributions in a rapidly changing and advancing field. This is a unique text since it is written *by* residents *for* residents, and each contributor has drawn upon extensive personal experience gained from the teaching rounds, conferences, and care rendered to patients in the surgical intensive care units at the Duke University Medical Center. Most important have been the personal observations of these contributors while working with patients in the units with 60 beds devoted solely to surgical intensive care in this hospital. The residents gain a thorough and in-depth experience from a wide variety of surgical problems, not only in general and cardiothoracic surgery, but those in neurosurgery, orthopaedics, otolaryngology, pediatric surgery, plastic and maxillofacial surgery, and urology as well.

One of the most meaningful rewards of the program director of a Surgical Residency Training Program is the achievements made by the *residents*. In this *Handbook* the editors and their colleagues have provided an extraordinary text that is clearly a *masterwork* in surgical intensive care. Among the most objective criteria of the significance of any text is its usage, and it is amazing that some 40,000 copies of the *second edition* have been printed, emphasizing its spectacular reception both in this country and abroad. Having read the contents of this current edition, it can be confidently predicted that it will actually exceed the astonishing record of its predecessor.

David C. Sabiston, Jr., M.D.
Chairman, Department of Surgery
Duke University Medical Center
Durham, North Carolina

PREFACE TO THE SECOND EDITION

It is readily apparent that an increasing number of complex surgical procedures are performed on patients who were not considered operative candidates in years past. This is due in large part to advances in perioperative management. Therapeutic, diagnostic, and supportive measures have advanced rapidly and a fundamental knowledge of each is a requisite for optimal management of surgical patients. Furthermore, the American Board of Surgery has emphasized that surgical residents must obtain the knowledge and skills to optimally manage the patient in the perioperative period, which includes postoperative care in the intensive care unit. Consequently Drs. Warren J. Kortz and Philip D. Lumb produced *Surgical Intensive Care: A Practical Guide*. This extremely usable text provided a concise and practical guide to the management of patients in the intensive care unit and was extensively used not only by the surgical house staff at Duke University Medical Center but at many training programs. However, as five years have passed since the first edition was published, a number of advances in critical care medicine and surgery have occurred. Therefore, it became clear that a revised and updated version of the manual was needed. Appropriate emphasis has been retained on providing a practical guide written by surgical residents with experience in the intensive care unit. Surgical considerations in the intensive care unit are stressed throughout each section, with special emphasis on patient management following major procedures.

Members of the surgical house staff at Duke University Medical Center have compiled the following second edition of *The Handbook of Surgical Intensive Care: Practices of the Surgery Residents at the Duke University Medical Center*. Its production was made possible only through the efforts and support of the previous editors. Although much of the text has been revised, the philosophy of a handbook for surgical intensive care has been maintained. From the preface to the first edition: "Surgical intensive care is titrated care and the knowledge of more experienced individuals should always be sought when dealing with multiple systems failure and the necessity to decide which organ system should be titrated against which pharmacologic intervention. This can be accomplished by careful attention to detail and by therapeutic management based on sound physiologic principles."

The information in this manual, although reflecting the opinions and experiences of the authors, should be used as a guide and utilized at the discretion of the physician in charge of each individual patient.

H. Kim Lyerly, M.D.

PREFACE TO THE THIRD EDITION

Care of the patient in the surgical intensive care unit has become increasingly complex and technologically oriented. Progress in therapeutic, diagnostic, and supportive measures has made complex surgical procedures possible today for patients who would not have been operative candidates just a few years ago. These rapid advances in technology have also led to the introduction of a variety of new therapeutic modalities, such as extracorporeal membrane oxygenation (ECMO) and devices for mechanical ventricular assistance.

The Handbook of Surgical Intensive Care: Practices of the Surgery Residents at the Duke University Medical Center is designed to provide a practical guide to the increasingly complex environment of the intensive care unit. Surgical considerations in the intensive care unit are stressed throughout each chapter, with a special emphasis on patient management in the perioperative period. A significant part of the educational experience of surgical training is provided by residents teaching residents. In this tradition, *The Handbook of Surgical Intensive Care* is a guide written by residents for residents. The goal of the authors is to organize practical knowledge useful in the intensive care unit with an emphasis on fundamental physiology.

The Handbook of Surgical Intensive Care has been extensively revised to reflect the increasingly rapid rate of change in technology and critical care medicine. New sections in this third edition include left ventricular assist devices, ECMO, pediatric surgery, and anesthesia.

The information in this manual, although representing the judgment and experience of the authors, should be viewed as suggestions and utilized at the discretion of the physician based upon the

needs of each individual patient. While every effort has been
made to ensure that recommended drug dosages are accurate,
product information should be double-checked prior to administration to ensure accuracy.

H. Kim Lyerly, M.D.
J. William Gaynor, M.D.

ACKNOWLEDGMENTS

This manual represents the information thought by each contributor to be most useful in the management of patients in the surgical intensive care unit. The enthusiasm of each of the authors was a critical component in this project and is gratefully acknowledged.

Several people reviewed portions of the text for its completeness and factual accuracy; we thank them for their efforts. These individuals include Herbert Chen, Kelly A. Alexander, Jennifer Parker, Eric Lillie, and W. Ben Vernon, M.D. Word processing for much of the manuscript was provided by Jane Delionbach, whose efforts are appreciated.

The chairman of the Department of Surgery at the Duke University Medical Center, Dr. David C. Sabiston, Jr., continues to set high standards for the house staff, and only with his support is the continuing production of this text possible. We thank him sincerely for his efforts on behalf of the editors and the contributors alike.

Nancy Chorpenning continues to play an increasingly supportive role in the development of these editions. Her guidance and assistance in the production of this book are gratefully acknowledged. We also thank Nancy Baker and Deborah Thorp for their efforts.

The support of the families of the authors is deeply appreciated, for it was their understanding and encouragement that allowed this work to be realized.

H. Kim Lyerly, M.D.
J. William Gaynor, M.D.

CONTENTS

LIST OF ABBREVIATIONS

AAA	abdominal aortic aneurysm
ABC	airway, breathing, circulation
ABG	arterial blood gas
ACE	angiotensin converting enzyme
ACS	American College of Surgeons
ACT	activated clotting time
ACTH	adrenocorticotropic hormone
ADH	antidiuretic hormone
ADP	adenosine diphosphate
AHA	American Heart Association
ALG	antilymphocyte globulin
APTT	activated partial thromboplastin time
ARF	acute renal failure
ARDS	adult respiratory distress syndrome
ASD	atrial septal defect
AT-III	antithrombin III
ATG	antithymocyte globulin
ATN	acute tubular necrosis
ATP	adenosine triphosphate
ATPase	adenosine triphosphatase
BP	blood pressure
BPH	benign prostatic hypertrophy
BUN	blood urea nitrogen
CAD	coronary artery disease
CaO$_2$	arterial oxygen content
CBC	complete blood count
CHF	Congestive heart failure
CI	cardiac index
CMR	cerebral metabolic rate
CMV	cytomegalovirus controlled mechanical ventilation

CO	cardiac output
COPD	chronic obstructive pulmonary disease
CPB	cardiopulmonary bypass
CPK	creatine phosphokinase
CRF	chronic renal failure
CSF	cerebrospinal fluid, colony stimulating factor
CVA	cerebrovascular accident
C$\bar{v}O_2$	mixed venous oxygen content
CVP	central venous pressure
CXR	chest x-ray
DI	diabetes insipidus
DIC	disseminated intravascular coagulation
DKA	diabetic ketoacidosis
DM	diabetes mellitus
DO$_2$	tissue oxygen delivery
2,3-DPG	2,3-diphosphoglycerol
DVT	deep vein thrombosis
EACA	epsilon-aminocaproic acid
EBV	Epstein-Barr virus
ECF	extracellular fluid
EDP	end-diastolic pressure
EDTA	ethylenediaminetetraacetic acid
EDV	end-diastolic volume
EF	ejection fraction
EFA	essential fatty acid
EMD	electromechanical dissociation
ERCP	endoscopic retrograde cholangiopancreatography
ESR	erythrocyte sedimentation rate
ET	end-tidal
FDP	fibrin/fibrinogen degradation products
FFA	free fatty acid
FFP	fresh frozen plasma
F$_I$O$_2$	fractional concentration of oxygen in inspired gas
GABA	γ-aminobutyric acid
GFR	glomerular filtration rate
GU	genitourinary
Hct	hematocrit
HIDA	lidofenin
HMW	high-molecular-weight
HR	heart rate

HSV	herpes simplex virus
HTLV	human T-cell lymphotropic virus
IVP	intravenous pyelogram
IABP	intraaortic balloon pump
ICP	intracranial pressure
IL	interleukin
IMA	inferior mesenteric artery
IMV	intermittent mandatory ventilation
I/O	input/output
IP	intraperitoneal
IPPB	intermittent positive pressure breathing
IVC	intravenous catheter
ITP	idiopathic thrombocytopenic purpura
JVD	jugular venous distention
KUB	kidney, ureter, bladder
LA	left atrium
LBBB	left bundle-branch block
LDH	lactate dehydrogenase
LFT	liver function test
LUQ	left upper quadrant
MAOI	monoamine oxidase inhibitor
MAP	mean arterial pressure
MAST	medical anti-shock trousers
MOFS	multiple organ failure syndrome
MOPP	methotrexate, Oncovin (vincristine), prednisone, procarbazine
MR	mitral regurgitation
MTX	methotrexate
MVR	mitral valve replacement
Nd:YAG	neodynium:yttrium-aluminum-garnet
NSAID	nonsteroidal anti-inflammatory agent
OR	operating room
PA	pulmonary artery; postereroanterior
$P(A-a)O_2$	arteriolar-arterial oxygen pressure difference
PaO_2	arterial oxygen partial pressure
$PaCO_2$	arterial carbon dioxide partial pressure
PCA	patient controlled analgesia
PCWP	pulmonary capillary wedge pressure
PE	pulmonary embolism
PEEP	positive end-expiratory pressure

PEG	percutaneous endoscopic gastrostomy
PFT	pulmonary function test
PG	prostaglandin
PIP	peak inspiratory pressure; proximal interphalangeal
PMI	point of maximal impulse
PMN	polymorphonuclear leukocyte
PND	paroxysmal nocturnal dyspnea
P$_{osm}$	plasma osmolality
PPD	purified protein derivative
PRBCs	packed red blood cells
PT	prothrombin time
PTA	percutaneous transluminal angioplasty
PTC	percutaneous transhepatic cholangiogram
PTH	parathyroid hormone
PTT	partial thromboplastin time
PVR	peripheral vascular resistance
PVC	premature ventricular contraction
RA	right atrium
RBBB	right bundle-branch block
RBC	red blood cell
RIA	radioimmunoassay
RNA	radionuclide angiocardiogram
R/O	rule out
RUQ	right upper quadrant
RV	residual volume; right ventricle
SAH	subarachnoid hemorrhage
SaO$_2$	saturation with oxygen, arterial blood
SBE	subacute bacterial endocarditis
SGOT	serum glutamic-oxaloacetic transaminase
SGPT	serum glutamic-pyruvic transaminase
SIADH	syndrome of inappropriate secretion of antidiuretic hormone
SLE	systemic lupus erythematosus
SMA	superior mesenteric artery
SV	stroke volume
SVC	stroke volume curve
SvO$_2$	saturation of hemoglobin with oxygen, mixed venous blood
SVR	systemic vascular resistance

SVT	supraventricular tachycardia
T$_3$	triidothyronine
T$_4$	thyroxine
TBG	thyroxine-binding globulin
^{99m}Tc DTPA	techetium 99m pentetate
TCT	thrombin clotting time
TIA	transient ischemic attack
TIBC	total iron-binding capacity
t-PA	tissue plasminogen activator
TPN	total parenteral nutrition
TRH	THYROTROPIN releasing hormone
TSH	thyroid stimulating hormone
TT	thrombin time
TTP	tissue thromboplastin
UO	urinary output
U$_{osm}$	urine osmolality
UPJ	ureteropelvic junction
UTI	urinary tract infection
V$_E$	exhaled minute volume
VF	ventricular fibrillation
V$_I$	inhaled minute volume
VSD	ventricular septal defect
V$_T$	tidal volume
VZV	varicella zoster virus
WBC	white blood cell

INTRODUCTION TO SURGICAL INTENSIVE CARE

1

I. **SURGICAL INTENSIVE CARE UNIT (SICU) ADMISSION.**

A. **Introduction.**

The SICU is that area of the hospital outside of the operating room (OR) where maximum personnel and technologic support are available to the patient. Not every surgical patient requires or benefits from intensive care. However, the support and interventions practicable in the SICU are absolutely essential to the survival of certain patients. The surgeon should decide if a patient would benefit from SICU admission from the emergency department, OR, or surgical ward.

B. **Admission Evaluation.**

The type of patient dictates the degree of monitoring and intervention required (Table 1–1). However, certain general considerations are applicable to all SICU admissions.

1. History.
   a. Diagnosis and operation.
   b. Anesthesia—agent and dosage.
   c. Intraoperative hemodynamic course.
   d. Blood loss.
   e. Blood and fluid replacement.
   f. Urine output.
   g. Intraoperative laboratories.
   h. Previous operations.
   i. Previous or chronic illness.
   j. Allergies.
   k. Preoperative medications.
   l. Bleeding disorders.

TABLE 1–1.

Reason for Admission Into SICU

Elective

Following complex operation or traumatic event (e.g., CABG, AAA, craniotomy, liver transplant).

Intensive nursing care required (e.g., burn, trauma, COPD, streptokinase infusion).

Monitoring and observation required.

Generally physiologically stable, even if chronic illness exists.

Mortality reflects physiologic reserve.

Emergent

Constant physical intervention required (e.g., postoperative MI with shock, respiratory insufficiency requiring intubation, GI hemorrhage with shock, S/P cardiac arrest).

Physiologically unstable.

Survival related to cardiorespiratory integrity and patient's capacity to respond to existing stress.

2. Physical examination.
   a. VS—baseline weight, temperature, BP, HR, rhythm.
   b. CNS—level of consciousness, orientation; movement of all extremities should be constantly reassessed, especially in a patient who is admitted with a depressed level of consciousness.
   c. Skin—color, mottling, piloerection.
   d. HEENT—pupils, NG and ET tube placement.
   e. Neck—JVD, central line placement.
   f. Chest—heart and lung sounds.
   g. Abdomen—girth, bowel sounds, NG tube placement.
   h. Extremities—skin color, temperature, pulses, movement, IV placement.
   i. Surgical dressing and drains—type, blood staining, or other output.
3. Baseline studies.
   a. ABC, electrolytes, creatinine, glucose, PT/PTT, UA, Ca, Mg, ABG.
   b. Portable CXR.
   c. ECG, 12-lead.
   d. Cardiac isoenzymes if indicated.

4. Documentation.
    a. ET tube placement, cuff inflation, ventilator settings, bilateral breath sounds.
    b. Indwelling catheters.
    c. Arterial line—waveform, evidence of distal arterial insufficiency.
    d. Pulmonary arterial line—waveform, location on CXR, balloon inflation.
    e. ECG monitor—rhythm.
    f. Drains.
    g. Chest tubes—location on CXR.
5. Admission orders.
    Example of SICU admission orders of complex patient.
    a. Admit—to SICU.
    b. S/P resection and grafting thoracoabdominal aortic aneurysm.
    c. Condition—stable.
    d. Diet—npo.
    e. Activity—bed rest, turn, cough q.h.
    f. Vital signs—continuous.
    g. Monitor:
        1) In and outs.
        2) Daily weights.
        3) Dextrostick q.6h.
        4) ECG, continuous.
        5) Arterial line—continuous pressure, flush q.2h.
        6) PA catheter—temperature, CO, and pressure q.h., continuous mixed venous O_2 saturation.
        7) Urine output q.h.
        8) Peripheral pulses q.h.
        9) Cutaneous O_2 monitor.
    h. IV—D5LR at 150 mL/hr.
    i. Medications.
        1) Morphine 1–4 mg IV q. 15 min prn.
        2) Sodium nitroprusside 250 mg in 250 mL NS through central line for BP > 160 mm Hg.
        3) Dopamine 250 mg in 250 mL NS at 5 μg/kg/min through central line.
        4) Cefazolin sodium (Ancef) 1 g IV q.6h. × three doses.

    j. Ventilator.
       1) Mode—IMV.
       2) FiO_2—50%.
       3) Tidal volume—1,000 mL.
       4) Respiratory rate—12/min.
       5) PEEP—5 cm H_2O.
    k. Drains.
       1) NG to low continuous wall suction; replace cc = cc with D5 ½ NS + 30 mEq KC1/L.
       2) Foley catheter to gravity drainage.
       3) Chest tube to 20 cm H_2O suction via PleurVac.
    l. Laboratory studies q.6h.
       1) ABC.
       2) ABG.
       3) Serum electrolytes, creatinine, glucose.
       4) PT/ PTT.
       5) UA.
       6) Ca^{2+}.
       7) Mg^{2+}.
       8) Cardiac isoenzymes.
    m. Portable CXR—R/O pneumothorax, check ET tube, CVP, and PA line placement.
    n. 12-lead ECG—R/O ischemia.

II. TRANSFER TO THE SICU.

Patients are often transferred to the SICU not only from the OR or ward but also from other institutions for definitive or long-term care. In the intrahospital transfer of unstable patients from the ward to the SICU, it is often most effective to transfer the patient as rapidly as possible. Although considerations regarding optimal timing for elective transfer are based on the nature of the disorder, certain factors are generally considered.

A. Preparation of Patient.

1. Replete intravascular volume if possible.
2. Optimize cardiac status.
3. Ventilation.
    a. Have an adequate supply of supplemental oxygen.
    b. Secure ET tube, if intubated.
    c. Careful attention to manual ventilation required to avoid significant blood gas alterations which might lead to hypotension or dysrhythmias.

4. Immobilize fractures and patients with possible neurologic injury.
5. Monitor:
   a. ECG.
   b. Arterial pressure.
   c. Pulse oximeter.
6. Communication.
   a. Confirm that SICU is ready to receive patient.
   b. Discuss with the receiving physician the patient's current status, clinical course, and active problems.
   c. All pertinent medical records should accompany the patient.

B. Interhospital Transport.
1. Indications.
   a. Need for more appropriate facilities or services.
   b. Major trauma (as defined by American College of Surgeons)
      1) Combined system injury.
      2) Open fracture.
      3) Uncontrolled hemorrhage.
      4) Blunt abdominal trauma with hypotension.
      5) Neurologic injuries—unconsciousness, posturing, paralysis.
      6) Severe maxillofacial injuries.
      7) Unstable chest injuries.
      8) Pelvic fractures.
      9) Penetrating abdominal wounds.
      10) Severe head, neck, and upper respiratory tract injuries.
   c. Critical burns.
   d. Amputations in potential replant candidates.
2. Contraindications.
   a. Adequate care available locally.
   b. Lack of personnel for safe travel.
   c. Patient not optimally stabilized (not always possible).
3. Preparation for transport—In addition to the guidelines mentioned previously, patients who are to be transported long distances, in confined spaces, and by air have additional considerations.
   a. Adequate IV access.
   b. Arterial catheter for pressure monitoring.

  c. Urinary catheter to monitor adequacy of volume replacement.
  d. NG tube for patient with ileus or altered mental status.
  e. Chest tube for any pneumothorax.
  f. Type-specific blood if available.
  g. Admission serum sample.
  h. Severed body parts in saline-moistened gauze inside a watertight container placed on ice.
 4. Special considerations for high-altitude transport.
  a. Have an adequate O_2 supply. The P_{O_2} at high altitudes may be half that at sea level.
  b. Decompress all trapped gas with chest tubes, NG tubes, drainage, etc. from the thorax, bowel, cranial vault, e.g., since gas expands with increasing altitude (Boyle's law).
  c. Monitor closely other sites of trapped gas such as ET tube cuff, MAST trousers, or air splints, for the same reason.
  d. Be aware of possible intracranial or intravascular fluid redistribution due to acceleration during transport.

III. DETERMINANTS OF PATIENT SURVIVAL IN SICU.
A. Introduction.
Various factors affect critically ill patients who require intensive care: The likelihood of survival for many different groups of patients can be approximated based upon these factors. This enables physicians to have a more realistic expectation of the outcome for a patient and allows for a more informed discussion of the severity of a patient's condition with the family. Quality control can be assured by comparing actual patient outcomes to those predicted, based on the determinants of survival. Limited medical resources can be directed toward those patients whom they would most benefit. However, the decision to deny or withdraw support should be made only following individualized patient assessment and not based solely on scoring systems designed to stratify illness severity. This is especially true as critical care expertise improves.

B. Scoring Systems.
 1. Acute physiology and chronic health evaluation (APACHE) (Table 1–2).

a. This system quantifies the severity of an acute illness based on:
   1) The weighted sum of 12 physiologic measurements.
   2) The age of patient.
   3) The chronic health of a patient.
2. Therapeutic intervention scoring system (TISS) (Table 1–3).
   a. This system classifies the severity of illness based upon the intensity of medical treatment by assigning points to 57 various therapeutic interventions.
3. System outcome scores (SOS) (Table 1–4).
   a. This system incorporates five objective components in a weighted sum that reflects the likelihood of death during hospital admission.

C. Other Important Factors.
1. Multiple organ failure—Patients with signs of decompensation of more than one organ system have the highest SICU mortality; the failure of multiple organs has a synergistic effect on outcome.
2. Cancer—Mortality in the SICU is not affected but these patients have a significant 1-year mortality rate following discharge.

D. Survival (Table 1–5).
These scoring systems attempt to quantify the severity of illness and predict outcome based on easily obtainable patient variables. They are based on retrospective statistical analyses of multiple factors and patient outcomes. These systems have limitations, however, resulting in significant false-classification rates. Unpredictable or unique events are frequently the only determinants of survival and many factors, excluded in the interest of simplicity, can affect survival. In addition, these systems were originally intended to assess medical patients and have not been validated for surgical patients. The systems are useful for obtaining a general appreciation for the severity of illness of an SICU patient and provide insight into those factors which are, in general, important in determining a patient's survival (Table 1–5).

TABLE 1–2.
APACHE II Severity of Disease Classification System*

Physiologic Variable	High Abnormal Range					Low Abnormal Range			
	+4	+3	+2	+1	0	+1	+2	+3	+4
Rectal temperature (°C)	≥41°	39.0°–40.9°		38.5°–38.9°	36.0°–38.4°	34.0°–35.9°	32.0°–33.9°	30.0°–31.9°	≤29.9°
Mean arterial pressure (mm Hg)	≥160	130–159	110–129		70–109		50–69		≤49
Heart rate (ventricular response)	≥180	140–179	110–139		70–109		55–69	40–54	≤39
Respiratory rate (nonventilated or ventilated)	≥50	35–49		25–34	12–24	10–11	6–9		≤5
Oxygenation									
$FiO_2 \geq 0.5$ (record P(A-a)O_2 [mm Hg])	≥500	350–499	200–349		<200				
$FiO_2 < 0.5$ (record only PaO_2 [mm Hg])					>70	61–70		55–60	<55
Arterial pH	≥7.7	7.60–7.69		7.50–7.59	7.33–7.49	7.25–7.32		7.15–7.24	<7.15
Serum Na (mmol/L)	≥180	160–179	155–159	150–154	130–149		120–129	111–119	≤110
Serum K (mmol/L)	≥7	6.6–9.0		5.5–5.9	3.5–5.4	3.0–3.4	2.5–2.9		<2.5
Serum creatinine (mg/dL) (double point score for ARF)	≥3.5	2.0–3.4	1.5–1.9		0.6–1.4		<0.6		
Hematocrit (%)	≥60		50.0–59.9	46.0–49.9	30.0–45.9		20.0–29.9		<20
WBC count (10^3/mm^3)	≥40		20.0–39.9	15.0–19.9	3.0–14.9		1.0–2.9		<1
Glasgow coma scale (GCS) score (score = 15 – actual GCS score)									

Age Points

Assign points to age as follows:

Age (yr)	Points
≤44	0
45−54	2
55−64	3
65−74	5
≥75	6

Chronic health points

If the patient has a history of severe organ system insufficiency or is immunocompromised assign points as follows:

a. For nonoperative or emergency postoperative patients— 5 points.

b. For elective postoperative patient— 2 points.

Definitions: Organ insufficiency or immunocompromised state must have been evident prior to this hospital admission and conform to the following criteria:

Liver: Biopsy-proven cirrhosis and documented portal hypertension, episodes of past upper GI bleeding attributed to portal hypertension, or prior episodes of heptic failure, encephalopathy, or coma.

Cardiovascular: NYHA class IV.

Respiratory: Chronic restrictive, obstructive, or vascular disease resulting in severe exercise restriction, i.e., unable to climb stairs or perform household duties, or documented chronic hypoxia, hypercapnia, secondary polycythemia, severe pulmonary hypertension (>40 mmHg), or respirator dependency.

Renal: Receiving chronic dialysis.

Immunocompromised: The patient has received therapy that suppresses resistance to infection, e.g. immunosuppression, chemotherapy, radiation, long-term or recent high-dose steroids, or has a disease that is sufficiently advanced to suppress resistance to infection, e.g., leukemia, lymphoma, AIDS.

*From Knaus WA, Draper EA, Wagner DP, et al: *Crit Care Med* 1985;13:818. Used by permission.

TABLE 1–3.

Therapeutic Intervention Scoring System (TISS)*

4 Points
  Cardiac arrest and/or countershock within 48 hr
  Controlled ventilation with or without PEEP
  Controlled ventilation with intermittent or continuous muscle relaxants
  Balloon tamponade of varices
  Continuous arterial infusion
  PA line
  Atrial or ventricular pacing
  Hemodialysis in unstable patient
  Peritoneal dialysis
  Induced hypothermia
  Pressure-activated blood infusion
  G suit
  Measurement of cardiac output
  Platelet transfusions
  Intra-aortic balloon assistance
  Membrane oxygenation
3 Points
  Hyperalimentation or renal failure fluid
  Pacemaker on standby
  Chest tubes
  Assisted respiration
  Spontaneous PEEP
  Concentrated K drip (>60 mEq/L)
  Nasotracheal or orotracheal intubation
  ET suctioning (nonintubated patient)
  Complex metabolic balance (frequent intake and output, Brookline scale)
  Multiple ABG, bleeding and STAT studies
  Frequent infusions of blood products
  Bolus IV medications
  Multiple (>3) parenteral lines
  Vasoactive drug infusion
  Continued antiarrhythmia infusions
  Cardioversion
  Hypothermia blanket
  Peripheral arterial line
  Acute digitalization
  Active diuresis for fluid overload or cerebral edema
  Active treatment for metabolic alkalosis or acidosis
2 Points
  CVP
  > 2 IV lines
  Hemodialysis for chronic renal failure
  Fresh tracheostomy (<48 hr)

Spontaneous respiration via ET tube or tracheostomy
Tracheostomy care
1 Point
ECG monitoring
Hourly VS or neuro-VS
"Keep open" IV route
Chronic anticoagulation
Standard intake and output
Frequent STAT chemistries
Intermittent IV medications
Multiple dressing changes
Complicated orthopedic traction
IV antimetabolite therapy
Decubitus ulcer treatment
Urinary catheter
Supplemental O_2 (nasal or mask)
IV antibiotics

*From Cullen DJ, Civetta JM, Briggs BA, et al: Therapeutic intervention scoring system: A method for quantitative comparison of patient care. *Crit Care Med* 1974; 2:57.

TABLE 1–4.

System Outcome Score (SOS)*

Component	Points
Vasopressor use	1.50
$Fio_2 > 0.5$	1.00
Oliguria	2.00
Coagulopathy	1.75
GCS score <5	3.75

*From McFee AS, Gilbert J: The outcome index: A method of quality assurance in the special care area. *Arch Surg* 1989; 124:825.

TABLE 1–5.

Predicted Mortality Based on Scoring Systems

System	Mortality				
	10%	15%	20%	35%	75%
APACHE	0–15	15–19	—	20–30	>30
TISS	5	11	23	—	43
SOS	0–2.75	—	3.0–4.75	—	5.0–0.75

IV. PREPARATION OF THE SICU PATIENT FOR OPERATION.

A. Volume Status (see Chapter 2).

1. Blood loss.
   a. Generally, 10 g hemoglobin/100 mL plasma are required prior to general anesthesia.
   b. Acute hemorrhage.
      1) Compensated for by increasing stroke volume and HR, mechanisms which are poorly tolerated on a chronic basis.
      2) Need to rapidly restore plasma volume.
      3) Correct hemoglobin concentration deficit more slowly: 1–2 units packed RBCs per day if time permits.
   c. Chronic anemia.
      1) Decreased RBC volume is compensated for by increasing plasma volume to maintain normal total blood volume.
      2) Generally, better tolerated than acute blood loss, even to a hemoglobin as low as 7 g/100mL.
2. Extravascular fluid deficits.
   a. Measurable losses—vomiting, NG suction, fistula or ileostomy output, diarrhea.
   b. Insensible and third-space losses—long bone fracture, burns, intestinal obstruction.
3. Assessment.
   a. VS—tachycardia, tachypnea, and hypotension suggest significant volume loss (> 40% total blood volume).
   b. Urine output—monitored with an indwelling catheter, this is the best measure of volume status in patients with normal renal function (desired minimal output is 0.5 mL/kg/hr).
   c. Skin turgor, mucous membranes, hematocrit, and BUN-creatinine ratio are late indicators of volume depletion.
4. Correction.
   a. Use isotonic solutions to first restore circulating volume as rapidly as possible and then correct electrolyte abnormalities.
   b. Overly rapid correction of hypovolemia in patients

with cardiovascular compromise may result in pulmonary edema.

B. Nutrition (see Chapter 12).
  1. Normal daily requirements.
     a. Protein—1.5 g/kg.
     b. Fat—2 g/kg.
     c. Carbohydrate—2 g/kg.
  2. Acute increase in metabolic needs increases requirements, e.g., trauma, sepsis, fever, thyrotoxicosis.
  3. Chronic malnutrition—poor intake, external losses (high intestinal fistulas, extensive surface burns, inflammatory bowel disease, protein-losing enteropathies), cancer cachexia, hypermetabolic states, short-bowel syndrome.
  4. Assessment.
     a. Weight loss of 10%–35% greatly impairs host defense mechanisms and wound healing.
     b. Weight loss >35% is life-threatening.
  5. Correction.
     a. Hyperalimentation—exceed basal requirements plus abnormal losses. Usually 7–10 days of hyperalimentation are required to be clinically beneficial.
     b. Route—enteral (preferred) or parenteral.
     c. Vitamins—both water-soluble and fat-soluble.
     d. Goal—restoration of recent weight loss and lean body mass prior to surgery, if possible, or at least achieve anabolic state.

C. Specific Organ Systems
  1. Cardiovascular (see Chapter 5).
     a. Myocardial infarction (MI).
        1) There is a significantly increased operative risk in patients who have suffered an MI within the previous 3 months.
        2) Elective procedures should be delayed at least 6 months.
     b. Atherosclerosis.
        1) Significant vascular disease at any site warrants careful cardiac evaluation.
        2) Patients with known heart disease should have maximal myocardial protection with consideration of coronary vasodilators, β-blockers, and CABG in certain situations.

    c. Congestive heart failure.
        1) Etiology should be identified (myocardial ischemia, valvular disease, dysrhythmias, hypertension, sepsis, hyperthyroidism) and treated.
        2) Optimal volume status should be established (preoperative PA pressure monitoring may be necessary).
    d. Hypertension
        1) Be sure that all preadmission medications are being continued.
        2) Systolic BP must be < 200 mm Hg prior to operation.
        3) Consider prazosin (Minipress) or clonidine. May need IV nitroprusside for hypertensive crisis.
2. Pulmonary (see Chapter 7).
    a. Pneumonia.
        1) Infections should be adequately treated with antibiotics before elective surgery.
        2) CXR, sputum, and WBC count should be assessed.
    b. Insufficiency.
        1) Severity should be documented with spirometry and ABG.
        2) Status should be optimized preoperatively with cessation of smoking, postural drainage, and instruction on coughing and deep breathing.
        3) Bronchodilators or steroids may be of benefit.
3. Renal (see Chapter 9).
    a. Bacteriuria.
        1) Can usually be treated by a single dose of antibiotics if there are no signs of upper tract infection or obstruction.
        2) Culture should be performed for postoperative antibiotic guidance, if needed.
        3) Sterilization of urine should be confirmed prior to planned use of prosthetic material.
    b. Volume status.
        1) Assess and optimize as described above.
        2) Patients requiring dialysis should be dialyzed the day prior to operation.

  c. Electrolyte abnormalities (see Chapter 10).
    1) Detect on routine preoperative laboratory studies and correct prior to surgery.
    2) Attention should be paid to preoperative medications and electrolyte disturbances they might cause.
  d. Chronic failure.
    1) If suspected, based on routine studies, creatinine clearance can be calculated to assess glomerular filtration and free water clearance to check tubular function.
    2) Careful adjustments of volume status and medications are required.
 4. Hepatic (see Chapter 11).
  a. Cirrhosis.
    1) Adjust dosages of medications and anesthetics for hepatic insufficiency.
    2) Correct coagulation abnormalities with fresh frozen plasma or vitamin K, if time permits.
    3) Significant operative risk is associated with liver failure patients.
 5. Immunologic (see Chapter 17).
  a. Anergy.
    1) Increased risk of infection.
    2) Impaired wound healing.
    3) May improve with improved nutrition.
  b. Neutropenia may require antibiotic prophylaxis.
 6. CNS (see Chapter 13).
  a. Altered mental status.
    1) More difficult to assess physical findings.
    2) Patient cannot communicate complaints or note changes in symptoms.
    3) Recent change requires evaluation prior to elective surgery.

D. Medications (see Chapter 23).
 1. Continue necessary preadmission medications.
 2. Preparation for surgery.
  a. General—antibiotic prophylaxis, bowel preparation, SBE prophylaxis, insulin adjustment.
  b. Specific—steroid prophylaxis (to avoid adrenal insufficiency), catecholamine blockade (for pheochromocy-

       toma), thyroid suppression (to avoid storm), immuno-
suppression (prior to transplant).

  c. Vasoactive drugs should be continued, as required.

  d. Anticoagulation—Patients taking warfarin sodium
(Coumadin) for prosthetic heart valves or other reasons should be converted to IV heparin. This can be
discontinued 6 hours preoperatively and restarted in
the postoperative period.

  e. TPN should be discontinued but D10W solution
should be given to avoid rebound hypoglycemia.

  3. Anesthetic premedications.

    a. Sedation.

    b. Tranquilization.

    c. Anticholinergics.

    d. Antihistamines.

SELECTED REFERENCES

Civetta JM, Hudson-Civetta JA, Nelson LD: Evaluation of
APACHE II for cost containment and quality assurance. *Ann
Surg* 1990; 212:266.

Cullen DJ, Civetta JM, Briggs BA, et al: Therapeutic intervention scoring system: A method for quantitative comparison of
patient care. *Crit Care Med* 1974; 2:57.

Jewell ER, Persson AV: Preoperative evaluation of the high-risk
patient. *Surg Clin North Am,* 1985; 65:3.

Knaus WA, Draper EA, Wagner DP, et al: APACHE II—A
severity of disease classification system. *Crit Care Med* 1985;
13:818.

McFee AS, Gilbert J: The outcome index: A method of quality
assurance in the special care area. *Arch Surg* 1989; 124:825.

HEMODYNAMIC MANAGEMENT

2

I. CARDIAC PHYSIOLOGY.

A thorough understanding of basic cardiac physiology is a prerequisite for the intelligent management of the critically ill patient. Cardiovascular management should **optimize myocardial performance and tissue perfusion at the lowest possible energy** cost in terms of myocardial O_2 consumption.

A. Cardiac Anatomy.

1. Basic anatomy and circulation.

   a. The heart is best understood as two separate volume pumps in series. The right atrium (RA) and right ventricle (RV) make up a low-pressure "bellows"-type pump while the left atrium (LA) and left ventricle (LV) make up a pressure-type pump. The in-series nature of these two pumps implies that the output of the right heart becomes the input of the left heart, and therefore the output of the left heart becomes the input of the right heart.

   b. Desaturated blood returning from systemic vessels to the RA via the two venae cavae is displaced passively and actively, by atrial contraction, through the tricuspid valve into the RV. Contraction of the RV ejects desaturated blood through the pulmonic valve into the low-pressure PA and subsequently through the pulmonary capillaries where gas exchange occurs. Blood saturated with O_2 is then returned to the LA where it is displaced passively and actively, via atrial contraction into the LV. LV contraction ejects blood through the aortic valve into the high-pressure aorta perfusing the coronary arteries, brain, kidneys, abdominal viscera, and extremities.

2. Myocardial blood flow.

   a. **Myocardial perfusion occurs primarily during dias-**

tole and is provided by the right and left coronary arteries which are the first branches of the aorta and arise from the sinuses of Valsalva.
b. The right coronary artery (RCA) generally supplies the RV free wall, sinus node, and atrioventricular (AV) node. In 90% of patients the RCA terminates as the posterior descending artery (right coronary dominance).
c. The left main coronary artery gives rise to the left anterior descending (LAD) and circumflex coronary arteries. The LAD is *usually* the largest of the coronary arteries and supplies the anterior and apical LV, the majority of the interventricular septum, and the left margin of the RV. The circumflex coronary artery supplies the lateral LV and in 10% of patients provides the posterior descending coronary artery (left coronary dominance).
d. The venous drainage of the heart occurs mainly via the coronary sinus which drains into the RA. Drainage also occurs via the anterior cardiac veins as well as thebesian and sinusoidal channels. Total coronary blood flow is normally 0.7–0.9 mL/min/g myocardium.

B. Biochemistry of Myocyte Contraction.
1. The heart converts chemical energy in the form of O_2 and substrate into mechanical energy in the form of circulatory pressure and flow. At the cellular level, electrical depolarization of the myocardial cell membrane allows ionized calcium flux into the cytoplasm, causing hydrolysis of ATP by myosin. This leads to a conformational change in the actin-myosin cross-bridge, producing sliding of myosin filaments relative to actin and shortening of the sarcomere (Fig 2–1). Calcium is then removed from the cell by active transport in the sarcoplasmic reticulum allowing relaxation, and ATP is regenerated by aerobic metabolism.
2. It appears that, over the physiologic range of sarcomere length (1.6–2.0 μm), the amount of metabolic energy converted to mechanical work is dependent on the surface area of available cross-bridge interactions and, therefore, directly proportional to end-diastolic sarcomere length. **The length dependency of cross-bridge interactions at the sarcomere level constitutes the fundamental basis for the Frank-Starling law.**

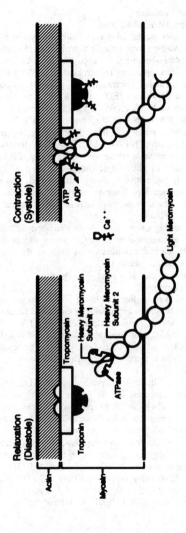

FIG 2–1.
Actin and myosin interaction with Ca^{2+} control of contractile proteins in cardiac muscle. (From Merin RG: *J Cardiac Surg* 1990; 5:266. Used by permission.)

C. Basic Cardiac Function.

1. Preload recruitable stroke work.

   a. In the experimental laboratory, plots of dynamic pressure vs. volume over a single heart beat yield characteristic pressure-volume (PV) loops (Fig 2–2,A). The area of each loop represents the stroke work (SW) produced by that particular contraction. At constant preload or end-diastolic volume (EDV) the PV loops are superimposed on each other. When EDV is decreased or increased, SW output or the area of the PV loop decreases or increases in a linear fashion (Fig 2–2,B).

   b. The relationship between SW and EDV, termed the *preload recruitable stroke work relationship* (PRSW) is independent of physiologic changes in afterload and is inherently insensitive to changes in preload. The slope of the relationship, however, increases with increasing inotropic state, signifying increased SW output at a constant preload.

   c. Based on this knowledge, a systematic approach to the cardiac management of the SICU patient can be undertaken by careful examination of each of the determinants of cardiac output (CO).

2. Determinants of cardiac output.

   a. Cardiac output.

   CO is defined as the amount of blood pumped by the heart per unit time and is usually expressed in liters per minute. Normal cardiac output is 3.5–8.5 L/min and is determined by four factors: **preload, afterload, heart rate (HR), and inotropic state.** Each can be separately manipulated to improve myocardial performance.

   b. Preload

   1) At the cellular level, preload is defined as end-diastolic sarcomere length, which is linearly related to EDV. The inability to monitor ventricular volume on a continuous basis in the SICU setting, however, makes this parameter impractical.

   2) LV end-diastolic pressure (LVEDP) represents the distending (filling) pressure of the ventricle and has been used as an index of EDV (preload). However, the relationship between LVEDP and EDV is exponential (Fig 2–2,B), not linear. LA pressure (LAP) correlates with LVEDP in normal hearts and is

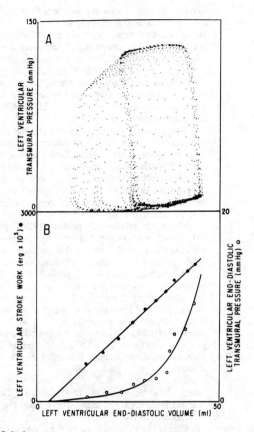

FIG 2–2.
A, pressure-volume loops during a vena caval occlusion. The area of each loop corresponds to the SW produced. **B,** the preload recruitable SW relationship *(straight line)* reveals the linear relationship between SW and EDV. Also illustrated is the exponential nature of the end-diastolic PV relationship.

therefore the closest approximation of preload available for continuous monitoring in the SICU. LAP can be measured directly by using an LA catheter.

3) In clinical practice, monitoring of pulmonary capillary wedge pressure (PCWP) is commonly utilized as an index of LAP and LVEDP. PCWP is a reflection of pulmonary venous and, hence, LAP. However, because of the exponential relationship between LVEDP (and thus PCWP) and EDV, PCWP is a less than optimal index of preload.

4) At filling pressures above 15–18 mm Hg, the ventricle operates on the very steep portion of the diastolic compliance curve, where further increments in PCWP produce very little change in EDV and little increase in CO (see Fig 2–2,B). Therefore, filling pressures should usually not be allowed to exceed this limit because of potential detrimental effects on cardiopulmonary performance.

5) In addition, **the relationship between PCWP and EDV is not constant** but is affected by changes in LV compliance, wall thickness, HR, ischemia and some medications. Clinically this implies that a PCWP which corresponds to a given EDV at one point in time may not correspond to the same EDV later as conditions change (Fig 2–3). Thus absolute values of PCWP are difficult to interpret and even trends in PCWP may be unreliable.

6) Right-sided filling pressures or the central venous pressure (CVP) have been utilized to estimate LV preload, but may be an unreliable index in critically ill patients.

c. Afterload.
1) Afterload can be defined as impedance to LV ejection and is usually estimated by the systemic vascular resistance (SVR).

a) Changes in afterload have no effect on the contractility of a normal heart. Thus, the SW performed for a given EDV is insensitive to changes in SVR.

b) The impaired ventricle represents a different situation, however, in which increasing afterload

CARDIAC MONITORING

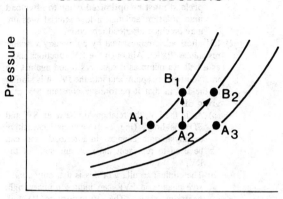

FIG 2–3.
A family of diastolic PV curves for the LV. A measure of LVEDP may represent quite different states of LV filling depending on compliance (A_1, A_2, A_3). Also, an increase in PAoP may indicate either a change in LV compliance without any change in LV filling (A_2/B_1) or may indicate a true increase in LV filling (A_2/B_2). (From Raper R, Sibbald W: *Chest* 1986; 89:427. Used by permission.)

                may decrease the SW output for a given EDV and thus impair myocardial performance.

    c) When faced with this clinical situation, afterload reduction therapy, usually with sodium nitroprusside (SNP) or use of the intra-aortic balloon pump (IABP), may increase CO by reducing the impedance to LV ejection.

    d) Decreasing afterload exchanges pressure work for flow work and serves to increase vital organ perfusion. Moreover, since pressure work is more costly than flow work in terms of myocardial O_2 consumption, decreasing afterload decreases myocardial energy requirement.

   e) It is important to keep in mind, however, that
      **preload must be optimized prior to afterload
      manipulation** and that a low arterial pressure
      may preclude afterload reduction.
2) RV afterload is represented by pulmonary vascular
   resistance (PVR). Although the RV functions more
   as a bellows pump as it squeezes blood against the
   interventricular septum and into the PA, it is similar
   to the LV in that it performs a constant SW at a
   given EDV.
   a) As in the LV, the relationship between SW and
      EDV is linear (Fig 2–4), appears insensitive
      to physiologic changes in afterload, and can
      be used to represent the inotropic state of the
      RV.
   b) The clinical corollary of this is that only a *massive* change in PVR can induce primary right
      heart dysfunction. The vast majority of RV failure is secondary to LV failure and generally re-

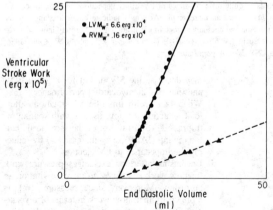

PRELOAD RECRUITABLE STROKE WORK RELATIONSHIPS

Ventricular
Stroke Work
(erg x 10^5)

- LV M_w = 6.6 erg x 10^4
▲ RV M_w = .16 erg x 10^4

End Diastolic Volume
(ml)

FIG 2–4.
Preload recruitable SW relationships of LV and RV.

    sponds to measures designed to improve LV performance.

  c) Isolated RV failure is rare but may result from massive pulmonary embolism, isolated RV infarction, or extremely high postoperative PVR secondary to severe COPD.

  d) In primary RV failure, PA perfusion results from the RV acting as "conduit" rather than a pump; therefore, RV preload should be adjusted to higher levels with vigorous volume infusion and a CVP ≥ 20 mm Hg may be required.

  e) The second line of therapy involves augmentation of RV contractility with simultaneous PVR reduction. Dobutamine or amrinone have both been advocated for this situation.

 3) Rarely, primary RV failure may be encountered in the postcardiotomy or postcardiac transplant patient. Some patients have been successfully managed with infusions of PGE_1 into the PA, with LA infusions of norepinephrine to counteract the systemic vasodilator effects. This regimen requires an LA catheter and is therefore reserved for postcardiac surgery patients.

d. Heart rate.

HR may influence cardiac function in a number of ways.

 1) Increasing the contraction frequency limits diastolic filling time, coronary perfusion time, and reduces EDV.

 2) Increasing rate increases the work output from the ventricle per unit time at a given EDV. Thus, increasing the HR can be considered an inotropic intervention.

 3) As would be expected, increasing the HR also increases myocardial O_2 consumption, an important consideration when attempting to optimize myocardial performance in the critically ill patient.

 4) The decreased length of diastole also decreases the time for coronary blood flow and may adversely affect coronary perfusion.

 5) The postoperative CABG patient with revascularized coronary arteries may be safely paced at HR of

100–110 bpm to increase CO. However, in the patient with known or suspected uncorrected coronary artery disease, pacing must be carefully instituted in order to avoid increased myocardial O_2 consumption and diminished coronary blood flow which might result in myocardial ischemia and worsening cardiac performance.

6) Brachycardia may significantly decrease CO and should be corrected as necessary with atropine, isoproterenol, or cardiac pacing.

e. Inotropic state.

1) Contractility is defined as an *intrinsic* property of myocardium which is manifest as a greater force of contraction for a given preload.

2) In terms of pressure and volume, the ventricle performs the same SW for a given EDV when inotropic state is held constant. When the inotropic state is augmented, more SW is produced at the same EDV.

3) Clinically, this translates into increased CO and mean arterial pressure (MAP) at a given filling pressure. Since both pressure work and flow work are increased with inotropic stimulation, the cost in myocardial O_2 consumption may be high.

4) There is evidence to suggest that an increased inotropic state may lead to a delay in recovery of function following myocardial ischemic injury. Therefore, **inotropic agents should be used with caution and only after preload, afterload, and HR have each been optimized.**

II. CARDIAC MONITORING.

A. Introduction.

Monitoring of critically ill patients has become increasingly invasive and complex. Invasive monitoring techniques provide insight into pathophysiology and allow accurate evaluation of therapeutic interventions. Nevertheless, noninvasive methods remain important. Frequent measurement of vital signs and repeated physical examination form the basis for all hemodynamic monitoring. It is important to avoid overreliance on technology as there is no substitute for calculated clinical decisions by experienced practitioners.

1. All data should be recorded on a flow sheet at the patient's bedside including vital signs, daily weight, fluid balance, and laboratory data, allowing early recognition of deterioration or improvement in the patient's status.
2. All patients should undergo continuous ECG monitoring of cardiac rate and rhythm. Modern systems can signal tachycardias, bradycardias, and various arrhythmias, including ventricular tachycardia, ventricular fibrillation, and asystole. Some systems also allow storage of recordings for later analysis.
3. **Changes in mental status, respiratory pattern, or peripheral perfusion may indicate impending shock, sepsis, or respiratory failure.** All critically ill patients should have frequent reassessment of neurologic status, respiratory patterns, urinary output, peripheral perfusion, etc. Examination of heart, lungs, and abdomen should also be performed.
4. Chest Radiography.
   a. A daily CXR should be obtained in all patients with endotracheal (ET) tubes or PA catheters and all patients who have undergone cardiac or noncardiac thoracic surgical procedures.
   b. A CXR is indicated in all patients in whom a deterioration of the clinical status has occurred to exclude problems such as pneumonia, congestive heart failure (CHF), and pneumothorax.
   c. A CXR must be obtained following ET intubation or placement of central venous catheters to assure proper positioning of all tubes and catheters.

B. Arterial Pressure.
Arterial pressure may be measured by a variety of invasive and noninvasive techniques and there may be a large discrepancy in the measured value in the same patient depending on the technique utilized.
1. Indirect measurement of arterial pressure.
   a. Auscultation.
      The auscultatory method (Riva-Rocci) utilizing a sphygmomanometer and stethoscope is the most commonly utilized technique. Flow in the large arteries is laminar and silent; however, a partial occlusion will produce turbulent flow which is audible. Auscultation over an occluded artery as the cuff is slowly released al-

lows determination of the pressure at which flow begins.

1) Pressure is usually measured in the brachial artery. It is important to use a BP cuff of the proper size (bladder length of at least 80% of arm circumference and cuff width of at least 40% of arm circumference). If the cuff is too small, the measured pressure will be falsely elevated. If the cuff is too large, the measured pressure will be falsely low.

2) The stethoscope is placed over the brachial artery and the cuff inflated to completely occlude the artery. The cuff is then slowly deflated (3 mm Hg/sec). The appearance of a "tapping" (Korotkoff) sound indicates the systolic pressure. The diastolic pressure is usually taken as the point at which the Korotkoff sounds muffle. Some authorities recommend defining diastolic pressure at the point of disappearance of Korotkoff sounds.

3) The BP must be measured in both arms in every patient. **A difference in systolic pressure > 15 mm Hg may indicate an obstructive arterial lesion or an aortic dissection.**

4) In patients with severe aortic regurgitation, the Korotkoff sounds may persist to 0 mm Hg. The diastolic pressure is then taken at the point of muffling of the sounds.

5) The arterial BP varies with respiration so that the systolic pressure falls with inspiration. Normally, this fall should be less than 10 mm Hg. **A difference of greater than 10 mm Hg is termed** *pulsus paradoxicus* **and may indicate cardiac tamponade or severe respiratory distress.**

6) The Riva-Rocci method measures blood flow and not true BP. In low-flow states, such as cardiac failure, hypovolemic shock, or pronounced vasoconstriction, the auscultatory method may be inaccurate. For example, in severe vasoconstriction secondary to norepinephrine infusion the directly measured BP may be very high, but actual blood flow is diminished and, as a result, the Korotkoff sounds are inaudible and a falsely low arterial pressure is obtained. In patients in whom these factors may be

active, direct measurement of BP should be obtained.

7) In some patients the Korotkoff sounds completely disappear between systolic and diastolic pressures, resulting in an auscultatory gap, and a falsely low systolic pressure might be assumed. This error can be avoided by inflating the BP cuff to 30 mm Hg above the pressure at which the radial pulse can no longer be palpated to assure complete occlusion of the artery.

8) Systolic BP can also be estimated by palpating the radial pulse, as the cuff is deflated, and noting the pressure at which the pulse can first be palpated. This method may underestimate the true systolic pressure but is useful when a quick rough estimate is sufficient. A handheld Doppler ultrasonic flow probe can be used to estimate the systolic pressure by listening for the onset of blood flow as the occluding cuff is deflated.

b. Automatic measuring devices.

1) A variety of automated devices for noninvasive measurement of arterial pressure are available and utilize an oscillometric technique. An automatic cuff placed around the upper arm is inflated and then slowly deflated. Pressure fluctuations in the brachial artery cause pulsations in the cuff pressure allowing determination of systolic and diastolic pressures. The same phenomenon also causes fluctuations in the mercury column when a sphygmomanometer is used to determine BP. Instruments are available which utilize a microphone to sense the audible turbulent flow as the cuff is deflated.

2) In stable patients, these devices are relatively accurate for measurement of MAP and can provide reasonable estimates of systolic and diastolic pressures. However, they are less accurate than the auscultatory or direct methods in hypotensive or unstable patients.

2. Direct measurement of arterial pressure.

a. In critically ill patients, it is often necessary to obtain continuous accurate monitoring of the arterial BP. **Indications for the use of direct BP monitoring include**

hemodynamic instability, use of vasoactive drugs (dopamine, norepinephrine, SNP, etc.) and intraoperative monitoring of selected patients. Direct measurement requires placement of an intraarterial catheter which is generally safe but may be associated with significant complications (Chapter 22).

b. Cannulation site.
  1) The radial artery is the usual site for cannulation. The hand is perfused by both the radial and ulnar arteries. The ulnar artery is dominant and communicates in most patients with the radial artery through deep and superficial palmar arches.
  2) Prior to cannulation of the radial artery, the patency of the ulnar artery must be demonstrated using the modified Allen's test. If the Allen's test is positive, another site of arterial cannulation should be chosen.
  3) In patients with severe atherosclerosis, Raynaud's disease, or other vasospastic diseases, cannulation of the radial artery must be carefully considered as ischemic necrosis of the hand has been reported.
  4) Alternate cannulation sites include the femoral artery, dorsalis pedis artery, axillary artery, and brachial arteries, although each of these sites is associated with complications (see Chapter 22).

c. Flush system.
  The catheter should be connected to a system (utilizing saline, not a dextrose-containing solution) which provides a continuous flush to the catheter at 3–5 mL/hr (Fig 2–5). The system should also allow intermittent flush boluses of 3–5 mL. Overly vigorous flushing of the system should be avoided as retrograde cerebral embolization can occur. Heparinized flush should also be avoided as heparin-induced thrombocytopenia and arterial thrombosis have been reported with even minimal exposure to heparin.

d. Transducing system.
  The transducing system converts the pressure transmitted by the fluid-filled catheter to an electronic signal (see Fig 2–5). Most errors in direct measurement of arterial pressure result from difficulties with the transducing and monitoring system.

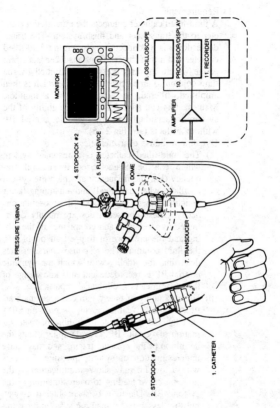

FIG 2–5.
The components used to directly monitor BP. The monitoring components are nearly the same independent of whether the catheter is in a radial, brachial, or femoral artery (or in the PA). The transducer size and plumbing components were enlarged for illustration purposes. (From Shoemaker WC, Ayers S, Grenvik A, et al: *Textbook of Critical Care Medicine,* ed 2. Philadelphia, WB Saunders, 1989. Used by permission.)

1) Requirements.

   A fluid-filled catheter connects the intraarterial catheter to the transducer and flush system. The transducer dome is a connection between the fluid-filled catheter and a transducer. The transducer is a strain gauge which converts pressure transmitted by the fluid column to an electronic impulse which is then amplified, filtered, and displayed on a monitor. Many factors can adversely affect the ability of the system to accurately record dynamic arterial BP without artifacts (see Fig 2–5).

2) Dynamic response characteristics.

   a) The fluid-filled catheter is a resonant system which can be characterized by natural frequency (Fn, the frequency at which the system oscillates when disturbed) and a damping factor which expresses how quickly these oscillations decay. These characteristics are mainly determined by the length and compliance of the tubing and the presence of trapped air bubbles in the fluid column. The response characteristics determine the fidelity with which the dynamic arterial BP is recorded, and thus knowledge of these parameters is clinically important.

   b) Underdamping of the system can accentuate artifacts such as "catheter whip" seen with a PA catheter and can result in significant overestimation of systolic BP. Overdamping blunts the definition of the pressure tracing and may cause underestimation of systolic pressure. Systems with a low Fn may show amplification of the pressure curve leading to overestimation of the systolic BP. Diastolic BPs are altered as well but to a lesser extent than are systolic measurements.

   c) Most currently available systems are underdamped and have a low Fn. Factors which further decrease the Fn include trapped air bubbles (in stopcocks, tubing, or transducer domes), long tubing lengths, compliant tubing, and clots on the catheter tip. These same factors also increase the damping coefficient of the system.

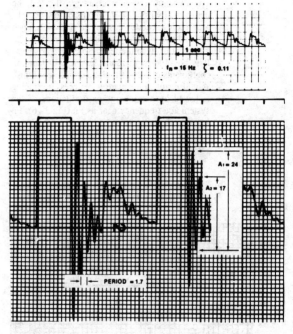

FIG 2–6.

The *upper panel* shows an arterial pulse waveform with two flushes. The natural frequency and damping coefficient can be determined from either flush. The *lower panel* shows the flush segment enlarged and marked to illustrate the method. The natural frequency (F_n) of the system is estimated by taking the period of one cycle *(PERIOD)*, in this case 1.7 mm, and dividing this into the paper speed, 25 mm/sec; Fn=25/1.7=15 Hz. The natural frequency can be more accurately determined by measuring multiple cycles. The damping coefficient is determined by taking the ratio of successive peaks of the oscillations, in this case A2/A1 = 17/24 = 0.71, then by using the equation in Figure 2–7, the damping coefficient z can be determined, in this case $z = 0.11$ (From Gardner RM: *Anesthesiology* 1981; 54:227. Used by permission.)

d) The dynamic response characteristics can be optimized by using short lengths of low-compliance tubing, careful flushing to remove trapped air, and use of tightly sealing connectors.

3) Measurement of dynamic response characteristics.

a) It is possible to measure the Fn and damping coefficients of a system clinically. A rapid flush should result in a square wave pressure tracing followed by a "ringing" or oscillations of the system at a frequency near its Fn (Fig 2–6). Fn is then calculated as:

$$\text{Fn (Hz)} = \frac{\text{paper speed (mm/sec)}}{\text{period (mm)}}$$

b) The damping coefficient is determined by taking the ratio of the amplitudes of two succes-

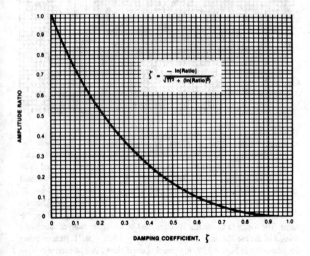

$$\zeta = \frac{-\ln(\text{Ratio})}{\sqrt{\pi^2 + (\ln(\text{Ratio})^2}}$$

FIG 2–7.
Graphical solution of the damping coefficient equation. (From Gardner RM: *Anesthesiology* 1981; 54:227. Used by permission.)

sive cycles (Fig 2–6) and using a graphical solution (Fig 2–7) to calculate the damping coefficient.

c) Fn should be optimized by eliminating unnecessary tubing and careful attention to purging the
system of air. Fn should be at least 12 Hz for a
HR > 60/min.

d) Optimal damping for waveform reproduc-
tion is present if a flush results in one undershoot of pressure followed by one small over-
shoot and then a return to the patient's natural
waveform (Fig 2–8).

e. Zero referencing and calibration.

1) When the system has been connected to the patient
and adequate dynamic response characteristics have
been assured, the system is zeroed and then calibrated.

a) To zero the transducer, the transducer is usually
placed at the level of the midaxillary line or the
cannulated artery (Fig 2–9,A).

b) The stopcock is then adjusted so that the transducer is closed to the patient and opened to air
at the level of the midaxillary line.

c) The monitor is then adjusted to a 0 mm Hg
baseline.

d) The stopcock is then closed to air and opened
to the patient.

e) It is not absolutely necessary for the transducer
to be at the level of the midaxillary line so long
as the stopcock which is opened to air during
the zero reference procedure is at that level (Fig
2–9,B).

2) Calibration is a separate procedure from zero referencing. The (Cal) button on monitor systems is an
electronic test of the amplifier system and does not
calibrate the transducer.

a) To calibrate the transducer, the stopcock is
again disconnected from the patient and connected to a mercury manometer.

b) The manometer is then pressurized to 200 mm
Hg and the gain of the amplifier and monitor is

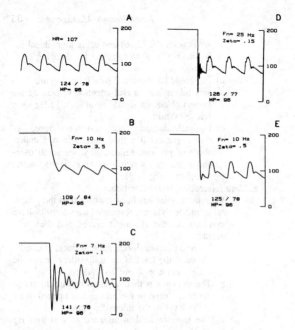

FIG 2–8.

Arterial pressure waveforms obtained from the same patient. **A** shows the patient's actual arterial pressure waveform as if recorded with a catheter-tipped transducer. The systolic pressure is 124 mm Hg, diastolic 78 mm Hg, and mean pressure *(MP)* 96 mm Hg. **B** shows the same patient's arterial waveform when recorded with an overdamped system. Note the fast-flush signal *(upper left)* returns slowly to the patient waveform. Systolic pressure is underestimated (109 mm Hg), diastolic is overestimated (84 mm Hg), and MP is unchanged. **C** shows an underdamped condition with low Fn (8 Hz). After the fast flush, the pressure signal oscillates rapidly (rings). Systolic pressure is overestimated (141 mm Hg), diastolic is slightly under-estimated (76 mm Hg), and MP is correct. **D** shows an underdamped condition but with high Fn (25 Hz). Note that the waveform is only slightly distorted and that the systolic pressure (128 mm Hg), diastolic pressure (77 mm Hg), and MP are close to the real pressures. **E** shows an ideally damped pressure-monitoring system. The undershoot after the fast flush is small and the original patient waveform is adequately reproduced. (From Shoemaker WC, Ayers S, Grenvik A, et al: *Textbook of Critical Care Medicine,* ed 2. Philadelphia, WB Saunders, 1989. Used by permission.)

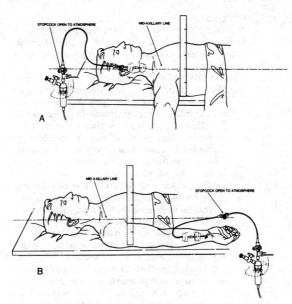

FIG 2–9.
Two methods of zeroing a pressure transducer. Note that the location at which the water-air interface occurs should always be at the midaxillary line when zeroing. **A,** the stopcock is placed near the transducer at the midaxillary line, or **B,** nearer the catheter at the midaxillary line. (From Shoemaker WC, Ayers S, Grenvik A, et al: *Textbook of Critical Care Medicine* ed 2. Philadelphia, WB Saunders, 1989. Used by permission.)

        adjusted so that the monitor indicates 200 mm Hg.
    c) Ideally, more than one pressure level should be tested (i.e., 50, 100, 150, 200 mm Hg) to ensure a linear response in the system.
  3) Zero referencing should be performed at least every shift and calibration should be performed a minimum of once daily.

  f. Complications.

    Arterial cannulation is subject to a variety of complications including ischemic necrosis of the hand. Complications increase markedly with increasing duration of cannulation.

    1) Thrombosis of the radial artery may occur in up to 38% of patients but is not necessarily associated with ischemic complications provided the ulnar artery and palmar arches are patent. Recanalization of the thrombosed artery almost always occurs.

      a) Ischemic complications may be increased by the use of vasopressors, the presence of occlusive vascular disease, or vasospastic disease (e.g., Raynaud's disease).

      b) The incidence of thrombosis may be decreased by the use of small (20-gauge) catheters, continuous flushing systems, Teflon catheters, and frequent rotation of cannulation sites.

    2) Infectious complications include local cellulitis at the insertion site and bacteremia with sepsis which may result from an infected catheter or from contamination of the fluid-filled monitoring system.

      a) Infectious complications increase markedly if the catheter is inserted via a surgical cutdown rather than a percutaneous technique and if the catheter is left in place for longer than 72 hours.

      b) Systemic antibiotics do not decrease the incidence of infectious complications. The insertion site should be inspected frequently.

      c) Flush systems should be changed at least every 48 hours (this is shown to be a safe interval in prospective trials).

      d) If local infection occurs, the catheter should be removed and the tip cultured. A new catheter can then be placed in a different site.

      e) If the patient develops signs of sepsis or bacteremia, the catheter should be removed and cultured and the patient placed on broad-spectrum antibiotic therapy (including an antistaphylococcal antibiotic).

3) Other complications include emboli from the catheter tip, hematoma at the insertion site, and hemorrhage if the catheter is inadvertently opened. Dysfunction of the catheter may occur if the catheter kinks or if the tip is resting against the vessel wall. Alternative cannulation sites, such as the axillary artery, dorsalis pedis artery, or femoral artery, are generally safe, but are associated with the same complications as radial artery cannulation. The brachial artery has been safely used for arterial pressure monitoring, but is generally avoided as occlusion may be associated with necrosis of the entire forearm and hand secondary to poor collateral circulation.

g. Removal of the catheter.

The catheter is removed and pressure held at the insertion site for 5–10 minutes until there is no evidence of bleeding. Prolonged pressure may be necessary in patients receiving anticoagulants or with coagulopathies. The site should be inspected for evidence of infection, hematoma, distal ischemia, and any motor or sensory change of the cannulated limb.

C. Central Venous Pressure.

1. The CVP provides an estimate of the RV filling pressure and can easily be assessed by using a central venous catheter with the tip in the RA and a fluid column manometer or measured through the RA lumen of a Swan-Ganz catheter.

   a. In normal individuals, changes in the CVP correlate directionally and quantitatively with changes in LV filling pressure.

   b. In individuals with preexisting cardiac or pulmonary disease, and patients with multisystem trauma, this correlation may not be valid.

   c. The CVP can be a misleading index of the patient's volume status and in critically ill patients any uncertainty should be resolved by insertion of a PA catheter to measure PCWP as an index of LV preload.

2. Measurement of the CVP remains useful in some clinical situations despite the poor correlation with LV preload. The CVP is a good estimate of RV preload and can be used

to guide volume therapy in patients with RV infarction. A disproportional rise in CVP when compared to PCWP is seen in these patients.

3. Measurement of CVP may also be useful in patients with suspected cardiac tamponade or constrictive pericarditis. Elevation of the CVP with equalization of the CVP, PA diastolic pressure (PAD), and PCWP is seen in these patients. A characteristic RA waveform (the square root sign) may be seen in patients with constrictive pericarditis.

D. Pulmonary Arterial Catheters.

The PA catheter is a 5F–7.5F flexible catheter with multiple lumen and an inflatable balloon (1.5 mL) at the tip to allow flow-directed insertion. A proximal lumen is used for measurement of RA pressure. A thermistor allows measurement of core temperature and CO by the thermodilution technique. A variety of modified catheters have been introduced including oximeter catheters to measure $S\overline{v}O_2$ and multielectrode catheters for cardiac pacing. The catheter is usually inserted via a central venous route and advanced to the PA (see Chapter 22). Use of the pulmonary artery catheter requires several assumptions concerning physiology and methodologic errors may make measurement of accurate pressures difficult. All data must be carefully correlated with the clinic situation before making therapeutic interventions.

1. Pulmonary arterial occlusion pressure.
   a. Physiology.
      PA catheters in the proper position allow measurement of PA systolic and diastolic pressures.
      1) When the balloon is inflated and "wedged," the distal vessels are separated from the proximal arterial pressure, and an unbroken fluid column exists along the pulmonary capillary bed and pulmonary veins to the LA. The pressure transmitted by this fluid column is a good estimate of LAP.
      2) In normal hearts, mean LAP is a good estimate of the LVEDP. The PCWP measured with balloon catheters has been shown to correlate well with the true wedge pressure measured by passing a small rigid catheter into the distal pulmonary vessels. This true wedge pressure has been shown in the cardiac catheterization laboratory to correlate well with directly measured LAP. Thus, the pulmonary

artery wedge pressure is an estimate of LVEDV which is used as an index of LV preload.

b. Assumptions.

1) The PA catheter estimates cavitary pressure with respect to atmospheric pressure as 0, not with respect to intrathoracic pressure, which is the pressure surrounding the heart.

   a) The transmural pressure (LV pressure − intrathoracic pressure) is the true distending pressure of the ventricle. Transmural pressure is affected by airway pressures, pleural pressures, intra-abdominal pressure, respiratory effort, mechanical ventilation, PEEP, etc.

   b) Transmural pressure can be calculated by actually measuring the surrounding pleural pressure and subtracting this value from the measured cavitary pressure. Clinical measurement of true pleural pressure is not possible (some centers use esophageal pressures as an estimate).

   c) Therefore, cavitary pressure alone must be used as an estimate of the true transmural pressure.

2) LV preload can be defined as sarcomere or muscle fiber length at end diastole.

   a) Both LVEDV and the end-diastolic minor axis diameter correlate linearly with fiber length.

   b) However, even if transmural pressure is measured, the relationship between EDV and pressure is exponential (Fig 2−2,B), not linear; consequently LVEDP is not a linear index of ventricular preload.

   c) Moreover, the relationship between end-diastolic pressure and volume is not constant. It is affected by ventricular compliance, wall thickness, HR, ischemia, and certain drugs.

   d) The LVEDP which corresponds to a given EDV at one point in time in a patient may not correspond to the same volume as clinical conditions change (see Fig 2−3). Thus, LVEDP and PCWP can be inaccurate indices of LV preload and must be continuously interpreted in the context of the clinical situation and overall cardiovascular performance.

3) It must be remembered that PCWP and LAP are only estimates of LVEDP and several factors can adversely affect the correlation between PCWP and LVEDP.

   a) Pulmonary veno-occlusive disease, arterial myxomas or tumors, atrial thrombus, mediastinal fibrosis, etc. may significantly alter the relationship between the PCWP and true LAP.

   b) Similarly, LAP does not necessarily correlate with LVEDP in all clinical settings. LAP in mitral stenosis and mitral regurgitation may overestimate the LVEDP (the latter can occasionally be diagnosed by the presence of v waves in the wedge pressure tracing) (Fig 2–10).

   c) Aortic regurgitation may cause early closure of the mitral valve while LV pressure continues to rise so that the LAP underestimates true LVEDP.

   d) In some patients with this diminished LV compliance, the "atrial kick" is responsible for a significant portion of ventricular filling. In these patients, mean LAP may underestimate LVEDP. If an a wave can be detected in the wedge pressure tracing, the height of this wave correlates better with LVEDP (Fig 2–10).

4) Despite the difficulties in the use of the PCWP as an index of LV preload, much useful information can be derived from the use of the PA catheter.

   a) PCWP can aid in the differentiation of cardiogenic from noncardiogenic pulmonary edema.

   b) PA catheters can also be used to measure thermodilution cardiac outputs and to obtain blood samples for measurement of $S\bar{v}O_2$, an index of tissue perfusion.

c. Positioning of PA catheters.

   1) Pulmonary capillary collapse occurs if alveolar pressure exceeds pulmonary venous pressure. Thus, to assure an unbroken fluid column between the distal catheter lumen and the LA, the catheter must lodge in a region of the lung where the venous pressure exceeds alveolar pressure.

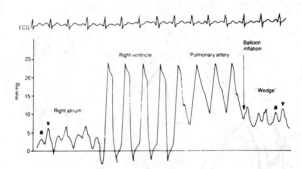

FIG 2–10.
Representative recording of pressures as a Swan-Ganz catheter is inserted through the right side of the heart into the PA. The first waveform is an RA tracing with characteristic a and v waves. The RV, PA, and PA wedge tracings follow in sequence. The pressures and waveforms shown here are normal. Note that the wedge tracing shows a and v waves transmitted from the LA. In addition, the wedge pressure (mean) is less than PA diastolic pressure. The wedge tracing is not always this distinct, but a very damped tracing or mean wedge pressure greater than PA diastolic pressure usually indicates some mechanical problem in the system (e.g., air bubble in the connecting tubing, catheter tip "overwedged," balloon inflated over distal orifice, catheter tip in zone I or zone II. etc.). In severe mitral regurgitation the large transmitted LA v waves occasionally may cause the wedge tracing to resemble a PA tracing. In such a case, careful analysis of the waveforms and attention to where the peak pressure occurs in relation to the ECG complex usually will avoid misinterpretation. (From Matthay MA: *Clin Chest Med* 1983; 4:233. Used by permission.)

2) West described three functional lung zones based on the distribution of pulmonary blood flow and ventilation (Fig 2–11). In zone I, alveolar pressure exceeds PA and venous pressures. In zone II, PA pressure is greater than alveolar pressure, which still exceeds pulmonary venous pressure. Only in zone III do both the PA and venous pressures exceed alveolar pressure.

3) In an upright patient, the apices represent zone I and the lung base is zone III, with zone II in be-

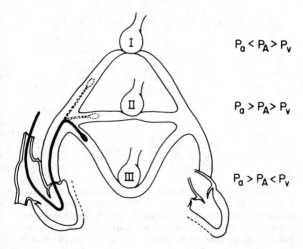

$P_a < P_A > P_v$

$P_a > P_A > P_v$

$P_a > P_A < P_v$

FIG 2–11.
Effect of catheter tip location and alveolar-vascular pressure relationships on wedge pressure (P_W). With increasing vertical distance above the LA plane, arterial (P_A) and venous (P_V) pressures decline relative to alveolar pressure (P_A), which is similar in all three zones. In either zone I or zone II, P_A exceeds P_V Hence, during balloon occlusion of the PA, alveolar capillaries collapse, causing P_W to reflect P_A rather than P_V pressure; P_W estimates P_V accurately only in zone III. (From O'Quinn R, Marini JJ: *Am Rev Respir Dis* 1983; 128:319. Used by permission.)

tween. In a supine patient, the zones are distributed from anterior to posterior. The distal lumen of the PA catheter must be in zone III to accurately estimate LAP.

4) Usually the greatest portion of blood flow is to zone III so the catheter normally migrates to this region. In the supine patient, the catheter tip is likely to be in zone III if it is positioned posteriorly beneath the level of the LA. This can be confirmed with a lateral CXR.

5) It is important to realize that the zones are not fixed anatomically. For example, diuresis or the addition

of PEEP can convert areas of lung in zone III to zone II while correction of hypovolemia may convert areas of lung in zone II to zone III.

6) Zone III positioning can also be tested by addition of an incremental level of PEEP. If the wedge pressure increases by greater than one half the increment of PEEP, zone III positioning is unlikely. However, failure to increase by greater than one half does not assure zone III positioning.

d. Zero and calibration procedures.

1) Measurement of the PA pressure requires a fluid-filled monitoring system and transducers identical to those used for direct measurement of arterial pressure (see Fig 2–5). To obtain accurate pressure recordings, it is necessary to optimize the dynamic response characteristics and to accurately zero and calibrate the transducers, as previously described.

2) The transducer is zeroed against atmospheric pressure. The reference level is the LA which is approximately at the fourth intercostal space in the midaxillary line (see Fig 2–9,A). The transducer itself does not have to be at this level when the zeroing procedure is performed so long as the catheter connected to the transducer dome is opened to the atmosphere at the appropriate level.

3) Calibration is performed with manometer pressurized to 40 mm Hg (this pressure may need to be increased in patients with significant pulmonary hypertension).

e. Measurement of PCWP.

1) After the PA catheter has been properly positioned and the transducer zeroed and calibrated, physiologic data may be recorded.

2) Prior to balloon inflation, RA pressure (RAP) and PA systolic, diastolic, and mean pressures should be recorded.

3) The balloon is inflated and allowed to wedge. If a wedge tracing appears, a mean PCWP is then recorded. Occasionally, the catheter migrates distally as it softens secondary to the body temperature. If less than a full balloon inflation produces a wedge trace, the catheter should be pulled back slightly. If

the catheter does not wedge it can be advanced slightly.
4) The catheter should never be advanced without the balloon fully inflated (Fig 2–12). Flexible sheaths are available which maintain sterility of the catheter during this manipulation. The balloon should be inflated for the shortest period of time possible to allow pressure measurement.
5) All pressure readings should be made from a graphical printout, not from the monitor display. The digital readouts from the monitors are based on

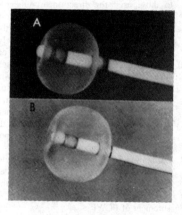

FIG 2–12.
Photographs of the balloon of a 7F Swan-Ganz catheter inflated with either 1.0 mL (**A**) or 1.5 mL (**B**) of air. Note that the catheter tip protrudes beyond the inflated balloon if less than the full recommended volume is used. The exposed catheter tip may cause endocardial damage, induce ventricular arrhythmias, or damage the PA. Also, using the recommended volume helps ensure a relatively proximal wedge position, which is important to lessen the risk of pulmonary infarction and to help maintain accuracy of thermodilution cardiac output and mixed venous PO_2 determinations. (From Sprung CL: *The Pulmonary Artery Catheter: Methodology and Clinical Applications.* Baltimore, Aspen Publishers, Inc, 1983. Used by permission.)

time-based averaging and do not accurately reflect measured pressures.

6) All readings should be made at end expiration when intrathoracic pressure is nearest atmospheric level. Normal inspiration will produce a negative deflection of tracing, positive pressure ventilation will produce a positive deflection during inspiration.

f. Positive end-expiratory pressure (PEEP).

1) The addition of PEEP may adversely affect the utility of the PCWP as an index of LV preload.

2) PEEP increases intrathoracic pressure and a portion of this increment is transmitted to the pulmonary vasculature (the amount is dependent on airway and lung compliance) and this increases the measured PCWP.

3) However, the increase in intrathoracic pressure produces increased pressure surrounding the heart and thus diminishes the transmural or true distending pressure of the ventricle. PCWP tends to overestimate LVEDP in the presence of PEEP.

4) Despite these difficulties, PCWP should be measured with the patient remaining on the ventilator without removal of the PEEP as this alters the patient's baseline status and may precipitate hypoxia.

g. PA diastolic pressure.

1) PAD may be used as an estimate of PCWP in patients without significant underlying pulmonary disease.

2) In patients with pulmonary hypertension PAD may be considerably greater than PCWP.

h. Cardiac tamponade.

Patients with cardiac tamponade may show equalization of right and left heart filling pressures (CVP, PAD, PCWP). Therefore, all pressures must be measured in any patient in whom tamponade is suspected (see Chapter 5).

i. Intracardiac shunts.

1) If a left-to-right shunt is suspected, blood samples for O_2 saturation should be obtained in superior vena cava (SVC), RA, RV, and PA during insertion of the catheter.

      2) A "step-up" or increase in O_2 saturation usually indicates a left-to-right shunt.

   j. Artifacts in measurement of PCWP.

     1) Catheter whip.

       a) Catheter whip is caused by acceleration of the fluid column in the catheter by contraction of the RV. Catheter whip may produce fluctuations in the pressure tracing causing inaccuracies in the estimate of PCWP.

     2) Overwedging and eccentric balloon inflation.

       a) Overwedging or continuous wedging occurs when the catheter migrates distally as it is softened by the body temperature.

         i) When a continuous flush system is used, overwedging is characterized by loss of the normal PA tracing and a progressive increase in the measured pressure.

         ii) The catheter should be withdrawn to a more proximal position as overwedging may lead to pulmonary infarction or hemorrhage.

         iii) If the CXR shows a peripheral location of the catheter tip (>5 cm from the mediastinum), the catheter should be withdrawn an appropriate distance.

         iv) Also, if the balloon volume needed to wedge the catheter decreases markedly, the position of the catheter should be corrected as this indicates distal migration.

       b) Eccentric balloon inflation can cause the catheter tip to enter a small side branch or to be forced against the vessel wall occluding the lumen and thus causing overwedging.

       c) Non-zone III positioning of the catheter may also cause the appearance of overwedging, especially in patients requiring mechanical ventilation.

2. Complications of PA catheters.

The reported incidence of significant morbidity is 20%–50% and mortality is reported to be 0%–4%. Placement of a PA catheter is subject to all the complications of central venous catheterization (see Chapter 22).

a. Thrombosis.
   1) Thrombosis of the internal jugular vein may occur in as many as 66% of patients requiring PA catheters.
   2) Occlusion of the SVC causing the SVC syndrome may also occur; however, it is usually asymptomatic.
   3) The incidence of pulmonary emboli secondary to PA catheters is uncertain.
   4) If clinical symptoms occur secondary to the thrombosis, low-dose thrombolytic therapy infusion has been utilized (streptokinase, urokinase, etc.).

b. Infection.
   1) Catheter sepsis may occur in as many as 2% of patients with PA catheters. Colonization of the catheter tip may occur even more commonly, especially in patients with other sites of infection.
   2) Catheter infection can be minimized by meticulous attention to aseptic technique, dressing changes, and removal of the catheter within 72 hours.
   3) Use of the antecubital venous cutdown for placement of the catheters is associated with an increased infection rate.
   4) If venous access is a problem and there is no evidence of infection, the catheters may be changed over a wire after 72 hours, although this has not been clearly shown to prevent infection.
   5) If sepsis occurs in a patient with a PA catheter, blood cultures should be obtained through the catheter, the catheter should be removed, and the tip sent for culture while continuing to evaluate other sites. After cultures have been obtained, broad-spectrum antibiotics should be begun. If a PA catheter is still necessary for management of the patient, a new catheter should be inserted at a different site.

c. Arrhythmias.
   1) Ventricular arrhythmias (PVCs and nonsustained ventricular tachycardia) are common during passage of the catheter through the RV. These are usually self-limited and resolve after the catheter passes into the PA, although ventricular fibrillation and

cardiac arrest have been reported. Lidocaine and a defibrillator should be available during the insertion procedure. Atrial arrhythmias have also been reported. Occasionally sustained ventricular arrhythmias occur necessitating removal of the catheter.

2) Transient RBBB has been reported following insertion of PA catheters. This is usually self-limiting and asymptomatic. In patients with preexisting LBBB, it has been suggested that a pacing catheter or prophylactic pacing wire be utilized because of the possibility of development of complete heart block.

d. Valvular damage.

1) Damage to the endothelium of the tricuspid and pulmonary valves, sterile vegetations, and bacterial endocarditis have all been reported in patients with PA catheters.

2) Rupture of the chordae tendineae of the tricuspid valve has also been reported as well as damage to the pulmonary valve causing pulmonary insufficiency.

e. Pulmonary infarction.

1) Pulmonary infarction may occur with distal migration of the catheter tip, possibly secondary to embolization of thrombus from the catheter tip.

2) Pulmonary infarction becomes manifest by appearance of a wedge-shaped infiltrate distal to the catheter tip on CXR. Hemoptysis may also occur.

f. Pulmonary arterial rupture.

1) PA rupture is a rare but often fatal complication. Mild hemoptysis may herald impending rupture which can result in exsanguinating hemoptysis or intrathoracic hemorrhage.

2) A variety of mechanisms have been postulated for PA rupture: (1) overinflation of the balloon, (2) eccentric balloon inflation forcing the tip through a side branch or vessel wall, and (3) advancing the catheter through the wall (balloon not inflated).

3) Pulmonary hypertension is a risk factor. Hemoptysis associated with a pulmonary infiltrate may signify pulmonary infarction but also may be a warning sign for impending rupture.

4) If hemoptysis develops, the catheter should be pulled back and, if at all possible, removed.

5) The development of exsanguinating hemoptysis or intrathoracic hemorrhage usually necessitates surgical intervention.

6) Tamponade of hemorrhage may be possible by placing a dual lumen ET tube and occluding the bronchus on the side of the rupture with a Fogarty balloon catheter. This will also prevent aspiration of blood in the other lung.

7) Suture ligature or repair of the perforation may be possible but often the lesion is deeper in the lung parenchyma, requiring lobectomy or pneumonectomy for adequate therapy.

8) To prevent pulmonary artery rupture, careful attention to correct catheter positioning is mandatory.

g. Knotting of the catheter.

1) Coiling of the catheter around itself or other catheters may result in a complete knot. This usually occurs in the RV but has been reported in the PA.

2) A tight knot in a small (5F) catheter can sometimes be safely withdrawn through the insertion site. If a larger catheter is used, or if significant resistance is met while removing the catheter, a venotomy must be performed.

3) In some cases it is possible to unknot the catheter by passing a flexible guidewire through the distal lumen, thus allowing safe removal of the catheter. A variety of other catheter techniques have been developed for unknotting and removing knotted catheters.

h. Rare complications.

These include intrathecal or intrapleural placement of the catheter, pneumoperitoneum, catheter production of systolic heart sounds, paradoxical arterial emboli, electrode displacement from pacing catheters, osteomyelitis of the clavicle, and suture of the catheter to a cardiac structure following cardiac operation.

E. Left Atrial Catheters.

1. Fluid-filled LA catheters may be placed via a pulmonary vein at the time of operation to determine LAP directly. These catheters obviate many of the difficulties in using

PCWP to estimate mean LAP; however, mean LAP is only an estimate of LVEDP. The relationship between LAP and LVEDP may be adversely affected by the presence of valvular heart disease, tachycardia, or changes in ventricular compliance.

2. **LA catheters must be used with great care to prevent embolization of thrombus or air.**

   a. LA catheters generally should not be used for fluid or drug administration.

   b. Rarely, during prostaglandin E (PGE), infusion for pulmonary hypertension, LA administration of norepinephrine is necessary to prevent systemic hypotension.

   c. *Catheters should always be aspirated prior to flushing and should never be flushed if the catheter is occluded.* Meticulous attention to detail is necessary to prevent arterial air emboli.

3. The catheter may remain in place for several days but should be removed prior to withdrawal of mediastinal drainage tubes. After the catheters are removed, the patient should remain at bed rest for 2 hours and a CXR should be obtained.

F. **Measurement of Cardiac Output.**

Measurement of the CO allows evaluation of the heart's ability to meet the metabolic demands of the body and the effects of therapeutic interventions. Blood flow is most commonly assessed clinically using indicator-dilution techniques. CO may be expressed as an absolute value in liters per minute or may be normalized for the patient's size by dividing by the patient's body surface area (BSA) (m^2) to derive a CI L/min/m^2.

1. Fick method.

   a. O_2 is utilized as an indicator. Calculation of CO requires accurate measurement of the patient's VO_2 and CaO_2 and $C\overline{v}O_2$.

   b. To measure VO_2, the patient must breathe from a Douglas bag containing a known volume of gas with a known concentration of O_2. Expired gas is also collected in a Douglas bag for a measured period of time.

   c. VO_2 is then calculated by the formula:

$$VO_2 = (F_IO_2 \times V_I) - (F_EO_2 \times V_E)$$

where F_IO_2 and F_EO_2 are the oxygen concentrations in the inhaled and exhaled gas, respectively, and V_I and V_E are the inhaled and exhaled minute volumes, respectively.

d. VO_2 may be measured indirectly using calorimetric methods.

e. When VO_2 is known, CO is calculated by the formula

$$CO = \frac{VO_2}{CaO_2 - C\bar{v}O_2}$$

f. For the Fick method to provide an accurate estimate of CO, VO_2 and blood flow must be constant. No arteriovenous shunting can occur and VO_2 as well as CaO_2 and $C\bar{v}O_2$ must be accurately measured.

2. Bolus indicator dilution methods.

  a. Introduction.

    1) Both dye-dilution and thermodilution techniques of measurement of CO involve injection of a bolus of an indicator solution and measurement of a change in temperature or concentration downstream.

    2) In a system with constant flow, a known concentration of indicator is injected and a continuous measurement of the concentration is made downstream.

    3) When a bolus is injected and complete mixing occurs, the concentration at the downstream point of measurement will rise from 0 to a maximum and then gradually decline, so that a continuous concentration curve over time can be generated.

    4) Flow can then be calculated as the amount of indicator injected divided by the area under this concentration curve.

  b. Dye-dilution technique.

    1) Indocyanine green dye is the standard dye for measurement of CO.

      a) 5 mg of dye are diluted in 1 mL of D5W and injected in a central vein.

      b) A continuous sample of arterial blood is withdrawn and the dye concentration measured, using an optical densitometer (8,050 Å).

    c) A concentration curve showing the rise and fall of the concentration of the dye over time is generated and CO can be calculated as above.

  2) The shape of the curve may also be useful in assessing the presence of shunts following correction of cardiac anomalies.

    a) With right-to-left intracardiac shunts, there is early appearance of the dye, altering the upstroke of the concentration curve.

    b) With left-to-right shunts, the dye is recirculated through the lungs, decreasing the peak and altering the downslope of the curve.

  3) Accurate estimation of CO using dye-dilution techniques requires constant blood flow, complete mixing of the dye, uniform sample withdrawal, and absence of air bubbles in the sample. Accumulation of dye secondary to repeated measurements may also lead to inaccurate estimation of CO.

 c. Thermodilution method.

  1) Thermodilution is by far the most frequently clinically used method for measurement of CO.

    a) A PA catheter is commonly utilized and a bolus of fluid (usually D5W) is injected through the proximal lumen and the temperature measured by a thermistor near the distal tip, resulting in a continuous curve of temperature change over time.

    b) Usually, cold injectate is used with a temperature of $0°-4°$ C, although room temperature injectate may be used.

    c) The thermodilution method has been shown to be accurate and to generally correlate well with CO determined by the Fick or dye-dilution methods, although a variation of as much as 10% between techniques may occur.

    d) Many factors adversely affect the accuracy of thermodilution CO.

      i) To obtain accurate measurements, core temperature in the PA and the injectate temperature must be accurately measured and the injection should be rapid and smooth.

ii) Heat gained by the injectate during injection, equilibration with vessel walls, and recirculation of heat may all diminish the accuracy of the measurement.

iii) Thermistor positioning against the vessel wall and respiratory variation can also cause errors.

iv) The presence of significant tricuspid or pulmonary valvular incompetence or intracardiac shunts render thermodilution techniques unreliable.

2) To measure CO:

a) A 10-mL syringe is filled with D5W cooled in an ice bath to 0° C. It is important that the injectate temperature be accurately measured either by placing a probe in a syringe in the ice bath or by a thermistor at the point of injection. Each catheter and CO computer has a calibration factor which must be accurately entered.

b) After assessing proper position of the catheter (an undamped PA tracing should be present), the indicator is rapidly (< 4 seconds) injected.

c) Ideally, the temperature curve measured by the thermistor should be displayed (Fig 2–13).

d) If the curve is irregular or if the initial change in temperatures slow, the measurement should be discarded.

e) CO should be measured three times and the average value recorded. If these vary by greater than 10%, or if the measured CO does not correlate with the observed clinical condition of the patient, all the previously discussed factors should be carefully rechecked and the measurements repeated.

3. Other techniques for CO measurement.

a. Intraoperatively, electromagnetic or Doppler flow probes can be placed directly on the aorta to measure CO.

b. Ultrasonography can be used to measure CO noninvasively. Aortic cross-sectional area may be measured using two-dimensional echocardiography and blood flow

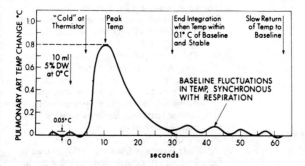

FIG 2–13.
Typical thermodilution curve. The peak of the thermodilution curve is 16 times higher than the baseline fluctuation, a good signal-to-noise ratio. Occasionally, baseline fluctuations reach 0.1° C, and in very high-flow states the peak temperature does not exceed 0.4° C. An iced injectate is essential under these circumstances to obtain an adequate curve. Integration should be continued until the curve returns to within the baseline fluctuations. Waiting for complete return to baseline will induce errors if the baseline shifts. (From Weisel RD, Vito L, Dennis RC, et al: Clinical applications of thermodilution cardiac output determination. *Am J Surg* 1975; 129: 449–454).

velocity in the aorta measured by Doppler echocardiography allowing calculation of CO.

G. Mixed Venous Oxygen Saturation ($S\bar{v}O_2$).

1. Assumptions.

   a. Mixed venous blood represents a perfusion-weighted average of blood draining from all of the body's organ systems. $S\bar{v}O_2$ provides an estimate of O_2 extracted and utilized by the body. It is important to realize that mixed venous blood represents an average of the entire body and no information can be derived concerning specific organ systems.

   b. An increase in $S\bar{v}O_2$ generally signifies an improvement in CO and DO_2 while a fall in $S\bar{v}O_2$ usually represents decreased DO_2 or increased VO_2 with greater tissue O_2 extraction.

   c. Mixed venous blood should be obtained from the PA to

ensure thorough mixing. The presence of a left-to-right intracardiac shunt will cause a "step-up" in oxygen saturation in the PA and invalidate the $S\overline{v}O_2$ as an index of tissue perfusion.

2. Measurement of $S\overline{v}O_2$.

   a. $S\overline{v}O_2$ may be measured directly from PA blood obtained from the distal lumen of a PA catheter or continuously using a fiberoptic oximeter incorporated into some Swan-Ganz catheters.

   b. If blood is withdrawn, the tip of the catheter must be in the nonwedged position and blood should be slowly withdrawn to prevent falsely "arterialized" samples. The first 2.5 mL withdrawn representing the dead space within the lumen of the catheter should be discarded.

   c. Because of regional differences in VO_2, blood obtained from the SVC, IVC, RA, and RV should not be used to determine $S\overline{v}O_2$ because of inadequate mixing.

3. Clinical utility.

   a. $S\overline{v}O_2$ may be continually monitored using PA oximetry catheters to provide information concerning trends in hemodynamic status and help evaluate the effects of therapeutic interventions.

   b. A decrease in $S\overline{v}O_2$ may indicate diminished CO with worsening tissue perfusion or increased VO_2 requiring increased oxygen extraction.

   c. An increase in $S\overline{v}O_2$ may signify improved tissue perfusion or increasing CO.

   d. Such trends must be carefully considered in critically ill patients and confirmed by other indices before therapeutic decisions are made. In patients with septic shock, O_2 extraction may be impaired and a rise in $S\overline{v}O_2$ may signal worsening O_2 extraction with increased tissue hypoxia rather than improved tissue perfusion.

   e. Continuous monitoring of $S\overline{v}O_2$ can provide information concerning the effect of routine interventions such as tracheal suctioning or turning of the patient, which may result in a precipitous fall in $S\overline{v}O_2$.

   f. Accurate measurement of $S\overline{v}O_2$ is necessary for calculation of CO by the Fick method, O_2 extraction ratio, VO_2, and intrapulmonary shunt ratios.

H. Transcutaneous Measurement of Oxygen Saturation.

1. Transcutaneous sensors are available which continuously

monitor peripheral O_2 saturation. These provide a useful index of tissue perfusion and cardiac performance and may be useful in following results of therapeutic interventions.

2. However, the sensors are not as accurate as saturations measured with standard ABGs and any increase or decrease in transcutaneous O_2 saturation should be confirmed by ABG before therapeutic intervention.

I. Derived Indices.

1. Mean Aortic Pressure (MAP)

$$MAP = \frac{DP + (SP - DP)}{3}$$

where SP and DP are systolic and diastolic BPs, respectively. Mean pulmonary artery pressure (MPAP) may be similarly calculated.

2. Systemic vascular resistance.

   a. SVR is an index of ventricular afterload or the impedance to LV ejection.

   $$SVR = \frac{(MAP - MRAP) \times 80}{CO}$$

   where MRAP is mean RAP and can be estimated by the CVP.

   b. The SVR index (SVRI) is a normalized value obtained by substituting CI for CO. The normal value for SVR is $900-1400$ dyne/sec/cm^{-5}.

   c. Similarly, a PVR index (PVRI) may be calculated as:

   $$PVRI = \frac{MPAP - MLAP \times 80}{CI}$$
   $$= \frac{(MPAP - PCWP) \times 80}{CI}$$

   where MLAP (mean LAP) can be approximated by PCWP. The normal range is $100-240$ dyne/sec/cm^{-5}/m^2.

3. Oxygen content of blood.

   The content of O_2 in CaO_2 may be calculated when the hemoglobin concentration (Hb) and SaO_2 are known.

$$CaO_2 = [Hb] \times SaO_2 \times 1.34 + PaO_2 \times 0.0031$$

where 0.0031 is the solubility coefficient of oxygen and 1.34 is O_2 (mL) bound to hemoglobin when the hemoglobin is fully saturated. PaO_2 and $P\overline{v}O_2$ are the arterial and mixed venous partial pressure of oxygen respectively. $C\overline{v}O_2$ is similarly calculated by substituting $S\overline{v}O_2$ for SaO_2 and $P\overline{v}O_2$ for PaO_2 $PO_2 \times 0.0031$ is small and is frequently ignored.

4. Alveolar Arterial Oxygen Difference (A-aDO$_2$)

The alveolar partial pressure of oxygen, or PAO_2, is calculated as:

$$PAO_2 = FIO_2 \times (\text{barometric pressure} - 47) - PACO_2$$

where FIO_2 is a fraction of inspired oxygen and $PACO_2$ is the alveolar partial pressure of CO_2 (approximated by the arterial partial pressure of CO_2, ($PaCO_2$)) and 47 mm Hg is the vapor pressure of water. The barometric pressure at sea level is 760 mm Hg. A-aDO$_2$ may be calculated as:

$$A\text{-}aDO_2 = PAO_2 - PaO_2$$

5. Intrapulmonary Shunt Fraction.

The intrapulmonary shunt fraction: QS/QT, where QS is the shunt flow and QT is the total flow (or cardiac output) may be calculated as:

$$\frac{QS}{QT} = \frac{CcO_2 - CaO_2)}{CcO_2 - C\overline{v}O_2} \times 100$$

where CcO_2 is the oxygen content of the pulmonary capillary blood. The CcO_2 may be calculated by assuming that the partial pressure of oxygen of the capillary blood is the same as PAO_2.

SELECTED REFERENCES

CARDIAC PHYSIOLOGY

Feneley MP, Elbeery JR, Gaynor JW, et al: Ellipsoidal shell subtraction model of right ventricular volume: Comparison with regional free wall dimensions as indices of right ventricular function. *Circ Res* 1990; 67:1427-1436.

Glower DD, Spratt JA, Snow ND, et al: Linearity of the Frank-Starling relationship in the intact heart: The concept of preload recruitable stroke work. *Circulation* 1985; 71:994–1009.

Rankin JS, Elbeery JR, Lucke JC, et al: An energetic analysis of myocardial performance, in Hori M, Suga H, Baan J, (eds): *Cardiac Mechanics and Function in the Normal and Diseased Heart*. Tokyo, Springer-Verlag, 1989, pp 165–188.

CARDIAC MONITORING

Bruner JMR, Krenis LJ, Kunsman JM, et al: Comparison of direct and indirect methods of measuring arterial blood pressure. *Med Instrum* 1981; 15:11.

Gardner RM: Direct blood pressure measurement—dynamic response requirements. *Anesthesiology* 1981; 54:227.

Hudson-Civetta J, Banner TEC: Intravascular catheters: Current guidelines for care and maintenance. *Heart Lung* 1983; 12:466.

Kirkendall WM, Feinleib M, Freis ED, et al: Recommendations for human blood pressure determination by sphygmomanometers. AHA committee report. Dallas, Subcommittee of the AHA Postgraduate Education Committee, 1980–1981.

Levett JM, Replogle RL: Thermodilution cardiac output: A critical analysis and review of the literature. *J Surg Res* 1979; 27:392.

Moser KM, Spragg RG: Use of the balloon-tipped pulmonary artery catheter in pulmonary disease. *Ann Intern Med* 1983; 98:53.

O'Quin R, Marini JJ: Pulmonary artery occlusion pressure: Clinical physiology, measurement and interpretation. *Am Rev Respir Dis* 1983; 128:319.

Raper R, Sibbald WJ: Misled by the wedge? The Swan-Ganz catheter and left ventricular preload. *Chest* 1986; 89:427.

Robin ED: The cult of the Swan-Ganz catheter. Overuse and abuse of pulmonary flow catheters. *Ann Intern Med* 1985; 103:445.

Swan HJC, Ganz W, Forrester J, et al: Catheterization of the heart in man with use of a flow-directed balloon-tipped catheter. *N Engl J Med* 1970; 283:447.

Swan HJC, Ganz W: Hemodynamic measurements in clinical practice: A decade in review. *J Am Coll Cardiol* 1983; 1:103.

West JB: *Respiratory Physiology: The Essentials,* ed 3. Baltimore, Williams & Wilkins, 1984.

Wiedemann HP, Matthay MA, Matthay RA: Cardiovascular-pulmonary monitoring in the intensive care unit (parts 1 and 2). *Chest* 1984; 85:537, 656.

SHOCK

3

I. PATHOPHYSIOLOGY OF SHOCK.
A. Introduction.
1. Shock is the state which exists when tissue perfusion, and thus tissue oxygen delivery (DO_2), is inadequate to sustain cellular metabolism.
2. The diagnosis and treatment of patients with shock remain major problems in the SICU.
3. Despite advances in understanding the pathophysiology of shock and marked improvements in therapy, mortality remains high.
4. In the early stages of shock, vigorous resuscitation may correct cellular hypoxia allowing reversal of the shock state. However, if diminished perfusion and DO_2 are allowed to persist, cellular injury may become irreversible.
5. Even if initial resuscitation appears successful, a state of hypermetabolism and organ failure (the multiple organ failure syndrome, MOFS) may ensue.
6. Successful management depends on early diagnosis, prompt resuscitation, and aggressive therapy of any underlying cause of the shock state.

B. Pathophysiologic Mechanism.
1. The basic pathophysiologic mechanism in shock is a defect of tissue perfusion and DO_2. In some forms of shock, especially septic shock and in advanced shock of etiologies, an inability of cells to utilize delivered O_2 may be present.
2. DO_2 depends on four factors; cardiac output (CO), hemoglobin concentration and saturation, and the peripheral microcirculation. DO_2 may be calculated using this formula:

$$DO_2 \text{ (mL } O_2/\text{min)} = CO \text{ (L/min)} \times CaO_2 \text{ (mL } O_2/100 \text{ mL blood)} \times 10$$

3. The amount of O_2 consumed (VO_2) is dependent not only on the amount delivered to the tissue but also the amount of O_2 extracted by the tissues. Oxygen extraction can be assessed by the $C(a-\overline{v})O_2$ which may be calculated using this formula:

$$C(a - \overline{v}) O_2 \text{ (mL } O_2/100 \text{ mL blood)}$$
$$= CaO_2 \text{ (mL } O_2/100 \text{ mL blood)}$$
$$- C\overline{v}O_2 \text{ (mL } O_2/100 \text{ mL blood)}$$

4. In addition to DO_2 it is important to assess actual VO_2, which may be measured or calculated using the Fick equation:

$$VO_2 \text{ (mL } O_2/\text{min)} = CO \text{ (L/min)}$$
$$\times C (a - \overline{v}) O_2 \text{ (mL } O_2/100 \text{ mL blood)} \times 10$$

5. The oxygen extraction ratio (OER) may also be utilized as an index of tissue O_2 extraction and is calculated using the following formula.

$$OER = \frac{C (a - \overline{v}) O_2 \text{ (mL } O_2/100 \text{ mL blood)}}{CaO_2 \text{ (mL } O_2/100 \text{ mL blood)}} \times 100$$

When DO_2 falls, or VO_2 rises, the initial compensatory mechanisms include an increase in CO and increased O_2 extraction. Some tissues (myocardium) normally extract essentially all available O_2 and can increase O_2 delivery to the cell only by increasing myocardial blood flow.

6. The normal value for $C(a-\overline{v})O_2$ is 4.0–5.5 mL $O_2/100$ mL blood. The OER is normally 22%–30%.
   a. An increase or widening of $C(a-\overline{v})O_2$ may indicate inadequate tissue perfusion with increased tissue O_2 extraction as compensation.
   b. Similarly, a narrowing of $C(a-\overline{v})O_2$ may indicate an improved DO_2.
   c. However, it is important to remember that some patients, especially those with septic shock, may exhibit an inability to extract and utilize O_2 in part due to peripheral shunting. In these patients a narrowing of $C(a-\overline{v})O_2$ or a fall in OER may actually imply a wors-

ening of the shock state and inability to extract and utilize DO_2.

C. **The Oxygen Supply–Consumption Relationship.**
1. In normal subjects, VO_2 is independent of DO_2. Supply exceeds demand so that over a certain range, VO_2 does not change with increases or decreases in DO_2 (Fig 3–1). However, if DO_2 decreases sufficiently, VO_2 will also decline, resulting in anaerobic metabolism.
2. In certain patients with shock, especially septic shock, the relationship between VO_2 and DO_2 changes and VO_2 becomes supply-dependent (Fig 3-1).
3. It has been suggested that supply dependence of VO_2 is a poor prognostic sign and often occurs in patients who are producing lactic acid. Lactate production results from anaerobic metabolism and implies that DO_2 is insufficient to meet the body's demands.
4. It is important to remember that the calculated VO_2 and DO_2 are representative of the whole body and no conclu-

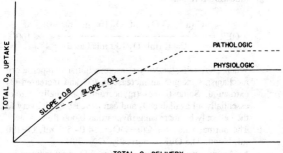

FIG 3–1.
A graphic representation of the relationship between VO_2 and DO_2 in normal and pathologic states. Normally VO_2 is independent of supply *(horizontal part of solid line)*. In sepsis or ARDS, oxygen extraction is abnormal *(slope of dotted line = 0.3)* and a much greater level of DO_2 is necessary to achieve supply independence *(horizontal part of dotted line)*. (From Kreuzer F, Cain SM: *Critical Care Clinics* 1985; 1:453–470).

sions can be made concerning each organ's regional DO_2 and VO_2.

5. Because the finding of supply dependency of VO_2 and lactate production indicates that DO_2 is not adequate to meet the body's demands, some investigators have suggested that therapy in these patients be directed at increasing DO_2 until VO_2 becomes supply-independent.

6. DO_2 can be increased by optimizing CO and CaO_2. CO can be increased by optimizing preload, decreasing afterload, and the use of inotropic agents. CaO_2 can be increased by transfusion and by increasing SaO_2.

7. No specific therapy is currently available to improve tissue O_2 extraction and utilization.

D. Oxygen Carrying Capacity.
1. Tissue O_2 availability is also dependent on the O_2 carrying capacity of hemoglobin.

2. The O_2 hemoglobin association-dissociation curve is sigmoid in shape. There is a high affinity for O_2 at high levels of PaO_2 which facilitates uptake of O_2 by hemoglobin in the lung. Conversely, there is a low affinity at the lower levels of PaO_2 which exist in the peripheral tissues facilitating release of O_2.

3. This curve is shifted to the right by increases in temperature and by decreases in pH, facilitating release of O_2 in the periphery.

4. Another important regulator of the release of oxygen from hemoglobin is 2,3-diphosphoglycerate (2,3-DPG) which is present in high concentration in RBCs.
   a. Higher concentrations of 2,3-DPG shift the association-dissociation curve to the right, decreasing the affinity of hemoglobin for O_2 and aiding the release of O_2.
   b. It is important to remember that 2,3-DPG levels are very low in banked blood, which may adversely affect DO_2 in patients following massive transfusions.

E. The Peripheral Microcirculation.
1. The peripheral microcirculation is also important in the regulation of DO_2.

2. In some patients with shock, especially hypovolemia or low CO, there is selective vasoconstriction with shunting of blood away from certain vascular beds to maintain cerebral and cardiac perfusion.

3. In patients with severe shock and disseminated intravascular coagulation (DIC), leukocyte plugging and microthrombi may occur.
4. Local control of the microcirculation is also abnormal in some patients, especially those with septic shock and may lead to arteriovenous shunting, further impairing DO_2.

II. CLASSIFICATION AND DIFFERENTIAL DIAGNOSIS OF THE SHOCK STATE.

A. Classification

Shock has traditionally been classified as cardiogenic, hypovolemic, or septic. Less common etiologies include neurogenic and anaphylactic shock. These classifications are useful but they are not mutually exclusive, e.g., an elderly patient with sepsis may also have significant underlying cardiac disease. In a particular patient a variety of factors may interact to impair DO_2.

B. Hypovolemic Shock.

1. The classic form of hypovolemic shock is hemorrhagic shock following trauma. Following hemorrhage, a decrease in LV preload and circulating RBC mass results in a diminished CO and impaired DO_2.
2. The body's compensatory mechanisms depend on the severity of blood loss (Table 3–1).
   a. With increasing blood loss, there is increasing sympathetic tone resulting in tachycardia, peripheral vasoconstriction, and shunting of blood away from the cutaneous, mesenteric, and skeletal muscle vascular beds, to maintain cerebral and cardiac perfusion.

TABLE 3–1.

Physiologic Changes in Hypovolemic Shock*

Blood loss (mL)	<750	750–1,250	1,250–2,000	2,000+
Blood loss (%)	<15%	15%–25%	25%–40%	>40%
Heart rate	Normal	↑	↑↑	↑↑↑
Blood pressure	Normal	Normal/↓	↓	↓↓
Respiratory rate	Normal	↑	↑↑	↑↑↑
Urine output	Normal	↓	Oliguria	Anuria
Mental status	Minimal anxiety	Mild anxiety	Confusion	Lethargy

    b. Another compensatory mechanism is secretion of a variety of hormones including cortisol, aldosterone, and vasopressin and other mediators.

    c. Fluid shifts from the interstitial and intracellular spaces occur to restore intravascular volume.

3. **Blood pressure is not a good indicator of the severity of hemorrhagic shock and may be maintained at normal levels by vasoconstriction.**

    a. Signs of end organ function such as perfusion of skin (capillary refill), mental status, and urinary output provide a more reliable assessment of the severity of the shock state.

    b. In the early stages hypovolemic shock is reversible by control of blood loss and appropriate restoration of intravascular volume. However, if tissue perfusion and DO_2 remain severely depressed, irreversible cellular injury may occur.

4. Any disease process which causes a loss of intravascular volume may result in shock. Common etiologies include GI bleeding, excessive diuresis, loss of fluid into the bowel lumen following bowel obstruction, and "third-spacing" of fluid in pancreatitis or following extensive surgery.

C. **Cardiogenic Shock.**

1. Cardiogenic shock results from the failure of the heart as a pump to deliver a CO sufficient to meet the body's needs.

    a. Classically, this is seen following myocardial infarction (MI) and may result from the loss of LV or RV myocardium or from complications of MI such as postinfarction ventricular septal defect or acute mitral regurgitation.

    b. Cardiomyopathies, chronic valvular disease, or arrhythmias all may adversely affect the ability of the heart to function as a pump.

    c. Cardiac tamponade represents a special form of cardiogenic shock in which there is inadequate filling of the heart secondary to compression of the cardiac chambers by pericardial fluid.

D. **Septic Shock.**

1. Pathophysiology.

    a. Septic shock is a complex pathophysiologic entity. Infections with a variety of organisms incite a host response with a number of humoral and cellular mediators including tumor necrosis factor (TNF), interleukins, arachidonic acid metabolites, platelet activating factor, and other cytokines.

b. In addition to the beneficial effects of this inflammatory response to infection, adverse effects including cellular injury may ensue.

2. Hemodynamic derangement.

a. The primary hemodynamic derangement in septic shock is loss of regulation of the peripheral microcirculation with vasodilation and arteriovenous shunting resulting in a low SVR.

b. Tissue O_2 extraction is abnormal, the relationship between DO_2 and VO_2 is altered and VO_2 may become supply-dependent (see Fig 3–1).

c. An actual defect in cellular or subcellular metabolism may be present and prevent the cell from utilizing O_2.

d. A circulating myocardial depressant factor may be present in patients with sepsis and the resultant cardiac dysfunction will further impair DO_2.

e. Early signs of septic shock include fever, tachycardia, tachypnea, and respiratory alkalosis.

f. CO is usually normal or elevated in the early stages and patients appear to be warm and well perfused although hypotension and oliguria may be present. SVR is low (Table 3–2).

g. If untreated early, septic shock may progress to a late irreversible stage characterized by multiple organ failure, low CO, and high peripheral resistance.

TABLE 3–2.
Clinical Parameters in Shock*

Shock Classification	Skin	Urine Output	JVD	CI	PCWP	SVR	C$\bar{v}O_2$
Hypovolemic	Cool, pale	↓	↓	↓	↓	↑	↓
Cardiogenic	Cool, pale	↓	↑	↓	↑	↑	↓
Early sepsis	Warm, pink	↓ ↑	↓ ↑	↑	↓	↓	↑ ↓
Late sepsis	Cool, pale	↓	↓	↓	↓	↑	↓ ↑
Neurogenic	Warm, pink	↓	↓	↓	↓	↓	↓

E. **Anaphylactic Shock.**
   1. Anaphylactoid reactions result from the interaction of antigen with IgE-bearing mast cells and basophils which have been previously sensitized.
   2. Anaphylactic shock may result from exposure to a wide variety of antigens including drugs, blood products, and insect bites.
   3. Hypotension, upper airway obstruction secondary to laryngospasm, bronchospasm, and urticaria may occur within seconds of exposure.
   4. Collapse and cardiac arrest follow if appropriate treatment is not instituted immediately (Table 3-3).

F. **Differential Diagnosis of the Shock State.**
   1. Differential diagnosis in patients with shock is aided by an understanding of the clinical situation (see Table 3-2). Obviously a young person seen immediately following a motor vehicle accident is more likely to be hypovolemic than septic.
   2. Once initial resuscitation has begun and the patient has been stabilized, more definitive diagnostic procedures can be undertaken as indicated.
   3. Evaluation should begin with a thorough history and physical examination and routine laboratory studies including a CXR and an ECG.
   4. Placement of a PA artery catheter can be very helpful and provide measurements of PCWP and CO. CaO_2 and $C\bar{v}O_2$ can be calculated and used to assess DO_2 and VO_2.
   5. After the patient has been stabilized, efforts should be made to find and treat any underlying cause of shock such as myocardial ischemia or infection.

III. MANAGEMENT OF THE SHOCK STATE.
A. **Initial Resuscitation.**
   1. Resuscitation of the patient with shock must begin with the standard "ABCs" (**Airway, Breathing, Circulation**). The first priority is to obtain a secure airway and make certain that the patient is ventilated adequately.
   2. IV access should be obtained and fluid resuscitation begun.
   3. CPR is instituted if necessary and any arrhythmia is treated appropriately.
   4. As the patient is being stabilized a search is made for im-

TABLE 3-3.

Anaphylactic Shock*

If anaphylaxis is suspected (history of recent injection or transfusion) begin therapy immediately.

Signs
  Laryngeal edema
  Hemolysis
  Bronchospasm
  Pulmonary hypertension
  Vascular collapse
  Pulmonary edema
  Urticaria
  Flushing
Treatment
  Stop administration of allergen
  Airway—intubation may be required; administer 100% O_2
  IV access—14- or 16-gauge IV
  IV fluid—500 mL LR
  Drugs
    Aqueous epinephrine
      IM—0.5-1.0 mg (0.5 mL 1:1,000 solution)
      IV—1.0-2.0 mL 1:10,000 solution (1 mL of 1:1,000 solution diluted
      with 9 mL NS gives a 1:10,000 solution) IV over 3-5 min if hypotensive
    Antihistamine (diphenhydramine)
      50 mg IV/IM
    Glucocorticoid
      Hydrocortisone 100-250 mg IV
      Methylprednisone 50-100 mg IM
    Aminophylline
      6 mg/kg IV loading dose
      0.5-1.0 mg/kg/hr infusion
    H_2 antagonist
      Cimetidine 300 mg IV

mediately life-threatening problems such as active hemorrhage, pneumothorax, or cardiac tamponade which are treated as indicated.

B. Stabilization.

1. After the initial resuscitation, routine laboratory studies and a CXR and a ECG are obtained. A Foley catheter should be inserted to monitor urinary output. A thorough

history is taken and a physical examination is performed to search for an underlying cause of the shock state.

2. The response to therapy should be assessed initially by clinical parameters including mental status, urinary output, peripheral perfusion (HR, BP, skin temperature, and capillary refill). If there has been no significant clinical improvement with the initial volume resuscitation (crystalloid 20 mL/kg or 500–1,000 mL), a second crystalloid bolus should be given and a search made for ongoing volume loss or other reasons for persistent hypotension and shock.

3. RBC transfusion should be begun if there is still evidence of hypovolemia after 2,000 mL of crystalloid.

4. **It is important to continually reassess the patient for adequacy and stability of ventilation and to continually monitor the circulation and peripheral perfusion.**

5. As the results of laboratory studies become available, abnormalities in acid-base state, oxygenation, and electrolytes must be corrected. Injuries should be treated as indicated.

6. If sepsis is felt to be an etiologic factor, cultures should be obtained and broad-spectrum antibiotic therapy initiated.

7. If the patient remains unstable, more aggressive measures are warranted including invasive monitoring and operative correction of injury or ongoing hemorrhage.

C. **Optimization of Tissue Oxygen Delivery.**

1. Introduction.

   a. The treatment goal of patients with shock is to restore DO_2 to normal (or supranormal) levels and to reverse the underlying cause of the shock state.

   b. Currently no therapy is available to improve cellular utilization of DO_2.

   c. Impaired DO_2 results in a tissue O_2 deficit. When this deficit is excessive, irreversible cellular injury occurs. Thus, aggressive therapy to restore DO_2 and "repay" the tissue O_2 deficit is indicated.

   d. Invasive monitoring is indicated with elderly patients, patients with significant underlying diseases, following multisystem trauma, and patients failing to respond appropriately to initial resuscitation so that the hemodynamic state and DO_2 can be optimized.

2. Cardiac output.

The optimal CO in patients with shock is uncertain, tissue O_2 needs must be met, yet myocardial work should not be increased to the point of myocardial ischemia (coronary blood flow and thus myocardial O_2 supply may be essentially fixed in patients with coronary artery disease).

a. Preload.

1) Preload should be optimized initially as CO can be increased with minimal myocardial O_2 consumption. Using the PA catheter as a guide, volume (crystalloid or colloid) should be infused to a PCWP of 15–18 mm Hg.

2) The optimal PCWP must be selected in each patient by careful volume expansion while monitoring CO.

b. Heart rate.

1) Significant bradycardia (HR<60) or tachycardia (HR>120) may adversely affect CO. Arrhythmias and bradycardia should be appropriately treated.

2) If necessary pacing at 100 bpm can be instituted to insure CO while allowing adequate diastolic time for coronary blood flow.

c. Afterload.

1) Afterload reduction may be useful, especially in patients with impaired ventricular function or valvular heart disease (mitral or aortic regurgitation). However in many patients with shock, SVR and MAP are decreased and careful consideration must be given to the use of a vasodilator.

2) Prior to using an afterload reducing agent, preload must be optimized or severe hypotension may result.

3) In the SICU, sodium nitroprusside (SNP) is the most commonly used agent. SNP is begun at an infusion of 0.5 μg/kg/min. The dosage is titrated to increase CO while maintaining an acceptable MAP (Table 3–4). The maximum infusion rate is usually 5.0–7.0 μg/kg/min. Occasionally, higher infusion rates are used.

4) If prolonged infusion of SNP is required, cyanide or thiocyanate toxicity may result. Evidence of a

TABLE 3–4.

Clinical Dose Ranges for Intravenous Cardiovascular Agents†

Agent	Starting Dose	Usual Dose	High Usual Dose	High Dose
Isoproterenol	0.01	0.025	0.05	0.2
Epinephrine	.03–.05	.05–0.1	0.2	0.4
Dopamine	2–4	6–10	15	25
Dobutamine	2–4	6–10	15	25
Amrinone	5	5	10–15	20
Norepinephrine	0.05	0.1	0.2	0.4
Phenylephrine	0.6	0.6–1.0	1–2	>2
Nitroglycerin	0.2	1	2	3
Nitroprusside	1	1–3	3–5	5–7

*Doses in μg/kg/min.
†Adapted from Smith PK: Postoperative Care in Cardiac Surgery, in Sabiston DC, Spencer FC (eds): *Surgery of the Chest*, ed 5. Philadelphia, WB Saunders, 1991.

lactic acidosis with rising $S\bar{v}O_2$ may indicate cyanide toxicity.

5) In certain patients (postcardiac surgery, acute mitral regurgitation, acute MI) institution of IABP support may be indicated to reduce afterload and improve coronary perfusion (see Chapter 6).

d. Inotropic state.

1) Inotropic agents may be used to augment myocardial contractility and increase CO. Some agents are also vasoconstrictors and may increase SVR and MAP. These agents may cause tachycardia, arrhythmias, and increase myocardial O_2 consumption (Table 3–4).

2) Dopamine is a naturally occurring catecholamine which is a precursor of norepinephrine.

a) At low doses (<3.0 μg/kg/min) it stimulates dopaminergic receptors, increasing renal and mesenteric flow.

b) At doses of 3–5 μg/kg/min, β-receptor effects predominate increasing CO and stroke volume (SV).

c) At high levels (>10 μg/kg/min) significant vasoconstriction may occur increasing SVR while decreasing renal and mesenteric blood flow.

d) Dopamine is the initial drug of choice for shock with low CO and low MAP, after preload has been optimized.

e) At low infusion rates, it is very useful to maintain renal blood flow (Tables 3–4, 3–5).

3) Dobutamine is a synthetic catecholamine with β_1, β_2, and weak α effects.

a) Infusion of dobutamine will increase CO and SV and may cause vasodilation resulting in decreased SVR.

b) Because of the vasodilation and increase in CO, the PCWP also usually decreases.

c) At higher doses there may be an increase in HR although the chronotropic effect is less than that seen with dopamine.

d) Dobutamine is useful in low CO states without significant hypotension, especially in the setting of CHF or acute MI.

e) Dobutamine may also dilate constricted vascular beds and improve peripheral perfusion and oxygen delivery (see Tables 3–4, 3–5).

4) Epinephrine is a naturally occurring catecholamine with α- and β-agonist effects.

a) β effects predominate (increased HR, CO, SV) at low dosages.

b) At higher dosages α effects predominate producing vasoconstriction and decreasing blood

TABLE 3–5.

Comparative Hemodynamic Effects of Vasoactive Drugs Used in Treating Shock*†

Drug	PCWP	SVR	SV	HR	PA Pressure	CO	Systolic BP
Dopamine	0–↑	0–↑	↑	↑		↑	0–↑
Dobutamine	↓	0–↑	↑	0–↑	0–↑	↑	0–↑
Norepinephrine	↑	↑	↓ or ↑	0–↑	↑	0–↓	↑

*Norepinephrine may ↓ SV by increasing afterload.
†Modified from Schuster D, Lefarak S: Shock, in Civetta JM (ed): *Critical Care.* Philadelphia, JB Lippincott, 1988.

flow to peripheral, mesenteric, and renal vascular beds.

   c) Continuous infusions of epinephrine are useful in low CO states, especially following cardiac surgery.

   d) Bolus infusions are useful in the treatment of anaphylactic shock and during CPR (Tables 3–1, 3–3).

5) Norepinephrine is a naturally occurring catecholamine with β_1- and α-agonist effects.

   a) It is a positive inotropic agent but the α-induced vasoconstriction markedly increases SVR while reducing renal and mesenteric perfusion.

   b) Norepinephrine is useful in the treatment of shock which does not respond to dopamine or dobutamine. However, the increased afterload secondary to vasoconstriction may lead to reduced CO in patients with impaired LV function.

   c) Norepinephrine may occasionally be used in patients with septic shock (high CO, low SVR) to increase perfusion pressures. An increased perfusion pressure may especially be useful in patients with critical peripheral vascular disease who require higher pressures to maintain flow (renal artery stenosis or carotid occlusive disease). However, the vasoconstriction of norepinephrine is nonspecific and may markedly decrease mesenteric and renal perfusion (Tables 3–4, 3–5).

6) Isoproterenol is a pure β-agonist which produces a marked increase in HR and may lower SVR and pulmonary vascular resistance (PVR).

   a) Infusions of isoproterenol are useful in symptomatic bradycardia and β-blocker toxicity.

   b) Isoproterenol may be useful in patients with primary RV failure (Table 3–4).

7) Phenylephrine is a pure α-agonist which causes vasoconstriction. Infusion of phenylephrine may be useful to maintain perfusion pressure in patients with septic shock (Table 3–4).

8) Amrinone is a noncatecholamine' pyridine derivative which is both a positive inotropic agent and a vasodilator.

   a) Amrinone increases cardiac output and decreases SVR.

   b) The use of amrinone may be limited by its long half-life (6 hours), vasodilation resulting in significant hypotension, and severe thrombocytopenia.

   c) Infusions of amrinone may be indicated in patients with RV dysfunction (see Table 3–4).

3. Other therapeutic modalities.

   a. In addition to optimization of CO, DO_2 can be improved by increasing the hematocrit (Hct) and SaO_2.

      1) The optimal Hct for DO_2 has not been determined and probably varies greatly in different patients and clinical situations. The benefits of increased O_2 carrying capacity must be weighed against the risk of transfusion. Also, increasing Hct results in increased blood viscosity and may worsen the microcirculation.

      2) Transfusion of packed RBCs should be used to obtain a Hct of at least 25%–30%. In some patients, a higher Hct may be beneficial, and the Hct should be adjusted to optimize DO_2.

      3) The SaO_2 should be maintained at a level greater than 90% and may require use of supplemental O_2, mechanical ventilation, and PEEP (Chapter 7).

   b. Steroids have been shown to have no beneficial effects on the course of septic shock and to possibly increase the risk of infection. Therefore, steroids should not be used in the therapy of septic shock.

   c. Naloxone has been used to treat patients with refractory septic shock. There are anecdotal reports of improved hemodynamics although no survival benefits have been documented. A wide range of dosages have been utilized and currently no specific recommendation covering the use of naloxone can be made. Its use in septic shock must be considered experimental.

D. Goals of Therapy.

1. The ultimate goal is reversal of the shock state and survival of the patient. Toward this end it is important to op-

timize tissue perfusion and DO_2, correct the acid-base status and electrolyte abnormalities, correct any underlying cause of the shock status (treat injuries, drain abscesses, treat infection with appropriate antibiotics, treat complications of the shock state [acute lung injury, acute renal failure]) and provide adequate nutrition.

2. The end point for optimization of DO_2 is uncertain. Normalization of DO_2 is probably insufficient in these hypermetabolic, catabolic patients. It has been suggested that achievement of "supranormal" values (CI >4.5 L/min/m^2, DO_2 >600 mL/min/m^2, VO_2 >170 mL/min/m^2) will increase survival. Because of the relationship between DO_2 and VO_2, DO_2 should be increased until supply independence of VO_2 is achieved and hyperlactatemia resolves.

E. Irreversible Shock and MOFS.

1. In some patients with shock an initial period of stability follows resuscitation. This brief phase may be followed by a period of hypermetabolism with progressive organ failure (lungs, kidneys, liver) (Table 3–6). There is continued deterioration with recurrent infections, sequential organ failure coagulopathy, and encephalopathy in the late stages. Mortality is very high and MOFS accounts for a large percentage of death in the SICU.

2. The etiology of MOFS is uncertain. It may be related to the degree of cellular hypoxia and injury with the initial episode of shock.
   a. There is increasing evidence that MOFS is the result of infection, especially with gut organisms. Shock with decreased mesenteric flow can alter the integrity of gut mucosa allowing translocation of bacteria into lymph nodes and the bloodstream.
   b. Repeated episodes of gram-negative sepsis develop, as well as nosocomial pneumonia and infection of invasive monitoring catheters.
   c. A variety of mediators including TNF, interleukins, prostaglandins, and cytokines may be important causes of cell injury.

3. No specific therapy for MOFS is available. Treatment should be directed at maintaining adequate DO_2, aggressive therapy of injuries and infections, appropriate treatment of pulmonary and renal failure, and early aggressive nutritional therapy (enteral feeding may help maintain gut

TABLE 3–6.

Multiple Organ Failure*

Organ System	Presentation	Syndrome
Lung	Hypoxemia + diffuse infiltrates	ARDS
Kidney	Creatinine >2mg/dL or 2 × admission	
	Urine output <500 mL/24 hr	Oliguric ARF
	Urine output >500 mL/24 hr	Nonoliguric ARF
Liver	Bilirubin 2 mg/dL, SGOT and LDH 2 × admission	Cholestatic jaundice
	Intractable hyperglycemia or hypoglycemia	Hepatocyte failure
	Cholecystitis with nonlithogenic bile	Acalculous cholecystitis
Gut	Upper GI bleed—2 units/24 hr	Stress ulceration
	Endoscopically confirmed superficial ulceration	
Coagulation	Thrombocytopenia, prolonged PT, PTT with FDP	DIC, hypofibrinogenemia
Heart	Hypotension, CI < 1.5 L/m^2, no MI	Myocardial failure
CNS	Response only to painful stimuli	Obtundation of sepsis

*Adapted from Civetta JN, Taylor RW, Kirby RR: *Critical Care.* Philadelphia, JB Lippincott, 1988.

mucosal integrity). Selective antibiotic decontamination of the gut has been advocated but its effect on survival remains controversial. Despite aggressive resuscitation and treatment, mortality remains high.

F. Treatment of Anaphylaxis.

1. Life-threatening airway obstruction may occur with anaphylaxis; thus immediate diagnosis and treatment is imperative. Epinephrine is the primary treatment and can be given SC(0.3–0.5 mL of 1:1,000 solution) or IV (1.0—2.0 mL of 1:10,000 solution).
2. If the laryngospasm fails to resolve, a stable airway must be obtained by either orotracheal intubation or cricothyroidotomy.

3. Because of the role of histamine in the pathogenesis of anaphylaxis therapy, H_1 (diphenhydramine, Benadryl) and H_2 (cimetidine, ranitidine) blockers should be initiated, and steroids may be necessary (Table 3–3).

SELECTED REFERENCES

American Heart Association: *Textbook of Advanced Cardiac Life Support*. Dallas, American Heart Association, 1987.

Astiz ME, Rackow EL, Fulk JL, et al: Oxygen delivery and consumption in patients with hyperdynamic septic shock. *Crit Care Med* 1987; 15:26.

Barton R, Cerra FB: The hypermetabolism, multiple organ failure syndrome. *Chest* 1989; 96:1153.

Cunnion, RE, Parrillo JE. Myocardial dysfunction in sepsis. *Chest* 1989; 95:941.

Kandel G, Aberman A: Mixed venous oxygen saturation: Its role in the assessment of the critically ill patient. *Arch Intern Med* 1983; 143:1400.

Schumacker PT, Cain, SM: The concept of a critical oxygen delivery. *Intensive Care Med* 1987; 13:223.

Shoemaker WC: Relation of oxygen transport patterns to the pathophysiology and therapy of shock states. *Intensive Care Med* 1987; 13:230.

Shoemaker WC, Kran HB, Appel PL: Therapy of shock based on pathophysiology, monitoring, and outcome prediction. *Crit Care Med* 1990; 18:519.

CARDIAC ARREST AND CARDIOPULMONARY RESUSCITATION $\quad$ **4**

I. CARDIAC ARREST.
A. Incidence.
1. Cardiac arrest is an emergency common to every medical specialty. While the frequency of cardiac arrest in the population at large is uncertain, it is generally agreed that the hospital population is at increased risk. Underlying medical and surgical problems, as well as the cardiovascular status of the individual surgical patient, may alter the risk of cardiac arrest.
2. There is a particular association between general anesthesia and cardiac arrest with a reported incidence as high as 1 in 1,700 cases.

B. Etiology.
Cardiac arrest may occur as a primary cardiac event, secondary to respiratory causes, or as a consequence of metabolic abnormalities.
1. Cardiac.
   a. Coronary artery disease is the single most frequent cause and is at least a contributing factor in the majority of cases. Many patients have a previous history of cardiac disease; however, cardiac arrest may be the first clinical manifestation of coronary artery disease.
   b. Structural abnormalities such as congenital anomalies, fibrosis, or hypertrophy may exist chronically which provide the anatomic substrate for a primary arrhythmia.
   c. Cardiac arrest also occurs in patients with no identifiable structural cardiac defect.

2. Respiratory.
   a. Acute respiratory failure may follow airway obstruction, upper or lower airway trauma, depression of the central respiratory drive, or the malfunction of mechanical ventilators. After respiratory arrest, effective circulation may continue for several minutes until hypoxemia and acidemia produce cardiac arrest, usually ventricular fibrillation.
   b. Even in the absence of acute respiratory failure, hypoxemia or hypercapnea, or both, may be contributing causes to cardiac arrest. These precipitating factors may occur in the clinical setting of severe atelectasis, chest trauma, pulmonary embolism, or severe intrinsic pulmonary disease with decreased gas exchange.
3. Metabolic.
   a. Cardiac arrest may be precipitated by disturbances in electrolytes, particularly K, resulting from acute or chronic losses of fluid and electrolytes that are inadequately or incorrectly replaced.
   b. In surgical patients, this may result from hyperthermic injury, prolonged febrility, or enteric losses (prolonged NG suction, enterocutaneous fistula, enterostomy, diarrhea). Moreover, nearly all patients undergo large fluid shifts perioperatively, and meticulous attention to detail is required for the maintenance of proper fluid-electrolyte balance.
   c. The use of diuretics without attention to K supplementation may result in significant hypokalemia and cardiac arrest.
   d. Extreme alterations in body temperature may cause cardiac arrest. In particular, patients are susceptible to ventricular dysrhythmias during hypothermic exposure as well as during the rewarming phase. These may occur due to environmental exposure but also occur on a daily basis in every hospital where hypothermia is induced during cardiopulmonary bypass. These patients frequently return to the SICU with a core temperature less than 35° C and require several hours to rewarm.

C. Pathophysiology.
1. Irrespective of the particular etiologic factors, the resulting cardiac arrest is evident as ventricular fibrillation or tachycardia, ventricular asystole, or cardiogenic shock of such

magnitude that no effective cardiac output (CO) or pressure is generated. This results in the cessation of flow of oxygenated blood to the body.

2. **The central nervous system (CNS) is most vulnerable in this situation and at normothermia will tolerate no more than 4–6 minutes of total ischemia.** After a longer period of arrest, resuscitation may result in recovery of other organ systems, but return of CNS function is unlikely.

D. Diagnosis.

1. In the unmonitored patient, the diagnosis of cardiac arrest is strongly suggested by the unexpected loss of consciousness and a lack of spontaneous respirations.

2. The definitive diagnosis of cardiac arrest is made by the loss of a previously palpable central arterial pulse.

   a. Audible heart sounds may be present in the absence of a palpable pulse, and a pressure wave may persist if the arterial pressure is being monitored.

   b. A nonpalpable carotid pulse (systolic pressure < 60 mm Hg) represents systemic pressure that is insufficient for coronary or cerebral perfusion and is an indication to begin CPR.

3. Respiratory arrest in a patient previously breathing spontaneously is diagnosed by loss of thoracic movements and absence of breath sounds bilaterally.

   a. In a mechanically ventilated patient, thoracic motion and breath sounds will persist after cardiac arrest and are not helpful in making the diagnosis.

   b. Ventilator failure may produce profound anoxia leading to cardiac arrest, despite continued inflation of the chest. A strong index of suspicion should be maintained, and the patient should be removed from the ventilator immediately and ventilated manually with 100% O_2.

   c. In the event of cardiac arrest in a mechanically ventilated patient, it is mandatory to immediately ascertain proper ET tube position and to rule out the presence of pneumothorax.

4. Syncope, seizures, vasovagal reactions, profound shock, and nonfatal arrhythmias may produce a clinical syndrome resembling cardiac arrest. However, the differential diagnosis should be considered only after resuscitation has begun, since the **complications of beginning basic life sup-**

port are far outweighed by the effect of any delay in treatment.

5. Specific diagnosis requires an ECG to differentiate between ventricular fibrillation, asystole, and ineffective output with persistent electrical activity (electromechanical dissociation, EMD). However, the initial treatment of each of these is the same and the initiation of therapy should precede any attempt at specific diagnosis.

II. CARDIOPULMONARY RESUSCITATION.

The treatment of cardiac arrest is divided into three phases: (1) **basic life support,** (2) **advanced life support,** and (3) **stabilization.** In the hospital setting, these phases are not clearly separated, and aspects of treatment from all three phases proceed simultaneously. For the sake of clarity, however, each is discussed separately as if each occurred sequentially.

A. Basic Life Support.

The goal of the initial treatment of cardiac arrest is to provide sufficient oxygenated blood to meet the body's metabolic demands until normal circulation can be restored. Basic life support is described by the letters ABC (airway, breathing, circulation).

1. Airway.
   a. Once apnea or pulselessness is established, resuscitation is initiated by establishing an airway.
      1) The mouth should be opened and inspected.
      2) Foreign objects, including chewing gum, tobacco, and dentures, should be removed.
      3) The airway then can be opened by extending the neck and lifting the jaw which lifts the tongue from the posterior pharynx (Fig 4–1).
      4) Mouth-to-mouth breathing is initiated and continued until other means of airway control and ventilation are available.
   b. Frequently, an oropharyngeal airway is utilized; however, care must be taken since this device itself can force the tongue posteriorly and obstruct the airway. This may be avoided by inserting the device with its blade reversed and sliding the tip across the hard palate, soft palate, and then the posterior wall of the oropharynx. After insertion, the device then is rotated 180 degrees into place so that its concave surface lies against

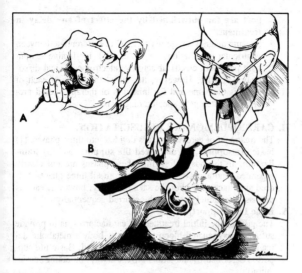

FIG 4–1.
A, the initial step in resuscitation requires opening the airway by tilting the head back and elevating the jaw if necessary to displace the tongue forward. **B,** the preparation for mouth-to-mouth resuscitation is to close the nose by compression and open the mouth. If the mouth cannot be opened, ventilation through the nose is possible if the lips are held closed. (From Sabiston DC Jr (ed): *Textbook of Surgery,* ed 13. Philadelphia, WB Saunders Co, 1986, p 2168. Used by permission.)

   the tongue anteriorly, maintaining patency of the airway.
  c. Alternatively, a nasopharyngeal tube may be used. This device is less likely to produce airway obstruction and is better tolerated than the oropharyngeal airway which can cause vomiting and aspiration in a responsive patient with an intact gag reflex.
  d. Many other devices are available to aid in establishing the airway, but most of these are cumbersome and should not be necessary in the hospital setting where ET

intubation should be performed by trained personnel as soon as possible.

e. **If spontaneous breathing is not immediately restored, or if the patient is unable to protect the airway, a more secure airway must be secured.** This may require orotracheal intubation, nasotracheal intubation, or cricothyroidotomy (see Chapter 22).

2. Breathing.

a. As soon as the airway is secured, ventilation of the patient should begin. Mouth-to-mouth breathing is applied first. Since exhaled air has an F_{IO_2} of approximately 0.15, this is adequate for the initial phase of the resuscitation.

b. Ventilation with 100% O_2 should be instituted rapidly to maximally saturate the arterial blood. This may be accomplished by a bag-valve-mask system when a laryngoscope and ET tube are not readily available.

c. Mask ventilation may require an oral or nasal airway to ensure patency of the airway. The technique of ventilation with a valved mask system should be mastered by all house officers since intubation may be difficult and at times impossible.

d. The rate of ventilation should be 12–15/min for an adult. Expansion of the chest should be evident and the presence of breath sounds bilaterally should be confirmed by auscultation.

e. The unilateral absence of breath sounds may be evidence of a collapsed lung, pneumothorax, or malposition of an ET tube.

f. The patient should be ventilated manually throughout the resuscitation including basic and advanced life support. Only after cardiac function has been restored and the patient is being stabilized should mechanical ventilation be instituted.

3. Circulation.

a. When there is only a single rescuer, external cardiac massage is begun after the airway is controlled and three breaths have been given; this continues with two breaths interposed after every 15 compressions.

b. In the hospital setting, there are usually multiple rescuers and one begins external cardiac massage while the other clears the airway and begins ventilation.

    c. The heel of one hand is placed over the other; the arms are straight with the elbows locked; and force is applied to the lower third of the sternum. A board should be placed beneath the patient, and the headboards of modern hospital beds have been adapted for this purpose. A compression rate of at least 80/min is recommended and a rate of 100/min is suggested. The compression phase should constitute 50% of the cycle (Fig 4–2).

  4. Physiology of external cardiac massage.

    a. Thoracic pump.

      1) The circulation of blood during external cardiac massage was believed initially to be caused by direct compression of the heart by the force applied to the sternum.

      2) Subsequently, this dogma was challenged by investigations which focused on the thoracic pump mechanism.

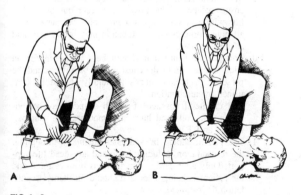

FIG 4–2.
A, the correct position of the hands for cardiac compression is determined by palpation of the xiphoid with one hand and placement of the other on the sternum above that level. **B,** external cardiac compression is accomplished by depression of the sternum for a distance of $1\frac{1}{2}$–2 in., using the heels of the hands and the weight of the rescuer at a rate of 80–100 bpm. (From Sabiston DC Jr (ed): *Textbook of Surgery,* ed 13, Philadelphia, WB Saunders Co, 1986, p 2169. Used by permission.)

a) According to this model, direct cardiac compression does not occur and blood flow during external compression is generated by the increase in intrathoracic pressure. The heart serves merely as a conduit, and regurgitant flow is prevented by venous valves at the thoracic inlet.

b) However, CO remains exceedingly low, less than 25% of controlled values. The aortic and all cardiac chamber pressures are equal according to this model. Thus, there is no pressure gradient to produce coronary blood flow.

c) Using the assumptions of this model, a rate of 60/min was demonstrated to be optimal in experimental animal studies.

b. High-impulse CPR.

1) Recently, this newer theory was challenged by experimental work which acknowledged the presence of a thoracic pump mechanism but demonstrated that high-impulse compression at faster rates significantly improved hemodynamic function during resuscitation. Since impulse is a function of force applied over time, high impulse is not solely dependent on increasing the force but can be achieved by the application of the same force over a briefer duration.

2) In these studies, measurements of LV dimensions provided evidence of direct cardiac compression. The peak LV pressure was consistently four to five times greater than the intrathoracic pressure. With increasing rate, stroke volume (SV) remained constant; thus, the CO increased, reaching approximately 50% of control values at a rate of 150/min.

3) Diastolic aortic pressure increased with the increasing CO, thus improving the coronary perfusion pressure. Moreover, coronary flow occurred during the diastolic or noncompressive phase and was inhibited during compression. With compressions of brief duration, the diastolic perfusion time was increased. Coronary blood flow increased up to a rate of 120/min, above which there appeared to be a critical limitation of perfusion time.

4) These studies suggested that a faster compression rate using high-impulse techniques provides the optimum combination of CO and coronary blood flow. Using this technique, increased survival was demonstrated in an animal model. It was on the basis of these and other data that the AHA increased the recommended compression rate.

5. Open chest cardiac massage.
   a. Indications.
      1) **In the overwhelming majority of cases, effective circulation may be achieved by external cardiac massage.**
      2) Open chest massage should be reserved for specific indications.
         a) In cases of cardiac arrest following known or suspected chest trauma when closed chest massage does not produce a palpable femoral arterial pulse, the chest should be opened so that the pericardium may be decompressed if tamponade is present. Emergent thoracotomy should be undertaken in all cases of cardiac arrest following penetrating thoracic trauma.
         b) Similarly, in patients in whom cardiac tamponade is strongly suspected, thoracotomy may be necessary. In certain of these cases, however, pericardiocentesis performed rapidly prior to actual cardiac arrest may allow cardiac filling sufficient to restore adequate hemodynamic function so that further therapy may be undertaken in a more controlled fashion (see pp 142–143).
         c) When inadequate blood pressure is generated using closed techniques the decision to perform thoracotomy and open cardiac massage should depend on the clinical situation and experience of the rescuer. Open massage may be indicated in patients with general chest wall deformities (scoliosis) or with an unstable chest wall following cardiac surgery.
   b. Techniques.
      1) When open chest massage is deemed necessary, a left anterior thoracotomy should be performed in

the fourth intercostal space and extended to the midaxillary line.

2) A chest retractor is inserted, the ribs spread, and the pericardium is opened.

3) Cardiac compression is performed, using the palm of the hand to compress the ventricles against the spine.

4) More complete emptying of the heart occurs with this technique and a longer noncompression period must be allowed for ventricular filling. Thus, a rate of 60–70/min is appropriate for open chest compression.

B. Advanced Life Support.

1. External cardiac massage and ventilation must continue and should not be interrupted for more than 5–10 seconds at a time while other maneuvers are performed. As soon as personnel are available, however, attention must be returned to restoring normal electrical and mechanical cardiac function. This is the purpose of advanced life support which involves (1) invasive and noninvasive monitoring, (2) electrical defibrillation, (3) pharmacologic therapy, and (4) cardiac pacing.

2. As initial resuscitation techniques and advanced life support are applied it is important to search for correctable difficulties such as dislodgement of an ET tube, tension pneumothorax, cardiac tamponade, etc.

3. Management of resuscitation efforts.

   a. Supervision.

      1) At this point, one person takes charge. This person may be a specific member of a designated resuscitation team or may be the senior physician present.

      2) Provided sufficient personnel are present, he should not actively participate in chest compression, ventilation of the patient, or the insertion of various catheters.

      3) He should direct the sequence of interventions during resuscitation and be responsible for terminating resuscitation efforts.

   b. Monitoring.

      1) The ECG provides the definitive diagnosis of the electrical status of the heart, directs the specific

therapy necessary, and allows evaluation of therapeutic maneuvers.

    a) Continual monitoring of the ECG should be obtained as soon as possible during resuscitation.

    b) Certain portable defibrillators which contain an oscilloscope and have paddles that serve as electrodes are particularly useful. These allow rapid assessment of the ECG early in the arrest; however, the standard limb leads should be applied as soon as possible.

2) While a central venous line may be placed for access, measurement of CVP is not helpful during resuscitation.

3) Frequent sampling of arterial blood is necessary and the femoral pulse should be palpable with adequate chest compression, making arterial puncture feasible. Occasionally, an indwelling arterial line may be useful to monitor arterial pressure during resuscitation.

  c. Venous access.

1) A large-bore (14–16 gauge) IV catheter should be placed in at least one antecubital fossa. The need for a central venous catheter during resuscitation is uncertain; moreover, the probability of complications due to the placement of central lines during chest compression is relatively high.

2) However, the drugs administered must reach the heart or the arterial side of the circulation, and there is legitimate concern over the quantity and velocity of peripheral venous flow owing to decreased perfusion of the extremities. This may be partially corrected by elevation of the arm and by rapid infusion of a large amount of fluid after administration of drugs. These maneuvers serve to increase the peripheral venous–RA pressure gradient.

3) The femoral vein offers an excellent site for access, perhaps the preferred site during CPR. A subclavian-type catheter inserted into the femoral vein will pass well up into the IVC.

4) If cannulation of the internal jugular or subclavian vein is necessary, chest compression should be halted for 10 seconds while the vein is entered and the guidewire or catheter passed. Chest compression then resumes while the catheter is threaded.

5) Cannulation of the saphenous vein under direct vision may be easily performed after exposure through a small incision (cutdown).

6) **Occasionally arterial lines will be inadvertently inserted while attempting to obtain venous access. This may be especially common while attempting to insert femoral venous lines. These lines can be used for volume resuscitation until adequate venous access is secured. Arterial lines should not be used for drug administration.**

7) Finally, drugs may be given directly into the heart using a long needle introduced via the subxiphoid approach. This approach should be used only when *absolutely necessary* because of the potential for direct damage to the heart or a coronary vessel.

8) Epinephrine may be administered via the ET tube with rapid absorption if no other access is available.

9) After drugs are given by any route, chest compression should continue for 10 seconds to allow circulation of the agent before defibrillation is attempted.

d. Intubation.

1) The placement of an ET tube secures the airway and should be performed as soon as possible. In addition to providing more effective ventilation and oxygenation, both gastric insufflation and aspiration of gastric contents are prevented (see Chapter 22).

2) The patient should be hyperventilated and oxygenated using a bag and mask prior to attempting ET intubation.

3) If not successful within 30 seconds, the attempted intubation must be interrupted and the patient must be ventilated between attempts.

    4) Occasionally in the presence of facial trauma, known or suspected cervical trauma, or repeated failure to intubate by experienced personnel, a cricothyroidotomy should be performed (see Chapter 22).

    5) High-frequency jet ventilation via a transtracheal catheter has become an accepted method of ventilatory support in the emergency setting.

e. Defibrillation.

    1) The development of closed chest defibrillation provided an effective, noninvasive technique of restoring normal electrical cardiac function. A single direct current (dc) countershock across the chest simultaneously depolarizes all myocardial cells, interrupting the reentry phenomena associated with ventricular tachycardia or the totally disorganized activity of ventricular fibrillation. After repolarization, the cells of the intrinsic conduction pathway should be the first to depolarize, initiating a coherent wave front of depolarization over the heart.

    2) The defibrillators most commonly used are the standard type with handheld paddles. These should be firmly applied to the chest with one paddle placed just to the right of the upper sternum and the other lateral to the left nipple and left anterior axillary line.

    3) To maximize the current delivered to the heart, a low-impedance gel or cream is used to decrease resistance at the paddle-skin interface.

    4) The strength of the first defibrillation should be 200 J. If this fails, the second attempt should be 200–300 J; the third and subsequent attempts should be 360 J if available.

    5) If ventricular tachycardia or fibrillation recurs after successful defibrillation, the strength of the previously successful shock should be selected for attempted defibrillation.

    6) Under most circumstances, basic life support should be initiated before defibrillation is attempted. However, after a witnessed arrest of a monitored patient, specifically the sudden conver-

sion of a relatively normal ECG to ventricular tachycardia or fibrillation, a single attempt at defibrillation may be justified if this can be performed immediately.

7) Myocardial hypoxia and acidosis can prevent successful defibrillation and should be corrected.

8) Defibrillation is of little use in true asystole, but correction of hypoxia and acidosis during a period of perfusion of the heart with oxygenated blood may restore some electrical activity. **Defibrillation may be attempted as in some cases it is difficult to differentiate asystole and fine ventricular fibrillation.**

9) Similarly, in the presence of fine ventricular fibrillation, it is wise to continue basic life support and use vasoconstrictors to increase the arterial pressure and thus the coronary perfusion pressure. These maneuvers may coarsen the fibrillation, increasing the likelihood of successful defibrillation.

10) Finally, if lethal ventricular arrhythmias recur rapidly after defibrillation, antiarrhythmic therapy should be instituted before another defibrillation is attempted.

f. Pharmacology.

Drug therapy in cardiac arrest is rational and aimed at correcting the causes and sequelae of the arrest, preventing a recurrence, and stabilizing hemodynamic function in the postresuscitation period. Major groups of drugs used in cardiac arrest are discussed briefly (Table 4-1).

1) Antiarrhythmic agents.

a) Despite optimal correction of hypoxemia, recurrent lethal dysrhythmias may occur early after successful defibrillation. This is most likely due to an area of regional ischemia or infarction which serves as an irritable focus and which either caused or was exacerbated by the arrest. In this situation, antiarrhythmic therapy should be instituted and continued through the stabilization period.

b) Lidocaine hydrochloride is successful in the majority of patients (1 mg/kg, then 0.5 mg/kg

TABLE 4–1.
Drugs Used in Cardiac Arrest and Resuscitation

Drug	Intravenous Bolus	Drug per 250 mL for Infusion	Infusion Rate
Amrinone	0.75 mg/kg over 2–3 min		5–10 µg/kg/min
Atropine	0.5–1.0 mg q. 5 min up to 2.0 mg		
Bretylium	5, then 10 mg/kg q. 30 min up to 30 mg/kg	2 g	1–2 mg/min
Calcium chloride	.5–1.0 g		
Dobutamine		500 mg	2–20 µg/kg/min
Dopamine		400 or 800 mg	1–20 µg/kg/min
Epinephrine	0.5–1.0 mg, repeat q. 5 min	1 mg	0.01–0.15 µg/kg/min
Isoproterenol		1 mg	0.01–0.1 µg/kg/min
Neosynephrine		10 mg	1–5 µg/kg/min
Nitroprusside		50–100 mg	1–10 µg/kg/min
Norepinephrine		4 mg	0.02–0.2 µg/kg/min
Procainamide	50 mg q. 5 min or 20 mg q. 1 min up to 1 g	2 g	1–3 mg/min
Sodium bicarbonate	1 mg/kg, then 0.5 mg/kg q. 10 min		
Xylocaine	1 mg/kg, then 0.5 mg/kg q. 5 min up to 3 mg/kg	2 g	1–4 mg/min

q.5 min up to 3 mg/kg). If severe ventricular dysrhythmias persist or if repetitive defibrillation is unsuccessful, any of the standard antiarrhythmics may be added to the lidocaine regimen. Currently, the choice is bretylium, despite the potential for adverse hemodynamic effects (5 mg/kg, then 10 mg/kg q. 30 min up to 30 mg/kg).

c) With either drug, only bolus doses should be administered during advanced life support with maintenance doses begun during the stabilization period.

d) Coronary perfusion pressure is an important determinant of myocardial perfusion, particularly of areas beyond critical stenoses which may act as arrhythmic foci due to pressure-dependent ischemia. Thus, in addition to antiarrhythmic drug therapy, adequate CO and arterial pressure are necessary to maintain a stable rhythm.

2) Atropine.

Parasympathetic tone may remain high during cardiac arrest and successful defibrillation may result in profound bradycardia or asystole. This is treated by the administration of atropine sulfate as an IV bolus which may be repeated as indicated (0.5–1.0 mg q. 5 min up to 2.0 mg). Atropine is also used in asystole to treat possible sinus node exit block.

3) Vasoconstrictors.

a) Vasodilation occurs with prolonged cardiac arrest, and the maintenance of BP during external chest compression is difficult.

b) Arterial pressure can be increased by vasoconstrictors, thus increasing cerebral, coronary, and renal perfusion.

c) Drugs such as methoxamine, neosynephrine, or norepinephrine may be used but the agent of choice is epinephrine (0.5–1.0 mg, repeat q. 5 min).

d) While epinephrine also has direct cardiac agonist effects, the change to a coarser pattern of ventricular fibrillation produced by this drug is most likely due to the increase in coronary blood flow secondary to the increased perfusion pressure.

4) Inotropic agents.
   a) Ineffective mechanical cardiac function may occur in the presence of a relatively normal cardiac rhythm. This defines electromechanical dissociation (EMD) and may occur as the primary diagnosis during advanced life support but may also occur after defibrillation.
   b) Epinephrine is the drug of choice in this situation and is used in an attempt to produce effective cardiac contractions. The drug is given IV as repetitive bolus doses. Epinephrine may also be used to sustain an adequate cardiac output in stabilization.
   c) Dopamine and dobutamine are also useful agents in this setting and isoproterenol may be useful, particularly when bradycardia is present. During stabilization, these drugs are given as a continuous infusion and titrated to effect.
   d) CaCl is the most potent inotropic agent known and formerly was a mainstay of the protocols in advanced life support. However, concern over reperfusion injury resulted in the deletion of CaCl from the formal protocols. However, this agent may be used at the discretion of the person in charge of the resuscitation team (2–4 mg/kg, repeat q. 10 min).

5) Sodium bicarbonate.
   a) The routine use of $NaHCO_3$ is no longer advocated in advanced life support. This resulted from the recognition that its use paradoxically increases intracellular acidosis and causes hypernatremia and hyperosmolality as well.
   b) Furthermore, it has been demonstrated that hyperventilation to reduce the arterial P_{CO_2} is more effective in preventing intracellular acidosis.
   c) However, preexisting metabolic acidosis, which may have caused the cardiac arrest, should be treated with $NaHCO_3$. Its use may be indicated in other specific clinical situations at the discretion of the person in charge of the

resuscitation team (1 mg/kg, then 0.5 mg/kg q. 10 min).

g. Pacing.

1) Occasionally, pacing may be effective in the absence of an intrinsic cardiac rhythm. Access may be obtained via the transvenous or transthoracic route, although the former is preferred.

2) A more common situation is the presence of complete heart block after defibrillation, for which temporary transvenous pacing is instituted. This can be discontinued with the return of normal conduction or converted to permanent pacing if necessary.

4. Therapeutic protocols.

a. Treatment of cardiac arrest is administered according to protocols developed by the AHA and based on the specific ECG diagnosis.

1) The protocols for ventricular fibrillation, asystole, and EMD are shown in Figure 4–3. (The protocol for ventricular tachycardia may be considered identical to that for ventricular fibrillation.) (see Appendix B).

2) The rhythm may change during resuscitation necessitating a change to another treatment protocol. Thus, **the ECG must be reassessed frequently.** This is best accomplished during brief periods of noncompression to avoid misinterpretation due to electrical artifacts resulting from chest compression.

b. Stabilization.

1) Every patient successfully resuscitated after a cardiac arrest should be placed in an SICU for at least 24 hours.

2) The previously healthy patient who sustains a cardiac arrest on induction of general anesthesia and is rapidly resuscitated may require only observation. However, patients with hemodynamic or electrical instability will require further therapy.

3) In addition to monitoring the ECG and the arterial pressure, virtually every patient should have a flow-directed PA catheter inserted to obtain measurements of PA and capillary wedge pressures.

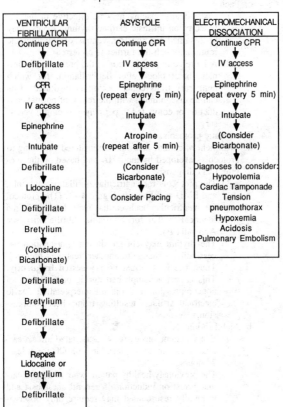

CARDIOPULMONARY RESUSCITATION
Specific Protocols*

VENTRICULAR FIBRILLATION	ASYSTOLE	ELECTROMECHANICAL DISSOCIATION
Continue CPR	Continue CPR	Continue CPR
Defibrillate	IV access	IV access
CPR	Epinephrine (repeat every 5 min)	Epinephrine (repeat every 5 min)
IV access	Intubate	Intubate
Epinephrine	Atropine (repeat after 5 min)	(Consider Bicarbonate)
Intubate	(Consider Bicarbonate)	Diagnoses to consider: Hypovolemia Cardiac Tamponade Tension pneumothorax Hypoxemia Acidosis Pulmonary Embolism
Defibrillate	Consider Pacing	
Lidocaine		
Defibrillate		
Bretylium		
(Consider Bicarbonate)		
Defibrillate		
Bretylium		
Defibrillate		
Repeat Lidocaine or Bretylium		
Defibrillate		

FIG 4–3.
Protocols for cardiopulmonary resuscitation. (Adapted from American Heart Association: *Textbook of Advanced Cardiac Life Support.* Dallas, American Heart Association, 1987.)

CARDIOPULMONARY RESUSCITATION

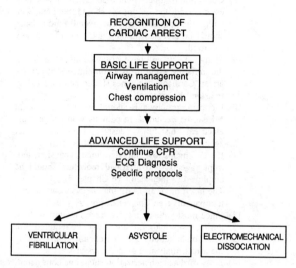

FIG 4–3 (cont.).

Only with such objective data can therapeutic decisions be made (see Chapter 2).

4) Upon admission to the SICU, the intubated patient may be converted to mechanical ventilation.

5) An NG tube should be passed to decompress the stomach and a Foley catheter should be inserted to empty the bladder so that urine output can be measured accurately.

6) A CXR should be obtained upon admission to the SICU to assess pulmonary status, the placement of central lines and the ET tube, and possible complications of resuscitation such as fractured ribs or pneumothorax.

7) Laboratory studies should be performed including evaluations of the hematocrit, electrolytes, glucose, and ABG.

8) Correction of a persistent base deficit may be necessary, and the serum K should be kept well within the normal range. The overall fluid balance should be assessed initially and thereafter closely followed.

9) Many patients will have sustained an MI, either as the initiating event or as a consequence of cardiac arrest. Cardiac isoenzymes should be evaluated by the standard protocol.

10) Lidocaine prophylaxis should be undertaken until MI can be excluded. In patients who demonstrate electrical instability despite lidocaine, other agents, such as bretylium, should be used.

11) If CO remains low, blood volume expansion, inotropic agents, and afterload reduction should be employed as indicated (see Chapter 3).

12) The insertion of an IABP may be necessary in certain patients (see Chapter 6, pp 199–204).

13) Since most patients receive large amounts of fluid during resuscitation, diuresis may be required. For acute renal failure due to ischemic injury during the arrest, dialysis may be necessary.

14) Early cardiac catheterization should be considered, particularly in the previously healthy individual whose arrest was the first manifestation of coronary artery disease.

5. Intraoperative arrest.
   a. Although the treatment is no different, an intraoperative arrest presents certain problems.
      1) Since patients are always monitored during surgery, the cardiac arrest and a specific ECG diagnosis should be immediately evident.
      2) Control of the airway will have been established previously and most patients will be intubated. When necessary, however, intubation can be performed expeditiously in this setting.
      3) Depending on the surgical procedure being performed, external chest compression may be under-

taken by the operative team or by anesthesia personnel without compromise of the sterile field.

4) Both sterile and nonsterile paddles should be available in every operating room for external defibrillation by either team.

5) Drugs can be given by the anesthesiologist through existing IV lines, and a central venous line may be established, if necessary.

b. During elective surgery, if cardiac arrest occurs on induction, the patient should be resuscitated and taken directly to an SICU with surgery postponed until cause and sequelae of the arrest are identified and treated. If the arrest occurs intraoperatively, the procedure should be terminated as rapidly as possible; when feasible, the wound should be closed immediately and the planned procedure aborted.

c. In emergency cases, the cause of arrest is frequently related to the condition for which surgery is undertaken. If the patient can be resuscitated, the operation must proceed with stabilization and further treatment of the underlying pathophysiology by the anesthesiologist.

C. Complications.

Besides mortality the complications of CPR are usually associated with the mechanical effects of intubation, compression, and invasive techniques.

1. Intubation.
   a. Intubation of esophagus with subsequent lack of ventilation.
   b. Tracheal laceration.
   c. Spinal cord compression in patients with cervical fracture (trauma).

2. Compression.
   a. Fractured rib.
   b. Pulmonary hemorrhage.
   c. Liver laceration.
   d. Splenic laceration.
   e. Cardiac contusion.
   f. Gastric rupture.

3. Invasive technique.
   a. Pneumothorax after line placement.
   b. Cardiac laceration with possible tamponade after subxiphoid injection.

D. Results.
   1. Approximately 50% of patients who sustain a cardiac arrest while in hospital can be resuscitated successfully and 50% of survivors discharged.
   2. As with out-of-hospital arrests, the time to initiation of resuscitation is a major determinant of survival.

SELECTED REFERENCES

Feneley MP, Maier GW, Gaynor JW, et al: Sequence of mitral valve motion and transmitral blood flow during manual cardiopulmonary resuscitation in dogs. *Circulation* 1987; 76:363.

Feneley MP, Maier GW, Kern KB, et al: Influence of compression rate on initial success of resuscitation and 24 hour survival after prolonged manual cardiopulmonary resuscitation in dogs. *Circulation* 1988; 77:240.

Kouwenhoven WB, Jude JR, Knickerbocker GG: Closed-chest cardiac massage. *JAMA* 1960; 173:1064.

Maier GW, Newton JR, Wolfe JA, et al: The influence of manual chest compression rate on hemodynamic support during cardiac arrest: High impulse cardiopulmonary resuscitation. *Circulation* 1986; 74:51.

Rankin JS, Maier GW: Cardiac arrest and resuscitation, in Sabiston DC, Spencer FC (eds): *Surgery of the Chest,* ed 5. Philadelphia, WB Saunders Co, 1990.

Rudikoff MT, Maughn WL, Effron M, et al: Mechanisms of blood flow during cardiopulmonary resuscitation. *Circulation* 1980; 61:345.

Standards and guidelines for cardiopulmonary resuscitation (CPR) and emergency cardiac care (ECC). *JAMA* 1986; 255:2905.

THE CARDIAC SYSTEM

5

I. ISCHEMIC HEART DISEASE.

The overall risk of myocardial infarction (MI) in the American adult undergoing a major surgical procedure is 0.2%. The mortality of postoperative MI approaches 50% in most series. Approximately 60% of perioperative MIs occur within the first 3 postoperative days with the majority of the remainder occurring between the fourth and sixth days. Patients identified as being at risk must be followed carefully for up to 6 days postoperatively for evidence of infarction or other complications.

A. Physiology.

Coronary artery disease secondary to atherosclerosis is the most common form of heart disease and accounts for most operative mortality due to heart disease. The imbalance between coronary blood flow and energy requirements may result in ischemia, usually manifested by chest discomfort.

B. Diagnosis.

1. The characteristic chest discomfort associated with ischemia is angina pectoris, which is usually described as a feeling of pressure, tightness, constriction, fullness, or heaviness. It is typically located in the anterior midchest region and there may be radiation to the neck, jaw, arms, or elbows. Angina pectoris usually lasts 3–5 minutes and is often produced by effort or emotional stress but may occur at rest.

2. Sharp chest pain is seldom due to myocardial ischemia.

3. The differential diagnosis of midsternal chest discomfort in the postoperative patient includes many disorders (Table 5–1).

TABLE 5–1.

Differential Diagnosis of Chest Pain

Myocardial ischemia
Pulmonary embolism
Pneumonia
Acute aortic dissection
Pericarditis
Esophageal spasm
Esophagitis
Peptic ulcer disease
Gastritis
Biliary disease
Pancreatitis
Incisional pain
Costochondritis

C. **Preoperative Management and Assessment of Ischemic Heart Disease.**
  1. Risk factors:
     a. Perioperative cardiac risk can be estimated based on a multifactoral analysis proposed by Goldman (Table 5–2).
     b. With increasing class, a higher proportion of patients develop life-threatening, or fatal complications. In Goldman's study, patients in class 4 accounted for half of the cardiac deaths.
     c. Several factors included in the index are potentially amenable to preoperative intervention. Perioperative hemodynamic monitoring to improve management is recommended in patients at high risk—NYHA class 3 or 4 angina with or without previous infarction, valvular heart disease, CHF, planned major vascular procedure, severe pulmonary disease, or operations involving major blood loss.
     d. Elective surgery should be delayed in patients with potentially controllable or reversible factors and careful postoperative observation to detect cardiac complications in an early stage is necessary.
  2. Evaluation:
     a. History, physical examination, CXR, and ECG are required. In selected patients further studies may be

TABLE 5–2.

Cardiac Risk Index Points*†

	Points
History	
Age >70 yr	5
Prior MI within 6 mo	10
Physical	
S_3 gallop or JVD	11
Important valvular aortic stenosis	3
ECG	
Rhythm other than sinus or PACs on last preoperative ECG	7
More than 5 PVCs per minute documented at any time prior to surgery	7
General status	
Po_2 <60 or PCO_2 >50 mm Hg	
K <3 or HCO_3 <20 mEq/L	
BUN >50 or creatinine >3 mg/dL	
Abnormal SGOT, cirrhosis, chronic liver disease, or patient bedridden from noncardiac causes	3
Operation	
IP, or intrathoracic operation	3
Emergency operation	4
Total possible	53

*Adapted from Goldman L: *Ann Surg* 1980;198:780–791.
†Class 1 = 0–5 points; class 2 = 6–12 points; class 3 = 13–25 points; class 4 = >26 points.

     indicated including exercise radionuclide angiography, IV dipyridamole-thallium imaging, or coronary angiography.

  b. Patients with chronic stable angina who are able to perform activities of daily living will probably tolerate the stresses of most noncardiac surgery. However, even in these patients, preoperative stress testing should be considered if major intrathoracic, upper abdominal, or vascular procedures are to be performed.

 3. Operations performed within 3 months of an MI have a 30% chance of resulting in recurrent MI or cardiac death. This risk falls to approximately 11% between 3–6 months. After 6 months, the risk is 5% and remains at this level.

4. Role of coronary artery bypass grafting:
   a. Patients with three-vessel or left main coronary disease, or disease refractory to medical therapy should be considered for revascularization prior to elective surgery.
   b. Operative mortality is significantly decreased in patients with coronary artery disease who have undergone prior coronary revascularization (0.9%) compared with those who have not (2%–4%) and is similar to mortality in patients without coronary artery disease (0.5%).
5. Medications: In general, cardiovascular medications should be continued to the morning of operation and then resumed as quickly postoperatively as possible using NG tube or IV administration as appropriate.

D. Myocardial Infarction.
   1. Diagnosis.
      a. MI should be suspected in any patient with unexplained hypotension; dysrhythmias, especially new onset; unexplained fevers; chest discomfort; development of a new murmur; development of an S_3 gallop; pulmonary edema on CXR or physical examination; new ECG changes; or changes in mentation. The physical examination may be completely normal in the patient with an evolving MI.
      b. Infarction in the postoperative patient may be painless in 50% of cases.
      c. Patients at high risk for ischemic events should be closely monitored including serial ECGs, cardiac isoenzymes, and invasive hemodynamic monitoring as indicated.
      d. The ECG may reveal ST-T wave abnormalities, isolated T wave changes, QRS changes, or no abnormalities at all. The postoperative patient with a suspected MI requires constant ECG monitoring.
      e. The measurement of creatine kinase (CK) and its isoenzyme CK-MB is the preferred method for detection of MI. An elevated CK-MB is virtually specific for myocardial injury. Elevations of CK can be found following surgery, IM injections, pulmonary embolus, trauma, and CPR. CK-MB increases by 4–6 hours following an MI, peaks at 24 hours, and returns

to normal over 3–4 days. If there is no significant elevation in the isoenzyme level by 12 hours and the ECG shows no evidence for myocardial ischemia, an acute MI is unlikely.

2. Management of MI:
   a. If myocardial ischemia or MI is suspected, the patient should be placed on bed rest with frequent monitoring of vital signs, an ECG obtained and continuous monitoring instituted.
   b. In the patient with chest pain, sublingual nitroglycerin should be administered. If the discomfort continues, nitroglycerin can be given twice more at 5-minute intervals.
   c. With ECG changes, persistent chest discomfort suspected to be angina, or other manifestations suspicious of myocardial ischemia, the patient should be transferred to the ICU.
   d. Prompt pain control is important.
      1) IV nitroglycerin (NTG) can be used with adequate monitoring. A continuous drip should be initiated at 5 μg/min and then increased by 5 μg/min until the pain resolves or MAP is reduced by 10%.
      2) Morphine should be given IV slowly in doses of 1–4 mg q.1–2 h. as indicated. Mild tranquilizers may be appropriate.
      3) If pain persists despite IV NTG, further therapy including heparin, treatment with calcium channel blockers, or institution of β-blockers may be necessary. IV propranolol or metoprolol may be used in the patient with evidence of increased sympathetic tone to decrease myocardial $\dot{V}O_2$. β-blockade must be carefully considered in the setting of hypovolemia or impaired ventricular function.
      4) If the pain fails to respond to these measures and in hemodynamically unstable patients, the IABP may be indicated (see Chapter 6, pp 199–204).
      5) Thrombolytic agents may be indicated in certain patients (see p 108).
      6) Urgent cardiac catheterization for diagnosis and angioplasty followed by coronary revasculariza-

tion as appropriate may be needed in patients failing to respond to other measures.

e. Supplemental O_2 is indicated to maintain O_2 saturation >90%.

f. Routine laboratory data and a CXR should be obtained. An ECG should be obtained immediately, at 6–8-hour intervals in the first 24 hours and then at least daily, especially if changes of infarction are not present on initial tracings. Cardiac isoenzymes should be measured q.8h. and LDH with isoenzymes q.12h. for up to 2–3 days.

g. Prophylactic lidocaine therapy is recommended to prevent potentially lethal ventricular dysrhythmias.

   1) Lidocaine should be administered as an initial bolus of 100 mg IV (or 1 mg/kg) and an IV infusion begun at 2 mg/min.

   2) In the setting of CHF, hypotension, or hepatic disease, the half life of lidocaine is prolonged and a smaller bolus dose and an infusion rate of 1 mg/min should be used.

   3) Older patients have a high risk of developing lidocaine toxicity. Toxicity is manifested predominantly by CNS stimulation and seizures. If indicated, serum levels should be monitored.

h. Reperfusion of the myocardium with IV or intracoronary thrombolytic agents (streptokinase [SK], urokinase [UK], or tissue plasminogen activator [t-PA]), or by surgical revascularization should be considered in all patients with acute MI. Clearly, these interventions may be contraindicated in the postoperative patient. Ischemic cell death begins within 20 minutes following coronary artery occlusion. If reperfusion is to be successful, it is important to intervene within 4–6 hours. The ability to perform prompt reperfusion depends on the availability of an interventional cardiologist and a cardiac surgeon.

i. The diet is dictated by the operative procedure but, if appropriate, it can be liquid or soft. Constipation is a common problem in patients with infarction and should be prevented by the use of stool softeners (docusate Na, 100 mg po b.i.d.) and mild laxatives.

   j. Anticoagulation is not routinely indicated.

      1) In patients with severe critical coronary stenosis, in which reocclusion is an issue, full systemic anticoagulation with IV heparin may be indicated.

      2) In patients with acute anterior infarction, there is a high (32%) risk of mural thrombus. Evaluation by echocardiography is indicated and if thrombus is present, anticoagulation should be considered. Documented systemic embolization is an absolute indication for full anticoagulation.

   k. In the patient with evidence of CHF or low CO, aggressive invasive monitoring including arterial line placement, monitoring of urinary output, and placement of a Swan-Ganz catheter should be utilized.

      1) Dopamine or dobutamine, β-adrenergic agonists, are used to increase CO. Side effects include tachycardia and vasoconstriction, (especially with dopamine in high doses). Therapy should be initiated at $2-3$ µg/kg/min and slowly increased until the desired hemodynamic response is obtained (Chapter 2).

      2) The use of the IABP may be lifesaving and reduces cardiac work by decreasing afterload while increasing diastolic pressure and coronary blood flow (see pp $199-204$).

   l. Hypertension increases myocardial O_2 demand and infarct size and should be controlled. If unresponsive to the previous outlined treatment of bed rest, pain relief, and sedation, the following approach is recommended:

      1) For mild diastolic hypertension (<105 mm Hg) oral agents can be helpful (β-adrenergic antagonists, clonidine, methyldopa). If hypertension is more severe or there are signs of continuing myocardial ischemia or dysfunction, parenteral therapy with hemodynamic monitoring is indicated.

      2) β-Adrenergic antagonists are the agents of choice when hypertension is associated with tachycardia, high CO, normovolemia, and normal or moderately elevated SVR. Labetolol $5-20$ mg IV may be administered initially, then titrated to the desired effect. Esmolol may be given as a 500 µg/

kg bolus followed by a continuous infusion of 50–300 μg/kg/hr.

3) IV sodium nitroprusside (SNP) or NTG is indicated in all patients with severe hypertension accompanied by reduced CO and high SVR.

    a) The initial dose of SNP is 0.5 μg/kg/min and should be increased in small increments with careful monitoring (Chapter 3).

    b) IV NTG is similar to SNP except that it has a more marked effect on venous capacitance. The initial dose is 10–20 μg/min and should be increased until control of pain or hypertension is achieved.

m. Hypotension may occur for a variety of reasons following MI.

1) Hypotension associated with bradycardia should be treated with atropine 0.5–1.0 mg IV. Pacing may be necessary for refracting bradycardia.

2) Persistent hypotension should be treated with inotropic agents and optimization of hemodynamics. Mechanical complications such as VSD or papillary muscle rupture must also be considered.

3. Complications of myocardial infarction.

a. Cardiogenic Shock (see Chapter 3):

1) Cardiogenic shock is suggested by hypotension (systolic BP <80 mm Hg or MAP < 60 mm Hg); oliguria; and elevated LA filling pressures (> 15 mm Hg). Shock may be present despite a normal BP.

2) Management includes the use of appropriate inotropic agents, IABP, and hemodynamic monitoring.

b. Dysrhythmias (see pp 143–168).

c. Rupture of the interventricular septum or papillary muscle:

1) The development of these complications is manifested by a new onset systolic murmur or CHF.

2) The diagnosis of VSD can be made by demonstrating a step-up in O_2 saturation from the RA to the RV utilizing a PA catheter.

3) With papillary muscle rupture and severe mitral regurgitation, the PA catheter may reveal a wedge pressure tracing with large v waves.

    4) Two-dimensional echocardiography with color flow Doppler is useful in the diagnosis of USD and MR.

    5) If hemodynamic compromise ensues, support with IABP and afterload reduction should be initiated. Urgent surgical repair may be indicated.

d. Right ventricular infarction (RVI):

    1) RVI is seen in patients with inferior MI. RV filling pressures are disproportionately increased when compared to LV pressure. The diagnosis can be difficult to distinguish from pericardial tamponade and echocardiography may be helpful.

    2) Therapy of RVI begins with fluid administration to support the failing RV. Following RVI, the RV functions primarily as a conduit and pulmonary blood flow is dependent on high right-sided filling pressures.

e. Ventricular aneurysm and rupture:

    1) Ventricular wall motion abnormalities are often seen with acute MI and usually improve with time.

    2) Ventricular aneurysm should be suspected in the patient with intractable heart failure, refractory ventricular dysrhythmias, or persistent ECG changes.

    3) Definitive diagnosis requires cardiac catheterization but echocardiography may be helpful.

    4) An important variant of ventricular aneurysm is pseudoaneurysm or ventricular rupture. In the latter entity, pericardial extravasation of blood is restricted locally by the pericardium. Urgent repair of a ventricular pseudoaneurysm or ventricular rupture is indicated.

f. Pericarditis (Dressler's syndrome):

    1) Pericarditis is common following acute infarction and is usually characterized by chest discomfort or pain and a pericardial rub. The syndrome is felt to be an autoimmune phenomenon. The pain is exacerbated by deep breathing or movement and may be relieved by sitting up.

    2) Therapy is usually symptomatic and includes aspirin, NSAIDs, or steroids.

3) It is important to differentiate the pain of postinfarction pericarditis from postinfarction angina or extension of MI. Presence of a rub and an elevated ESR suggests the diagnosis of pericarditis.

II. VALVULAR HEART DISEASE

The spectrum of symptoms and signs of valvular heart disease ranges from asymptomatic to acute cardiovascular collapse. Valvular lesions amplify the hemodynamic fluctuations of anesthesia and shock.

A. Aortic Stenosis (AS).

1. Etiology:
   a. *Congenital AS* may be supravalvular, valvular, or subvalvular.
   b. *Acquired AS* is most commonly degenerative calcific (senile) valvular AS.

2. Pathophysiology:
   a. LV output is maintained by the development of concentric hypertrophy which can generate adequate output CO against increased afterload for years before LV decompensation. Elevated LVEDP is caused by decreased LV compliance (secondary to hypertrophy), LV failure, or both.
   b. AS is considered to be critical when the aortic valve area is <0.4 cm^2/m^2 BSA (¼ of normal orifice).
   c. Atrial contraction is important in severe AS to maintain adequate CO. Therefore, complete heart block or atrial fibrillation may be poorly tolerated.

3. History:
   a. The natural history of acquired AS is a long latent period with onset of symptoms most commonly in the sixth decade. **The most important lesion to identify preoperatively is the presence of *severe* aortic stenosis, which is associated with a 13% perioperative mortality.**
   b. There are three cardinal symptoms: angina pectoris, syncope, and CHF.
   c. Angina pectoris is present in two thirds of patients with severe or critical AS, and 50% of these have concomitant coronary artery disease.
   d. Syncope occurs secondary to attenuated cerebral blood flow during activity when arterial perfusion

pressures drop with peripheral vasodilation in the setting of a fixed CO.

   e. CHF occurs when LV hypertrophy can no longer generate an adequate CO in the presence of markedly increased afterload.

4. Physical examination:
   a. Small volume and sustained pulse with delayed upstroke (pulsus parvus et tardus).
   b. Sustained LV lift.
   c. Respiratory variation in pressure (pulsus alternans).
   d. Normal S_1, paradoxically split S_2 (LV dysfunction).
   e. A crescendo/decrescendo systolic murmur, completed before A_2, heard best at the base, and often transmitted along the carotids and to the apex. An ejection click may be heard in noncalcific disease.

5. ECG:
   a. LV hypertrophy (LVH) is frequently seen with LA enlargement (LAE) in 80% of severe cases.
   b. Left anterior fascicular hemiblock may be seen in 10% of cases.

6. CXR:
   a. Most have a normal cardiac silhouette, cardiomegaly is a later finding.
   b. Poststenotic dilation may be present.
   c. A calcified valve may be seen on the lateral film.

7. Echocardiography:
   a. Helpful in determining site of stenosis and leaflet anatomy.
   b. Doppler allows calculation of aortic gradient using a modified Bernoulli equation.
   c. Best objective noninvasive method of following disease progression.

8. Treatment:
   a. Symptomatic patients have a 40% 5-year and 20% 10-year survival with medical therapy. Symptomatic patients with severe AS have a 1-year mortality of 25%. Average survival with angina is 5 years; with syncope, 3 years; and with CHF, 1–2 years.
   b. Medical therapy is restricted to *asymptomatic* patients and includes chemoprophylaxis against infective endocarditis (Table 5–3), treatment of dysrhythmias,

TABLE 5–3.

Differential Diagnosis of Mitral Regurgitation, VSD, Tricuspid Regurgitation, and Aortic Stenosis*†

Physical, Roentgenographic, or Electrocardiographic Feature	Mitral Regurgitation	VSD	Tricuspid Regurgitation	Aortic Stenosis
Systolic murmur	Harsh and pansystolic	Harsh and pansystolic	Pansystolic	Ejection, crescendo-decrescendo
Primary location of murmur	Apex	Left sternal border	Left sternal border	Base of heart; occasionally apical
Radiation of murmur	Axilla; occasionally base and neck	Left precordium	Little	Carotids
Thrill	Occasionally present at apex	Usually present at left sternal border	Rare	Occasionally present at base
Murmur with inspiration	No change	No change	Increases	No change
Valsalva maneuver	May increase	Increases or no change	No change	Decreases

Venous pressure	Often normal	Slightly elevated with prominent A and V waves	Elevated, with very prominent V waves	Usually normal
Pulsatile liver	No	No	Yes	No
Pulmonary component of S_2	Normal; occasionally increased	Normal or loud; usually delayed	Usually increased	Normal
Apical impulse	Hyperkinetic; occasional heaving	Hyperkinetic	Weak or normal	Forceful and sustained
ECG	Left ventricular hypertrophy; left atrial hypertrophy	Biventricular hypertrophy (Katz-Wachtel phenomenon)	Right ventricular hypertrophy, occasional right atrial hypertrophy	Left ventricular hypertrophy with associated ST-T changes
Chest roentgenogram	Moderately enlarged heart, marked left atrial enlargement	Enlarged left and right ventricle	Enlarged right ventricle	Often normal heart size or left ventricular hypertrophy

*From Braunwald E: *Heart Disease; A Textbook of Cardiovascular Medicine.* Philadelphia, WB Saunders Co, 1988, p. 1014.

†√SD = ventricular septal defect.

and surveillance of disease progression (6–12-month intervals).

c. Surgery is indicated in symptomatic patients and in asymptomatic patients with critical AS or LV dysfunction. The procedure of choice is aortic valve replacement (AVR).

d. Balloon valvuloplasty remains investigational, and is currently restricted to use in children, patients who refuse surgery, or those deemed too ill or debilitated for AVR.

9. Idiopathic hypertrophic subaortic stenosis (IHSS):

a. IHSS involves the interventricular septum in a nondilated ventricle to the heart.

1) The most characteristic abnormality is not systolic but diastolic dysfunction due to decreased LV compliance.

2) The most common symptoms are dyspnea (90% of symptomatic patients) and angina (75%).

3) Physical examination may reveal a systolic murmur (Table 5–4).

4) The ECG may be normal or have LVH and prominent Q waves laterally suggestive of infarction ("pseudoinfarct").

5) Diagnosis is best made with two-dimensional echocardiography.

6) Treatment includes β-blockade to decrease contractility relieving LV outflow obstruction. Positive inotropic agents should be avoided. Surgery is reserved for those refractory to β-blockade. Chemoprophylaxis against infective endocarditis is necessary.

B. Aortic Insufficiency (AI).

1. AI may result from a defect in the valve leaflets or from dilation of valve annulus.

2. Pathophysiology:

a. The SV of the LV is ejected into the aorta with some fraction returning during diastole which decreases the effective CO and increases the preload of the LV. The increased preload leads to increased diastolic wall tension. Compensation occurs by dilation and hypertrophy. Severe chronic AI may be well tolerated for long periods of time.

TABLE 5–4.
Effects of Various Interventions on Systolic Murmurs*†

Intervention	Hypertrophic Obstructive Cardiomyopathy	Aortic Stenosis	Mitral Regurgitation	Mitral Prolapse
Valsalva	↑	↓ or unchanged	↓	↓ or ↑
Standing	↑	↓ or unchanged	↓	↑
Handgrip or squatting	↓	↓ or unchanged	↑	↔ ↑ ↓
Supine position with legs elevated	↓	↑ or unchanged	Unchanged	
Exercise	↑	↑ or unchanged	↓	
Amyl nitrite	↑↑	↑	↓	↓ ↓ ↓
Isoproterenol	↑↑	↑	↓	

*From Braunwald E: Heart Disease; A Textbook of Cardiovascular Medicine. Philadelphia, WB Saunders Co, 1988, p. 1041.
†↑ ↑↑ = markedly increased.

b. The ejection fraction (EF) is often normal until LV function deteriorates. LV end-systolic volume is a sensitive index of LV function and correlates well with operative mortality and postoperative LV function.

c. *Acute AI,* commonly caused by infective endocarditis, aortic dissection, or trauma, is poorly tolerated because the regurgitant fraction is filling a normal-sized ventricle. Since the SV cannot adequately augment acutely, forward flow diminishes and LVEDP rises rapidly to high levels.

3. History:

a. Patients with *chronic, severe AI* may be asymptomatic. When symptoms develop, they are exertional dyspnea, orthopnea, and paroxysmal nocturnal dyspnea (PND). Syncope is rare.

b. *Acute AI* may present with CHF, pulmonary edema, and shock, if severe.

4. Physical examination:

a. Palpation of the pulse reveals a brisk upstroke and rapid collapse best noted in the radial artery with arm elevated (water-hammer pulse, Corrigan's pulse). The pulse pressure is widened.

b. The apical impulse is diffuse, hyperdynamic, and displaced laterally and inferiorly.

c. Capillary pulsations are noted by pressing a glass slide against the patient's lip or transilluminating the fingertips (Quincke's pulse).

d. Cardiac auscultation reveals a high-frequency diastolic decrescendo murmur, best heard when the patient is leaning forward in full expiration. A systolic murmur may be secondary to concomitant AS or a flow murmur in pure AI. A mid- to late diastolic rumble (Austin Flint murmur) is common in severe AI and is heard at the apex.

e. With *acute AI,* patients appear severely ill, are tachycardic, and show evidence of peripheral vasoconstriction (cool, pale, cyanotic). Pulmonary edema may be present. The peripheral signs are generally more subtle or absent. The diastolic murmur is lower-pitched and shorter in duration.

5. ECG.
   a. Chronic AI: left axis deviation, LVH, and intraventricular conduction defects (late).
   b. Acute AI: nonspecific ST-T wave changes.
6. CXR.
   a. Chronic AI: Cardiomegaly is related to AI duration and severity, as well as LV function. Chronic severe AI may lead to massive cardiomegaly (cor bovinum). The aortic root may be dilated.
   b. Acute AI: usually normal cardiac silhouette; pulmonary edema may be present.
7. Echocardiography:
   a. Very helpful in assessing and following LV function.
   b. May show thickening of the valve cusps, prolapsing or flail leaflets, vegetations, or aortic root dilation.
   c. Doppler ultrasound is the most sensitive and accurate technique in the detection of AI.
8. Treatment:
   a. Patients with moderately severe or severe AI have a 75% 5-year and 50% 10-year survival when treated medically. Once symptomatic, patients deteriorate rapidly.
   b. Medical management is indicated in mild to moderate AI. Patients should be followed on semiannual basis to assess clinical status as well as LV function. Afterload reduction should be given if there is evidence of increased diastolic pressure. Chemoprophylaxis against infective endocarditis is indicated.
   c. Patients who are asymptomatic with good LV function do not need surgery even if AI is severe and LV function is preserved; however, it is important to treat patients surgically when symptoms develop and before significant LV dysfunction occurs. Aortic valve replacement (AVR) is the procedure of choice.
   d. Prompt surgical therapy is usually required in *acute AI*. In preparation for surgery, afterload reduction and inotropic support may be necessary. If the etiology is infective and the patient is not hemodynamically compromised, 10–14 days of systemic antibiotics should precede surgery. Surgery to AVR should be performed when hemodynamic instability develops,

there is diastolic closure of the mitral valve, or upon completion of a 2-week course of antibiotics.

e. Patients with severe LV dysfunction preoperatively often improve little following AVR; however, their clinical course is improved compared with medical therapy alone.

C. Mitral Stenosis (MS).

1. Etiology:
   a. The most common cause is rheumatic heart disease (RHD).
   b. Lesions that simulate MS physiologically include LA myxoma or thrombus causing a ball valve effect.

2. Pathophysiology:
   a. The mitral valve area (MVA) is 4–6 cm^2 in normal adults. A gradient is measurable when the MVA is reduced to 2 cm^2 (6–8 mm Hg). Severe compromise in flow is noted when MVA <1 cm^2 and this is associated with $\geq$ 25 mm Hg gradient (critical MS). An MVA near 0.5 cm^2 is said to be the smallest size compatible with life.
   b. Increasing LA pressures lead to pulmonary venous congestion and pulmonary edema. The consequent symptom of dyspnea occurs initially with stress, infection, and atrial fibrillation, all of which increase LA pressure.
   c. Mitral valve flow depends on HR and CO; therefore, if HR increases, diastolic filling time decreases, leading to increased LA pressures (e.g., atrial fibrillation with rapid ventricular response). According to hydraulic principles, the transvalvular gradient is a function of the square of the flow. If the HR is doubled, LA pressure will increase fourfold. Atrial contraction increases presystolic transvalvular gradient by ~30% in MS. Withdrawal of atrial contraction may decrease CO by 20%. Therefore, maintaining normal sinus rhythm is important in optimizing hemodynamics.

3. History:
   a. The principal symptom is dyspnea.
   b. Other symptoms include fatigue, orthopnea, PND, hemoptysis, atypical angina (rest pain which may be indistinguishable from angina pectoris), thromboem-

bolism (rare since advent of surgical therapy), and even cardiac cachexia.

4. Physical examination:
   a. An RV lift may be palpated along the LSB.
   b. A staccato accentuated S_1 occurs when a flexible mitral valve is present.
   c. An opening snap (OS) is heard just after the second heart sound and heard best at the apex with the diaphragm. The OS is less audible with increased valve calcification.
   d. The diastolic murmur of MS is low-pitched and best heard with the bell at the apex with the patient in left lateral position. It may be barely audible if CO is low.
   e. If concomitant mitral regurgitation (MR) is present, a systolic murmur is heard, along with a soft S_1 and no OS.

5. ECG:
   a. Atrial fibrillation is common.
   b. If in normal sinus rhythm (NSR), LA enlargement is present in 90% of patients.
   c. With elevated right-sided pressures, RV hypertrophy (RVH) may be present.

6. CXR:
   a. CXR usually reveals a normal heart size. If cardiomegaly is present, it is secondary to RVH.
   b. LA enlargement (LAE) is seen either as a double density or a concave indentation of the middle third of the esophagus on lateral film exposed during barium swallow.
   c. Cephalad redistribution of pulmonary flow, interstitial edema, and Kerley's B lines indicate pulmonary venous congestion.
   d. Mitral valve calcification may be seen.

7. Echocardiography:
   a. The mitral valve orifice size is accurately measured.
   b. Provides visualization of the extent of calcification and pliability of the leaflets and therefore helps determine suitability for valvotomy (commissurotomy).
   c. LA thrombus can be identified.
   d. Doppler analysis allows quantification of mitral valve gradient

8. Treatment:
   a. Following a 20–25-year latent period after rheumatic fever, a 5-year period of progression from mild to severe symptoms occurs. Patients who are asymptomatic or minimally symptomatic may be stable for years; however, once symptoms occur, rapid deterioration generally occurs. This is usually associated with a MVA of ≤ 1.0 cm^2. Five-year survival in symptomatic patients with MS or combined MS and MR is 45% with medical therapy alone.
   b. Considerable symptomatic relief is experienced with diuresis and sodium restriction. Digoxin is of limited benefit, except in patients in atrial fibrillation, who benefit from control of the ventricular response.
   c. If hemoptysis develops, sedation, upright positioning, and diuresis are usually adequate to control bleeding.
   d. Anticoagulation is important in patients with atrial fibrillation. If the patient is in NSR and has a history of either CHF or systemic embolization, anticoagulation is indicated as well.
   e. β-Blockade may increase exercise tolerance by decreasing HR, whether the patient is in atrial fibrillation or NSR.
   f. Surgery is indicated in patients with NYHA classes 3 and 4. Class 1 and 2 patients should be individualized with consideration for mitral valve annulus size, lifestyle limitations, and history of systemic embolization. Because of the high rate of recurrence after systemic embolization, mitral valve replacement (MVR) is indicated, even if no other symptoms are present.
   g. Balloon valvuloplasty is not as effective as the surgical options, and should be used only in patients who refuse surgery, or when open correction carries an exceedingly high risk.

D. **Mitral Regurgitation (MR).**
   1. Etiology:
      a. *Chronic MR* usually results from RHD, myocardial ischemia, or degeneration of leaflets.
      b. *Acute MR* may be spontaneous or caused by trauma, ischemia or infarction, endocarditis, RHD, or prosthetic valve dysfunction.

2. Pathophysiology:
   a. The mitral valve orifice is in parallel with the aortic valve and therefore impedance to ventricular emptying is reduced in MR by bidirectional decompression into the aorta and LA. The volume of regurgitant flow is dependent upon the LV-LA pressure gradient, the mitral valve orifice dimensions, and SVR.
   b. As LV function deteriorates, the LV dilates with subsequent annular dilation leading to worsening MR.
   c. Severe CHF may be associated with a normal EF or mildly decreased EF. When the EF <40%, LV dysfunction has become much worse. This population represents a high-risk group whose clinical status unlikely to improve after mitral valve replacement (MVR).
   d. Effective (forward) flow is usually depressed in seriously ill patients whereas total CO (forward plus regurgitant) may be very high (10–20 L/min).
3. History:
   a. The natural history of MR is variable and depends on the severity of the lesion and the etiology (rapid progression is more common in connective tissue diseases). The 5-year survival with symptomatic MR, medically treated, is approximately 45%.
   b. Symptoms arise as a manifestation of the severity and rate of progression of MR, associated coronary artery disease, and concomitant valvular disease. Many patients are asymptomatic with mild MR for life.
   c. Fatigue is generally the first symptom and usually connotes a decreased CO.
4. Physical examination:
   a. The pulse has a brisk upstroke (helpful in differentiation from AS, which has a delayed upstroke).
   b. The point of maximal impulse (PMI) is displaced to the left.
   c. The murmur is high-pitched, holosystolic, and must be differentiated from AS, VSD, and tricuspid regurgitation (Tables 5–3 and 5–4). It is usually best heard at the apex with radiation to the left axilla.
   d. There is little correlation between the intensity of the murmur and the severity of the MR

5. ECG:
   a. Atrial fibrillation is common
   b. If NSR, LAE is frequently seen.
   c. LV enlargement (⅓ of patients with severe MR).
6. CXR:
   a. Cardiomegaly with LVH and LAE is common.
   b. There is little correlation between LAE and LA pressures.
   c. Lungs are usually clear (vs. MS). Interstitial edema signifies concomitant AI or LV failure.
   d. Calcification of the annulus is best seen on lateral or RAO views, usually C-shaped.
7. Left ventriculography:
   a. Regurgitant volume can be assessed accurately by Fick's method.
   b. Estimation of severity can be assessed based on degree of LA and pulmonary venous opacification.
   c. Etiology may be determined (mitral valve prolapse, flail leaflet, annular dilation).
8. Echocardiography:
   a. Helpful in determining etiology and hemodynamic significance of MR.
   b. Not as accurate as ventriculography in determining severity of MR, unless color flow Doppler is used (correlates well with Fick's method).
9. Treatment:
   a. Medical therapy is aimed at treatment of CHF with afterload reduction and diuresis. Sodium nitroprusside or IABP may be required in setting of acute MR. Chronic MR is best treated with angiotensin converting enzyme (ACE) inhibitors or hydralazine and a diuretic. Digoxin may be needed to treat atrial fibrillation. Chemoprophylaxis against infective endocarditis is necessary.
   b. Surgery is indicated in patients with NYHA class 2 (especially if LV end-systolic volume > 30 mL/m^2), 3, and 4 CHF. There is increasing support for surgery in class 1 patients with 4+ MR if mitral valve repair can be performed.
   c. Surgical options are mitral valve repair or MVR.
   d. If ischemic MR is unresponsive to medical therapy, it is best treated with MVR with or without CABG.

e. Acute MR should be treated surgically as an emergency when it is secondary to trauma, SBE, or papillary muscle rupture. With ischemic MR not associated with papillary muscle rupture or CHF, it is best to wait 4–6 weeks prior to MVR, if possible.

E. Prosthetic Valves.

1. *Tissue:*

   a. Currently, porcine valves are the most commonly implanted xenografts (Hancock, Carpentier). Their hemodynamic profiles are similar to the comparably sized low-profile mechanical valves (see below). Bovine pericardium xenografts (Ionescu-Shiley) have had a high rate of failure in the aortic and mitral positions.

   b. Homografts are used increasingly as procurement and preservation techniques improve. Hemodynamics are excellent, even in small sizes, and thromboembolic complications are rare.

   c. Tissue valves have the advantage of not requiring anticoagulants. However, there is some evidence warfarin for 3 months following MVR is beneficial.

   d. Tissue valves are generally less durable than mechanical valves. The durability of homografts may be comparable.

2. *Mechanical:*

   a. The Starr-Edwards (bull-cage) valve has been implanted more than any other and long-term data (30-year) are available. The current models are very durable. The disadvantage is in the bulky design (not suitable for mitral position in small LV or for small aortic annulus) and the inferior flow dynamics (vs. low-profile valves), which produce more turbulent flow.

   b. There are many low-profile valves available. The tilting disc valves include Omniscience, Medtronic-Hall, and Bjork-Shiley. The Bjork-Shiley is no longer available in the United States because of durability problems. Bileaflet valves (St. Jude, Duromedics) have excellent flow dynamics, and their early durability data are promising.

   c. *All* mechanical valves, regardless of position, require long-term anticoagulation with warfarin.

3. Valve selection:
   a. A bioprosthesis is generally chosen for patients in whom long-term anticoagulation is not possible, including elderly patients, noncompliant patients, and coexisting diseases which preclude anticoagulation, and alcoholics.
   b. In women contemplating pregnancy, a bioprosthesis should be chosen to avoid the necessity of anticoagulation.
   c. Mechanical prostheses are generally chosen for other patients.
4. Anticoagulation:
   a. Long-term anticoagulation is associated with a 1%–2% per year risk of hemorrhagic complications.
   b. In patients who require surgery, warfarin should be discontinued 2–3 days preoperatively.
   c. Surgery can be done after the PT has fallen to within 1–2 seconds of control.
   d. If the prosthetic valve is in the mitral position, heparin infusion should begin as soon as the warfarin is discontinued (24 hours after last dose), and continued until 6 hours before surgery.
   e. Once hemostasis is achieved (approximately 12–24 hours after surgery) IV heparin is initiated and continued until anticoagulation with warfarin is adequate.

F. **Infective Endocarditis.**
1. Native valve endocarditis is classified as either acute or subacute depending upon the clinical presentation and the etiologic organism.
   a. Acute: *Staphylococcus aureus, Streptococcus pneumoniae, Streptococcus pyogenes, Neisseria meningitidis, Neisseria gonorrhoeae, Haemophilus influenzae.*
   b. Subacute: *Streptococcus viridans, Staphylococcus epidermidis.*
   c. The two groups are associated with distinctly different manifestations, clinical course, and complications.
   d. This classification is not absolute. Some cases of acute infective endocarditis have been caused by *S. viridans,* and some cases of subacute infective endocarditis by *S. aureus.*

2. Diagnosis:
   a. Fever is the most common sign (85%–97%).
   b. Murmur (90%), especially new onset.
   c. Peripheral stigmata (petechiae, subungual hemorrhages, Osler's nodes, Janeway's lesions, Roth's spots).
   d. Blood cultures (sine qua non for diagnosis).
   e. Echocardiography.
3. Treatment:
   a. The mainstay is IV antibiotic and symptomatic therapy (antipyretics, etc.).
   b. Surgery is indicated in the following:
      1) No response to antibiotics after 1 week of IV antibiotic therapy.
      2) Recurrent embolic events.
      3) Relapse of infection.
      4) Fungal endocarditis.
      5) Endocarditis involving the sinus of Valsalva or AV nodal tissue.
      6) Abscess of the interventricular septum usually manifested by a conduction defect or heart block.
      7) Right-sided endocarditis.
      8) CHF nonresponsive to medical therapy.
4. Prosthetic valve endocarditis (PVE) (Table 5–5).
   a. *Early PVE* (<60 days after implantation) is secondary to surgical contamination and is most commonly caused by staphylococcus.
   b. *Late PVE* (>60 days after implantation) like native valve endocarditis, is usually secondary to transient bacteremia, and most commonly caused by *S. viridans*.
   c. Medical therapy alone usually fails. Mortality approaches 100% in medically treated patients with CHF, ongoing sepsis, fungal PVE, valve obstruction, unstable prosthesis, or new onset heart block.
   d. The relative and absolute indications for surgery are listed in Table 5–5.
5. Chemoprophylaxis:
   a. Prophylaxis is indicated in any patient with congenital heart disease (before and after operation), valvular heart disease, IHSS, pacemakers, or ventriculoatrial shunts (for treatment of hydrocephalus). The excep-

TABLE 5-5.

Features of Prosthetic Valve Endocarditis (PVE)*

Microbiology	(%)
Early PVE	
Staphylococci	45
Staph. epidermidis	25
Staph. aureus	20
Gram-negative	20
Fungi	10
Diphtheroids	10
Streptococci	10
Other	5
Late PVE	
Streptococci	40
S. viridans	30
Group D, *S. pneumoniae*	10
Staphylococci	35
S. epidermidis	25
S. aureus	10
Gram-negative	10
Fungi	5
Other	5

Clinical manifestations	(%)
Fever	97
Murmur (new/changing)	56
Petechiae	33
Splenomegaly	33
Emboli	33
Roth spots	5
Osler's nodes	5
Janeway lesions	5

Indications for surgery

Absolute	Relative
Congestive heart failure	Mild congestive heart failure
Ongoing sepsis	Nonstreptococcal organism
Fungal etiology	Early PVE
Valve obstruction	Embolism
Unstable prosthesis by fluoroscopy	Paravalvular leak
New-onset heart block	Vegetations by echocardiography
	Relapse
	Culture-negative without response

*Modified from Braunwald E: *Heart Disease; A Textbook of Cardiovascular Medicine.* Philadelphia, WB Saunders Co, 1988, p 1125.

tions include those with isolated ostium secundum ASD, patients >6 months after *primary* (without prosthetic material) closure of secundum ASD, and patients >6 months after ligation of a patent ductus arteriosus.

b. Recommendations for prophylaxis are listed in Table 5–6.

III. PULMONARY EDEMA AND CONGESTIVE HEART FAILURE.

A. Pulmonary Edema.

1. Pathophysiology.
   a. Pulmonary edema results in increased extravascular lung water, leading to the clinical syndrome of hypoxia, dyspnea, and chest rales.
   b. Pulmonary edema can be either cardiogenic or noncardiogenic.
      1) Cardiogenic pulmonary edema is the consequence of increased hydrostatic intercapillary pressure due to increased LV EDP seen in heart failure.
      2) Noncardiogenic pulmonary edema can be due to either altered alveolar capillary membrane permeability (ARDS, sepsis, O_2 toxicity) or a decrease in plasma oncotic pressure (low serum albumin).
2. Diagnosis:
   a. Symptoms include dyspnea, orthopnea, PND, fatigue, nausea, diaphoresis, cough, agitation, altered mental status.
   b. Physical signs are chest rales, tachypnea, cyanosis, tachycardia. JVD and peripheral edema may be present.
   c. Laboratory findings reveal hypoxemia in the face of adequate ventilation as evidenced by a markedly decreased PaO_2 with a normal or low $PaCO_2$. The CXR shows interstitial PE with cephalization of the vasculature and enlarged hilar vessels.
3. Treatment:
   a. Initial clinical maneuvers are directed at stabilization and resuscitation. The second stage involves identification and treatment of the precipitating factors.

b. Initial treatment:
   1) An adequate airway must be secured. ET intubation may be indicated. Supplemental O_2 should be administered.
   2) The circulation must be assessed to assure tissue perfusion and O_2 delivery.
      a) Perfusion and DO_2 may be assessed clinically by mental status, urinary output, skin temperature, capillary refill, and BP. If perfusion is inadequate, invasive monitoring techniques and inotropic therapy may be necessary (Chapter 2 and Chapter 3).
      b) Tachyarrhythmias may cause pulmonary edema and can respond quickly to appropriate therapy.

TABLE 5-6.

Infective Endocarditis Prophylaxis

Dental Procedures	
Category	Antibiotic Regimen
Local anesthesia	
Not allergic to penicillin	A. Amoxicillin 3 g PO 1 hr before
Allergic to penicillin or had penicillin recently	B. Erythromycin 1.5 g PO 1 hr before; 0.5 g 6 hr later
General anesthesia	
No special risk	C. Amoxicillin 1 g IM or IV; 0.5 g PO or IM 6 hr later
Patients at special risk†	
Not allergic to penicillin	D. Amoxicillin 1 g IM or IV plus gentamicin 120 mg IM or IV: amoxicillin 0.5 g orally or IM 7 hr later
Allergic to penicillin	E. Vancomycin 1 g IV plus gentamicin 120 mg IM or IV

Surgery or Instrumentation of the Upper Respiratory Tract	
Category	Antibiotic Regimen
No special risk	Recommendation C (above)
Special risk	Recommendation D or E (above)

Genitourinary Surgery or Instrumentation	
Category	Antibiotic Regimen
Not allergic to penicillin	Recommendation D (above)
Allergic to penicillin	Recommendation E (above)
Patient with infected urine	Regimen to cover organisms isolated

Obstetrical and Gynecological Procedures

Endocarditis is very uncommon after these procedures; however, patients at special risk of infection should receive antibiotic cover as for genitourinary surgery.

Pediatric Doses

Amoxicillin: Children under 10 years—half the adult dose
Erythromycin: Children under 5 years—one quarter the adult dose
Gentamicin: 2 mg/kg
Vancomycin: 20 mg/kg

*From Braunwald E: *Heart Disease; A Textbook of Cardiovascular Medicine.* Philadelphia, WB Saunders Co, 1988, p 1127.

†Patients at special risk include those with prosthetic valves, those who have a past history of endocarditis, or those who require general anesthesia and are allergic to penicillin. The latter group requires vancomycin, which must be administered IV over a 30-minute period. IM administration of 1 gm of amoxicillin may be painful. It is recommended that it be given in 2.5 mg of 1% lidocaine. Patients at special risk should always undergo procedures within the hospital.

   c) Malignant hypertension may result in acute pulmonary edema secondary to increase in LV afterload.

   d) Pulmonary edema may result from acute or chronic valvular disease and the presence of a murmur should be ascertained.

3) Establish IV access and place a Foley catheter.

4) Elevate the head of the bed.

5) Obtain ABG, CBC, electrolytes, glucose, creatinine, CXR, ECG.

6) Begin continuous ECG monitoring.

7) Decrease pulmonary congestion.

   a) Morphine:

     i) Morphine causes significant venous pooling in the splanchnic bed, decreasing venous return and LV preload.

   ii) The dosage is 1–4 mg IV, repeated q.10 min as indicated. The patient should be in a well-monitored setting with careful attention to vital signs to avoid respiratory depression.

b) Diuretics: An initial dose of furosemide 10–40 mg can be given IV.

c) Vasodilator drugs:

   i) Vasodilators act by decreasing SVR, which results in lowering of LVEDP, thus lowering pulmonary hydrostatic pressure.

   ii) Venodilators, such as NTG, are the most effective in lowering right-sided pressures. However, they can augment the effect of furosemide and should be used cautiously.

   iii) IV NTG may be required. NTG has a half-life of 1–3 minutes. The starting dose is 10 μg/min and can be increased by 5–10 μg/min to a maximum of 200 μg/min. Hypotension is the most common side effect.

   iv) In patients with pulmonary edema and low CO or impaired ventricular function, afterload reduction with sodium nitroprusside may be indicated. The infusion should begin at 0.5 μg/kg/min and is titrated until the desired effect or hypotension occurs.

d) Mechanical reduction of pulmonary congestion.

   i) Phlebotomy: 250–500 mL of blood can be removed. This technique is occasionally helpful in patients with fixed intravascular volume (i.e., renal failure).

   ii) Rotating tourniquets can be applied to all but one extremity and rotated every 15–20 minutes to the free extremity.

   iii) Hemodialysis and ultrafiltration.

8) Improve cardiac function.
   a) Parenteral inotropic therapy may be needed in severe cases when left ventricular failure is present.
      i) The initial agents of choice are dopamine or dobutamine, or both.
      ii) Digoxin is of use when atrial tachycardias are present but is of no benefit in the patient in sinus rhythm.
      iii) Dobutamine may be preferred if the BP is normal. It improves hemodynamics (CO) and decreases total peripheral resistance and PCWP. With dobutamine, side effects (increases in BP, HR, and ventricular irritability) are unlikely at infusion rates < 10 µg/kg/min.
      iv) Dopamine is preferred in hypotensive patients. At low doses (<5 µg/kg/min), dopamine has a selective renal vasodilating effect. At doses >10 µg/kg/min, dopamine is an α-agonist and may cause undersirable increases in total peripheral resistance.
      v) Dobutamine or dopamine can be started at 2 µg/kg/min and increased as necessary.
      vi) Amrinone represents an entirely new class of inotropic agents, bipyridine phosphodiesterase inhibitors. It is a direct arterial dilator, and has direct inotropic effect as well. The initial dose is 0.75 mg/kg given over 2–3 minutes followed by an infusion of 5–10 µg/kg/min. Amrinone may be particularly useful when RV failure is also present.
   b) Afterload reduction with SNP or IABP may be necessary in cases of severe LV dysfunction.
4. Precipitating factors such as arrhythmias, fluid overload, severe hypertension, acute MI, SBE, and hypermetabolic conditions should be diagnosed and treated. Operation may be required for acute valvular insufficiency or the mechanical complications of MI.

     5. Reassessment of the chronic underlying causes, is necessary to reevaluate the efficacy of past treatment, the presence of surgically correctable lesions, or the development of a new etiology.

B. Congestive Heart Failure.

  1. Pathophysiology:

    a. CHF represents failure of the heart as a pump and in its most severe form results in cardiogenic shock.

    b. CHF may result from loss of functional myocardium due to ischemic heart disease, cardiomyopathy, or chronic valvular heart disease.

  2. Diagnosis:

    a. The symptoms of CHF can be grouped as those of pulmonary congestion (peripheral edema, PND, orthopnea, exertional dyspnea, nocturia) and those resulting from decreased CO (fatigue, weakness, confusion, cold clammy extremities, anorexia, poor exercise tolerance).

    b. Physical findings include pulmonary congestion (basilar rales, expiratory wheezes, tachypnea), decreased peripheral pulses, tachycardia, S_3 gallop, peripheral cyanosis, pallor, JVD, hepatojugular reflux, hepatomegaly, and peripheral edema.

    c. The CXR shows PE, cardiomegaly, and vascular cephalization. Abnormal ventricular function can be assessed by radionuclide angiography, MUGA scanning, echocardiography, or cardiac catheterization.

    d. The cause should be quickly established. Hypertension is by far the most common causative factor, (approximately 75% of cases). Coronary artery disease is the next most common (approximately 10%).

      1) Surgically correctable cases include coronary artery disease, congenital or valvular heart disease, constrictive pericarditis or tamponade, ventricular aneurysm, endocarditis, coarctation of the aorta, and large systemic arteriovenous fistulas.

      2) Commonly, surgeons must treat decompensation of previously diagnosed CHF. Precipitating factors include pulmonary embolus (PE), infection, anemia, hyper- or hypothyroidism, arrhythmias, hypertension, excessive sodium load secondary to

inappropriate diet or IV fluid administration, failure to take cardiac medications, silent MI, administration of sodium-retaining or cardiac depressant medication, or emotional stress. Less frequently seen causes are pregnancy and alcohol abuse.

3. Treatment:

   a. Management is focused on decreasing the cardiac work load, increasing myocardial contractile performance, decreasing ventricular afterload, and relieving congestive symptoms by reducing the excess fluid accumulation.

   b. *Reduction of cardiac work* is accomplished by restricting physical activity up to and including strict bed rest.

   c. Digitalis is the mainstay of treatment. Digitalis is most helpful when CHF is precipitated by supraventricular tachycardia, particularly atrial fibrillation. It should be avoided in patients with idiopathic hypertrophic subaortic stenosis, Wolff-Parkinson-White syndrome, sick sinus syndrome (SSS), and evidence of AV block on ECG.

      1) The method of digitalization is often determined by the clinical setting. A loading dose of approximately 12–15 µg/kg lean body weight should be given. This dose should be reduced to 10 µg/kg in patients with renal insufficiency. This dose usually ranges between 1.0 and 1.5 mg and is administered by giving one half the calculated dose initially and one fourth of the dose q.2–4h. × 2.

      2) Alternatively, in stable patients with atrial fibrillation, digoxin 0.50 mg IV can be given followed by 0.25 mg IV after 2–4 hours. Additional doses are then titrated by the ventricular response.

      3) The normal maintenance dose is 0.125–0.375 mg/day. This can be given either IV or po, depending on the patient's condition.

      4) Careful monitoring of digoxin serum levels is mandatory. Steady state is reached 5–7 days following initiation of therapy. The half-life in patients with normal renal function is 1.5 days and increases pro-

gressively as the C_{CR} decreases. Sampling times should be q.7–10ds. Toxicity is usually manifest at levels >3.0 ng/mL.

5) Digitalis toxicity is frequently manifested by paroxysmal atrial tachycardia with block or junctional rhythms. Toxicity may be treated by administration of digitalis antibodies.

d. Reduction of symptoms of CHF:

1) Dietary sodium should be restricted to <2 g/day.

2) Fluid restriction to approximately 2 L/day is indicated in some patients.

3) Diuretic agents promote salt and water excretion and have intrinsic vasodilating properties. Furosemide is the drug of choice in patients with decreased GFR and who are critically ill.

a) The initial dose in patients with normal renal function is 20 mg po.

b) The IV dose is roughly half of this oral dose and should be given slowly over 1–2 minutes. The dose should be doubled and administered q.4–6h. until a satisfactory diuresis is initiated.

c) Single doses >200 mg are rarely indicated, infrequently augment the response, and are associated with significant toxicity (ototoxicity, electrolyte disturbances, jaundice, pancreatitis, nausea, vomiting, etc.).

d) Ethacrynic acid is a loop diuretic comparable to furosemide. The usual starting dose is 25 mg IV. This can be increased in 25-mg increments to a maximum of 100 mg.

e. Afterload reduction:

1) Vasodilator therapy is well established. It is most effective in the setting of decreased CO, pulmonary congestion, and high SVR. With normal or decreased PCWP, vasodilators are not indicated. They are particularly useful in patients with hypertension and regurgitant valvular disease.

2) Hydralazine and minoxidil are two direct-acting arterial vasodilators. They are usually used for long-term oral therapy.

3) Venodilators:
   a) Nitrates decrease ventricular preload by increasing venous capacitance.
   b) They are useful in patients with elevated atrial pressure and low CO. However, in the absence of increased atrial pressures, these agents may actually decrease CO.
4) Mixed vasodilators:
   a) Captopril (Capoten) has a beneficial effect in approximately two thirds of patients.
      i) The mechanism of action is inhibition of ACE, thus decreasing levels of angiotensin II.
      ii) A starting dose of 6.25-12.5mg po t.i.d. should be increased gradually.
      iii) Doses >25 mg po t.i.d. are rarely indicated.
   b) Nifedipine (Procardia), a calcium channel blocker, is useful in treating hypertension and decreasing afterload.
      i) The initial dose is 10 mg po q.6–8 h. (may also be given sublingually).
      ii) The usual maximum dose is 120 mg/day.
   c) Prazosin, an α-adrenergic blocking agent, is primarily an arterial vasodilator. The initial dose is 1 mg po q.6–12h. titrated to maximum dose of 20 mg/day.
   d) Frequently, vasodilator therapy is initiated in the acute setting using SNP and invasive monitoring. After cardiac function has been optimized, the patient is converted to oral therapy while continuing invasive monitoring.

IV. CARDIAC TAMPONADE.
A. Etiology.
The causes of cardiac tamponade are numerous, and reflect any pathologic process that may result in a pericardial effusion (Table 5–7), most commonly neoplastic and idiopathic.
B. Pathophysiology.
   1. Pericardium.
      a. The pericardium, a fibrous sac enclosing the heart and proximal great vessels, normally contains 15–35 mL of serous fluid.

TABLE 5-7.

Etiologies of Cardiac Tamponade

Neoplastic (lung, breast, lymphoma, melanoma)
Idiopathic
Infectious (viral, bacterial, mycobacterial, fungal)
Connective tissue diseases (SLE, scleroderma, rheumatoid arthritis, acute rheumatic fever)
Metabolic (uremia, myxedema, coagulopathy)
Cardiovascular (postinfarction effusion or rupture, CHF, dissecting aortic aneurysm)
Pharmacologic (anticoagulants, hydralazine, phenytoin, procainamide)
Traumatic (penetrating trauma, cardiac catheterization, pacing wires, pericardiocentesis, intracardiac injections, blunt trauma, CPR, postoperative)
Other (Loeffler's, Reiter's, Behçet's syndromes, pancreatitis, amyloidosis, serum sickness, chylous effusion, radiation)

---

      b. As the intrapericardial fluid volume increases, the first 80–120 mL are tolerated well with a minimal rise in intrapericardial pressure, and maintenance of systemic arterial BP. However, when the rate of additional pericardial fluid accumulation is brisk, the poorly compliant pericardium cannot accommodate, and cardiac tamponade may occur with as little as 200 mL of pericardial fluid.

      c. In contrast, when pericardial fluid increases gradually, the pericardium becomes distensible, and tamponade may not ensue until 2,000 mL or more has accumulated.

  2. Cardiac filling.

      a. Normal cardiac filling is bimodal (Fig 5–1). Initially, venous return increases with the onset of ventricular ejection and the resultant decrease in intrapericardial pressure (the x descent of the CVP). Later, RV filling occurs in diastole with the opening of the tricuspid valve (the y descent). The latter stage is markedly diminished or absent in pericardial tamponade, as diastolic filling is markedly impaired.

      b. When intrapericardial pressure rises, the thin-walled RV is selectively compressed, thereby limiting pulmonary flow, and ultimately LV preload. Increased adrenergic stimulation occurs to compensate, as evidenced by resultant tachycardia and vasoconstriction.

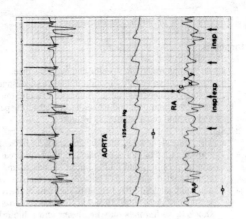

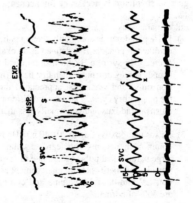

FIG 5–1.

Left (turn book), normal bimodal cardiac filling in a patient with mild CHF. Superior vena caval velocity *(V SVC)* and pressure *(P SVC)* tracings are shown (V_O represents sero flow). The predominant peak *(S)* accompanies ventricular systole. The smaller peak *(D)* occurs during ventricular diastole[2]. *Right,* right atrial *(RA)* and aortic pressure tracings from a patient with pericardial tamponade. The aortic pressure declines by 20 mm Hg during inspiration (pulsus paradoxus). The RA pressure declines normally during inspiration *(INSP)*. The x descent is dominant, and no y descent is present. *EXP* = expiration. (Modified from Shabetai R: *The Pericardium.* New York, Grune & Stratton, 1981, p 69; and Sharking SW: *Am J Med* 1983; 83:111–122).

C. Diagnosis.

1. Symptoms:
   a. The symptoms are nonspecific and may be vague.
   b. An oppressive or full sensation in the chest, dyspnea, air hunger, head and neck "fullness," extreme thirst, and abdominal pain and nausea (secondary to hepatic and visceral congestion) may be present

2. Signs:
   a. The clinical findings may be impressive. Beck described a triad of increased venous pressure, decreased arterial pressure, and muffled heart sounds, found in approximately one third of patients with traumatic cardiac tamponade. Ninety percent of such patients have at least one of these signs. **However, in some patients in shock these findings may be absent and a high degree of suspicion is necessary for accurate diagnosis.**
   b. Pulsus paradoxus.
      1) Pulse paradoxus is commonly seen in patients with cardiac tamponade. It is defined as an exaggerated decrease in systolic BP on inspiration. Korotkoff sounds are documented when first heard (in expiration only) and when first appreciated throughout the respiratory cycle. The pressure difference is the pulsus paradoxus and is normally less than 10 mm Hg.
      2) Pulsus paradoxus of up to 20–40 mm Hg is not uncommon in patients with cardiac tamponade. A large paradoxical pulse occurs late in cardiac tamponade, but merits prompt management as concurrent LV end-diastolic volume and coronary flow are 50% of normal.
      3) As patients with cardiac tamponade become hypotensive, pulsus paradoxus becomes more difficult to diagnose.
      4) Pulsus paradoxus is not pathognomonic as it may be seen in patients with asthma, cardiac failure, constrictive pericarditis, chronic lung disease, PE, obesity, MS with right heart failure, tense ascites, RV infarction. In contrast, patients with aortic insufficiency, underlying elevated EDP, extreme hypotension, or an ASD may develop cardiac tamponade and not have pulsus paradoxus.

    c. Jugular venous distention reflects increased CVP. Equalization of central venous, RA, and PA diastolic pressures, when combined with progressive hypotension, is suggestive of cardiac tamponade, particularly in the trauma victim.

3. CXR:
    a. Nontraumatic causes usually reveal a water bottle, pear-shaped, or globular heart.
    b. In traumatic tamponade, the CXR may reveal associated injuries, but rarely shows significant cardiac silhouette enlargement.

4. ECG:
    a. An ECG demonstrating total electrical alternans (both P and QRS waves) is a rare but pathognomonic finding.
    b. Electrical alternans of the QRS complex only is more common, but less specific.
    c. Decreased QRS voltage, altered ST segments, and T wave abnormalities are often present, but nonspecific.

5. Echocardiography:
    a. Echocardiography is the most accurate noninvasive method of diagnosis of pericardial effusion, and should be instituted in hemodynamically stable patients. However, appropriate management, particularly in the trauma patient, should not be delayed for echocardiographic confirmation of cardiac tamponade.
    b. Abnormally increased respiratory variation in transvalvular flow velocities, and diastolic posterior motion of the anterior RV wall are sensitive indicators for the echocardiographic diagnosis. With decreased LV volume and mitral valve anterior diastolic excursion, and concomitant increased RV dimensions with inspiration, the interventricular septum may bulge toward the LV. Diastolic collapse of the RV may be seen.

6. Differential diagnosis (Table 5–8):
    a. The onset may be insidious or sudden.
    b. In patients with life-threatening hypotension or shock, treatable causes (such as cardiac tamponade) must be immediately excluded.
    c. Cardiac tamponade may present as EMD.
    d. **The diagnosis requires a high degree of clinical suspicion and careful history and physical examination.**
    e. Patients with cardiac arrest or EMD of unclear etiology

TABLE 5–8.

Differential Diagnosis of Cardiac
Tamponade

Tension pneumothorax
Constrictive pericarditis
Superior vena cava syndrome
Hypovolemic shock
Acute right heart failure (usually
    pulmonary embolism)
Myocardial infarction
Congestive heart failure

who fail to respond to initial resuscitation measures
may require emergent pericardiocentesis to rule out
cardiac tamponade.

D. Treatment.

1. Therapeutic interventions include intravascular volume
   administration, sympathomimetics, dialysis in the uremic
   patient, pericardiocentesis, subxiphoid pericardial window, and thoracotomy.

   a. IV volume administration is critical in resuscitation. It
      will increase venous pressure in an attempt to over-
      come intrapericardial pressure, and increase CO.

   b. Sympathomimetic agents should be used judiciously.
      Intense vasoconstriction is present in severe cases of
      tamponade, and inotropic support with concomitant
      α-adrenergic agonist activity will only further impair
      systemic circulation.

   c. Several authors recommend isoproterenol, an ino-
      trope, chronotrope, and vasodilator.

2. Urgent dialysis in the patient with known renal failure may
   be lifesaving and obviate surgical intervention. However,
   in the hemodynamically unstable patient with renal insufficiency, time may not permit dialysis and more aggressive measures should be considered.

3. Pericardiocentesis may be diagnostic as well as therapeutic in patients with nontraumatic cardiac tamponade
   (Chapter 22).

   a. Traumatic cardiac tamponade usually necessitates
      emergent thoracotomy in a moribund patient for relief

of tamponade, and provision of internal cardiac massage.

b. Echocardiographic guidance is helpful in pericardiocentesis, but must not delay the procedure in unstable patients.

c. Diagnostic pericardiocentesis is being performed less often for at least two reasons: (1) in a series of 120 patients, only 24% of procedures yielded a specific diagnosis, despite obtaining fluid in 90% of attempts; (2) the subxiphoid window has emerged as a safer technique that provides a definitive diagnosis in virtually all patients.

V. CARDIAC ARRHYTHMIAS.
A. Diagnostic Methods.

1. Following a thorough history and physical examination, laboratory analysis may be helpful in revealing the cause of an arrhythmia. Standard evaluation must include a CXR, 12-lead surface ECG, ABG analysis, CBC, and measurement of serum electrolytes. When appropriate, serum drug levels are measured.

   a. The CXR may reveal pneumothorax, pericardial disease, or pulmonary pathology.

   b. The ECG may reveal evidence of myocardial ischemia or pericarditis.

   c. Disturbances in arterial pH, Pco_2, or Po_2 as well as a variety of electrolyte abnormalities may all predispose to cardiac arrhythmias. Of particular importance is the serum potassium level, especially in patients following cardiac surgery and in those taking digitalis. Serum magnesium and calcium are routinely measured. Anemia is treated when appropriate.

2. Temporary pacing electrodes.

   a. Temporary atrial and ventricular epicardial pacing wires are routinely placed after most cardiac surgical procedures. These are sutured to the midbody of the RA and the RV free wall and are exited through the patient's chest wall. Atrial wires conventionally exit the skin to the right of the midline and ventricular wires to the left of the midline.

   b. Temporary epicardial wires are helpful in both diagnosis and treatment of various arrhythmias.

1) Atrial electrograms are obtained by attaching the atrial wires to the right arm and left arm leads of the surface ECG using alligator clips.

2) Leads I, II, and III are then examined. This will yield a bipolar atrial electrogram in lead I and unipolar atrial electrograms in leads II and III.

3) Atrial activity will be especially prominent on the bipolar electrogram and its relationship to ventricular activity easily discernible from the unipolar recordings. The usefulness of this maneuver cannot be overemphasized.

4) Epicardial wires provide a direct low-resistance electrical pathway to both the atria and ventricles and therefore must be handled *cautiously*. The therapeutic role of temporary epicardial wires is discussed in section V.C.

3. Carotid sinus massage:

a. Carotid sinus massage may also be useful in evaluating and treating certain arrhythmias. By increasing refractoriness in the AV node, the ventricular response to SVTs is often slowed, aiding in diagnosis. Occasionally, this results in interruption of the arrhythmia.

b. Carotid artery disease is a relative contraindication to carotid sinus massage. Profound bradycardia and hypotension can result which one must be prepared to treat.

B. Cardiac Conduction System.

1. Myocardial cellular depolarization resulting in mechanical contraction is caused by action potentials traveling from myocyte to myocyte.

a. The cardiac action potential is the result of the movement of ions across the plasma membrane. These ion fluxes are responsible for the configuration of the action potential.

b. The action potential will vary slightly from region to region in the heart. The associated phases of the action potential and related membrane excitability and refractoriness will therefore vary among cells of the specialized conduction system, the atria, and the ventricles.

2. The classification of antiarrhythmic drugs is based primarily on effects produced on normal His-Purkinje tissue.

1) The effect of antiarrhythmic drugs may vary in different portions of the heart and may also vary between healthy and diseased tissue.

2) Clinical effects result not only from direct actions on cardiac cells but also through effects on the autonomic nervous system.

3. The two basic mechanisms responsible for arrhythmias are enhanced automaticity and reentry.

   a. In enhanced automaticity there is an abnormality in pacemaker activity.

   b. The mechanism of reentry is perpetuated by circus movement at either the microscopic or macroscopic level. The basic prerequisites for reentry include an abnormality in conduction and inhomogeneity of repolarization.

C. **Arrhythmias**

   Antiarrhythmic drugs are summarized in Table 5–9.

   1. Sinus Tachycardia.

      a. Diagnosis:

         1) Sinus tachycardia is a physiologic response to pain, stress, hypovolemia, anemia, hypoxia, hyperthermia, hypoglycemia and other abnormalities.

         2) In the adult, sinus tachycardia is defined as a sinus rhythm with a rate >100 bpm.

         3) The normal HR varies with age. A rate of up to 150 bpm is normal in the neonate, 125 bpm is normal for children up to 2 years of age, and 115 bpm is normal for a child 4 years old.

         4) In sinus tachycardia, the R-R interval is constant between beats and there is 1:1 AV conduction.

      b. *Treatment is aimed at the underlying problem.* Pain is treated with appropriate medication. If indicated, volume repletion and transfusion of blood products is performed. Supplemental O_2 is administered and electrolyte abnormalities corrected.

   2. Sinus bradycardia. Sinus bradycardia is a common finding in well-trained athletes. Pathologic conditions resulting in sinus bradycardia include SSS, hypothermia, hypothyroidism, and increased intracranial pressure (Cushing response).

TABLE 5–9.
Antiarrhythmic Drugs

Class	Medication	Route of Delivery	Dosage	Therapeutic Plasma Concentration	Comments
Ia.	Quinidine gluconate Quinidine sulfate	po	324–648 mg q.8–12h.	1.5–5.0 μg/mL	Increase plasma digoxin level
	Procainamide	po	L: 750–1,000 mg M: 250–500 mg q.4h. or 500–1,000 mg q.6h. (SR preparation)	4–10 μg/mL	Rapid loading may cause hypotension
		IV	L: 500–1,000 mg over 30–60 min M: 1–4 mg/min		
	Disopyramide	po	100–200 mg q.6h.	3–8 μcg/mL	Anticholinergic side effects are common
Ib.	Lidocaine	IV	L: 1 mg/kg bolus M: 1–4 mg/min	2–5 μcg/mL	Watch for CNS toxicity, especially with hepatic disease
	Phenytoin	po	100 mg t.i.d.–q.i.d.	10–20 μcg/mL	Hepatic clearance
		IV	L: 10–15 mg/kg over 20–30 min M: 100 mg IV t.i.d.–q.i.d.		
	Mexiletine	po	L: 400 mg M: 200–400 mg q.8h. to maximum of 1,200 mg in 24 hr		Hepatic clearance
Ic.	Encainide	po	25–50 mg q.8h.		Used under electrophysiologic guidance
	Flecainide	po	100–200 mg q.12h.	0.2–1.0 μcg/mL	Used under electrophysiologic guidance

		Route	Dosage	Level	Comments
	Propafenone	po	150–300 mg q.8h.		Dose should not be increased more frequently than every three days
1d.	Moricizine	po	200–300 mg q.8h.		Dose should not be increased more frequently than every three days
II.	Propranolol	po	10–60 mg q.6h.		Nonselective β-blocker
		IV	0.5–1.0 mg q.15–30 min up to a maximum 5 mg total		
	Atenolol	po	50–200 mg/day		Cardioselective
III.	Amiodarone	po	L: 800–1,600 mg/day M: 400–600 mg/day		Used under electrophysiologic guidance only; significant toxicity
	Bretylium	IV	L: 5–10 mg/kg over 10–20 min M: 1–2 mg/min		Hypotension associated with administration
IV.	Verapamil	po	40–120 mg q.6h.		Do not give with β-blocker concomitantly
		IV	2.5–5.0 mg over 2 min up to maximum of 15 mg total in 15 min		
V.	Digoxin	po	L: 0.5 mg, then 0.25 mg q.2–4h. × 2 doses M: 0.125–0.5 q.d.	0.8–2.0 ng/mL	May need to adjust dosage with quinidine, verapamil, and amiodarone
		IV	L: 0.5 mg, then 0.25 mg q.2–4h. × 2 doses M: 0.125–0.25 q.d.		
VI.	Adenosine	IV	6 mg as bolus over 1–2 sec; if unsuccessful 12 mg as bolus over 1–2 sec (may repeat × 1)		Effect is very short-lived

*Adult dosages only. L = load; M = maintenance; SR = slow release.

    a. Diagnosis:

        1) The diagnosis is made when a sinus rhythm with a rate <60 bpm is observed on the surface ECG.

        2) Often a sinus arrhythmia is present with varying R-R intervals.

    b. Treatment:

        1) If the patient is asymptomatic, no treatment is necessary.

        2) If the patient is symptomatic with manifestations of hypoperfusion and low CO (altered mental status, hypotension, signs and symptoms of CHF, myocardial ischemia, or low urinary output), treatment is indicated.

        3) The initial drug of choice is atropine 0.5–1.0 mg IV, repeated every several minutes as needed.

        4) If the patient fails to respond to atropine or if prolonged treatment is required, isoproterenol (1 mg in 250 mL D5W) can be administered as a continuous infusion beginning at 1 µg/min titrated to an appropriate HR.

        5) In the patient following cardiac surgery where temporary epicardial pacing wires are present, atrial pacing is a simple and effective way to increase HR and improve cardiac performance.

        6) Transcutaneous pacing (Zoll pacemaker) may be indicated in patients not responding to medical therapy.

        7) In symptomatic patients failing to respond to medical therapy, emergent transvenous or transthoracic pacing may be lifesaving.

  3. Premature contractions.

    a. Presentation:

        1) Premature contractions are initiated either in the supraventricular, junctional, or ventricular regions of the heart and are commonly encountered in surgical patients. They may be either insignificant or the harbinger of a serious and potentially lethal arrhythmia.

        2) Premature contractions must be interpreted in the setting in which they occur.

           a) In the clinic, premature contractions are often seen in the young patient with no underlying

cardiac disease. If asymptomatic, they may require no treatment.
b) In elderly patients, they commonly reflect an underlying cardiac abnormality and may be exacerbated by concurrent pathologic conditions.

3) Common etiologic factors include myocardial or pericardial disease, electrolyte and acid-base disturbances, instrumentation (central venous and PA catheters), and pathologic conditions of other major organ systems.

b. Diagnosis:

The surface ECG is essential in determining whether premature contractions initiate in the atria (PAC), junctional region (PJC), or ventricular region (PVC).

1) PACs are characterized by a P wave with different morphology from that of sinus rhythm, usually followed by a normal QRS complex.
   a) Depending upon the interval between the last sinus beat and the premature complex, AV conduction is variable.
   b) PACs can be completely blocked in the AV node or may exhibit aberrant conduction with a long PR interval and wide QRS complex.
   c) The site of block with aberrant conduction is usually in the His-Purkinje system. The QRS complex in aberrantly conducted beats commonly exhibits a RBBB pattern.

2) PJCs result in a premature QRS complex with a normal contour.
   a) They are not preceded by a P wave but may activate the atria retrograde.
   b) Retrograde activation is dependent upon the coupling interval to the prior sinus beat and is upon the relative speeds of antegrade and retrograde conduction. The resulting P wave therefore can either precede, be concurrent with, or follow the QRS complex.
   c) Retrograde P waves are by definition abnormal in contour.

3) PVCs originate distal to the bundle of His and are characterized by a wide, abnormal QRS complex that is not preceded by a P wave.

   a) The QRS complex is usually characterized as
      bizarre and >0.12 second in duration.
   b) The presence of fusion beats on the ECG is also
      substantial evidence of PVC.
c. Treatment:
   1) In asymptomatic individuals with no underlying
      heart disease, no treatment is necessary.
   2) In elderly patients or those with known cardiac dis-
      ease, premature contractions may be the harbinger
      of tachyarrhythmias.
      a) Standard evaluation is instituted and abnormal-
         ities such as myocardial ischemia, and electro-
         lyte and acid-base disturbances are sought and
         treated.
      b) Patients with frequent PACs are treated with
         digoxin and occasionally a class Ia antiarrhyth-
         mic agent (Table 5–10). Prior treatment with
         digoxin is necessary because class Ia antiar-
         rhythmics have a vagolytic effect and may en-
         hance conduction through the AV node and in-
         crease the ventricular response.
      c) PJCs may progress to junctional tachycardias
         which are seen primarily in infants and chil-
         dren, particularly following open heart sur-
         gery.
         i) In the adult, junctional tachycardias are
            frequently due to digitalis toxicity. Ap-
            propriate therapy is aimed at prevention
            of PJC deteriorating into tachycardias.
         ii) Digitalis toxicity with refractory arrhyth-
            mias may require therapy with specific
            antidigitalis antibodies.
         iii) PJCs may often be suppressed by over-
            drive atrial pacing (in patients with tem-
            porary epicardial pacing wires) or by the
            administration of propranolol.
      d) PVCs require treatment when they are fre-
         quent (≥6–8/min), multifocal (exhibiting var-
         ious morphologies), occur in couplets, or ex-
         hibit the "R on T phenomenon." The latter is
         known to initiate VF.

TABLE 5–10.
Tachyarrhythmias[*]

Arrhythmia	Mechanism	Ventricular Rate (bpm)	Acute Treatment		Chronic Treatment	Comment
			Unstable	Stable		
Sinus tachycardia	EA of SA Node	>100		Relieve underlying problem, rarely β-blocker		Usually due to stress or trauma
Atrial fibrillation	Intraatrial micro-RE	80–180	dcCV	Digoxin, verapamil, propranolol	Add type Ia agent	Common after cardiac surgery
Atrial flutter	Intraatrial RE	80–160	dcCV	Rapid atrial pacing, digoxin, verapamil, propranolol	Add type Ia agent	Carotid massage may aid in diagnosis
AV nodal reentry tachycardia	RE within the AV node	140–200	dcCV	Adenosine, verapamil, vagotonic maneuver	Digoxin, verapamil, propranolol, type Ia agent	Carotid massage may terminate
AV reentry tachycardia using concealed pathway	Macro-RE involving atria, AV node, ventricles, and accessory pathway	140–240	dcCV	Adenosine, type Ia agent	Type Ia, Ic agent, amiodarone	Avoid digoxin and verapamil

(Continued.)

TABLE 5–10 (cont.)

Arrhythmia	Mechanism	Ventricular Rate (bpm)	Acute Treatment		Chronic Treatment	Comment
			Unstable	Stable		
Intraatrial reentry tachycardia	Intraatrial RE	100–150	dcCV	Verapamil, type Ia agent	Verapamil, type Ia agent	Usually underlying cardiac disease
SA nodal reentry tachycardia	RE within SA node	80–200	dcCV	Verapamil, propranolol, vagotonic maneuver	Digoxin, verapamil, propranolol	Must differentiate from sinus tachycardia; carotid massage may terminate
Automatic atrial tachycardia	EA of atrial focus	100–200	dcCV†	Verapamil, type Ia agent	Verapamil, type Ia agent	May be seen with digitalis toxicity
Atrial tachycardia with block	EA of atrial focus	Atrial rate 150–200; ventricular rate variable	dcCV†	(1) Stop digoxin (if taking digoxin), phenytoin, propranolol, Digi-Bind (2) Digoxin (if not taking digoxin), type Ia agent	Digoxin, type Ia agent	Usually due to digitalis toxicity

Arrhythmia	Mechanism	Rate		Treatment		Comments
Multifocal atrial tachycardia	EA of atrial foci	100–130	dcCV†	Treat underlying disorder, verapamil	Treat underlying disorder, verapamil	Common with COPD and drug toxicity
Nonparoxysmal junctional tachycardia	EA of AV junction	70–130	dcCV†	Treat underlying disorder; stop digoxin	Treat underlying disorder	May be due to digitalis toxicity
Paroxysmal junctional tachycardia	EA of AV junction	120–250	dcCV†	Propranolol, amiodarone, propafenone	Amiodarone	Rare in adults
Ventricular tachycardia	Ventricular RE	100–220	dcCV	Lidocaine, type Ia agent, bretylium	Type Ia, Ic agent, amiodarone	AV dissociation and fusion beats
Torsades de pointes	Unknown	200–250	dcCV	Stop offending drug, lidocaine, overdrive pacing, isoproterenol, $MgSO_4$	Stop offending drug	Suspect type Ia, III agents; occurs with long QT interval

*EA = enhanced automaticity; RE = reentry; dcCV = direct current cardioversion.
†Often unsuccessful in terminating.

      i) Treatment begins with the standard evaluation. All abnormalities are corrected and, if the arrhythmia persists, antiarrhythmic therapy begun.

      ii) Malfunction of a temporary pacemaker placed to a "back-up" mode is also a cause of PVCs. In this setting, turning the pacemaker off cures the arrhythmia.

      iii) Acute medical treatment is lidocaine or procainamide (Table 5–10). Both are given as an IV loading dose followed by continuous infusion. Chronic treatment consists of suppression therapy when indicated. This usually consists of administration of type Ia, Ic, or III agents. Again, chronic therapy is dependent upon the setting in which the PVCs occur and any underlying cardiac abnormality.

4. Atrial fibrillation (AF).

  a. Introduction.

    1) AF is an extremely common arrhythmia. AF may occur in up to 20% of adults undergoing cardiac surgery.

    2) AF may be either an acute or chronic problem. Common causes include valvular, ischemic, and congenital heart disease; pericardial disease; PE; endocrine disorders; and acid-base or electrolyte disorder.

    3) Patients may be either asymptomatic or exhibit severe hemodynamic impairment.

      a) The primary determinants of the patient's hemodynamics are the underlying cardiac condition and the ventricular rate response.

      b) Loss of organized atrial contraction and shortened diastolic filling time associated with a high ventricular rate can result in a profound reduction in effective CO.

    4) Patients with chronic atrial fibrillation are prone to formation of thrombi within the diseased atria which can lead to systemic thromboembolism.

b. Diagnosis:

1) In atrial fibrillation there is a complete lack of organized atrial activity caused by multiple, intraatrial microreentry circuits.

2) The ventricular rate is typically irregularly irregular, between 100 and 180 bpm in the untreated patient. Because of the multiple reentrant circuits within the atria which may depolarize the AV node, there is variable penetration of impulses with block occurring within the AV node.

3) The surface ECG therefore reveals no discernible P waves and irregularly occurring QRS complexes.

4) Atrial epicardial and esophageal leads reveal disorganized atrial activity.

5) Carotid sinus massage may temporarily slow ventricular response, but will have no impact on the arrhythmia itself.

c. Treatment.

1) **Hemodynamic instability**:

a) With hemodynamic instability, treatment consists of *synchronized* electrical cardioversion. Care must always be taken in cardioverting patients receiving digitalis but can be performed safely in patients with no evidence of digitalis toxicity.

b) For atrial fibrillation, an initial shock of 50–100 J is delivered. If the initial shock is unsuccessful, the energy level is increased and the shock repeated.

2) **Hemodynamic stability**:

a) If the patient is hemodynamically stable, medical treatment is aimed at slowing the ventricular rate and achieving chemical cardioversion.

b) Control of ventricular rate is achieved by slowing conduction through the AV node.

i) Treatment is begun with the administration of IV digoxin.

ii) A dose of 0.5 mg IV followed by repeat doses of 0.125–0.25 mg IV q.2–4h. up to 1.25–1.50 mg total dose within 24 hours.

        iii) The digitalis dose is titrated to the ventricular response.

    c) If a more prompt slowing of the ventricular rate is desirable, IV propranolol 0.5–1.0 mg or verapamil 2.5–10 mg may be administered.

        i) β-Blockers and verapamil should not be given to patients with CHF because of their negative inotropic effects.

        ii) Calcium channel and β-blockers should not be administered concomitantly because of the risk of precipitating complete heart block.

    d) Once satisfactory control of the ventricular rate is obtained, chemical cardioversion is attempted. Treatment is begun with class Ia agents. Because of their vagolytic effect on the AV node, it is essential to control ventricular response prior to their administration.

    e) Rapid atrial pacing has no role in the treatment of atrial fibrillation.

    f) If patients fail to convert to normal sinus rhythm after achieving therapeutic levels of an appropriate class Ia agent, electrical cardioversion may be indicated. Anticoagulation for 6 weeks is often instituted prior to electrical cardioversion.

5. Atrial flutter:

  a. Introduction.

    1) The pathophysiologic mechanism underlying atrial flutter is intraatrial reentry.

    2) Atrial flutter has been subdivided into two types based upon atrial rate, probable site of reentry within the atria, and response to rapid atrial pacing. The atrial rate is typically between 250 and 350 bpm in type I flutter and between 350 and 430 bpm in type II flutter.

    3) The arrhythmia may be paroxysmal or chronic in nature.

    4) The etiologic factors are identical to those of atrial fibrillation and the hemodynamic consequences depend upon underlying heart disease and ventricular rate response.

b. Diagnosis:
   1) Atrial flutter waves can usually be identified on the surface ECG and are best seen in the inferior leads. There is generally 2:1 or 4:1 AV conduction present.
   2) Carotid sinus massage is frequently helpful in diagnosis by slowing AV conduction and unmasking flutter waves.
   3) Esophageal and epicardial electrograms are extremely helpful in diagnosis and are useful in treatment.

c. Treatment:
   1) **Hemodynamic instability**:
      a) If hemodynamic compromise is present, *synchronized* dc cardioversion is the treatment of choice.
      b) For atrial flutter, one should begin with a shock in the range of 25–50 J. If unsuccessful, the energy level is increased and the shock repeated.
   2) **Hemodynamic stability**.
      a) Rapid atrial pacing:
         i) In the hemodynamically stable patient, rapid atrial pacing is extremely useful in converting atrial flutter to sinus rhythm. Temporary atrial epicardial pacing wires left following open heart surgery and esophageal pacing can be used for this purpose.
         ii) The atria are paced at a rate greater than the intrinsic flutter rate and after entrainment of the atria, the pacing stimulus is either abruptly terminated or gradually slowed.
         iii) Frequently this is successful in converting the rhythm to sinus rhythm or in converting atrial flutter to atrial fibrillation. It is generally easier to control the ventricular response in the latter.
      b) Medical treatment:
         i) Medical treatment consists of slowing the ventricular rate response and achieving

chemical cardioversion. The ventricular rate is controlled with IV digoxin 0.5 mg IV followed by 0.125–0.25 mg IV q.2–4h. to a maximum of 1.25–1.50 mg over 24 hours.

   ii) If more rapid control of the ventricular rate is desired, either IV verapamil 2.5–10 mg or propranolol 0.5–1.0 mg.

   iii) Following control of the ventricular rate, chemical cardioversion is attempted using type Ia antiarrhythmic agents. This should be instituted only after control of the ventricular rate because of the possibility of these agents causing enhanced conduction through the AV node.

6. AV nodal reentry tachycardia (AVNRT).
  a. Introduction.
    1) AV nodal reentry tachycardia (AVNRT) is the cause of >50% of the arrhythmias collectively known as *paroxysmal supraventricular tachycardias*.
    2) The cause is a reentry circuit within the AV node itself, characterized by sudden onset and termination.
    3) The surface ECG is extremely helpful in the differentiation of AVNRT from other types of paroxysmal supraventricular tachycardia.
    4) AVNRT frequently occurs in otherwise healthy patients with no known organic heart disease.
  b. Diagnosis:
    1) The ECG typically reveals a narrow QRS complex tachycardia with a rate between 140 and 200 bpm.
    2) As the arrhythmia is initiated within the AV node, the atria are depolarized retrograde and the ventricles antegrade simultaneously. P waves occur concurrently with the QRS complex and are therefore frequently not visible on the ECG.
    3) Carotid sinus massage often results in abrupt termination of the arrhythmia. A functional bundle-branch block pattern during the tachycardia can be seen but does not affect the rate.

c. Treatment.
   1) **Hemodynamic instability**:
      If hemodynamic compromise is present, *synchronized* dc cardioversion is the treatment of choice. Initial attempts are begun at 10–50 J and increased if unsuccessful.
   2) **Hemodynamic stability**:
      a) If no hemodynamic compromise is present, maneuvers and medications that increase refractoriness of the AV node are the mainstay of treatment.
      b) Vagotonic maneuvers (carotid sinus massage, the Valsalva maneuver) are frequently successful.
      c) Acute medical therapy consists of administering adenosine 6–12 mg IV. Adenosine is successful in terminating AVNRT in >90% of cases and has minimal and short-lived side effects.
      d) IV verapamil 2.5–5.0 mg IV is the second drug of choice.
      e) Digoxin and propranolol IV may also be effective.
      f) Atrial or esophageal pacing has been effective in some patients.
      g) Chronic therapy is indicated in patients with refractory, recurrent attacks and consists of digoxin, verapamil, propranolol, or a type Ia antiarrhythmic agent. Patients refractory to medical therapy have been successfully treated surgically.
7. AV reentry tachycardia with a concealed pathway.
   a. Introduction.
      1) This arrhythmia constitutes approximately one third of the paroxysmal supraventricular tachycardias. An anomalous pathway directly connecting the atria and ventricles is present bypassing the AV node.
      2) The mechanism underlying this arrhythmia is macroreentry involving atria, AV node, accessory pathway, and ventricles. The arrhythmia may be either orthodromic or antidromic.

    a) The orthodromic is the more common of the re-
       ciprocating tachycardias in which the AV node
       serves as the antegrade limb and the bypass
       tract as the retrograde limb of the macroreen-
       trant circuit.
    b) In the antidromic variety, the accessory path-
       way serves as the antegrade limb and the AV
       node as the retrograde limb.
  b. Diagnosis:
    1) The rate of AV reciprocating tachycardia using a
       concealed extranodal pathway ranges from
       140–240 bpm.
    2) The surface ECG generally reveals a narrow QRS
       complex tachycardia with a P wave following the
       QRS complex. The P wave is typically inverted in
       the inferior leads and morphology may be helpful
       in localizing the bypass tract site.
    3) By definition, AV block cannot occur since both
       atria and ventricles are necessary parts of the mac-
       roreentrant circuit.
    4) With antidromic AV reentrant tachycardia using a
       concealed pathway, the ECG reveals a wide com-
       plex tachycardia because ventricular activation oc-
       curs via the accessory pathway. This can be ex-
       tremely difficult to differentiate from ventricular
       tachycardia.
  c. Treatment:
    1) **Hemodynamic instability**:
       With hemodynamic compromise, *synchronized* dc
       cardioversion is utilized beginning with energy lev-
       els of 10–50 J and increased if unsuccessful.
    2) **Hemodynamic stability**:
       If hemodynamically stable, acute medical therapy
       may be aimed at any site within the macroreentrant
       circuit.
       a) Vagal maneuvers may interrupt the arrhythmia
          by prolonging AV node refractoriness.
       b) For orthodromic tachycardia either lidocaine
          or a type Ia antiarrhythmic agent is chosen as
          the initial course of medical therapy. These
          lengthen the refractory period of the bypass
          tract.

    c) Adenosine and propranolol may interrupt the arrhythmia by prolonging refractoriness in the AV node.

    d) Digitalis is contraindicated because of the possibility of development of atrial fibrillation with conduction over the bypass tract resulting in VF. **Digitalis preparations are absolutely contraindicated in patients with atrial fibrillation in the presence of preexcitation.** Verapamil also may increase conduction over accessory pathway, and is contraindicated.

    e) Chronic medical therapy consists of type Ia agents, type Ic agents, type III agents (amiodarone), and β-blockers. Most chronic drug regimens are prescribed under the guidance of electrophysiologic drug testing. In drug-resistant cases, options include surgical and nonsurgical ablation of accessory pathways as well as pacemaker therapy.

8. Intraaterial reentry tachycardia.

  a. Introduction: Intraatrial reentry tachycardia is caused by a reentrant circuit confined to the atria. The majority of patients have underlying organic heart disease.

  b. Diagnosis:

    1) Since the reentrant circuit is confined to the atria, ventricular activation occurs via the AV node and narrow QRS complexes are present on the ECG.

    2) The HR usually ranges from 100–150 bpm. P waves are often biphasic and occur before the QRS complexes as atrial conduction is antegrade. Atrial epicardial and esophageal electrograms reveal similar findings.

  c. Treatment:

    1) **Hemodynamic instability**: With hemodynamic instability *synchronized* dc cardioversion beginning with 10–50 J is recommended. If unsuccessful, the dose is increased and the shock repeated.

    2) **Hemodynamic stability**: In stable patients, type Ia antiarrhythmic agents are the treatment of choice. Verapamil is occasionally successful.

9. Sinoatrial nodal reentry tachycardia (SNRT).
   a. Introduction:
      1) SNRT is a relatively rare form of SVT, constituting only 5%–10% of cases.
      2) The arrhythmia results from a reentrant circuit within the SA node and usually is seen in patients with underlying organic heart disease.
   b. Diagnosis:
      1) SNRT may be extremely difficult to distinguish from sinus tachycardia. Surface ECG reveals a narrow QRS complex with P waves which are upright and precede the QRS complex. The rate is usually 80–200 bpm.
      2) Vagal maneuvers may be useful in the diagnosis of SA nodal reentry tachycardia in that they may abruptly terminate the arrhythmia.
   c. Treatment:
      The reentrant circuit, confined to the SA node, is influenced by changes in autonomic tone. Vagotonic maneuvers may therefore interrupt the arrhythmia. Medical treatment and prophylaxis consist of propranolol, verapamil, and digitalis.
10. Automatic atrial tachycardia (AAT).
    a. Introduction:
       1) AAT is due to enhanced automaticity of an atrial focus distinct from the SA node.
       2) AAT is generally associated with chronic disease such as COPD, cardiomyopathy, or drug toxicity (especially digitalis).
    b. Diagnosis:
       1) Characteristically, there is a warm-up phenomenon present with a gradual progressive increase in HR before the arrhythmia reaches its stable rate. The HR usually ranges from 100–200 bpm.
       2) The surface ECG reveals upright P waves with a different morphology from those seen during sinus rhythm. QRS complexes are narrow and in the absence of AV nodal block there is 1:1 AV conduction. Atrial epicardial and esophageal electrograms reveal the same findings.

    c. Treatment:
- 1) Type Ia antiarrhythmic agents are the treatment of choice.
- 2) If digitalis toxicity is suspected, withhold the drug and take appropriate measures.
- 3) Phenytoin and propranolol may be effective in suppressing this arrhythmia in selected patients.
- 4) In patients with severe manifestations of digitalis toxicity, antidigoxin antibody is available.

11. Multifocal atrial tachycardia (MAT).
- a. Introduction.
  - 1) MAT results from several automatic atrial foci.
  - 2) MAT is commonly seen in patients with COPD.
  - 3) Other causes include cardiomyopathy, diabetes mellitus, and drug toxicity (digitalis and theophylline).
- b. Diagnosis:

  The surface ECG reveals a narrow QRS complex tachycardia with P waves of at least three different morphologies.
- c. Treatment:
  - 1) Correct underlying acid-base and electrolyte disturbances.
  - 2) Drug toxicities should be suspected and treated when appropriate.
  - 3) Verapamil has been used successfully.

12. Atrial tachycardia with block.
- a. Introduction: Atrial tachycardia with block occurs primarily in patients with digitalis toxicity. The rhythm is due to an automatic atrial focus and generally is associated with 2:1 AV block.
- b. Diagnosis:
  - 1) The ECG reveals positive P waves with uniform morphology and 2:1 or greater AV block.
  - 2) The atrial rate is usually 150–200 bpm and the ventricular response is dependent upon the degree of block within the AV node.
  - 3) The key to differentiating this arrhythmia from atrial flutter is the finding of isoelectric intervals between P waves on the 12-lead ECG and the slower rate. Carotid sinus massage generally will

increase the degree of AV block but will not terminate the arrhythmia.

c. Treatment:

1) In patients not receiving digitalis, digoxin can be used to control ventricular response and a type 1a antiarrhythmic agent used to treat the arrhythmia itself.

2) In patients receiving digitalis, toxicity must be assumed and the medication withheld. Electrolyte disturbances are corrected and in cases of severe toxicity, antidigoxin antibody administered.

3) Phenytoin or propranolol are occasionally useful in the digitalis-toxic patient.

13. Nonparoxysmal junctional tachycardia.

a. Introduction:

1) Nonparoxysmal junctional tachycardia occurs secondary to enhanced automaticity of the AV junction.

2) As in other arrhythmias due to enhanced automaticity, there is usually gradual onset and termination of nonparoxysmal AV junctional tachycardia.

3) This arrhythmia also may be due to digitalis toxicity.

b. Diagnosis:

1) This arrhythmia typically occurs in patients with underlying pulmonary and cardiac disease. The HR is typically 70–130 bpm. Impulses originating in the AV node cause ventricular depolarization. Atrial activation may occur either retrograde from the AV junctional tissue or antegrade via the SA node or an ectopic focus.

2) The ECG may reveal P waves which precede, coincide with, or follow the QRS complex and are of varying morphology. There may be complete AV dissociation.

3) Epicardial and esophageal electrograms will confirm the ECG findings.

c. Treatment:

1) Treatment is aimed at the underlying problem. In the patient not receiving digitalis who is **hemodynamically unstable**, *synchronized* dc cardioversion is the treatment of choice. An initial shock of

50–100 J should be administered and increased and repeated as necessary.

2) In the patient suspected of having digitalis toxicity, the arrhythmia is unlikely to respond to electrocardioversion and the risk of precipitating a severe ventricular arrhythmia is present. Therefore treatment consists of withholding digitalis and administering phenytoin or propranolol. Administration of antidigoxin antibody may be necessary.

14. Paroxysmal junctional ectopic tachycardia.
  a. Introduction: Paroxysmal junctional ectopic tachycardia is rare in adults and is seen usually in neonates and infants following cardiac surgical procedures.
  b. Diagnosis:
    1) The ECG reveals a narrow complex tachycardia with AV dissociation. This is confirmed by epicardial and transesophageal electrograms.
    2) The typical HR is 120–250 bpm. With rapid rates, there may be aberrant ventricular conduction resulting in a wide complex tachycardia which is difficult to differentiate from ventricular tachycardia.
  c. Treatment:
    1) In the **hemodynamically unstable** patient, *synchronized* dc cardioversion is performed beginning with 50–100 J and repeated as necessary.
    2) Propranolol may help in the acute setting, especially in adults. Amiodarone and propafenone may be useful.
    3) In children the tachycardias frequently are refractory to medical therapy and measures such as ablation of the AV nodal tissue must be performed.

15. Ventricular tachycardia.
  a. Introduction.
    1) Three or more consecutive premature ventricular complexes at a rate >100 bpm constitutes ventricular tachycardia. The arrhythmia is due to a reentry circuit within the ventricles and is of particular concern because of its propensity to deteriorate into VF.
    2) A clinical dilemma is distinguishing ventricular tachycardia from a supraventricular arrhythmia with aberrant ventricular conduction. This can be

extremely difficult and require sophisticated electrophysiologic studies with the capability of recording His bundle electrograms. A SVT with either bundle branch block or conduction over an accessory bypass tract may closely mimic ventricular tachycardia.

b. Diagnosis:

1) Findings on the ECG diagnostic of ventricular tachycardia include a wide complex (QRS > 0.16 sec) tachycardia (>100 bpm), AV dissociation, and the presence of fusion beats.

2) Findings suggestive of ventricular tachycardia include a QRS complex with duration >0.14 second, left axis deviation, and a mono- or biphasic RBBB-shaped QRS in lead Vl.

3) A triphasic QRS complex with a RBBB configuration in lead VI suggests SVT with aberrant conduction.

4) Epicardial lead and transesophageal electrograms may help to differentiate between the two types of arrhythmias by making the presence of AV dissociation more clearly definable.

c. Treatment:

Rapid recognition and initiation of appropriate intervention is important in successful treatment of ventricular tachycardia. The risk of deterioration into ventricular fibrillation is always present.

1) **Hemodynamic instability:**

a) With hemodynamic instability, *synchronized* dc cardioversion is the treatment of choice beginning with a shock of 50–100 J. If unsuccessful, the energy level is doubled and cardioversion repeated. Occasionally, multiple attempts are required. If cardioversion is unsuccessful, lidocaine, procainamide, or bretylium should be administered and cardioversion repeated.

b) A precordial thump may be administered while the patient is being prepared for synchronized dc cardioversion and occasionally is successful in terminating the arrhythmia.

2) **Hemodynamic stability**:
   a) In patients who are only minimally symptomatic or who are tolerating the arrhythmia well, treatment consists of IV lidocaine as a 75–100 mg bolus followed by continuous infusion of 1–4 mg/min.
   b) If lidocaine infusion is unsuccessful, the next drug of choice is IV bretylium as a loading dose of 5–10 mg/kg over 10–15 minutes followed by a continuous infusion of 1–2 mg/min.
   c) If bretylium is unsuccessful, IV procainamide is given in a loading dose of 1,000 mg over 15–20 minutes (so as to avoid systemic hypotension) followed by a continuous infusion of 1–4 mg/min.
   d) When the possibility exists that the wide complex tachycardia is due to a supraventricular arrhythmia with conduction over an accessory AV bypass tract, it is important to recall that digoxin and verapamil may shorten the refractory period of the bypass tract and lead to a more rapid ventricular response with the risk of deterioration into VF.
   e) In patients with recurrent, difficult-to-control ventricular tachycardia, class Ic, and class Id and class III agents are frequently administered on a chronic basis.
   f) Numerous surgical procedures are available to patients with medically refractory ventricular tachycardias.
16. Torsades de pointes (polymorphic ventricular tachycardia).
   a. Introduction:
      1) Torsades de pointes (polymorphic ventricular tachycardia) is characterized by wide QRS complexes which vary in amplitude and alternate in polarity about the isoelectric point on the surface ECG.
      2) The risk of degeneration into VF is present. The arrhythmia typically occurs with prolongation of the QT interval and may be secondary to a congenital

abnormality or, more typically, result from administration of antiarrhythmic agents. Most commonly, class Ia and Ib agents are the causative drugs. Numerous agents, including antibiotics and psychotropic drugs, have also been implicated.

b. Diagnosis:
1) The diagnosis is made from recognizing the classic finding on the ECG. The HR is typically 200–250 bpm.
2) Frequently, QT prolongation can be found on ECG recordings prior to the occurrence of the arrhythmia.
3) Torsades de pointes generally occurs in the setting of the administration of antiarrhythmic agents.

c. Treatment:
1) Treatment consists of withholding any possible causative agents and in the presence of **hemodynamic instability**, synchronized dc cardioversion beginning with 50–100 J. If unsuccessful, the energy level is doubled and the shock repeated.
2) In stable patients, the treatment of choice is overdrive pacing. Both atrial and ventricular pacing can be successful.
3) Lidocaine and bretylium have been used successfully in other cases. These are administered as noted above.
4) Case reports exist suggesting that magnesium sulfate may be useful. This is administered as a 1–2-g IV bolus.

17. Ventricular fibrillation:
a. VF results from multiple microreetrant circuits within the ventricles. The surface ECG reveals only chaotic undulations without organized electrical activation.
b. Treatment consists of *nonsynchronized* defibrillation beginning with an energy level of 200 J and the institution of standard CPR measures (Chapter 4). If the initial shock is unsuccessful, CPR is continued, the energy level increased to 360 J, and the shock repeated.
c. Patients who are successfully defibrillated should be maintained on an infusion of an appropriate class Ib or Ia antiarrhythmic agent.

VI. CARDIAC PACEMAKERS.

A. Inter-Society Commission for Heart Disease Code for Cardiac Pacing Modes.

1. In this system, the first letter represents the cardiac chamber being paced; the second letter identifies the cardiac chamber being sensed; and the third letter denotes the mode of pacemaker response to the sensed activity.

   a. Chamber paced: The code uses the letter *A* for atrium, *V* for ventricle, and *D* for dual (both chambers). Thus, the first letter may be A, V, or D.

   b. Chamber sensed: The letter *A* stands for atrium, *V* for ventricle, and *D* for dual. The letter *O* is used when no chamber is sensed; however, an asynchronous mode of pacing is rarely used.

   c. Mode of response: The pacemaker may respond to sensed activity by either inhibiting *(I)* or triggering *(T)* its electrical output. A dual response *(D)* indicates that the atrium is triggered and the ventricle is inhibited. The third position therefore may be represented by A, V, or D.

2. The most frequently used pacemakers are shown in Table 5–11. As an example, the AAI pacemaker paces the atrium only, senses atrial activity only, and its pacing output is inhibited by the presence of native atrial electrical signals.

B. Indications for Cardiac Pacing.

1. Cardiac pacemakers may be temporary or permanent. The indications for both significantly overlap, and therefore the choice of short- vs. long-term pacing usually depends on the nature of the underlying disease. In surgical practice temporary pacemakers are most frequently used either to

TABLE 5–11.

Types of Pacemaker

Mode	Description
AAI	Atrial demand
VVI	Ventricular demand
DVI	AV sequential fixed rate
VDD	Atrial synchronous
DDD	AV universal

TABLE 5–12.

Major Indications for Cardiac Pacing

Temporary	Permanent
Symptomatic bradycardia after acute myocardial infarction	Sick sinus syndrome
Bifascicular or trifascicular block after acute anterior myocardial infarction	Mobitz type II AV block
Bridge to permanent pacing	Third-degree heart block
Following cardiac surgery	Medically refractory low cardiac output syndrome improved by temporary pacing
Low cardiac output syndrome	Persistent bifascicular block following acute myocardial infarction
	Symptomatic bilateral bundle-branch block

treat conduction block secondary to perioperative MI or
routinely following cardiac surgery (Table 5–12).

2. Sick sinus syndrome. usually presents as symptoms of dizziness or presyncope secondary to severe sinus bradycardia with intermittent sinus pauses and is the most common
   indication for permanent pacemaker placement.
   a. Atrial demand pacing (AAI) is suitable for this syn-
      drome, but many patients have coexisting AV conduc-
      tion abnormalities.
   b. Ventricular demand pacing (VVI) is required when AV
      node or bundle-branch conduction delay is present.
   c. AV synchronous or dual-chamber pacing (DDD) is in-
      dicated in patients who require the "atrial kick" to
      maintain cardiac output.

3. Mobitz type II and complete AV block generally require
   pacing, with either ventricular demand or dual-chamber
   modes.
   a. Etiology.
      1) Sclerodegenerative change:
         a) Typically seen in the elderly.
         b) Often preceded by LBBB or RBBB.
         c) Progression to advanced heart block necessi-
            tates permanent pacing
      2) Conduction defects secondary to cardiomyopathy
         usually represent permanent injury from any of a

number of causes and therefore require permanent pacing
3) Ischemic cardiac disease.
   a) Anterior MI:
      i) The conduction disturbance is generally not reversible.
      ii) Permanent pacemaking is the rule, not the exception.
   b) Inferior MI:
      i) Usually a reversible insult to conduction.
      ii) Permanent pacing is indicated for disturbances which persist over 2–3 weeks.
4. Cardiac surgery.
   a. Treatment of conduction block.
      1) AV block may be seen following valve replacement or repair of septal defects, and may be related to pre- or intraoperative ischemia, or may be a side effect of cardioplegia.
      2) Temporary pacing during first postoperative week is the initial therapy.
      3) Permanent pacing is indicated for heart block >1 week's duration.
   b. Treatment of low cardiac output.
      1) Low CO is not uncommon following cardiac operations.
      2) Atrial pacing at 100 bpm is simple and may significantly increase CO without adversely affecting myocardial $\dot{V}_{O_2}$.
      3) AV sequential pacing may be needed to optimize hemodynamics in patients with conduction delay and poor cardiac reserve.
   c. Conversion of atrial flutter (rapid atrial pacing).
      1) The atrium is paced at 350 bpm or faster.
      2) If atrial capture occurs, the pacing rate is slowly reduced to 100 bpm or may be rapidly terminated.
      3) Normal sinus rhythm may be maintained or patients may convert to atrial fibrillation with slower ventricular response.

C. Pacemaker Implantation.
1. Most permanent pacemakers currently are placed transvenously under local anesthesia using fluoroscopic guidance. This technique provides the best long-term thresh-

olds and diminishes both fracture and dislocation of the electrode lead.

2. Preoperative antibiotics with staphylococcal coverage are administered and continued for 24 hours postoperatively.

3. A pacemaker pocket is fashioned on the anterior chest; a medial location helps reduce generator migration.

4. After venous cannulation through the incision, a floppy J wire is inserted and passed into the RA, a tear-away sheath is passed over the wire, and the wire withdrawn.

5. The pacemaker lead is then passed through the sheath directed toward the atrium or ventricular apex under fluoroscopic guidance and gently embedded into the myocardium.

6. Following lead placement, acceptable positioning is confirmed by functional testing and the sheath removed.

7. The lead is secured to the venous entrance site or pectoral fascia, connected to the pacemaker generator, and the wound is closed.

D. Functional Assessment

1. Thorough evaluation of pacemaker function must include both pacing and sensing capabilities. A pacing system analyzer is used to simulate the output and sensing circuits to measure a pacemaker's voltage, current, rate, interval pulse width, sensitivity, and refractory period. These determinations are critical during pacemaker placement and during evaluation of pacemaker malfunction.

2. Stimulation threshold is defined as the lowest voltage or current delivered to the heart at a given pulse width resulting in depolarization of the myocardium.

   a. RV thresholds of ≤ 0.5 V should be obtained with a pulse width of 0.5 ms.

   b. RV thresholds >1 V are unacceptable.

   c. Atrial thresholds should approach those of the ventricle; thresholds >2 V are unacceptable.

3. Resistance is equal to voltage divided by current. Resistance values between 300 and 800 Ω are acceptable at 5 V.

   a. Low resistance levels result in excess current and may be due to poor lead placement. Decreased battery life may result.

   b. High resistance levels decrease current which may result in failure to capture

4. R wave sensitivity measures the ability of the pacemaker to detect spontaneous myocardial depolarizations and is determined by both amplitude and frequency of the electrical signal.
   a. Amplitudes of >4 mV for ventricular electrograms and 1.5 mV for atrial electrograms are satisfactory.
   b. The slew rate is the change in amplitude over time (>0.5 mV/msec is acceptable).

E. Pacemaker Complications.
   1. Complications of insertion:
      a. Pneumothorax, most frequently due to subclavian cannulation (Chapter 22).
      b. Air embolism.
      c. Vascular injury.
      d. PVCs and even ventricular tachycardia may result from stimulation of the pulmonary outflow tract and will usually cease after withdrawal of the guidewire
      e. Ventricular perforation may occur and is rarely of clinical significance, but tamponade can occur.
      f. Catheter dislodgment can be minimized by testing stability of placement intraoperatively by having patient cough.
   2. Postoperative complications:
      a. The incidence of pocket hematoma can be decreased by meticulous hemostasis during placement.
      b. Infection is an unusual complication with the use of prophylactic antibiotics and careful sterile techniques.
         1) Etiologic organisms are most commonly gram-positive, either staphylococcus or streptococcus.
         2) Treatment of pacemaker infection:
            a) Removal of the entire pacemaker system.
            b) Wound cultures.
            c) IV antibiotics.
            d) Use of temporary pacemaker.
            e) Reimplantation of a permanent pacemaker using a different access site once the infection is completely eradicated.
   3. Late complications:
      a. Pacemaker migration may be reduced by medial positioning of generator pocket.
      b. The incidence of skin erosion is decreased by deep subcutaneous pockets or subfascial pockets in thin patients.

c. Venous thrombosis may occur and is a rare cause of fatal PE.

d. Twiddler's syndrome represents fracture or dislodgment of the pacemaker lead by habitual twisting of the generator by the patient.

4. Pacemaker malfunctions are infrequent. Long-term patient follow-up with complete pacemaker testing is mandatory. Inappropriate pacing or failure to pace may be secondary to electrode lead or generator malfunction, underlying cardiac disease, drug toxicity, or electrolyte abnormalities.

a. Failure to capture:

1) Failure to capture is often manifested by dizziness or syncope

2) Etiology:

a) Lead displacement—most frequent during first month after implantation.

b) Lead fracture—may result from Twiddler's syndrome.

c) Perielectrode fibrosis may result in high thresholds.

d) Antiarrhythmic medications (particularly toxic levels of procainamide and quinidine).

e) Electrolyte disturbance, particularly hyperkalemia or hypokalemia.

3) Evaluation of possible dysfunction:

a) ECG monitoring to determine the status of pacemaker signal and effectiveness of capture.

b) Serum potassium level and antiarrhythmic drug levels should be checked to exclude underlying nonpacemaker cause of malfunction.

c) Plain radiographs or fluoroscopy should be obtained to identify lead fracture or dislodgment, the most frequent reason for noncapture.

d) Test generator output.

4) Treatment is based on the underlying cause of malfunction. In symptomatic patients with true pacemaker malfunction (lead fracture or dislodgment) immediate temporary pacing is imperative. This may be accomplished by insertion of a pacing Swan-Ganz catheter, a temporary pacing electrode, or application of a noninvasive temporary cardiac pacer (Zoll device).

b. Runaway pacemaker represents ventricular tachycardia caused by sudden increase in pacing rate.
  1) Complication of fixed-rate pacemakers.
  2) May progress to VF.
  3) Requires urgent replacement of the impulse generator.
c. "Pacemaker syndrome" is manifested by syncope and hypotension after implantation of a ventricular pacemaker.
  1) This syndrome is attributed to inadequate CO in patients who require atrial component to EDV. The loss of AV synchrony adversely affects LV preload.
  2) Treatment is AV sequential pacing by dual-chamber devices to restore AV synchrony and the contribution of atrial systole to ventricular filling.

SELECTED REFERENCES

ISCHEMIC CARDIAC DISEASE

Charlson ME, MacRenzie CR, Ales K, et al: Surveillance for postoperative myocardial infarction after noncardiac operations. *Surg Gynecol Obstet* 1988; 167:407–414.

Goldman L: Cardiac risks and complications of noncardiac surgery. *Ann Surg* 1983; 198:780–791.

Salem DN, Isner JM: Management of cardiac disease in the general surgical patient. *Curr Probl Cardiol* 1980; 5:1.

VALVULAR HEART DISEASE

Braunwald E: *Heart Disease; A Textbook of Cardiovascular Medicine.* Philadelphia, WB Saunders Co, 1988.

Sabiston DC, Spencer FC: *Surgery of the Chest,* ed 5. Philadelphia, WB Saunders Co, 1990.

Weitz HH, Goldman L: Noncardiac surgery in the patient with heart disease. *Med Clin North Am* 1987; 71:413.

PULMONARY EDEMA AND CONGESTIVE HEART DISEASE

Salam DN, Isner JM: Management of cardiac disease in the general surgical patient. *Curr Probl Cardiol* 1980; 5:1.

Sibbald WH, Calvin JE, Holliday RL, et al: Concepts in the pharmacologic and nonpharmacologic support of cardiovascular function in critically ill surgical patients. *Surg Clin North Am* 1983; 63:455.

Smith WM: Epidemiology of congestive heart failure. *Am J Cardiol* 1985; 55:3A.

Staub NC: Pulmonary edema. *Physiol Rev* 1974; 54:678.

CARDIAC TAMPONADE

Beck CA: Two cardiac compression triads. *JAMA* 1935; 104:715–718.

Callaham ML: Pericardiocentesis in traumatic and nontraumatic cardiac tamponade. *Ann Emerg Med* 1984; 13:924–945.

Shabetai R, Mangiardi L, Bhargava V, et al: The pericardium and cardiac function. *Prog Cardiovasc Dis* 1979; 22:107–134.

Spodick DH: Pericarditis, pericardial effusion, cardiac tamponade, and constriction. *Crit Care Clin* 1989; 5:455–476.

CARDIAC ARRHYTHMIA

Gillette PC, Garson A: *Pediatric Arrhythmias: Electrophysiology and Pacing,* Philadelphia, WB Saunders Co, 1990.

Manolis AS, Estes NAM: Supraventricular tachycardia: Mechanisms and therapy. *Arch Intern Med* 1987; 147:1706–1716.

Waldo AL, MacLean WAH: *Diagnosis and Treatment of Cardiac Arrhythmias Following Open Heart Surgery,* Mount Kisco, NY, Futura Publishing Co, 1980

Walsh KA, Ezri MD, Denes P: Emergency treatment of tachyarrhythmias. *Med Clin North Am* 1986; 70:791–811.

CARDIAC PACING

Del Negro AA, Fletcher RD: Cardiac pacemaker emergencies. *Cardiovasc Clin* 1986; 16:135.

Dreifus IS, Michelson EL, Kaplinsky E: Bradyarrhythmias: Clinical significance and management. *J Am Coll Cardiol* 1983; 1:327.

Hauser RG: Multiprogrammable cardiac pacemakers: Applications, results, and follow-up *Am J Surg* 1983; 195:740.

Luceri RM, Castellanos A, Zaman L, et al: The arrhythmias of dual-chamber cardiac pacemakers and their management. *Ann Intern Med* 1983; 99:354.

Medina R, Michelson EL: Update in cardiac pacemakers: Description, complications, indications, and follow-up. *Cardiovasc Clin* 1985; 16:177.

Zoll PM, Zoll RH, Faulk RH, et al: External noninvasive temporary cardiac pacing: Clinical trials. *Circulation* 1985; 71:937.

CARDIAC SURGERY 6

I. PERIOPERATIVE MANAGEMENT.

A. Preoperative Evaluation.

1. **Cardiac**:
   a. The patient must be evaluated for history of MI, CHF, symptoms of ischemic heart disease (angina), history of arrhythmia or pacemaker insertion, congenital heart defects, and valvular disease.
   b. The results of all invasive (catheterization), and noninvasive (echocardiogram, exercise tolerance testing [ETT], radionuclide angiocardiogram [RNA]) testing must be carefully assessed.
   c. Any previous cardiac interventions such as thrombolysis, percutaneous transluminal coronary angioplasty (PTCA), or cardiac surgery should be noted.

2. **Pulmonary**:
   a. The patient must be evaluated for evidence of pulmonary disease including COPD, history of PE, recent pneumonia, and smoking history. Any previous thoracic surgery should also be noted.
   b. Evaluation must include a CXR and preoperative ABG. Pulmonary function testing may be indicated in high-risk patients.

3. **Neurologic**:
   a. Patients with signs and symptoms of cerebrovascular disease, should be completely evaluated preoperatively.
   b. In patients with significant extracranial carotid disease, the performance of preoperative carotid endarterectomy or, rarely, concomitant endarterectomy may be indicated.

4. **Hematologic**:
   a. The presence of any coagulopathy is particularly important in those patients undergoing cardiopulmonary bypass (CPB).
      1) Bleeding disorders.
      2) Anticoagulant therapy (including antiplatelet therapy).
      3) Hemoglobinopathy.
      4) History of heparin-induced thrombocytopenia.
   b. In patients with unstable angina undergoing cardiac surgery it is usually preferable to continue heparin therapy until the time of surgery.
   c. Frequently, patients will receive thrombolytic therapy prior to cardiac surgery resulting in an increased risk of postoperative hemorrhage.

5. **Vascular disease**:
   a. Assess for any signs or symptoms of peripheral vascular disease including a careful examination of the femoral and pedal pulses. This is extremely important in patients who may need IABP insertion.
   b. A history of previous venous thrombosis, venous insufficiency, or vein stripping is important in patients undergoing CABG with saphenous vein grafts.

6. **Urinary tract disorders**:
   a. Previous nephrectomy or renal failure.
   b. Previous or current urinary tract infection (UTI).
   c. In patients with a history of prostate disease or bladder outlet obstruction, a urology consult may be indicated.

7. **Oral and alimentary tract disorders**:
   a. An assessment of dentition is particularly important, especially in those about to undergo valve replacement. Dental procedures should be carried out preoperatively.
   b. History of previous peptic ulcer disease, gastritis, hepatitis or cirrhosis, pancreatitis, or cholelithiasis.
   c. History of previous abdominal surgery.

8. **Endocrine disorders**:
   a. Each patient must be carefully assessed for diabetes mellitus, and for evidence of thyroid, parathyroid and adrenal insufficiency or hyperactivity.

9. **Drug history**:
   a. Current medications.
   b. Allergies.
   c. History of drug or ethanol abuse.

B. Preoperative Laboratory Tests and Studies.
1. Routine laboratory studies should include CBC with differential, electrolytes, glucose, BUN, creatinine, calcium, PT, APTT, and urinalysis.
2. If hepatic dysfunction is suspected, liver function tests (SGOT, SGPT, alkali phosphates, bilirubin) are necessary.
3. A CXR is obtained on every patient.
4. Preoperative ECG.
5. A type and crossmatch, for 6 units of PRBCs, 4 units of FFP, and 10 units of platelets.

C. Preoperative Preparation.
1. Aspirin should be discontinued 2–3 weeks prior to elective operation. In patients with unstable angina or critical coronary disease, heparin should be continued.
2. Monamine oxidase inhibitor (MAOI) and tricyclic antidepressants should be withheld 1 week prior to surgery.
3. For patients taking steroids, cortisone acetate or hydrocortisone 100 mg IM or IV should be administered on the evening before and the morning of surgery, providing protection against hypoadrenalism. Postoperatively, steroids 100 mg q.6–8 h. are continued until the patient can be tapered or converted to the preoperative regimen.
4. Patients are kept NPO after midnight for elective surgery when the patient has DM. The morning insulin dose is held and the blood glucose is controlled intraoperatively and immediately postoperatively with a continuous insulin infusion.
5. Nitrates, β-blocking agents, calcium antagonists, and other antianginal agents are usually continued until the time of surgery.
6. In patients undergoing anti-arrhythmic procedures, all antiarrhythmic agents should be discontinued prior to operation. These agents may make it impossible to initiate and map the arrhythmias intraoperatively.
7. The patient should take a preoperative shower with Hibiclens or phisohex and should be shaved from the chin to ankles bilaterally.
8. A broad-spectrum antibiotic, generally cephalosporin (cefazolin, cefamandole) should be given on call to the OR. If the patient is penicillin-allergic, vancomycin may be used.
9. Preoperative sedation should be ordered (frequently by cardiac anesthesia), usually a narcotic (methadone 5–15 mg po)

and a benzodiazepine (diazepam 5–10 mg po) are given. A sleeping medication (secobarbital 100–200 mg po q.hs.) is ordered for the night prior to surgery.

D. Postoperative Care.

1. **Initial assessment:**

   As soon as the patient arrives in the SICU, a rapid and thorough assessment is necessary. All hemodynamic monitoring catheters are calibrated immediately. **LA lines should be handled with great care because of the danger of air embolism.** These lines should be aspirated and flushed by the resident.

   a. **Determination of vital signs:**

      1) BP.
      2) HR.
      3) Respiratory rate.
      4) Intracardiac pressures and CO.
      5) Temperature.

   b. **Neurologic assessment:**

      1) Level of consciousness.
      2) Motor and/or sensory deficits.
      3) Examination of the pupils.

   c. **Respiratory assessment:**

      1) Auscultation of breath sounds.
      2) Examination for chest wall symmetry.
      3) Assessment of tracheal position.
      4) Assessment of mediastinal and chest tubes for presence of an air leak or active hemorrhage.
      5) A volume ventilator is usually employed. A TV of 12–15 mL/kg with an initial F_1O_2 of 1.0 (100% O_2) should be used with a PEEP of $\geq$ 5 cm H_2O. An initial IMV rate of 8–12/min is usually adequate.

   d. **Cardiac status:**

      1) The HR and rhythm or paced rate should be noted. Any arrhythmias or conduction defects should be treated.
      2) The atrial (usually exiting from right side of the chest) and ventricular (usually exiting from left side of the chest) temporary pacing wires should be connected to a pacemaker. If the patient does not require pacing, the pacemaker should be left in the ventricular "demand" position. A back-up rate of 60 bpm is acceptable. The pacing thresholds should be

tested daily. Pacemaker batteries should also be checked.
   3) Auscultation of heart.
e. **GI examination**:
   1) Auscultation and palpation of abdomen.
   2) The NG tube should be checked for patency and position.
f. **Vascular examination:**
   1) Palpate all peripheral pulses and evaluate peripheral perfusion (capillary refill, skin temperature, cyanosis).
   2) Evaluate the legs for signs of ischemia, especially in patients with an IABP.
g. Record initial physiologic data including core temperature, CO, mean BP, HR, CVP, PA systolic and diastolic pressure, PCWP, and LAP when available.
h. The dosages of IV inotropic drugs and afterload reducing agents should be noted.
i. If an IABP has been inserted, its timing and efficacy should be assessed. It is timed either off the arterial pressure tracing or the ECG.
j. Quantitate patient output:
   1) The chest tube output should be checked q 30 min for the first 4–6 hours, then hourly.
   2) The urinary output should be checked every hour.
k. Obtain blood for routine laboratory evaluation including CBC with differential, platelet count, electrolytes, glucose, BUN, creatinine, ABG, DIC screen (fibrinogen, fibrin split products, PT, PTT), ionized calcium, urinalysis.
l. Obtain a CXR and ECG.
m. The ACT is obtained to assess reversal of intraoperative heparin.

2. **Postoperative orders**: Standard postoperative orders should include:
   a. Frequency of vital signs, intracardiac pressure, and CO determinations.
   b. Strict input and output determination including measurement of NG, urinary, and chest tube output.
   c. NPO, NG tube to continuous low wall suction.
   d. Foley catheter to straight drain

   e. Bed rest.
   f. Ventilator settings should be specified including FiO_2, TV, rate, PEEP, and mode.
   g. Chest tube to 20 cm of wall suction.
   h. Autotransfusion guidelines (if utilized).
   i. Sedatives and narcotics: morphine 1–4 mg IV q 1h. prn pain; medazolam 2.5–5.0 mg IV q 1–2h. prn agitation.
   j. Pacemaker settings including type (atrial, ventricular, AV sequential), mode (synchronous or asynchronous), and rate of pacing must be specified (see p 169).
   k. Dosages of IV medications including inotropic, after-load reducing, and antiarrhythmic agents. Calculated dosage sheets for inotropic and afterload reducing agents are necessary and should be attached to the chart or flow sheet.
   l. Usually the preoperative antibiotic is continued until the chest tubes are removed.
   m. Postoperative laboratory data and frequency.
   n. Mylanta II 15–30 mL via NG tube prn gastric pH < 6. Use of the H_2 blocker (ranitidine 50 mg IV q 8h. or cimetidine 300 mg IV q 6h.) may be indicated.
   o. Acetaminophen 650–1300 mg suppository q 2h. prn temperature > 38.2° C.
   p. Diabetic management, if indicated, should include insulin administration, Dextrostix frequency, and urine monitoring. In the immediate postoperative period a continuous infusion of regular human insulin and hourly blood glucose determinations are utilized.
E. **Complications.**
   1. **Arrhythmias** (Chapter 5, pp 145–168):
      a. Arrhythmias following cardiac surgery occur in up to 48% of patients. They usually appear within the first 3 postoperative days.
      b. The most critically ill patients usually have the most serious arrhythmias. Precipitating factors include intraoperative ischemia, inadequate myocardial protection, cardioplegia, low CO, surgical trauma, catecholamines, anesthetic agents, tracheal stimulation, electrolyte and acid-base abnormalities, hypoxia, hypercarbia, and underlying heart disease.
      c. The most common postoperative arrythmias are atrial fi-

brillation and atrial flutter. Ventricular ectopy occurs less commonly.

d. Bradycardia, cardiac heart block, and even asystole may be seen in the immediate postoperative period and require cardiac pacing.

e. β-Blockade with atenolol 25–50 mg po q.d. or propranolol 10 mg po q.i.d. has been used prophylactically to prevent atrial arrythmias. Impaired LV function, COPD, and heart block are contraindications to β-blockade (Chapter 5, pp 154–164).

2. **Hemorrhage**:

a. Bleeding is a common postoperative complication.

   1) Reduction of blood loss to a minimum is imperative and can be facilitated by careful opening of the chest, limiting unnecessary dissection, obtaining meticulous hemostasis, and adequate reversal of anticoagulants.

   2) Bleeding is a problem especially following prolonged periods of CPB, reoperations, deep hypothermia with circulatory arrest, and in patients receiving antiplatelet or thrombolytic agents.

   3) To minimize postoperative transfusion, all shed blood is collected and autotransfused (p. 602–604).

   4) An ACT is obtained to establish total neutralization of the intraoperative heparin.

b. Postoperative hemorrhage may result from mechanical factors or from a defect in the coagulation system.

   1) **Patients who are hemodynamically unstable or who manifest high rates of bleeding (>400–500 mL/hr) should be urgently returned to the OR to rule out a mechanical source.**

   2) Patients who are hemodynamically stable with evidence of a coagulopathy are initially managed by correction of the coagulation abnormalities, so long as the hemorrhage is not excessive.

   3) If hemorrhage persists following correction of the coagulopathy, the patient is returned to the OR for reexploration.

c. Correction of abnormalities in coagulation factors.

   1) If ACT is prolonged, protamine sulfate may be required to reverse the heparin effect and the dosage can be determined from a plot calculated intraopera-

tively. Protamine sulfate is administered by slow IV infusion. If given too rapidly, protamine can cause hypotension. If given in excess, it can cause peripheral vasodilation and increased bleeding.

2) Prolongation of PT and PTT may be seen. The ACT should be corrected with protamine before the PT and PTT can be adequately interpreted. With a normal ACT, FFP can be administered. Usually 2 units of FFP are given and the values remeasured.

3) Thrombocytopenia or platelet dysfunction is a universal finding following CPB. Platelets adhere to any foreign surface (i.e., pump lines, oxygenators, filters). There is evidence that the platelets that remain are not maximally competent. They aggregate poorly and do not perform normally on glass bead retention tests. Platelet dysfunction may also be seen in patients receiving preoperative aspirin therapy.

   a) For a platelet count < 50,000, a pooled pack of six to ten platelet concentrates should be administered and the platelet count remeasured.

   b) For a platelet count < 100,000, with persistent bleeding, platelets should be administered.

   c) For patients with massive bleeding, platelets are administered regardless of platelet count.

   d) Patients with cyanotic heart disease are particularly apt to have abnormal platelet function.

4) If the fibrinogen level is <100 mg/dL, cryoprecipitate should be administered (10–20 units) and the fibrinogen level remeasured.

5) Fibrinolysis is occasionally seen following CPB and is characterized by decreased fibrinogen, thrombocytopenia, increased fibrin split products, and an accelerated euglobulin clot lysis time (<30 minutes) and may be treated with ε-aminocaproic acid (Amican) 4 g IV, and then 1 g/hr for 4 hours.

6) Disseminated intravascular coagulation (DIC) is a consequence of activation of both the coagulation and fibrinolytic systems, and occurs rarely following cardiac procedures, usually in the presence of low CO and poor tissue perfusion. Laboratory findings include thrombocytopenia, decreased fibrinogen, elevated fibrin split products, prolonged PT and

PTT, and a prolonged euglobulin clot lysis time (>2 hours). This may be difficult to distinguish from primary fibrinolysis. If suspected, a hematologist should be consulted.

   a) The major therapeutic approach to DIC is the treatment of the *underlying* cause. Unless severe hemorrhagic or thrombotic complications are present, treatment of the coagulation abnormalities should be withheld.

   b) Cryoprecipitate and FFP may be given if bleeding is the major complication. However, both anticoagulation and factor replacement therapy are potentially dangerous.

   c) Amicar may lead to widespread thrombosis in this condition and its use should be discouraged.

   d) Heparin therapy for thrombotic complications should be initiated only after expert consultation and begun at low doses.

7) Chelation of calcium by citrate in banked blood may occur. In cases of multiple transfusions, 500 mg $CaCl_2$ is administered for every 4 units PRBCs transfused. Ionized calcium levels should be used to guide replacement.

8) Hypothermia is common following cardiac surgery and leads to clotting dysfunction. Aggressive efforts to correct hypothermia include overhead heaters, warm IV fluids, blood warmers, and ventilator heaters.

d. PEEP is sometimes effective in decreasing the amount of postoperative drainage.

   1) While its benefit is controversial, PEEP should be used before reexploration in hemodynamically stable patients. PEEP is instituted at 5 cm, and increased in increments of 5 cm up to a maximum of 20 cm H_2O.

   2) Careful titration of PEEP must be used because of its possible adverse affects on CO. If CO is impaired with high levels of PEEP, it should be discontinued.

e. Postoperative hypertension may lead to increased hemorrhage.

   1) Sodium nitroprusside is the drug of choice to maintain a low MAP by reducing afterload.

2) β-Blockade with labatelol 2.5–5.0 mg IV or esmolol 50–300 µg/kg/min may be used in patients with an adequate CO and persistent hypertension.

3) Sufficient pain medications are given to help control BP and the intrinsic catecholamine response.

f. Signs and symptoms of transfusion reactions include fever, allergic manifestations varying from urticaria and rash up to severe bronchospasm and vascular collapse, hemolysis, hematuria. If a reaction occurs, the blood transfusion should be stopped and the unit returned to the blood bank with a blood sample from the patient (Chapter 3, p 70).

1) Antihistamines (diphenhydramine HCl 25–50 mg IV) are given.

2) H_2 antagonists (cimetidine 300 mg IV or ranitidine 50 mg IV) are given.

3) Aminophylline is indicated for bronchospasm (6 mg/kg IV over 1 hour as a loading dose followed by 0.3–0.7 mg/kg/hr as a continuous infusion).

4) Corticosteroids (methylprednisolone 1 gm IV) may be necessary.

5) Catecholamines (epinephrine) may be necessary if true anaphylaxis occurs.

g. Reexploration is usually indicated if bleeding persists at a rate > 200 mL/hr for 4–6 hours without signs of abatement following correction of any coagulopathy.

1) There are no precise rules when a patient should be reexplored.

2) In patients with massive bleeding (>500 mL/hr), or hemodynamic compromise immediate reexploration is indicated.

3) Cardiac tamponade may require urgent reexploration in the SICU.

4) Early reexploration is associated with less blood replacement and fewer complications.

3. **Cardiac tamponade** (see pp 137–143).

a. When a patient becomes hemodynamically unstable following a cardiac operation, cardiac tamponade must be excluded especially in the presence of low CO, elevated and equal venous filling pressures, oliguria, and enlargement of the cardiac silhouette on CXR. In patients who have been bleeding and have a sudden decrease in chest tube output, tamponade is the primary diagnosis and must be excluded.

b. Hemodynamic evaluation includes determination of CO, CVP, RV pressure, PA pressure, and PCWP. These are often elevated and there is an equalization of the patient's venous filling pressures. However, failure to find equalization does not rule out tamponade.

c. The patency of chest tubes should be ascertained. The tube should be stripped vigorously and, if not patent, a 4F or 5F Fogarty catheter can be passed using sterile technique to remove any obstructing clot.

d. The CXR is examined for enlargement of the cardiac silhouette.

e. Vigorous volume resuscitation and, when indicated, inotropic support is initiated. PEEP can aggravate the hemodynamic decompensation of tamponade and should be discontinued.

f. **In the unstable patient, immediate reexploration is indicated.**

    1) Ideally reexploration is performed in the OR but can be performed in the SICU.

    2) All SICUs should have a sterile set of instruments, retractors, suction tips, and drapes to rapidly perform a thoracotomy or median sternotomy.

    3) The lower end of the sternum can be opened quickly and drainage established while the remainder of the sternum is opened.

    4) Following sternotomy the patient should be taken to the OR for definitive treatment and closure once the condition is stabilized.

    5) The risk of infection is surprisingly low following emergent reexploration in the SICU.

g. Echocardiography confirms the diagnosis in stable patients and can be performed using a portable unit in the SICU. However, reexploration should not be delayed in an unstable patient to obtain an echocardiogram.

h. Late cardiac tamponade may occur in up to 6% of patients following cardiac procedures and can follow any type of procedure regardless of whether the pericardium has been left opened or closed.

    1) Delayed tamponade should be suspected in patients with a gradual decrement in postoperative cardiac function.

    2) It usually has an insidious onset and occurs between 5–14 days postoperatively.

    3) If the effusion is small and the patient is asymptomatic, it can be followed with CXR and echocardiogram.

    4) If the effusion is large, a pericardiocentesis can be performed. This may be the only treatment necessary if the fluid is serosanguinous.

    5) Occasionally, there is a large amount of clot present and reexploration and drainage may be necessary. The preferred approach is a subxiphoid incision. If this is not possible, a thoracotomy or repeat median sternotomy can be performed.

4. Postoperative low cardiac output:

   a. Maintenance of an adequate CO is essential to patient survival. It is not uncommon for CO to be depressed postoperatively for several days. Studies have shown that a CI <2 L/min/m^2 indicates severe dysfunction and an increased probability of acute cardiac death. Whereas the cardiac index must be individualized somewhat for the patient's condition (in a hypothermic patient with known preoperative cardiac dysfunction, a CI <2 L/min/m^2 may be acceptable), it is important to promptly treat low output to avoid mortality (Table 6–1).

   b. CO is defined by (1) **HR**, (2) **preload**, (3) **afterload**, (4) **myocardial contractility**. The treatment of low CO involves the manipulation of these four variables (see pp 109 and 171).

    1) **Heart rate**:

      a) HR should be maintained between 90–100 bpm to maximize CO. While rates of 50–80 bpm may be tolerated preoperatively without difficulty, they can be associated with postoperative arrhythmias and low output. Rate augmentation to 90–100 bpm is usually beneficial.

      b) In patients with normal conduction, atrial pacing is the procedure of choice. The optimal rate can be determined by repetitive measurements of CO at different HRs.

      c) If the patient is in heart block, AV sequential pacing may be utilized to maximize CO. An AV

TABLE 6–1.

Management Schema for the Treatment of Postoperative Cardiac Dysfunction

Mean Left Atrial Pressure (mm Hg)	Mean Systemic Pressure (mm Hg)	Cardiac Index (L/min/m²)*		
		<2.0	2.0–3.0	>3.0
≤7	Any	VE	VE	NT
8–14	<100	VE	VE	NT
	>100	VE + SNP	VE plus NP	NT
15–19	<80	VE + D, Do, or E	VE plus D, Do or E	NT
	>80	D,Do, or E + SNP or NG	NT	NT
>20	<80	D, Do, or E	D, Do or E	NT
	>80	D,Do, or E + NP or NG	NP, NG or NT	NP, NG, or NT

*VE = volume expansion;NT = no treatment if UO adequate; SNP = sodium nitroprusside; D = dopamine; Do = dobutamine; E = epinephrine; NG = nitroglycerin.

interval of 150 ms is employed in most adult patients.

  d) While not as hemodynamically beneficial as normal sinus rhythm or atrial pacing, AV sequential pacing is preferable to ventricular pacing.

  e) In patients with bradycardia and atrial flutter or fibrillation, where atrial pacing is impossible, ventricular pacing will often markedly improve CO and reduce LV filling pressures.

2) **Preload**:

  a) Most postoperative hypotension is secondary to hypovolemia.

  b) In the postoperative cardiac patient, the filling pressures are the most reliable indicators of volume status.

  c) The exact filling pressures required for adequate CO are subject to great individual variation.

  d) Knowledge of both right- and left-sided filling

pressures are essential in the treatment of post-operative patients.

e) Left-sided filling pressures are best assessed by an LA line. However, when this is not present, a PA catheter should be positioned to measure PCWP.

f) Optimizing ventricular preload is one of the primary methods of improving CO and is preferable to catecholamine administration, even in the absence of marked hypovolemia, because of its few side effects.

g) Postoperative cardiac patients usually require higher filling pressures than normal adults, secondary to either decreased ventricular compliance following operation or intrinsic myocardial dysfunction.

3) **Afterload**:

a) Cardiac function can be markedly improved by reducing impedance to LV ejection (especially in patients with impaired ventricular function). Patients following cardiac procedures are usually vasoconstricted with elevated SVR. When CO is decreased in this situation, reduction of afterload is usually of great benefit. The two major means of afterload reduction are pharmacologic agents (vasodilators) and the IABP.

b) Vasodilators fall into three major groups:

   i) Primary venodilators (nitroglycerin).

   ii) Primary arterial vasodilators (hydralazine and methyldopa).

   iii) Mixed arterial and venodilators (sodium nitroprusside [SNP] and prazosin).

c) In the postoperative period with low CO and elevated SVR or systemic hypertension, SNP is the drug of choice.

   i) SNP is preferred for its balanced vasodilating effects, rapid onset and brief duration, and ability to precisely titrate dosages.

   ii) Extreme care should be taken in employing SNP when the arterial pressure is low.

   iii) In many patients, it is necessary to administer volume with SNP to maintain preload at the desired level.

iv) If prolonged treatment with SNP is required it is important to monitor for cyanide or thiocyanate toxicity, especially in patients with renal dysfunction.

d) Some patients with impaired ventricular function will require chronic afterload reduction therapy.

4) **Myocardial contractility**:

a) While rate, rhythm, preload, and afterload can be optimized without excessive physiologic costs, the enhancement of myocardial contractility requires pharmacologic agents which increase myocardial VO_2 and energy expenditure. Thus, while the use of these drugs is often critical in the postoperative period, they should be used with caution and only after optimizing the other determinants of cardiac performance.

b) Dopamine and dobutamine are usually the first drugs employed in patients with normal cardiac rate and a normal MAP. Dopamine is more commonly used following cardiac surgery and is useful when the MAP is low.

i) Both drugs have positive inotropic effects without significant α-receptor-mediated vasoconstriction at moderate dosages (2–10 μg/kg/min).

ii) At low dosages (2–5 μg/kg/min), dopamine also causes mild vasodilation and improves renal blood flow.

iii) The chronotropic effects of dopamine may cause untoward effects and necessitate the cessation of the drug. Dobutamine has less chronotropic effect than dopamine.

c) Epinephrine:

i) This drug is helpful when there is systemic arterial hypotension because of its α-vasoconstricting effects. It is both an α-receptor and β-receptor agonist.

ii) It has both positive inotropic and chronotropic effects.

iii) It is especially useful in patients with impaired ventricular function and persistent low CO despite use of dopamine.

   d) Isoproterenol:
      i) This is a β-receptor agonist that decreases both SVR and pulmonary vascular resistance while increasing myocardial contractility.
      ii) Its positive inotropic effect is accompanied by significant chronotropic effects and an increase in myocardial irritability which limits its usefulness.
      iii) It is a helpful drug in RV failure and in patients with β-blocker toxicity.
   e) Norepinephrine:
      i) An extremely potent α-receptor and β-receptor agonist, norepinephrine produces intense vasoconstriction along with its inotropic activity. It has minimal chronotropic effect.
      ii) The significant vasoconstriction with resultant increase in afterload may decrease CO and impair peripheral perfusion.
   f) Amrinone:
      i) Amrinone represents a new class of inotropic agents, the bipyridine phosphodiesterase inhibitors. It is a direct arterial dilator, which may be more important than its weak inotropic effect in increasing cardiac performance. It is useful in patients with RV dysfunction.
      ii) It has mild positive chronotropic effects, but is less likely than dobutamine to cause tachycardia.
      iii) Side effects include GI upset, thrombocytopenia, myalgia, fever, hepatic dysfunction, and ventricular irritability.
5. **Sudden hypotension**:
   a. A precipitous fall in systemic BP must be immediately corrected in postoperative cardiac patients.
   b. Rapid assessment and treatment are mandatory.
   c. Causes of hypotension include cardiac tamponade, arrhythmia, hypovolemia, peripheral vasodilation, and ventricular dysfunction. The treatment varies according to the diagnosis (Table 6–2).

TABLE 6–2.

Causes of Sudden Hypotension Following Cardiac Surgery

Hypovolemia	Massive bleeding
	Rapid vasodilation with inadequate volume replacement
Peripheral vasodilation	Inadvertent vasodilator bolus
	Rapid rewarming
	Transfusion or drug reaction
	Steroid or morphine administration
	Fever
Ventricular dysfunction	Tamponade
	Tension pneumothorax
	Arrhythmias
	Myocardial infarction
	Hypoxemia
	Discontinuation of intropic agent
	Pacemaker malfunction

6. **Postoperative fever and infection**.
   a. Acute postoperative fever:
      1) Many patients are febrile following CPB. Fever increases the metabolic rate and causes a shift in the hemoglobin dissociation curve such that a given PaO_2 results in a lower hemoglobin saturation.
      2) In the immediate postoperative period, a variety of therapeutic interventions are useful.
         a) Acetaminophen and enteric-coated aspirin suppositories, 650–1300 mg per rectum q 3–4h. prn.
         b) Sponge baths and fans.
         c) Cooling blankets.
         d) Vigorous pulmonary toilet and ET suctioning to avoid atelectasis.
         e) When these fail, methylprednisolone 125–250 mg IV is administered.
      3) Shivering results in a dramatic increase in O_2 consumption and should be controlled with sedation (meperidine 12.5–25 mg IV) and, if necessary, pa-

ralysis with pancuronium bromide 2–4 mg IV and ventilatory support. Incremental doses of pancuronium bromide 0.01 mg/kg may be used to maintain neuromuscular blockade.

4) Pyrexia causes peripheral vasodilation and may aggravate hypovolemia and cause hypotension. Appropriate volume should be administered to maintain adequate preload.

b. Persistent postoperative fever:

1) A fever that persists for several days is worrisome.

2) Major concerns in the postoperative cardiac surgical patient include pneumonia, UTI, wound infection, and endocarditis (especially with cardiac prostheses).

3) Endocarditis in the presence of any type of cardiac prosthesis or patch implies that the prosthesis is infected. This is an extremely serious complication with a high mortality rate. The diagnosis is suggested by fever, a new murmur, and is confirmed by positive blood cultures. Echocardiography can be useful in the diagnosis of endocarditis and may show valvular insufficiency, negative or periprosthetic leak.

7. **Wound infections**:

a. Superficial or subcutaneous infections can occur either in chest or leg incisions.

1) Superficial infections involving a chest incision specifically do not involve the sternum and are manifest by serosanguinous or purulent drainage and local inflammation.

2) Treatment involves removal of overlying skin sutures, incision and drainage, culture of the drainage, local dressing changes, and antibiotics if a significant cellulitis is present.

b. Deep infections involving the sternum and mediastinum (mediastinitis) have a high mortality and should be suspected clinically in a patient with fever, especially in the presence of an unstable sternum.

1) Sternal wound drainage often occurs.

2) The CXR may reveal a sternal air stripe (separation of the sternal edges), displacement of a sternal wire (sternal dehiscence), or retrosternal air.

3) Early mediastinal reexploration with irrigation and debridement is mandatory.

4) Excellent results have been obtained with initial debridement followed by daily open dressing changes and in several days closure with placement of a pedicled muscle or omental flap to the mediastinal space. This method has produced a dramatic increase in survival from mediastinitis with up to an 80% success rate and appears to be the procedure of choice in the treatment of sternal and mediastinal infections.

5) In selected patients the sternum can be rewired and a closed irrigation of the substernal space performed for 1–3 weeks with 0.5% providone-iodine solution.

   c. Infection of the vein harvest site may occur, especially in patients with diabetes or peripheral vascular disease. Therapy includes opening of the wound, debridement, frequent dressing changes, and, occasionally, antibiotics. In some patients skin grafting may be necessary.

8. **Postpericardiotomy syndrome** is usually encountered during the second to third postoperative week and is an inflammation of the pericardium that is felt to be an autoimmune phenomenon.

   a. The syndrome is characterized by pleuritic chest pain, low-grade fever, malaise, and a pleuropericardial rub.

   b. Laboratory tests reveal leukocytosis and an elevated ESR.

   c. Treatment involves steroids (oral prednisone) and other anti-inflammatory medications (aspirin, indomethacin).

   d. It is mandatory that this syndrome be differentiated from infection before steroidal and anti-inflammatory therapy.

   e. Pericardial effusions can develop as a serious complication of postpericardiotomy syndrome and may require specific therapy.

9. **Renal failure**:

   a. Urinary output is critical in the immediate postoperative period following CPB. Patients often exhibit interstitial volume excess. Urinary output in this situation is dependent on CO, blood volume, state of hydration, and condition of the kidneys. ARF is unusual (1%–2%) follow-

      ing cardiac surgery, however, oliguria is a common find-
ing, occurring in 10%–20% of patients.

  b. Because of the interstitial and total body volume excess,
diuretics are frequently utilized in the immediate postoperative period to maintain diuresis (>100 mL/hr) and to
mobilize interstitial fluid. Careful attention to intravascular volume status is necessary to avoid overdiuresis.

  c. If oliguria occurs, CO and filling pressures should be optimized.

     1) If intravascular filling pressures are low, volume in-
fusion may be necessary to maintain urinary output,
even in the presence of total extravascular volume
excess.

     2) In patients with adequate filling pressures, improve-
ment in CO and ultimately urinary output can be
achieved by low-dose dopamine (2–3 μg/kg/min),
afterload reduction, and maintenance of an optimal
cardiac rhythm and rate.

     3) Patients with significant hypertension or renal artery
stenosis preoperatively may require a high MAP to
maintain renal function.

F. Specific Operations.

  1. Coronary artery bypass grafting.

    a. In most centers, CABG is the most common cardiotho-
racic operation performed.

     1) Approximately 250,000 CABGs are performed in
the United States per year.

     2) The principle indications are disabling angina pecto-
ris not controlled by medical therapy, left main and
triple-vessel coronary artery disease, and unstable
angina.

     3) Present mortality rates for elective CABG are <1%.

    b. The general care of a patient following CABG is dis-
cussed above. There are a few specific concerns:

     1) Perioperative MI occurs in approximately 2%–
5% of patients and can cause hypotension and cardiac conduction defects. Generally, such infarctions
are limited and do not cause serious myocardial dysfunction.

     2) Other complications include bleeding, tamponade,
hypotension, hypertension, pulmonary or renal insufficiency, and postpericardiotomy syndrome.

     3) Chest tubes are removed when drainage has de-

creased to <30 mL/hr. Most surgeons leave the chest and mediastinal tubes until the morning of the second postoperative day in patients who have had an internal mammary artery bypass graft.

4) Temporary pacing wires are placed for diagnosis and treatment and are removed on postoperative day 5 unless an electrophysiologic study is planned or the wires are needed for treatment of an arrhythmia.

5) Late complications include infections (leg wounds, sternal wounds), postpericardiotomy syndrome, thrombophlebitis, persistent leg edema.

6) The late development of chest pain or recurrent angina is ominous. An ECG, CXR, ABG, and electrolytes should be immediately obtained. Recurrent angina may be the result of graft closure and early recatheterization may be indicated.

2. **Valvular replacement**:

There has been a recent increase in attempts to perform reparative rather than ablative procedures on the cardiac valves, particularly in the mitral position.

a. Cerebral complications are more common following valve replacement.

1) This is due to several factors including an increased incidence of embolization from manipulation and debridement of the calcified and degenerative valves, and from air trapped in the LV and aorta following operation.

2) A complete neurologic examination is mandatory as soon as the patient regains consciousness.

3) In the presence of neurologic impairment, a neurology consult should be obtained and an EEG and CT scan obtained when appropriate.

b. Anticoagulation is routinely administered to all patients receiving mechanical valves and many patients with chronic atrial fibrillation.

1) The timing of the initiation of treatment varies among surgeons. Anticoagulation is usually begun soon after all pacing wires and intracardiac catheters are removed.

2) Patients are begun on sodium warfarin and the PT is carefully followed. The PT is maintained at 1.5–2.0 times control.

3) Chronic anticoagulation is not indicated in patients with tissue valves unless the patients are in chronic atrial fibrillation although some surgeons will anticoagulate these patients for 3 months.

4) Most surgeons place patients with tissue valves on enteric-coated aspirin or dipyridamole, or both.

5) The hemorrhagic complications of anticoagulation are significant and these patients need to be carefully followed on a long-term basis.

c. Hypertension following aortic valve replacement can be significant. BP should be carefully controlled to minimize potential bleeding from the aortic suture line. SNP is the drug of choice.

d. Patients with mitral valve disease present some specific challenges in their postoperative management.

1) These patients often have pulmonary hypertension and LV dysfunction preoperatively. Moreover, they usually manifest symptoms and signs of CHF.

2) After surgery, these patients may need inotropic support for several days. They usually require moderate to high filling pressures and afterload reduction to maintain optimal CO.

3) Gradual diuresis of excess extravascular volume is beneficial over the first several days.

4) Valvular dysfunction can be demonstrated by the left atrial trace or the PCWP. A large v wave is seen with residual MR.

5) The assessment of postoperative valvular function is best performed with echocardiography.

3. **Surgical treatment of arrhythmias**:

Most operations involve either the isolation or ablation of the arrhythmogenic substrate. This usually involves intraoperative epicardial or endocardial mapping of the arrhythmia.

a. All patients should have continuous ECG monitoring postoperatively and frequent ECGs.

b. Atrial and ventricular wires are placed prior to chest closure and used for both treatment and diagnosis. These are used postoperatively for diagnostic studies and should not be removed until these studies are completed and evaluated.

c. Patients undergoing procedures for ventricular tachycardia tend to be older patients with severe ischemic heart disease, LV dysfunction, and LV aneurysms. These are high-risk patients who often require prolonged inotropic support and careful hemodynamic monitoring.

d. Patients undergoing procedures for SVT are usually young and without cardiac disease. However, in patients with secondary cardiomyopathies or those having taken amiodarone preoperatively, profound myocardial depression may occur postoperatively. Amiodarone should be discontinued 6–8 weeks preoperatively. The postoperative dysfunction seen in patients on amiodarone requires-high-dose catecholamine (epinephrine) support.

II. VENTRICULAR ASSIST DEVICES.
A. Intraaortic Balloon Pumps.

1. The IABP assists the circulation directly by decreasing the afterload during systole and increasing aortic pressure during diastole thereby facilitating coronary artery perfusion (Fig 6–1). It assists the circulation indirectly by decreasing LVEDP and volume (Frank-Starling mechanism) resulting in decreased wall tension (law of Laplace) (see Fig 6–1). Both direct and indirect assistance result in decreased myocardial $\dot{V}O_2$.

2. **Indications for IABP** (Table 6–3):
   a. The major indication in the SICU is the inability to wean the patient from CPB without mechanical support.
   b. Pump failure with subsequent inadequate perfusion (CI < 1.8 L/min/m^2 in the context of maximal augmentation of preload and maximal inotropic support) is also a common indication.
   c. Use of the IABP should be considered when angina persists despite maximal therapy with nitroglycerin, β-blockade, and calcium channel blockade (unstable angina).
   d. The only absolute contraindication to IABP insertion is aortic insufficiency which is markedly exacerbated by diastolic counterpulsation.
   e. For details of the insertion technique, see Chapter 22.

3. **Technique of assistance and weaning**:
   a. Timing of the IABP should be adjusted so that deflation occurs during ejection to decrease afterload and inflation occurs during diastole to augment forward flow and especially coronary perfusion.

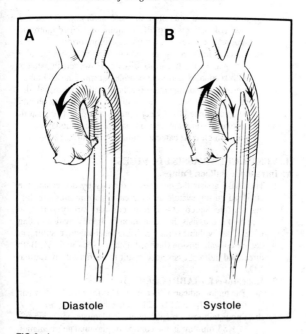

FIG 6–1.
Diagramatic representation of IABP. **A,** balloon inflated during diastole resulting in increased coronary blood flow. **B,** balloon deflated during systole (ejection) thereby reducing afterload.

    b. To optimize ventricular assistance the IABP should inflate synchronous with aortic valve closure. If the apparatus is phased with the ECG, inflation would occur during the peak of the T wave. If the apparatus is phased with central aortic pressure, inflation would be timed with the dicrotic notch. Finally, if the apparatus is phased with peripheral (radial) pressure, inflation would be timed 50 ms before the dicrotic notch (Fig 6–2).

TABLE 6–3.

Indications for IABP

Inability to wean from cardiopulmonary
  bypass
Cardiogenic shock
  Myocardial infarction
  Acute mitral regurgitation
  Acute ventricular septal defect
Myocardial ischemia
  Unstable angina
  Postinfarction angina
  Failed percutaneous coronary
    angioplasty
Bridge to cardiac transplantation

   c. To further optimize ventricular assistance and coronary
      artery perfusion, the IABP should deflate such that mean
      diastolic pressures are 10–15 mm Hg greater than the
      trough of an unaugmented diastole. Deflation is set to
      provide the maximal decrease in aortic pressure at the be-
      ginning of ejection which requires that the balloon defla-

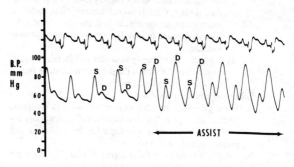

FIG 6–2.
ECG and aortic pressure tracings showing diastolic augmentation during
ventricular assist with IABP. (From Shoemaker WC, Ayres S, Grenvik A:
Textbook of Critical Care Medicine. Philadelphia, WB Saunders Co, 1989,
p. 421).

tion begin before the R wave and be completed prior to the onset of ejection (see Fig 6–2).

d. Manipulations of the apparatus (inflation, deflation) are performed with the balloon at half-volume and the mode set at 1:2 (one inflation per two cardiac cycles).

e. Once the optimal timing has been determined, the balloon volume may be fully inflated and the mode increased to 1:1.

f. Since the onset of both deflation and inflation occur at points in time predicted on the basis of data obtained from previous cardiac cycles, historical timing requires a stable cardiac rhythm. Thus, accurate timing is frequently difficult during dysrhythmias.

   1) During a chaotic rhythm, counterpulsation may cease owing to fail-safe mechanisms which prevent balloon inflation during ejection.

   2) Recent work demonstates clearly the superiority of controlling the IABP using real-time analysis of electromechanical data. With deflation triggered by the R wave, timing of the IABP for each cardiac cycle is set by events in that cycle. This method is virtually unaffected by cardiac dysrhythmias. Although deflation occurs slightly later than with standard timing, there is no deleterious effect on SV or mean ejection pressure. In fact, the slightly later deflation appears to provide superior hemodynamic function.

   3) Virtually, all currently available IABPs utilize "real-time control" either as the primary time mode or as a selective option for arrhythmias.

4. **Failure of counterpulsation**:

a. Since constant, accurate counterpulsation is essential, particularly in the "balloon-dependent" patient, any interruption in pumping must quickly be evaluated and proper pump function restored.

b. Loss of an adequate ECG signal is probably the most common cause of interrupted IABP function.

   1) This may be rectified by switching to a different ECG lead with a better signal-noise ratio, by replacement of the adhesive ECG pads on the patient, eliminating causes of electrical interference in the ECG

signal, or by changing the timing mode to trigger the IABP from the arterial pressure waveform.

   2) Interference due to AV sequential pacing generally may be avoided by keeping the atrial pacing signal as low as possible.

   3) Conversion to timing by aortic pressure may be necessary.

c. A poor pressure tracing from the arterial line may also result in interruption of IABP function. Flushing or repositioning the catheter may result in an improved waveform and allow appropriate timing. If the waveform remains inadequate it may be necessary to switch to the ECG for timing.

d. Adequate gas flow to the balloon must be maintained.

   1) The supply tank must be replaced when its volume is low, and kinks in the tubing must be avoided.

   2) A leak in the balloon may develop during counter pulsation, but more commonly results from a tear during insertion.

   3) Excessive loss of gas may require removal of the balloon, followed by replacement with another, if necessary.

e. If no specific problem can be identified it is often helpful to exchange the balloon pump for another.

f. Cardiogenic shock with very low CO may not improve with IABP and no effect of the counterpulsation will be seen.

5. **Weaning from IABP support**:

a. Guidelines for weaning or continuation of assistance in the postoperative patient include CI, urinary output, ABG, PCWP, and need for inotropic agents.

b. Weaning is attempted when these parameters indicate an improvement in ventricular function and inotropic agents have been discontinued or the dosages significantly reduced. Sequential reductions of the assistance mode are made over a 6–12-hour period. When little hemodynamic deterioration occurs in the 1:3 mode, assistance may be discontinued. Coagulation studies and the platelet count should be normal (see chapter 22 for removal technique).

6. **Complications of IABP**:

a. The incidence of complications ranges from 10%–30%.

b. The most frequent complication is ipsilateral limb ischemia. Limb perfusion can frequently be reestablished by simple manipulation of the sheath. If the limb remains severely ischemic it may be necessary to remove the IABP and choose an alternative insertion site.

c. Thrombocytopenia secondary to platelet consumption may be seen and resolves following balloon removal. Platelet transfusion may be necessary prior to removal of the IABP.

d. Infection at the insertion site may occur. Although prophylactic systemic antibiotics are not recommended, they are frequently used to prevent bacteremia. Infection may occur locally at the insertion site or systemically owing to the balloon catheter traversing the skin to enter the bloodstream. Meticulous attention to sterile technique during insertion and dressing changes is mandatory.

e. Localized dissection of the artery and emboli are less common. They have been linked to the development of mesenteric, renal, and spinal cord ischemia, as well as CVAs. Insertion of the balloon under fluoroscopic guidance may prevent injury to the intima by the balloon catheter.

f. Hematoma formation or retroperitoneal hemorrhage occasionally occurs and requires surgical intervention.

g. The formation of a pseudoaneurysm at the arteriotomy site following removal requires surgical correction.

B. Other Ventricular Assist Devices.

1. Introduction.

a. There are some circumstances of pump failure where the IABP is unable to adequately augment the circulation. In these situations more invasive extracorporeal or implantable ventricular assist devices (VADs) are sometimes employed.

b. VADs divert the patient's circulation so as to completely unload the ventricle (blood is removed from the atrium or directly from the injured ventricle and reperfused into the aorta or PA).

c. Their use of results in reduction of ventricular work and $\dot{V}O_2$, augmentation of the effective CO, and a complete phase shifting of the peak arterial pressure contour into diastole, facilitating coronary artery perfusion. Myocardial $\dot{V}O_2$ is markedly decreased owing to the reduction in ventricular volumes and pressures as well as a reduction in chamber diameter and wall tension.

      d. Assist devices are broadly categorized as either centrifugal or pulsatile pumps. They may be used as either a bridge to tranplantation or as temporizing measures to allow a "stunned" ventricle to recover from an ischemic insult. The choice of support system is made intraoperatively.

2. Centrifugal pumps:
   Centrifugal pumps (e.g., Bio-medicus) are by far the most common assist devices and may be utilized for either univentricular or biventricular support.

      a. They are readily available, inexpensive, and relatively simple to use. However, they do require manual operation (a perfusionist).

      b. To prevent potential thromboembolic complications, it is recommended that these patients be anticoagulated (ACT two times control) which may lead to significant bleeding and associated complications

3. Pulsatile pumps:

      a. These devices require systemic anticoagulation. However, owing to pulsatile flow, the risk of thromboembolism may be less. These devices are more expensive, require considerable training to use, and are not readily available. They are, however, automatically controlled and very durable. There is a significant risk of infection. Nevertheless, the pulsatile pumps, may be used for longer-term support than the centrifugal devices, permitting time for a heart allograft to become available.

      b. One pulsatile pump warrants particular mention—the Anstadt cup. This experimental device supports the circulation by direct mechanical ventricular actuation. Since it is applied to the epicardial surface, there is no blood–foreign body interface and anticoagulation is not required. This VAD is simple to use and generates physiologic flow.

4. Contraindications to ventricular assist:
   A flaccid noncontractile ventricle, prolonged CPR, uncontrolled bleeding, and pulmonary hemorrhage are all relative contraindications to VAD insertion. Increased use of the Anstadt cup may change some of these criteria from absolute to relative.

5. Weaning from ventricular assist:

      a. As described with the IABP, a variety of parameters are evaluated to determine if and when circulatory support may be discontinued. Additional studies may be indicated in the case of the VAD. These include evaluation of ventricular function by transesophageal echocardiography and nuclear scanning (MUGA). These devices, if shown to be redundant, (i.e., ventricular recovery) are removed in the OR under sterile precautions.

b. There remains further experimental research and more clinical trials before extra- or intracorporeal circulatory assist devices become commonplace. At present, patient selection is an extremely important determinant of outcome. The patient should have either a salvageable ventricle or be a good transplant candidate (no other organ failure).

SELECTED REFERENCES

Behrendt DM, Austin WG: *Patient Care in Cardiac Surgery,* ed 4. Boston, Little, Brown & Co, 1985.

Borkon AM, Schaff HV, Gardner TJ, et al: Diagnosis and management of postoperative pericardial effusions and late cardiac tamponade following open heart surgery. *Ann Thorac Surg* 1980; 31:512.

Davdon P, Corcos T, Gandjbakhch I, et al: Prevention of atrial fibrillation or flutter by acebutolol after coronary bypass grafting. *Am J Cardiol* 1986; 58:933.

Gailiunas P Jr, Chawlar R, Lazarus JM, et al: Acute renal failure following cardiac operations. *J Thorac Cardiovasc Surg* 1980; 79:241.

Jurkiewicz MJ, Bostwick J, Hester TR, et al: Infected median sternotomy wound: Successful treatment by muscle flaps. *Ann Surg* 1990; 191:738.

Litwalk RS, Jurado RT: *Care of the Cardiac Surgical Patient.* Norwalk, Conn, Appleton-Century-Crofts, 1982.

Mills NL: Postoperative hemorrhage after cardiopulmonary bypass. *Ann Thorac Surg* 1982; 34:607.

Sabiston DC. *Textbook of Surgery,* ed 13. Philadelphia, WB Saunders Co, 1986.

Silverman NA, Wright R, Levitsky S: Efficacy of low-dose propranolol in preventing postoperative supraventricular tachycardia. *Ann Surg* 1982; 196:194.

THE PULMONARY SYSTEM 7

I. PULMONARY PHYSIOLOGY.

A. Ventilation.

1. *Ventilation* is the movement of air in and out of the lungs.

2. **Airway anatomy:** The airway is divided into conducting airways and the respiratory zone.

   a. Conducting airways (Fig 7–1).

      1) The conducting airways consist of the trachea, bronchi, lobar and segmental bronchi.

      2) Terminal bronchioles are the smallest airways without alveoli.

      3) The conducting airways do not take part in gas exchange and represent the anatomic dead space.

   b. Respiratory zone (see Fig 7–1).

      1) The respiratory zone consists of the airways distal to the terminal bronchiole, lined by alveoli, which take part in gas exchange (called an acinus or lobule).

      2) The respiratory zone is composed of respiratory bronchioles, alveolar ducts, and alveolar sacs.

      3) Normally there are approximately 300 million alveoli (0.5 mm diameter). The alveolar surface area for diffusion is 50-100 m^2 and the diffusion barrier between blood and gas is very thin (0.5 μm), (Fig 7-2).

      4) Surfactant is a substance secreted by Type II alveolar cells that contain dipalmitoyl phosphatidylcholine. Surfactant lines the alveolar suface and reduces the surface tension thus increasing compliance of the lung and decreasing the work

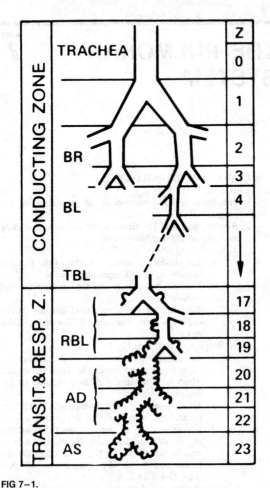

FIG 7–1.
Schematic diagram of airway. *BR* = bronchus; *BL* bronchiole; *TBL* = terminal bronchiole; *RBL* = respiratory bronchiole; AD = alveolar duct; AS = alveolar sac. (From Weibul ER: *Morphology of the Human Lung.* Berlin, Springer-Verlag, 1963, p 1i1. Used by permission.)

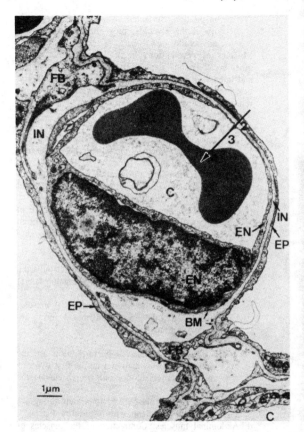

FIG 7–2.
Electron micrograph showing blood-gas diffusion barrier. The *large arrow* denotes the path for diffusion of gas from the alveolus. C = pulmonary capillarys; EC = erythrocyte; EP = alveolar epithelium; IN = interstitium; EN = capillary endothelium; FB = fibroblast; BM = basement membrane (From Weibul ER: *Respir Physiol* 1970; 11:54. Used by permission.)

inspiration. Surfactant also increases the stability of the alveolus, preventing atelectasis and airway closure.

3. **Muscles of respiration:** Inspiration is active during quiet breathing and depends mainly on the diaphragm and intercostal muscles. During quiet breathing, expiration is passive. Deflation occurs as lung and chest wall return to resting position by elastic recoil.

   a. Diaphragm:
      1) The diaphragm originates from the lower ribs, separating the thoracic and abdominal viscera, and is innervated by the phrenic nerve (cervical roots 3, 4, and 5).
      2) Contraction during inspiration forces the abdominal contents downward increasing the vertical dimension of the thoracic cavity.
      3) If the diaphragm is paralyzed, the decrease in intrathoracic pressure with inspiration results in a paradoxical upward movement of the diaphragm.

   b. Intercostal muscles:
      1) Contraction of the external intercostal pulls the ribs upward and outward increasing the lateral and AP dimensions of the chest.
      2) Contraction of the internal intercostal muscles pulls the ribs downward and inward during active expiration.

   c. Accessory muscles:
      1) The accessory muscles of inspiration are the scalene muscles which elevate the first two ribs and the sternocleidomastoids which elevate the sternum.
      2) The accessory muscles are important during exercise and in patients with respiratory distress.

   d. Abdominal muscles: Contraction of the muscles of the abdominal wall increases the intraabdominal pressure pushing the diaphragm upward. The abdominal muscles contribute to active expiration and cough.

4. **Lung volumes** (Fig 7–3):
   a. *Tidal volume* (TV) is the volume of air inspired during normal inspiration following a normal expiration.

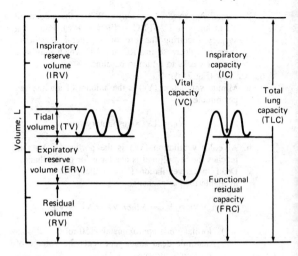

FIG 7–3.
The subdivisions of lung volumes.

 b. *Inspiratory reserve volume* (IRV) is the volume of air representing the difference between maximal inspiration and the peak inspiratory TV.

 c. *Expiratory reserve volume* (ERV) is the volume of air representing the difference between maximal expiration and the end expiratory TV.

 d. *Residual volume* (RV) is the volume of air remaining in lung after maximal expiration.

5. **Lung capacities** (Fig 7–3):

 a. *Total lung capacity* (TLC) is the amount of air in the lungs after maximal inspiration (TLC = RV + ERV +TV + IRV).

 b. *Vital capacity* (VC) is the amount of air expired from maximal inspiration to maximal expiration (VC = IRV + TV + ERV).

 c. *Inspiratory capacity* (IC) is the amount of air inspired from end expiratory TV point to maximal inspiration (IC = IRV + the end expiratory TV point).

    d. *Functional residual capacity* (FRC) is the amount of air in lungs at TV (FRC = ERV + RV). Following surgery requiring the use of a general anesthetic, there is a decrease in FRC and VC which may take days or weeks to return to baseline.

6. Air flow (Fig 7–4):
    a. Minute ventilation ($\dot{V}_E$) is the amount of air inspired per minute.

$$\dot{V}_E = TV \times \text{respiratory rate}$$

    b. Alveolar ventilation ($\dot{V}_A$) is the portion of $\dot{V}_E$ that reaches the alveoli and is available for gas exchange.
    c. Dead space ventilation (V_D) is the part of $\dot{V}_E$ not available for gas exchange.

$$\dot{V}_E = \dot{V}_A + V_D \ or \ \dot{V}_A = \dot{V}_E - V_D$$

    1) Normal V_D is approximately 150 mL.
    2) Anatomic dead space represents the volume of conducting airways.
    3) Physiologic (or alveolar) dead space represents the volume of alveoli which do not take part in gas exchange (ventilated but not perfused).

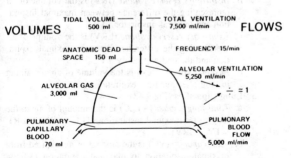

FIG 7–4.
Diagram of a lung showing typical volumes and flows (From West JB: *Respiratory Physiology—the Essentials*, ed 3, Baltimore, Williams & Wilkins Co, 1985. Used by permission.)

7. Distribution of ventilation.
   a. Gravity is responsible for the normal distribution of ventilation. The most dependent portion receives the greatest ventilation.
      1) In the upright position the ventilation to the base of the lung is greater than to the apex.
      2) In the supine position the posterior (dependent) portion receives more ventilation than the anterior (superior) portion.
   b. The distribution of ventilation is altered by changes in lung volume.
      1) With inhalation from a lung volume >FRC, distribution is normal.
      2) When inhalation begins at a lung volume < FRC, ventilation is preferentially distributed to the apex.
   c. Airway closure:
      1) Airway closure refers to collapse of small airways during expiration at low lung volumes (approaching RV) trapping gas in distal alveoli.
      2) In young patients airway closure occurs only at very low lung volumes (<FRC).
      3) The volume at which airway closure occurs *(closing volume [CV])* increases with age owing to loss of elastic recoil.
      4) Alveoli distal to "closed airways" which are perfused but only intermittently ventilated create a ventilation-perfusion mismatch resulting in hypoxemia
      5) Loss of surfactant increases alveolar instability, thus potentiating airway closure.
   d. Lung diseases affecting distribution of ventilation:
      1) Localized: bullae, cysts, bronchiectasis, fibrosis.
      2) Generalized: emphysema (decreased basal ventilation).
8. Lung compliance (Fig 7–5).
   a. *Compliance (C)* refers to lung expansibility and is defined as the volume (V) change per unit pressure (P):

$$C = \frac{\Delta V}{\Delta P}$$

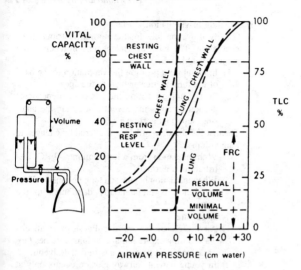

FIG 7-5.
Relaxation pressure-volume curve of the lung and chest wall. The subject inspires (or expires) to a certain volume from the spirometer, the top is closed, and he then relaxes his chest. The curve for lung and chest wall can be explained by the additions of the individual lung and chest wall curves. (From West JB: *Respiratory Physiology—the Essentials,* ed 3. Baltimore, Williams & Wilkins Co, 1985. Used by permission.)

1) Normally the lung is very compliant implying that a large change in volume results in only a small change in pressure. At large lung volumes the lung becomes less compliant or stiffer.
2) The lung is elastic and tends to collapse while the chest wall tends to expand outward. The chest wall is pulled inward by the elastic recoil of the lung and the lung is pulled outward by the chest wall.
3) FRC is the lung volume at which these two opposing forces are in equilibrium.

b. Total compliance (CT) reflects the combined compliances of the lung (CL) and chest wall (Ccw).

$$1/C_T = 1/C_L + 1/C_{cw}$$

c. Dynamic compliance (Cdyn) is compliance during movement of air:

$$Cdyn = TV/\text{peak transpulmonary pressure}$$

d. Static compliance (Cstat) is compliance at end inspiration when there is no air flow.

$$Cstat = TV/\text{plateau pressure} = 1/\text{elastic recoil}$$

    1) Cstat measures the elastic recoil properties of the lung.
    2) The plateau pressure is the transpulmonary pressure measured at end inspiration.
e. Disease states affecting compliance:
    1) Emphysema increases compliance.
    2) Fibrosis decreases compliance.
    3) Increasing age increases compliance.

9. Airway resistance:
    a. Airway resistance is the pressure difference between the mouth and the alveoli divided by the flow rate.
    b. The resistance to flow is dependent on the length and especially the radius of the airway.
    c. Although the peripheral airways are narrow, because of branching they are numerous and the total cross-sectional area is large (Fig 7–6).
    d. Most of the pressure drop occurs at the level of the medium-sized bronchioles.

10. Work of breathing may be divided into three components: compliance work, tissue resistance work, and airway resistance work. The work of breathing normally accounts for 2%–3% of total energy expenditure but it may increase significantly in disease states (up to 30%).

11. Respiratory quotient (RQ):
    a. RQ is the ratio of CO_2 produced ($\dot{V}CO_2$) to O_2 uptake ($\dot{V}O_2$),

$$RQ = \dot{V}CO_2/\dot{V}O_2$$

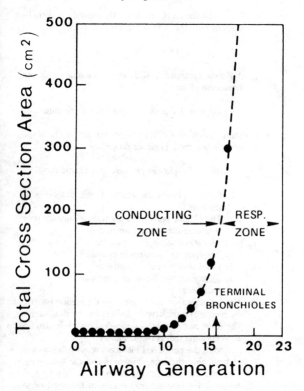

FIG 7-6.
Diagram showing the rapid increase in total cross-sectional area of the airways. (From West JB: *Respiratory Physiology—the Essentials,* ed 3. Baltimore, Williams & Wilkins Co, 1985. Used by permission.)

    b. Normally $\dot{V}CO_2$ is approximately 200 mL/min and $\dot{V}O_2$ is approximately 250 mL/min resulting in an RQ of 0.8.

    c. A high carbohydrate diet may increase $\dot{V}CO_2$ and elevate RQ to 1.0

B. Pulmonary Perfusion.
  1. Anatomic considerations.
     a. Pulmonary circulation:
        1) The pulmonary vascular bed receives the entire CO (5 L/min) at a very low pressure (mean = 15 mm Hg).
        2) A dense network of capillaries surrounds the alveoli increasing the surface area available for gas exchange (50–100 m^2).
     b. Bronchial circulation:
        1) The bronchial arteries arise from the aorta and supply the larger airways.
        2) Desaturated bronchial blood returns to the heart through the pulmonary veins and forms a natural shunt accounting for 1%–2% of total CO.
  2. Distribution of pulmonary perfusion:
     a. Blood flow to the alveoli increases linearly from apex to base and is determined by hydrostatic pressure differences within the lung.
     b. Four physiologic zones describe the distribution of blood flow based on the alveolar (PA), arterial (Pa) and venous (Pv) pressure (Fig 7–7).
        1) Zone 1: PA > Pa > Pv. PA > Pa, collapsing the capillaries. Zone 1 is not perfused. Under normal conditions the PA pressure is great enough so that no zone 1 exists.
        2) Zone 2: Pa > PA > Pv.
           a) Blood flow to the alveoli is determined by the difference between Pa and PA. Pv does not affect flow.
           b) As arterial pressure increases down zone 2, blood flow to the alveoli also increases. This process is known as *recruitment*.
           c) Blood flow in zone 2 varies as PA varies during the respiratory cycle.
        3) Zone 3: Pa > Pv > PA.
           a) Pv >PA and blood flow is determined by the arteriovenous pressure difference.
           b) Blood flow to the alveoli occurs throughout the respiratory cycle in zone 3.
        4) Zone 4: Low lung volume (<FRC): Low lung volumes with atelectasis result in a decrease in

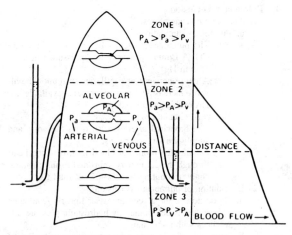

FIG 7–7.
Diagram showing the uneven distribution of blood flow in the lung based on the pressures affecting the capillaries. (From West JB, et al: *J Appl Physiol* 1964; 19:713. Used by permission.)

blood flow at the bases due to increased vascular resistance which is secondary to collapse of extraalveolar vessels which are normally held open by expanded lung parenchyma.

5) In the upright patient zone 1 is at the apex and zone 3 is at the base. In a supine patient, zone 1 is anterior and zone 2 is posterior.

3. Factors influencing distribution of perfusion.
   a. Supine position and exercise increase apical flow without decreasing basilar flow.
   b. Lung volume:
      1) At volumes >FRC, distribution is normal.
      2) At volumes <FRC, distribution is more uniform.
      3) At volumes near RV, there is reversal of distribution with apex > base.
   c. Alveolar hypoxia (PO_2 < 70 mm Hg) causes pulmo-

nary vasoconstriction and increases pulmonary vascular resistance. This causes a more uniform distribution of blood flow.

   d. Acidosis also causes pulmonary vasoconstriction thereby increasing pulmonary vascular resistance and redistribution of blood flow.

   e. Increasing age causes a more uniform distribution of blood flow.

4. Disease states altering pulmonary blood flow.

   a. Localized lung disease (pulmonary emboli, bullae, cysts, bronchiectasis, carcinoma) may alter blood flow.

   b. Generalized disease (pulmonary hypertension, emphysema) results in a loss of the normal blood flow pattern with more uniform distribution usually seen.

5. Pulmonary water balance:

   a. Fluid balance across the capillary and alveolar membrane is determined by the Starling forces of capillary hydrostatic pressure (Pc), interstitial hydrostatic pressure (Pi), capillary osmotic pressure (Πc), and interstitial osmotic pressure (Πi).

   b. Pc $-$ Pi represents the force driving fluid out of the capillary while Πc $-$ Πi represents the force driving fluid into the capillary.

   c. The ability of the capillary membrane to prevent the passage of plasma protein is important in maintaining Πc. In certain disease states (ARDS), the membrane is compromised and a "leak" of plasma protein into the interstitium can occur.

   d. Normally there is a small net flux of fluid out of the capillary which is drained by lymphatics.

   e. In patients with elevated pulmonary capillary pressure this flux of fluid may greatly increase. When the capacity of the pulmonary lymphatics is exceeded, pulmonary edema results.

   f. Initially, there is only interstitial edema. In the late stages of pulmonary edema the alveoli fill with fluid and oxygenation of blood is significantly impaired.

C. **Matching of Ventilation and Perfusion.**

Gas exchange is dependent upon the ratio of ventilation ($\dot{V}$) to perfusion (Q) in each alveolar unit.

1. Normal $\dot{V}/Q$ matching.
   a. Usually the distribution of ventilation closely parallels perfusion.
   b. The concentration of gases in the blood leaving the alveolus reflects the partial pressure of gases within the alveolus and is primarily determined by $\dot{V}/Q$.
2. $\dot{V}/Q$ mismatch.
   a. $\dot{V}/Q$ mismatch is the most common cause of hypoxemia (decreased PaO_2). $\dot{V}/Q$ mismatch affects O_2 exchange to a greater degree than CO_2 exchange.
   b. Variations in $\dot{V}/Q$ (Fig 7–8):
      1) A $\dot{V}/Q$ of 0 implies alveolar units are perfused but not ventilated; therefore no gas exchange can occur. If alveoli are not ventilated, the concentration of O_2 and CO_2 in the alveolus is equal to the concentration in venous blood (normally $PO_2 = 40$ mm Hg, $PCO_2 = 45$ mm Hg).
      2) $\dot{V}/Q < 1$ implies ventilation is less than perfusion and limited gas exchange does occur. The concentrations of O_2 and CO_2 in the alveolus is

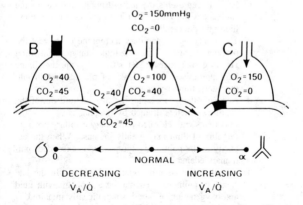

FIG 7–8.
Effect of altering the $\dot{V}/Q$ on PO_2 and PCO_2 in a lung unit. (From West JB: *Ventilation/Blood Flow and Gas Exchange*, ed 3. Oxford, England, Blackwell Scientific Publications, Inc, 1977. Used by permission.)

between those of mixed venous blood and those of normal arterial blood (PO_2 40–100 mm Hg, PCO_2 = 40–45 mm Hg).

3) $\dot{V}/Q$ of 1 implies that ventilation and perfusion are well matched and normal gas exchange may occur. The concentration of O_2 and CO_2 in the alveolus is normal (PO_2 = 100 mm Hg, PCO_2 = 40).

4) $\dot{V}/Q$ >1 implies ventilation exceeds perfusion; only a fraction of ventilated gas can take part in gas exchange.

    a) The concentration of O_2 and CO_2 in the alveolus is between normal arterial concentration and that of inspired gas (PO_2 = 100–150 mm Hg, PCO_2 = 0–40 mm Hg).

    b) The fraction of ventilation that does not take part in gas exchange is part of the physiologic dead space.

5) A $\dot{V}/Q$ of infinity implies that alveolar units are ventilated but not perfused; no gas exchange can occur.

    a) The concentration of O_2 and CO_2 in the alveolus is that of inspired air (PO_2 = 150 mm Hg, PCO_2 = 0 mm Hg).

    b) These alveolar units also represent physiologic dead space or wasted ventilation.

3. Shunt.
  a. Definition:

1) *Shunt* refers to mixed venous blood that enters the arterial circulation without undergoing gas exchange. Venous admixture refers to a mixture of venous and arterial blood.

2) Under normal conditions, 1%–2% of CO is shunted via the bronchial circulation.

3) Anatomic shunting usually occurs as a result of a congenital cardiac defect resulting in a right-to-left shunt.

4) Physiologic shunting refers to blood that passes through the pulmonary circulation without undergoing gas exchange.

  b. Shunt fraction:

1) Shunt fraction is the ratio of blood flow through the shunt (Qs) to the total blood flow (Qt) (p 63).

$$Qs/Qt = \text{shunt fraction} = (CcO_2 - CaO_2)/(CcO_2 - C\overline{v}O_2)$$

where CcO_2 is the O_2 content of pulmonary capillary blood, CaO_2 is the O_2 content of arterial blood, and $C\overline{v}O_2$ is the oxygen content of mixed venous blood.

2) CcO_2 cannot be measured directly but can be estimated from a blood specimen obtained from a PA catheter.

c. Shunts cause a decrease in arterial O_2 concentration with little change in CO_2. This decrease cannot be completely corrected by ventilation with 100% O_2.

4. CO_2 removal and $\dot{V}/Q$ mismatch:
   a. Decreased CO_2 removal results from a decreased $\dot{V}E$ or an increased VD.
   b. Increased VD is most commonly caused by an elevated $\dot{V}/Q$. If VE does not increase to compensate for the wasted alveolar ventilation, PCO_2 will rise. When VE increases in appropriately, PCO_2 returns to normal.

D. Oxygen and Carbon Dioxide Diffusion and Transport.

1. Normal tensions (mm Hg):
   a. Inspired air (Pi): $O_2 = 150$, $CO_2 = 0$.
   b. Alveoli (PA): $O_2 = 100$, $CO_2 = 40$.
   c. Mixed venous blood (P$\overline{v}$): $O_2 = 40$, $CO_2 = 45$.
   d. Arterial blood (Pa): $O_2 = 80 - 100$, $CO_2 = 40$.
   e. Mitochondria (Pm): $O_2 = 1$.

2. Pulmonary gas transfer:
   a. Gases move across the alveolar-capillary barrier by passive diffusion driven by concentration gradients.
   b. Fick's law states that the rate of gas transfer (V gas) is proportional to the tissue area (A) and the difference in partial pressures ($P_1 - P_2$) and inversely proportional to the thickness of the diffusion barrier (T).

$$V \text{ gas} = (A/T)k(P_1 - P_2)$$

where k is proportional to (solubility/molecular weight$^{1/2}$), $A = 50-100$ m^2, and $T = 0.5$ μm.

1) CO_2 diffuses 20 times faster than O_2 owing to its increased solubility.

2) O_2 diffusion is decreased if PaO_2 is decreased (high altitude), alveolar wall thickness is increased (pulmonary edema), or RBC transit time is decreased (exercise).

3) There are enormous diffusion reserves under normal conditions. The large $PaO_2 - P\overline{v}O_2$ gradient favors rapid O_2 diffusion while increased solubility favors CO_2 diffusion. Gas equilibrium occurs well before the end of the 0.75-second capillary transit time.

  c. Diffusing capacity DLCO.

1) DLCO is usually measured by the single-breath carbon monoxide (CO) test.

$$DLCO = VCO/(P_ACO - P_CCO)$$

where DLCO is the diffusing capacity of CO (in mL/min/mm Hg), VCO is the rate of CO transfer (mL/min), P_ACO is the alveolar partial pressure of CO (mm Hg), and P_CCO is the capillary partial pressure of CO (negligible). The normal value for D is 20–25 mL/min/mm Hg.

3. Lung O_2 transfer.

  a. The alveolar air equation allows estimation of P_AO_2 and gives an indication of what PaO_2 should be if lungs are functioning normally.

$$P_AO_2 = PiO_2 - (P_ACO_2/R) + [F]$$
$$P_AO_2 = F_IO_2 (PB - 47) - (PaCO_2/R)$$

where PB is atmospheric pressure, 47 is the correction for water vapor pressure at sea level, F_IO_2 is the fraction of inspired O_2, P_ACO_2 may be estimated by $PaCO_2$, R is the respiratory quotient, and F is a correction factor which is small if room air is breathed and may be ignored. This calculation is most accurate at room air ($F_IO_2 = 0.21$) and is age-independent.

  b. Arterial O_2 concentration.

1) PaO_2 reflects P_AO_2 and the overall $\dot{V}/Q$ and is measured directly from ABGs.

2) PaO_2 is age-dependent and may be estimated as $PaO_2 = 109 - 0.43$ (age in years). This de-

crease results from age-dependent changes in $\dot{V}/Q$.

   3) Causes of decreased PaO_2 include $\dot{V}/Q$ mismatch, shunt, hypoventilation, and a decreased DLCO (increased diffusion barrier).

  c. The alveolar-arterial O_2 pressure difference $P(A-a)O_2$ is the difference between calculated PAO_2 and measured PaO_2.

   1) An increase in $P(A-a)O_2$ represents an abnormality in O_2 transfer.

   2) The normal range of values is 10–20 mm Hg, and >25 is considered abnormal

   3) Respiratory causes of an increased $P(A-a)O_2$ include diffusion barrier, right-to-left intrapulmonary shunt, and $\dot{V}/Q$ mismatch. Nonrespiratory causes are right-to-left intracardiac shunts and hyperthermia.

   4) A decreased PaO_2 with normal $P(A-a)O_2$ is seen with high altitude, decreased R, and central hypoventilation.

4. The hemoglobin-O_2 dissociation curve.

  a. O_2 in the blood may be dissolved in solution or bound to hemoglobin in a reversible fashion. Most O_2 is bound to hemoglobin.

  b. Each hemoglobin molecule may bind up to four O_2 molecules and the affinity of hemoglobin for O_2 is affected by a variety of factors including the amount of O_2 already bound to the molecule, temperature, pH, PCO_2, and the concentration of diphosphoglyerol (2, 3-DPG).

  c. The hemoglobin-O_2 dissociation curve is sigmoid (Fig 7–9).

   1) The greatest affinity for O_2 occurs when O_2 concentration is high, and the hemoglobin molecule has already bound three molecules of O_2. Thus the high concentration of O_2 present in the lung facilitates the saturation of all binding sites on the hemoglobin molecule.

   2) The affinity of hemoglobin for oxygen is decreased with lower O_2 concentration, thus facilitating O_2 release in the peripheral tissues.

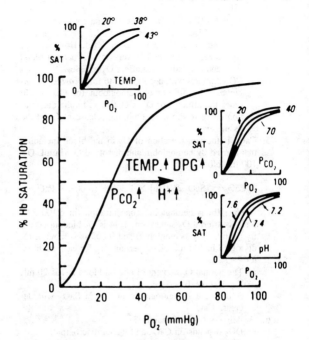

FIG 7-9.
The hemoglobin-O_2 association-dissociation curve. Note the sigmoid shape of the curve, and the shift of the curve by pH, PCO_2, temperature, and 2,3-DPG. (From West JB: *Respiratory Physiology—the Essentials,* ed 3. Baltimore, Williams & Wilkins Co, 1985. Used by permission.)

        d. The affinity is altered by local conditions (see Fig 7-9).
            1) A fall in pH, rise in PCO_2 or increased temperature, as occurs at the tissue level, will shift the curve to the right facilitating the unloading of O_2.
            2) A rise in pH, fall in PCO_2, or decreased temperature, as occurs in the lung will shift the curve to the left, increasing binding of O_2.

3) 2,3-DPG is formed during anaerobic glycolysis in RBCs. The presence of 2,3-DPG facilitates release of O_2 at the tissue level. However, the level of 2,3-DPG is very low in banked blood and may adversely affect O_2 release.

e. CO combines with hemoglobin to form *carboxyhemoglobin*. The affinity of hemoglobin for CO is 240 times the affinity for O_2. CO also shifts the dissociation curve to the left, inhibiting release of O_2 at the tissue level.

5. CaO_2 is the concentration of O_2 in the blood including that carried by hemoglobin and dissolved O_2 (in mL O_2/100 mL blood).

$$CaO_2 = (SaO_2 \times [Hb] \times 1.34) + (0.003 \times PaO_2)$$

where [Hb] is hemoglobin concentration (in g/100 ml), SaO_2 is arterial O_2 saturation, 1.34 is O_2 binding capacity (in mL O_2/g hemoglobin) and 0.003 is volume of O_2 dissolved in 100 mL blood per mm Hg for each millimeter PaO_2.

a. The normal O_2 content of arterial blood is 16–20 mL O_2/100 mL blood.

b. A decrease in hemoglobin or fall in SaO_2 will decrease CaO_2.

6. O_2 delivery (DO_2) (Chapter 3).

a. DO_2 depends on CaO_2 and the cardiac output:

$$DO_2 \text{ (mL/min)} = \text{cardiac output (L/min)} \times CaO_2 \times 10$$

1) Normal DO_2 is 800–1,000 mL/min.
2) Normal ($\dot{V}O_2$) is 250 mL/min.

b. Inadequate DO_2 can occur despite a normal CaO_2 secondary to decreased cardiac output.

7. CO_2 transport and elimination.

a. CO_2 transport:

1) CO_2 is the waste product of aerobic metabolism. The normal CO_2 production is approximately 200 mL/min.

2) The majority of CO_2 in arterial blood (90%) is carried as bicarbonate:

$$CO_2 + H_2O \rightarrow H_2CO_3 \rightarrow H^+ + HCO_3^-$$

    3) CO_2 binds to hemoglobin (carbaminohemoglobin) and is also dissolved in the blood. These forms are important for CO_2 transport.

  b. CO_2 Elimination:

    1) CO_2 is eliminated only by ventilation.

    2) All expired CO_2 comes from alveolar gas where $PACO_2$ approximates $PaCO_2$.

    3) A diffusion gradient exists between venous blood ($PvCO_2 = 45$) and alveolar gas ($PACO_2 = 40$). As $PvCO_2$ decreases, CO_2 stored as bicarbonate becomes available.

$$HCO_3^- + H^+ \rightarrow H_2CO_3 \rightarrow H_2O + CO_2$$

  c. $PaCO_2$ is a direct measure of $\dot{V}A$ and reflects the balance between CO_2 production in the tissues and CO_2 elimination in the lungs.

II. PULMONARY EVALUATION.

A. History and Physical Examination.

  1. History:

    a. Risk factors and environmental exposure associated with pulmonary disease including smoking history.

    b. Past medical history of chronic pulmonary disease including previous and current medications and allergies.

    c. Exercise tolerance and severity of debilitation secondary to pulmonary diseases.

    d. Surgical history of thoracic procedures, previous difficulties with intubation, and history of pulmonary embolism (PE) or pulmonary insufficiency.

  2. Physical examination:

    a. The surface anatomy examination must assess body habitus, thoracic deformities, degenerative spinal disease, symmetry of chest wall expansion, and use of accessory muscles for breathing.

    b. The auscultatory examination assesses air movement airway secretion (rhonchi), airway constriction (wheezing), pleural scarring (pleural rubs), pulmonary edema (rales), and areas of hypoventilation.

B. **Chest Radiograph.**
   1. The CXR allows assessment of chronic and acute pathologic changes and must be compared with previous films to fully evaluate changes.
   2. Identify bony structural abnormalities and thoracic morphology.
   3. Assess cardiac silhouette and vascular changes associated with pulmonary hypertension or acquired and congenital cardiovascular disease.
   4. Assess parenchymal lung disease, mass lesions, infiltrative processes, pleural processes.
   5. Identify abnormalities of diaphragm and large airways.
C. **Laboratory Evaluation.**
   1. Routine laboratory data:
      a. CBC may identify anemia or polycythemia, leukocytosis and differential shifts, and platelet abnormalities.
      b. Serum chemistry should be checked to identify electrolyte abnormalities often associated with acid-base derangements.
   2. Sputum evaluation:
      a. Describe gross appearance, tenacity, daily volume.
      b. Evaluate by culture and sensitivity, Gram stain, acid-fast bacteria (AFB) stain, KOH preparation, and cytology.
      c. Serial A.M. samples are optimal.
   3. Additional tests:
      a. The response to skin testing with PPD must be assessed to evaluate exposure to TB and controls must be used to assess anergy.
      b. The α_1-antitrypsin levels should be checked in patients with emphysema and a suggestive family history.
      c. The sweat chloride concentration should be assessed in patients suspected of having cystic fibrosis.
D. **Pulmonary Function Tests.**
   1. Spirometry.
      a. Static mechanics (see Fig 7–3).
         1) Volumes:
            a) *Tidal volume* (TV) is the normal inspiratory volume beginning with cessation of normal expiration.

    b) *Inspiratory reserve volume* (IRV) is the volume measured between peak TV and maximal inspiration.
    c) *Expiratory reserve volume* (ERV) is the volume measured between end TV and maximal expiration.
    d) *Residual volume* (RV) is the volume remaining in lungs at maximal expiration (not measured by spirometry). RV must be measured by a gas dilution technique (helium).
  2) Capacities:
    a) *Functional residual capacity* (FRC) is the amount of air remaining in lungs at end of TV (RV + ERV = FRC). FRC may be measured by body plethysmography.
    b) *Inspiratory capacity* (IC) is the amount of air expired from maximal inspiration to end TV (IRV + TV = IC).
    c) *Vital capacity* (VC) is the amount of air expired from maximal inspiration to maximal expiration (IRV + TV + ERV = VC).
    d) *Total lung capacity* (TLC) is the amount of air in the lungs following maximal inspiration (IRV + TV + ERV + RV = TLC).
2. Dynamic mechanics:
  a. *Maximum breathing capacity* (MBC) is the largest volume of air that can be moved in and out of the chest in 1 minute.
  b. *Maximum voluntary ventilation* (MVV) is the maximum volume of gas breathed per unit time under given testing conditions.
  c. MBC and MVV correlate with subjective symptoms of dyspnea. MBC is markedly reduced in obstructive disease
  d. Flow rates can be determined by spirometry (Fig 7–10) and the clinical utility is based upon the principle that more effort is required to move air in the patient with airway obstruction (bronchitis, emphysema).
    1) FEV_1 is the forced expiratory volume during the first second of forced expiration. The value of FEV_1 is dependent on patient effort during testing.

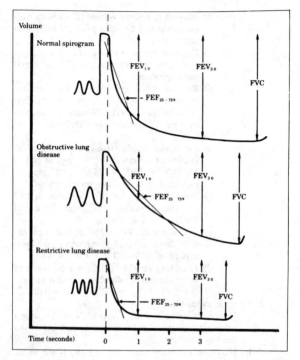

FIG 7–10.
Spirometry usually allows differentiation of obstructive and restrictive patterns. In both patterns the FVC is reduced. However, flows are reduced in obstructed and are normal or "supernormal" in restrictive patterns. See text for definition of terms.

        2) FEF 25%–75% is forced expiratory flow measured during expiration of 25%–75% of VC and is termed the maximal mid-expiratory flow rates (MMEFR). This measurement is useful for evaluation of mild obstructive disease and small air-

way disease <2 mm diameter. The MMEFR is independent of patient effort and cooperation.

3) FVC is forced VC, measured during forced expiration.

4) FEV_1/FVC represents the fraction of the FVC maximally expired in 1 second. FEV_1/FVC is useful in differentiating restrictive (normal or increased) and obstructive (decreased) disease.

3. Diffusing capacity:

a. Multiple factors affect DLCO in alveoli.

b. DLCO may be measured by single-breath CO test and is useful in dyspneic patients with normal VC, MMEFR, and ABGs.

c. DLCO is decreased in collagen diseases, sarcoidosis, asbestosis, PE.

d. DLCO is increased in left heart failure, polycythemia, mitral valve disease.

e. Serial determinations may be useful in evaluating response to therapy in disease process.

4. Patient evaluation:

a. In obstructive lung disease, lung volumes (TLC, FRC) are increased while flow ($FEV_{25\%-75\%}$, FEV_1) is decreased. FEV_1/FVC is decreased.

b. In restrictive lung disease, lung volumes are decreased, while flow is normal or increased. FEV_1/FVC is normal or increased.

c. An FEV_1 >2.0 L is associated with minimal operative risk; between 2.0–1.0 L, moderate risk; and <0.8 L, high risk.

d. MBC or MVV < 50% predicted value indicates increased operative risk.

e. TLC and all subdivisions of lung capacities are reduced following abdominal or thoracic operations.

5. Evaluation for pulmonary resection (Table 7–1):

a. Hypercarbia at rest on room air is a contraindication to resection ($PaCO_2$ > 45 mm Hg).

b. PFTs can be used to estimate the effect of resection on postoperative pulmonary function.

1) The product of the fraction of pulmonary parenchyma to be resected and preoperative FEV_1 subtracted from the preoperative FEV_1 gives an estimate of postoperative FEV_1.

TABLE 7–1.

Operative Criteria for Pulmonary Resection*

Function	Test	Patient at Risk	Prohibitive Risk
Dynamic mechanics	FEV$_1$ postoperatively, FVC preoperatively, MBC preoperatively	<1.0 L/sec <2.0 L/sec <55%	<0.8 L/sec <1.5 L/sec <35%
Ventilatory	PO$_2$ preoperatively, resting	50–65 mm Hg	<50 mm Hg
	PCO$_2$ preoperatively, resting	40–44 mm Hg	>45 mm Hg
Cardiac	ECG, resting; ETT (Exercise Tolerance Testing) tube	Ischemia, atrial arrhythmias	Acute MI, ventricular arrhythmias
	Rest/exercise RNA or MUGA	EF <50% or fall with exercise	EF <30%
Hematologic	Hemoglobin level, chronic	>17 g/dL	>20 g/dL
Clinical assessment	Stair walking	Unable to walk up 2 flights	Unable to walk up 1 flight
	Postexercise ABG	Fall in PO$_2$, CO$_2$ retention	Fall in PO$_2$ <50 mm Hg

  2) Minimal criteria for pulmonary resection:
     a) Minimal requirements for lobectomy are an
        estimated postoperative MVV > 40% pre-
        dicted and FEV$_1$ > 0.8 L.
     b) Minimal requirements for pneumonectomy
        are a postoperative MVV >55% predicted
        and a postoperative FEV$_1$ >0.8 L (60 years)
        and >1.0 L (65 years). The calculated post-
        operative FVC should be >1.5 L (decrease
        of FVC for right lung, 45%–50%, and left
        lung, 35%–40%) (see Table 7–1).
  c. The final decision concerning operability includes
     evaluation of resectability as well as associated medi-
     cal problems and surgical risk. This risk-benefit anal-
     ysis must be applied to each patient individually.
E. Arterial Blood Gas Determination.
  ABG determinations measure PaO$_2$ and PaCO$_2$ as well as
  pH, HCO$_3$, base excess or deficit, SaO$_2$, carboxyhemoglobin

and methemoglobin saturation, reduced hemoglobin, and total O_2 content.

1. PaO_2:
   a. PaO_2 reflects alveolar oxygen pressure and the overall $\dot{V}/\dot{Q}$.
   b. PaO_2 is age-dependent, declining from a normal of 100 mm Hg at age 20 to 80 mm Hg at age 70 years.
   c. A variety of pathologic processes interfere with O_2 transfer resulting in low PaO_2:
      1) Respiratory causes include diffusion barrier, right-to-left intrapulmonary shunt (vascular, parenchymal, or both), and $\dot{V}/\dot{Q}$ mismatch.
      2) Nonrespiratory causes include right-to-left intracardiac shunt, and patient hyperthermia. A low $C\overline{v}O_2$ magnifies the effect of a $\dot{V}/\dot{Q}$ mismatch or intrapulmonary shunt.
      3) Causes of low PaO_2 without an increased $P(A-a)O_2$ include low FIO_2, altitude (lowers barometric pressure, P_B), decreased R, and central hypoventilation causing hypoxemia and hypercarbia. If a patient with pure hypoventilation has an increased $P(A-a)O_2$, a superimposed respiratory cause should be sought.
2. $PaCO_2$ and $\dot{V}A$:
   a. $PaCO_2$ is a direct measurement of $\dot{V}A$ and reflects the balance between CO_2 production (tissue) and CO_2 excretion (lungs).
   b. Normal $PaCO_2$ is 38–42 mm Hg.
   c. Room air $PaCO_2$ >45 mm Hg indicates significant hypoventilation.
3. Acid-Base Balance (see p. 430):
   a. ABGs must be drawn properly, stored anaerobically, and analyzed within several minutes of being drawn. In practice, pH and $PaCO_2$ are usually measured, and the HCO_3^- is calculated.

F. Ventilation-Perfusion Scans.

$\dot{V}/\dot{Q}$ scans are used to evaluate anatomic and physiologic shunting of pulmonary blood flow and $\dot{V}/\dot{Q}$ mismatch such as seen with chronic or acute PE and are most useful when correlated with findings on CXR.

1. Ventilation scan: [131] Xe gas inhalation study identifies areas of decreased alveolar ventilation and is useful to

    assess airway obstruction or parenchymal destruction secondary to underlying disease.

2. Perfusion scan: ^{131}I, ^{51}Cr, or ^{99m}Tc IV perfusion scans identify areas of decreased pulmonary blood flow, and are useful to assess areas of decreased vascularity, vascular constriction, or vascular occlusion from acute or chronic processes.

3. General principles: Ventilation defects may be seen with pneumonia, emphysema, or tumors. COPD may lead to defects in both scans. A perfusion scan defect with a normal ventilation scan indicates a high probability of PE.

G. Bronchoscopy.

IV access is necessary, standard intubation equipment, cardiac monitoring, and resuscitation equipment should be readily available. Topical lidocaine anesthesia and IV sedation with benzodiazepine (Valium) are standard premedications. O_2 therapy and IV atropine are helpful to increase PaO_2 and reduce pulmonary secretions. Bronchodilators may be beneficial in patients with reactive airway disease.

1. *Diagnosis:* Useful for evaluation of airway obstruction, biopsy of mass lesions, aspiration of cystic lesions, and localization of bleeding sites.

2. *Therapy:* Useful for laser tumor ablation, relief of airway obstruction, coagulation of bleeding sites, dilation of stenoses, and intubation in difficult patients.

3. *Rigid bronchoscopy:* Removal of foreign bodies, biopsy of large airway lesions, and management of massive hemoptysis usually require general anesthesia.

4. *Flexible bronchoscopy:* The flexible bronchoscope is more comfortable, can be used for bedside procedures, and allows easier access to segmental and subsegmental airways, particularly of the upper lobes.

5. *Complications:*
   a. Bronchoscopy can be accomplished with a low major complication rate (0.08%) and an extremely low mortality (0.01%).
   b. Therapeutic interventions add a small increment of risk.
   c. Bronchoscopy may be complicated by bronchospasm, hypoxia, aspiration, infection, perforation, pharyngeal spasm, vocal cord damage, and hemorrhage.

d. One-half of major complications and deaths are results of either respiratory depression caused by excessive premedication or adverse reactions to topical anesthetics.

III. RESPIRATORY FAILURE.

Respiratory failure is defined as a condition where changes in ventilation and/or perfusion result in inadequate CO_2 removal, acidemia, or arterial hypoxemia (Tables 7-2 and 7-3).

A. Responses of the Lung to Injury.

1. The pulmonary system has a limited variety of responses to noxious stimuli. The large airways and bronchioles respond with changes in tone and secretions while the alveoli respond by altering pulmonary blood flow in response to alveolar gas concentrations and pH. Pulmonary epithelium and endothelium both become "leaky" in response to a wide variety of inflammatory mediators, allowing accumulation of interstitial fluid (interstitial edema) and, secondarily, alveolar fluid (alveolar edema). Interstitial and alveolar edema critically affect alveolar ventilation, perfusion, and diffusion.

TABLE 7-2.

Indices of Respiratory Failure

Measure	Normal	Respiratory Failure
Vital Capacity (mL/kg)	60-75	10
Functional residual capacity (mL/kg)	30-40	<60% predicted
VD/VT	0.3	0.6
Compliance (L/cm H_2O)	0.1	0.02
Inspiratory force (cm H_2O)	-80 to -100	-20
Shunt (Qs/Qt)	5%	15%
Room air PaO_2 (mm Hg)	90-95	60
$PaCO_2$ (mm Hg)	40	60
Arterial pH	7.40	7.25
Respiration rate (breaths/min)	12-18	>30
Work of breathing	Negligible	Excessively increased

TABLE 7-3.

Etiologies and Conditions Resulting in Acute Respiratory Failure

Failure of Ventilation, Etiology	General Terms	Specific Conditions
Decreased respiratory drive, altered mental status	Decreased CO_2 sensitivity in obesity, COPD, and under effect of anesthesia; hypoxic drive is limited after anesthesia or bilateral carotid endarterectomy	Sedatives/hypnotics, neurosurgical procedures, hypernatremia, hyperosmolarity, increased ICP
Decreased muscle strength	Hypothermia delays washout of neuromuscular blockers from neuromuscular junction	Incomplete reversal of neuromuscular blocking agents, predisposition to aspiration, phrenic nerve paralysis, topical cardiac cooling, C2-4 spinal cord transection, neuromuscular disease
Restrictive disease (decreased compliance decreases FRC, decreases tidal volume, increases work of breathing)	**Diaphragmatic dysfunction:** chest wall and abdominal wall are interdependent; upper abdominal surgery increases abdominal muscle tone, limiting abdominal and, via diaphragm, chest compliance	Upper abdominal surgery, supine position, obesity, pregnancy, ascites, abdominal malignancy, gastric dilatation subdiaphragmatic abscess
	Chest wall dysfunction	Thoracotomy, flail chest, postoperative splinting, encircling burn, obesity, occlusive dressings

Failure of Ventilation, Etiology	General Terms	Specific Conditions
	Parenchymal dysfunction: PEEP may increase total extravascular lung water; FRC is diminished and airway closing occurs at larger volume; airway closing may limit expiration as FRC approaches CV	Edema—(increased extravascular lung water) hydrostatic: CHF, volume overload; permeability: hypoproteinemia, sepsis, aspiration, ARDS, pneumonia, contusion
Airway obstruction, increased airway resistance	**Larynx, pharynx**	Loss of muscle tone, obesity, hematoma, vomitus/foreign bodies, laryngospasm, epiglottal inflammation/edema
	Bronchioles: small decreases in diameter effect large increase in airway resistance; edema is not distinguishable from bronchospasm	Reactive airways/ bronchospasm, allergic reaction, asthma Decreased mucus clearance, plugging Intubation, suctioning Loss of anesthetic-induced bronchodilation Bronchitis, emphysema, loss of radial elastic support, excessive secretions Edema Intraluminal obstruction—cancer, blood

(Continued.)

TABLE 7-3 (cont.).

Failure of Ventilation, Etiology	General Terms	Specific Conditions
Primary decrease in FRC	Anesthesia decreases outward recoil of chest wall, increase lung elastic recoil; compromises surfactant	Hemo-, hydro-, pneumothorax atelectasis, emphysema, flail chest
Increased dead space	Normal VD/VT = 0.3	Emboli, thrombus, air, fat, air trapping-emphysema, excessive TV, breath-stacking
Inadequate ventilation	Increased demand Excess carbohydrates transformed to fat and CO_2 Hypothermia and neuromuscular blockade decrease production of CO_2	Malignant hyperthermia Starved patient on TPN Increased sympathetic tone, exercise, burns
Inadequate perfusion	Normally alveolar to arterial oxygen equilibration after 30% of capillary length traversed	Anemia, altered hemoglobin, sickle cell disease, carbon monoxide increases, apparent shunt Cardiac failure Decreased PaO_2 NO_2 offloading-diffusion hypoxia
V/Q mismatch	Increased shunt, venous admixture	Contusion Bronchoconstriction Alveolar collapse—atelectasis
Impaired diffusion	Increased alveolar capillary distance	Pulmonary edema Aspiration, hemoptysis Late ARDS, alveolar fibrosis

2. **Intrapulmonary shunting:**
   a. Mixing of shunted, low SaO_2 with oxygenated blood produces a reduction in PaO_2 that responds poorly to increased FiO_2.
   b. Shunts may occur secondary to true arteriovenous anastomoses, in regions of lung collapse or consolidation, or secondary to regions of low $\dot{V}/Q$.
   c. Individual pulmonary units contribute to physiologic shunting, or wasted perfusion, as $\dot{V}A$ is decreased and becomes increasingly inhomogeneous. $\dot{V}A$ may be inadequate when dead space is increased; when muscle weakness or diminished respiratory drive limit VT or reduce respiratory rate; or when atelectasis is present.
   d. Hypoxic pulmonary vasoconstriction (HPV) partially compensates for $\dot{V}/Q$ mismatching; however, bronchioles are not able to alter ventilation to low $\dot{V}/Q$ units.
   e. Therapy is therefore primarily directed at improving ventilation. Increasing cardiac output may keep more pulmonary vascular beds open and paradoxically increase Qs/Qt.

3. **Decreased FRC:**
   a. Surgical procedures impose a variety of insults that result in perioperative loss of FRC. Thoracic volume loss, altered pulmonary compliance, or chronic disease also diminish FRC.
   b. Decreased FRC becomes pathologic when FRC approaches CV at which closure of small airways occurs.
   c. End-expiratory flow is limited when CV is met before FRC, aggravating alveolar hypoventilation as airways collapse at each end expiration. These airways have a markedly increased resistance, require much more work to ventilate than open airways, and thus may reduce TV.

4. **Increased airway resistance:**
   a. Acute mucosal responses to noxious stimuli are hemorrhage, edema, changes in secretions, sloughing.
   b. Laryngeal and bronchial muscles usually react by increased tone or spasm.
   c. Mechanical factors that attenuate the normal bronchiolar radial expanding forces (loss of FRC is most

commonly due to atelectasis or loss of elastic tissue) also reduce airway diameter. Small changes in diameter dramatically alter airway resistance and work of breathing.

d. Interstitial and alveolar edema also increase the work of breathing by decreasing pulmonary compliance.

e. As the work of breathing is increased by stiffer lungs, TV is diminished, limiting $\dot{V}_A$.

B. Therapy for Acute Respiratory Failure

1. Airway obstruction must be relieved and a stable means of ventilating the patient secured. *(Remember ABC.)*

   a. Head tilt, jaw thrust, and chin lift may adequately open the supraglottic airway.

   b. Oral obstructions and foreign bodies must be removed.

   c. An oropharyngeal airway may be inserted.

      1) The correct size is the distance from tragus of ear to corner of mouth.

      2) The airway provides a bite block but may induce gagging or vomiting in a lightly anesthetized patient.

      3) The airway must be positioned posterior to the tongue.

   d. Nasopharyngeal airways are better tolerated by alert patients and may be inserted despite clenched teeth.

   e. ET intubation (see Chapter 22).

   f. ET suctioning: The patient should be hyperventilated prior to suctioning and afterward with 100% O_2, and 5 mL NS via the ET tube may be used to loosen secretions.

2. **Supplemental O_2 therapy:**

   a. Will not completely correct hypoxia in the presence of a true shunt.

   b. Hypoxia secondary to alveolar hypoventilation must be treated by improving ventilation.

   c. Useful in the setting of decreased oxygen-loading capability:

      1) Decreased cardiac output.

      2) Impaired carrying capacity.

      3) Impaired diffusion capacity.

   d. **Toxicity:**

      1) O_2 therapy may result in resorption of alveolar gas and collapse of poorly ventilated units ($\dot{V}$/

Q<0.1) and may limit or reverse local hypoxic pulmonary vasoconstriction, thus worsening physiologic shunting, resulting in a variable effect on PaO_2.

2) Use of 100% O_2 for >6 hours leads to decreased macrophage activity and decreased mucus velocity. There may be a progressive decrease in VC and lung compliance with progressive increase in $P(A-a)O_2$.

3) Use of 100% O_2 for >60 hours or >60% for a prolonged period may result in irreversible injury.

4) Toxicity is mediated by surfactant degradation and alveolar inflammation.

3. **Continuous positive airways pressure (CPAP):**
   a. CPAP increases FRC.
   b. CPAP may be administered by nasal prongs, mask, or ventilator, and may hasten recovery of FRC after extubation.
   c. **Risks:**
      1) Levels of 5–10 cm H_2O are unlikely to depress CO in adequately hydrated patients. However, CPAP >10 cm H_2O may decrease CO.
      2) If FRC is normal, CPAP may impair pulmonary function by forcing TV into stiffer portion of compliance curve.
      3) VD may be increased and limit alveolar ventilation if TV is not also increased.
      4) CPAP may be difficult to administer and requires patient cooperation.

4. **Bronchodilators** (Table 7–4).
   a. β_2-Adrenergic agonists:
      1) Increase mucociliary transport.
      2) Have a decreased effectiveness in acidemia.
      3) In resistant bronchospasm, a trial of increased dose and frequency may break bronchospasm.
      4) No evidence that tachyphylaxis occurs.
      5) Steroids may improve receptor responsiveness.
   b. Parasympatholytics:
      1) Have strong bronchodilating potential.
      2) Atropine has the side effect of drying and decreasing volume of secretions.
      3) Systemic absorption and tachycardia may occur.

TABLE 7-4.
Bronchodilators

Medication	Adult Dosage, Route	Benefits	Contraindications/Risks
Metaproterenol	2 mL of 1% solution for 15 min aerosol	Minimal system effect	May cause tachycardia
Terbutaline	0.2 mg MDI q. 4–6 h. 0.25 mg SC q. 4–6 h.	Minimal system effect	May cause tachycardia
Albuterol	0.09 mg MDI q. 4–6 h. 0.1–0.4 mg aerosol q. 4–6 h.	Minimal system effect	May cause tachycardia
Epinephrine	0.3 mL 1:1,000 SC	Activity not limited by mucus plugging where aerosols may fail	Tachycardia and cardiac arrhythmias
Racemic epinephrine	1:8 dilution of 2.25% solution for 15 min aerosol	Reduces edema and dilates airways, particularly postintubation and in croup	Not for routine use because of risk of paroxysmal supraventricular tachycardia
Atropine	1–4 mg aerosol q. 4–6 h.	May thicken large, thin secretions	Decreased GI motility, sweating, salivation, bronchial secretions CNS overstimulation

Drug	Dose	Effects	Comments
Ipratropium bromide (Atrovent)	0.08–0.5 mg MDI* q. 3–4 h.	Lack of systemic side effects. No adverse effect on ciliary motility. No adverse effect on mucus velocity, viscosity, volume. No side effects at doses 20 times greater than maximal physiologic response. Maximum effect for 2 hr	
Isoproterenol	1–2 mL of 1% solution over 15 min q. 3–5 h.	Increases mucociliary transport rate	IV route limited to children secondary to cardiovascular toxicity; duration of activity may only be 1–1.5 hr
Phenylephrine	0.25–0.5 mL of 1% solution over 15 min q 4–6 h.	Increases mucus gland secretion. Prolongs activity of concomitantly administered medications by vasoconstriction. Limits postintubation nasal congestion	

*MDI = metered dose inhaler.

    c. Methylxanthines:
        1) Inhibit phosphodiesterase and adenosine.
        2) Augment hypoxic ventilatory drive.
        3) Improve diaphragmatic contractility.
        4) Significant bronchodilation may not occur immediately and may require 90–120 minutes of therapy.
  5. Aerosol therapy.
    a. Humidification prevents water loss from the respiratory tract, mucosal drying and desquamation, and drying of secretions.
    b. Bronchomucotropism:
        1) Excessively thin or thick secretions cannot be mobilized while excessively thick secretions also produce plugging and casts.
        2) Cholinergics increase mucus production while β-adrenergic agonists increase mucociliary transport.
        3) Aerosolized H_2O does not decrease mucus viscosity.
    c. Medications:
        1) Aerosol administration of β-agonists and parasympatholytics is generally superior to parenteral route.
        2) If severe bronchospasm is present, aerosol may not reach distal bronchi.
        3) **Continuous nebulization is superior to metered dose inhaler.**
        4) IPPB has no added benefit and may risk barotrauma.
        5) Only 10%–15% of total dose is retained by lung.
        6) Systemic absorption of drugs may occur.

C. Specific Conditions.
  1. **General considerations of perioperative care:**
    a. To limit atelectasis, maintain FRC, and avoid pneumonia.
    b. Smoking should be stopped 2 weeks prior to surgery.
    c. Preoperative teaching of proper coughing technique is important.
    d. For decreased TV or respiratory rate in the recovery room:

    1) Stimulate the patient to deep-breathe and cough.

    2) Use naloxone to reverse excessive sedation.

    3) Reversal of residual neuromuscular blockade may be necessary.

    4) Use narcotics to relieve pain and reduce splinting.

    5) Elevate the head 30 degrees to increase FRC.

  e. For decreased PaO_2:

    1) Supplemental O_2 may be administered.

    2) Improve posture, reduce gastric dilation.

    3) Mobilize secretions. If cough is ineffective, ET suctioning will directly remove secretions and stimulate coughing.

    4) CPAP to limit end-expiratory small airway collapse.

    5) Consider intubation and mechanical support.

  f. Mobilize as soon as possible postoperatively.

2. **Reactive airways disease (bronchospasm, asthma).**

  a. **Pathophysiology:**

    1) Potential etiologies include aspiration, anaphylaxis, central obstruction, carcinoid, cystic fibrosis, sarcoid, PE, bronchiolitis, cardiac failure, ARDS, toxin exposure.

    2) The central problem is mucus plugging, mucosal edema, and bronchospasm which result in airway obstruction.

    3) Acute exacerbations may be secondary to infection (bronchitis, pneumonia), allergies, pneumothorax, PE, or oversedation.

  b. **Evaluation:**

    1) Signs of impending respiratory failure include agitation, anxiety, upright posture, increased use of accessory muscles, fright, sweating, shortness of breath, pulsus paradoxus, increased cough with effort, labile expiratory flow rates.

    2) ABG:

      a) Normally, hyperventilation secondary to low PaO_2 will result in hypocapnia.

      b) **Normocapnia or hypercapnia may signal fatigue and impending respiratory failure.**

3) PA and lateral chest films are obtained to exclude pneumothorax and cardiogenic pulmonary edema.

4) Bedside spirometry (FEV_1) may be useful to monitor the effects of therapy.

c. **Therapy:**

1) Treat or remove aggravating injury or underlying condition.

2) Supplemental O_2:

   a) Administer O_2 by face mask in gradually increasing increments until an appropriate PaO_2 is reached.

   b) Carefully monitor patients with COPD who may have limited hypoxic drive.

   c) Face tent administration provides humidification without increasing anxiety.

   d) Nasal cannula O_2 should be avoided as many patients in distress mouth-breathe resulting in a highly variable FiO_2.

3) Start aerosolized β-agonist bronchodilatation. May require repeated treatments q. 20–30 min initially (albuterol 0.4 mL in 4 mL NS).

4) Obtain IV access, begin fluids, and maintain hydration.

5) IV theophylline:

   a) Loading dose of 6 mg/kg IV over 1 hour.

   b) Infuse 0.6–1.0 mg/kg/hr, adjust to serum levels of 10–20 µg/mL.

   c) Maintenance infusion must be reduced (0.3–0.5 mg/kg/hr) in nonsmokers, elderly patients, and patients with CHF or liver disease because of reduced theophylline metabolism.

   d) In patients already receiving theophylline, maintenance infusion may be started without a loading dose.

   e) Side effects include nausea, vomiting, tachycardia.

6) SC epinephrine (0.3–0.5 mL of 1:1,000 solution) is not effective in acidemia and may have adverse cardiac effects, especially in the elderly.

7) IV steroids are critical in severe asthma.
   a) Restore bronchial muscle responsiveness to catecholamines.
   b) Improvement may not be apparent before 6 hours.
   c) Hydrocortisone 100 mg IV q.6h. is commonly used. Methylprednisolone may also be used.
   d) The patient may be converted to a tapered dose of oral prednisone after resolution of the acute event.
   e) Inhaled steriods (Beclamethasone-MDI) are useful in chronic therapy, but are not as helpful during acute exacerbation and parenteral steroids should be used.
8) If $\dot{V}_A$, or PaO_2 remain inadequate, intubation with mechanical ventilation is indicated.
   a) ET suctioning, deep suctioned sputum sample for culture.
   b) PEEP to open closed alveoli and improve $\dot{V}/Q$ matching.
   c) FiO_2 of 1.0 worsens $\dot{V}/Q$ by abolishing collateral ventilation to units otherwise plugged by secretions and worsens shunt by reversing HPV in poorly ventilated areas.
   d) May require sedation and neuromuscular blockade
   e) Consider reverse inspiration-expiration (I/E) ratio to allow adequate exhalation time and avoid air trapping.

3. **Pneumothorax.**
   a. **Diagnosis:**
      1) Pneumothorax may need to be >40% for healthy patients to be symptomatic.
      2) **Symptoms:**
         a) Ipsilateral pleural pain occurs in 98% of patients.
         b) Tachypnea.
         c) Dyspnea.
      3) **Signs:**
         a) Decreased ipsilateral chest wall motion.
         b) Contralateral tracheal deviation.

c) Increased tympany.

d) Breath sounds decreased or absent.

4) **CXR:**

a) The supine AP CXR does not exclude pneumothorax.

b) Upright inspiratory and expiratory films may be necessary.

5) If the patient is unstable, perform a thoracentesis in second interspace anteriorly in the midclavicular line to exclude tension penumothorax.

b. **Therapy.**

1) Isolated pneumothorax, <15%, asymptomatic, and stable:

a) Observation, bed rest for 7–10 days.

b) Daily CXRs.

c) Administration of 100% O_2 may speed resorption.

2) Pneumothorax: recurrent, >15%, enlarging, or symptomatic with dyspnea or mediastinal shift.

a) Tube thoracostomy (see Chapter 22).

b) Simple aspiration may occasionally be sufficient.

3) **Tension pneumothorax:**

a) **Tension pneumothorax is a life-threatening medical emergency.**

b) **The diagnosis is made clinically and therapy usually instituted before a CXR is obtained.**

c) **The usual clinical setting is sudden hemodynamic deterioration in a patient on mechanical ventilation, following central venous puncture or thoracentesis.**

d) Tension pneumothorax is frequently seen following penetrating and nonpenetrating thoracic trauma.

e) The diagnosis is suggested by the findings of absent breath sounds over the hemithorax, contralateral shift of the trachea and mediastinal structures, hyperresonance to percussion, and JVD.

f) The diagnosis of tension pneumothorax is confirmed by needle aspiration (usually through the second intercostal space anteriorly). If tension pneumothorax is present there should be a rush of air and immediate hemodynamic improvement will occur.

g) A tube thoracostomy should be performed (see Chapter 22).

h) **Tension pneumothorax must be considered in the differential diagnosis of cardiac arrest and EMD (see pp 80–83).**

4) Any patient with a pneumothorax of any size should have a prophylactic tube thoracostomy prior to undergoing general anesthesia or positive pressure ventilation to prevent development of a tension pneumothorax.

4. **Hemothorax:**
   a. Trauma and surgery are the most common causes.
   b. A small hemothorax in an otherwise stable patient may be treated with observation and serial CXRs.
   c. Hemothorax following trauma usually requires tube thoracostomy to prevent fibrothorax.
   d. Following tube thoracostomy a continued output of 150–200 mL/hr for >6 hours is an indication for thoracotomy.

5. **Pleural effusion** (Table 7–5):
   a. Imbalance between lymphatic drainage and fluid production.
   b. Thoracentesis for diagnosis, may adequately treat.
   c. Tube thoracostomy if >500 mL, recurrent, or symptomatic.
   d. Send fluid for culture and sensitivity, cytology, pH, glucose, LDH, protein, amylase, WBC, RBC, AFB smear, Gram's stain.
   e. After 1,000 mL drainage, clamp tube and delay continued drainage for several hours to prevent reexpansion pulmonary edema.

6. **Esophageal perforation:**
   a. Iatrogenic perforations are common (endoscopy, dilation of strictures, placement of stents, passage of NG or orogastric tubes, following resection). Other causes include swallowed foreign bodies, esophageal cancer, caustic injuries, and forceful vomiting (Boerhaave's syndrome).

TABLE 7–5.
Constituents of Pleural Effusions*

	Transudate	Exudate
Routine tests		
Protein	<3.0 g/dL	>3.0 g/dL
LDH	Low	High
Pleural fluid–serum LDH ratio	<0.6	>0.6
Special tests		
RBC	<10,000/mm³	>100,000/mm³ suggests neoplasm, infarction, trauma; 10,000–100,000/mm³ indeterminate
WBC	<1000/mm³	Usually >1,000/mm³
Differential WBC	Usually >50% lymphocytes or mononuclear cells	>50% lymphocytes (tuberculosis, neoplasm) >50% polymorphonuclear cells (acute inflammation)
pH	>7.3	<7.3 (inflammatory)
Glucose	Same as blood (±)	Low (infection) Extremely low (rheumatoid arthritis, occasionally neoplasm)
Amylase		>500 units/mL (pancreatitis; occasionally neoplasm and infection; esophageal perforation)
Specific proteins		Low C3, C4 components of complement (SLE, rheumatoid arthritis) Rheumatoid factor Antinuclear factor

*(Modified from Braunwald E, et al: *Harrison's Principles of Internal Medicine*, ed 11. New York, McGraw-Hill Book Co, 1987).

    b. Clinical features include fever, pain on swallowing, cervical mediastinal crepitus, and chest pain.

    c. Diagnosis is suggested by the presence of air in mediastinal or cervical tissue on plain films. Contrast studies of the esophagus with Gastrograffin should be performed to localize the perforation. If no perforation is seen, a barium esophagogram should be obtained. Occasionally, esophagoscopy is useful to locate small leaks.

    d. A pleural effusion with an elevated amylase is worrisome for esophageal perforation.

    e. Early recognition and institution of therapy is vital. Initial therapy consists of IV fluids, broad-spectrum antibiotics, NPO, NG suction and tube thoracostomy to prepare the patient for operative repair which should be undertaken on an urgent basis.

7. **Aspiration.**

    a. Risk factors.

       1) Decreased level of consciousness:

          a) Alcohol, sedatives.

          b) Residual anaesthesia.

          c) Seizures.

          d) Narcotics.

          e) CVA.

       2) Diminished defenses:

          a) NG tube.

          b) Tracheostomy

          c) ET tube.

          d) CPR.

          e) Protracted vomiting.

       3) Esophageal disorders:

          a) Zenker's diverticulum.

          b) Achalasia.

          c) Hiatal hernia.

          d) Stricture.

       4) Gastric disorders:

          a) Delayed emptying.

          b) Outlet obstruction.

    b. Severity of injury is proportional to volume and acidity of aspirated gastric secretions.

1) Aspiration of acid produces a variable clinical course:
   a) Rapid respiratory failure with death in 24 hours (12%).
   b) Benign course with clearing of CXR in 4–5 days (62%).
   c) Initial rapid recovery but later infection and respiratory failure (26%, 60% mortality).
2) Aspiration of food may occlude airway with large particles, while smaller particles migrate to bronchioles to produce atelectasis and granulomas. These particles may provide culture medium for bacterial growth.

c. Prevention of perioperative aspiration:
1) NPO 6–8 hours preoperatively.
2) Reduce gastric acidity to pH >2.5.
   a) Histamine blockers (cimetidine 300 mg IV, ranitidine 50 mg IV) q. hs and on call to OR.
   b) Sodium citrate po on call to OR.
3) Reduce volume of gastric contents.
   a) Metoclopromide 10 mg po or IV q. hs and on call to OR.
   b) Preoperative NG suction for emergent surgery or patients with gastric outlet obstruction.
4) Sellick (cricoid pressure) manuever during intubation.
5) Suction above ET cuff prior to extubation.

d. Treatment of aspiration:
1) Put head down and turn patient into lateral position. Suction mouth and oropharynx.
2) ET suctioning. *Do not lavage.* Do not instill alkaline agents (also toxic to respiratory epithelium). If large particles or large volume is obstructing the airway, consider bronchoscopy.
3) Supplemental O_2 to increase PaO_2.
4) Administer bronchodilators to counter reflex bronchospasm.
5) Antibiotic therapy is based on deep-suctioned culture specimens. Antibiotics are administered only if pneumonia develops. There is no benefit

to prophylactic antibiotic therapy unless aspirated material is heavily infected.

6) Aspiration of oropharyngeal organism may result in a mixed aerobic-anaerobic pneumonia or lung abscess.

7) Monitor intravascular volume status. Pulmonary third-spacing from injury may cause hypovolemia.

8) Steroids are of no benefit and may cause harm.

8. **Pneumonia.**

   a. Pneumonia is an infection of the lung parenchyma and may present as a consolidated pulmonary infection.

      1) Symptoms:
         a) Pleuritic chest pain.
         b) Dyspnea.
         c) Productive cough.
         d) Hemoptysis.

      2) Signs:
         a) Fever.
         b) Tachypnea.
         c) Diminished breath sounds.
         d) Dullness to percussion.
         e) Egophony.

      3) The radiograph manifestations are variable.
         a) Alveolar pneumonia—dense consolidation with air bronchograms.
         b) Bronchopneumonia—streaky segmental infiltrates without air bronchograms.
         c) Interstitial pneumonia—reticular infiltrate which may be bilateral.

      4) Patients with preexisting pulmonary disease (COPD), smokers, and mechanically ventilated patients are at higher risk.

      5) Consolidation decreases compliance and FRC, increases $\dot{V}/Q$ mismatching, and worsens venous admixture (Qs/Qt).

   b. Antimicrobial therapy is the cornerstone of treatment.

      1) The choice is dependent on accurate identification of causative organism.

      2) Tracheal aspirates may not reflect true etiology; sputum from distal bronchial tree is more accurate.

3) *Streptococcus pneumoniae, Haemophilus influenzae,* and *Mycoplasma pneumoniae* are common causes of community-acquired pneumonias.

4) Gram-negative organisms such as *Eschirichia coli, Klebsiella,* and *Proteus* are frequent causes of nosocomial pneumonia.

5) Protected-tip bronchoscopic brushings give most accurate sample.

c. Supplemental O_2 maintains PaO_2.

d. Adjunctive treatment is primarily aimed at improving reduced lung volumes.

1) Humidification of inspired gas, bronchodilators, postural drainage, incentive spirometry, cough, and deep breath all improve ventilation.

2) Bronchoscopy may be required to obtain cultures as well as to directly remove mucus plugs and allow reexpansion of collapsed lung. Bronchoscopy can also evaluate possible obstructing endobronchial lesions resulting in a postobstructive pneumonia.

9. **COPD** (Table 7–6):

a. Acute respiratory failure is the product of acute illness or insult in the setting of chronic pulmonary dysfunction.

1) Compensation for loss of elastic lung recoil (loss of FRC) such as barrel chest, low flow rates, small tidal volumes at higher inspiratory reserve capacity, and flattened diaphragms may fail with added insult of infection, bronchoconstriction, PE, oversedation, or fever.

2) Mortality of acute respiratory failure in this group is approximately 5%.

b. Exacerbating factors include infection, CHF, noncompliance with medications, allergies, smoking, pneumothorax, and PE. In every patient with an exacerbation, an exacerbating factor should be sought.

c. Evaluation should include CXR, ABG, routine laboratory data (CBC, chemistries), spirometry.

d. In patients with purulent sputum, initial antibiotic therapy should be guided by the sputum gram stain.

e. Supplemental O_2 is administered to obtain an SaO_2 of 90% if possible.

TABLE 7–6.

Chronic Obstructive Lung Disease: Salient Features of the Two Types*

	Predominant Emphysema	Predominant Bronchitis
Age at time of diagnosis (yr)	60±	50±
Dyspnea	Severe	Mild
Cough	After dyspnea starts	Before dyspnea starts
Sputum	Scanty, mucoid	Copious, purulent
Bronchial infections	Less frequent	More frequent
Respiratory insufficiency episodes	Often terminal	Repeated
Chest film	"Hyperinflation" ± bullous changes, small heart	Increased bronchovascular markings at bases, large heart
Chronic $PaCO_2$ (mm Hg)	35–40	50–60
Chronic PaO_2	65–75	45–60
Hct (%)	35–45	50–55
Pulmonary hypertension		
Rest	None to mild	Moderate to severe
Exercise	Moderate	Worsens
Cor pulmonale	Rare, except terminally	Common
Elastic recoil	Severely decreased	Normal
Resistance	Normal to slight increase	High
Diffusing capacity	Decreased	Normal to slight decrease

*Modified from: Braunwald E, et al: *Harrison's Principles of Internal Medicine*, ed 11. New York, McGraw-Hill Book Co, 1987, 1090.

      1) Administer O_2 carefully in patients with chronic hypercapnia who may be dependent on a hypoxic drive for ventilation.

      2) Administer O_2 by face mask in gradually increasing increments until an appropriate saturates SaO_2 is achieved.

      3) Nasal cannula administration is avoided because many patients in distress mouth-breathe.

    f. Inhaled bronchodilators or IV steroids may diminish tracheobronchial inflammation and edema.

    g. Patients with obtundation, increasing fatigue, severe respiratory acidosis (pH<7.2), or failing to improve with therapy may require mechanical ventilation.

10. **ARDS.**
   a. ARDS results from a wide variety of diseases (Table 7–7).
      1) Endotoxic shock and trauma are the most common precipitating factors
      2) ARDS may follow aspiration, viral or fungal pneumonia, transfusion, uremia, inhaled toxin exposure, fat embolism, shock, eclampsia, or drug exposures.
      3) Falling PaO_2 and respiratory distress are indicators that ARDS may follow an injury.
      4) During recovery, DLCO is the best indicator of residual damage from fibrosis.
   b. **Pathologic changes:**
      1) Specific changes in the acute stage (24–48 hours) include interstitial and alveolar edema that result from epithelial and endothelial damage.
      2) The consequence of these effects is **noncardiogenic pulmonary edema.**
      3) Interstitial edema occurs first as capillary endothelial junctions widen, increasing vascular per-

TABLE 7–7.

Conditions Which May Lead to the Adult Respiratory Distress Syndrome (ARDS)*

1. Diffuse pulmonary infections (e.g., viral, bacterial, fungal, *Pneumocystis*)
2. Aspiration (e.g., gastric contents with Mendelson's syndrome, water with near drowning)
3. Inhalation of toxins and irritants (e.g., chlorine gas, NO_2, smoke, ozone, high concentration of O_2)
4. Narcotic overdose pulmonary edema (e.g., heroin, methadone, morphine, dextropropoxyphene)
5. Nonnarcotic drug effects (e.g., nitrofurantoin)
6. Immunologic response to host antigens (e.g., Goodpasture's syndrome, systemic lupus erythematosus)
7. Effects of nonthoracic trauma with hypotension ("shock lung")
8. In association with systemic reactions to processes initiated outside the lung (e.g., gram-negative septicemia, hemorrhagic pancreatitis, amniotic fluid embolism, fat embolism)
9. Postcardiopulmonary bypass ("pump lung," "postperfusion lung")

*Adapted from Braunwald E, et al: *Harrison's Principles of Internal Medicine*, ed 11. New York, McGraw-Hill, 1987, p. 1135.

meability allowing unimpeded egress of protein, thus increasing the interstitial osmotic pressure which leads to fluid shifts from capillaries into interstitium.

4) When the capacitance of the interstitial space is exceeded and lymphatic flow is insufficient to remove excess fluid, alveolar edema results.

5) Direct alveolar epithelial damage also causes a luminal exudate, filling the terminal air sacs.

6) In the chronic stage (>48 hours) intra-alveolar fluid consolidation leads to fibrosis.

7) Cellular proliferation and infiltration result in alveolar septal thickening and fibrosis.

c. These changes have a complex effect on pulmonary physiology, resulting in congestive atelectasis and inadequate oxygenation. The goal of therapy is to maximize tissue oxygenation using a minimal FiO_2 so that repair proceeds as rapidly as possible without O_2 toxicity.

d. **Criteria for diagnosis.**

1) Clinical setting:
   a) Frequently a catastrophic event.
   b) Chronic pulmonary disease and cardiogenic pulmonary edema must be excluded as the cause of the patients repiratory difficulties.

2) The CVR may reveal a variety of patterns:
   a) Clear.
   b) Fine reticular infiltrates.
   c) Diffuse alveolar and interstitial infiltrates.

3) Physiologic effects:
   a) $PaO_2 < 50$ mm Hg on $FiO_2 > 0.6$.
   b) $C_{TL} < 50$ mL/cm H_2O.
   c) Increased Qs/Qt and VD/TV.

4) Pathologic anatomy:
   a) Heavy lungs (>1,000 g)
   b) Congestive atelectasis.
   c) Hyaline membranes.
   d) Fibrosis.

e. Pathophysiology.

1) Ventilation.
   a) Edema:
      i) Increases stiffness, increasing work of breathing.

    ii) Bronchiolar narrowing, increased resistance to air flow.
   b) Atelectatic alveoli:
    i) FRC is decreased to limits of closing volume.
    ii) Inadequate number of ventilation units to exchange CO_2.
   c) Increased $\dot{V}/Q$ mismatch as regional ventilation is lost.
  2) Oxygenation.
   a) Edema:
    i) Decreased diffusion capability.
    ii) Increased pulmonary vascular resistance.
   b) Atelectatic alveoli:
    i) Increased physiologic shunt, Qs/Qt.
    ii) Increased Qs/Qt prevents adequate PaO_2.
    iii) Oxygen toxicity with increased FiO_2.
 f. Treatment:
  1) Remove injurious stimuli.
  2) Use minimal FiO_2 necessary to support PaO_2 at 60–80 mm Hg (SaO_2 = 90%).
   i) O_2 may have enhanced toxicity in this disorder.
   ii) Optimize DO_2 by maintaining Hct at 25%–35% and maximizing CO (see p 76).
  3) Initiation of mechanical ventilation and use of PEEP may be necessary to maintain adequate oxygenation.
  4) Invasive monitoring with a PA catheter may be necessary to exclude cardiogenic pulmonary edema and optimize PEEP. **The optimal level of PEEP is that associated with the greatest DO_2.**
  5) Supportive care until lungs can repair themselves.
  6) Aggressively treat sources of sepsis
  7) If sepsis occurs after onset of ARDS, the source is likely pulmonary. If sepsis is the cause of ARDS, the source is likely abdominal.
  8) Steroids have no demonstrated benefit and increase the risk of infection.

9) Pulmonary hypertension is an expected finding.
10) Manage the patient with the lowest pulmonary capillary pressures compatible with an adequate CO and DO_2 in order to decrease the driving force for the accumulation of pulmonary edema.

11. **Hemoptysis:**
   a. Etiologies include trauma, neoplasm, infections, foreign bodies.
   b. Obtain CXR to evaluate for pneumonia and neoplasm.
   c. Obtain coagulation studies including platelet count, fibrinogen, PT, PTT, Hct.
   d. Order blood replacement, FFP, cryoprecipitate.
   e. Cough suppression with codeine and humidified air.
   f. Most hemoptysis is not life-threatening and will stop with conservative therapy.
   g. **Massive hemoptysis** (>600–1,000 mL/24 hr):
      1) Massive hemoptysis was traditionally caused by tuberculosis and bronchiectasis. Malignancy, cystic fibrosis, fungal infections, and anticoagulation have become more common causes in the United States.
      2) Bronchoscopy provides an anatomic diagnosis and localization of the hemorrhage. Initial control may be obtained by balloon tamponade, iced saline lavage, laser photocoagulation, or isolation techniques using selective mainstem bronchial intubation or dual-lumen ET tubes and selectively placed Fogarty catheters.
      3) Resection of the involved section of lung is indicated for bleeding not controlled with less invasive techniques, bleeding from tuberculosis, bronchiectasis, or resectable lung tumors.

12. **Pulmonary embolism.**
   a. Diagnosis:
      1) The sudden onset of dyspnea with or without chest pain and tachycardia should suggest the diagnosis of PE.
      2) The clinical diagnosis of PE is neither sensitive nor specific.
      3) Signs and symptoms range from mild dyspnea to cardiovascular collapse.
      4) The majority of PE are silent.

     5) Physical signs are nonspecific but are likely to be signs of RV failure or pulmonary hypertension.

     6) Hemoptysis is a relatively uncommon manifestation of PE.

     7) Generally <25% of patients have physical findings.

  b. Initial evaluation:

     1) ABG.

     2) ECG.

     3) CXR.

     4) A V/Q scan should be performed.

       a) If the scan indicates a high probability of PE, treatment should be initiated.

       b) If the scan indicates a low probability of PE with a clear CXR, treatment is not indicated.

       c) If the scan is indeterminate or unobtainable, proceed to pulmonary angiography. Pulmonary angiography will document PE.

       d) If the scan is not obtainable, consider venography or MRI scanning. The presence of MRI or venographic evidence of pelvic or femoral thrombosis is an indication for anticoagulation.

  c. Therapy consists of systemic anticoagulation with heparin.

     1) Heparin 10,000–20,000 units IV followed by infusion of 1,000 units/hr.

     2) Adjust dosages to maintain APTT at least 2 to 2½ times control levels.

     3) Obtain serial platelet counts. Heparin-induced thrombocytopenia and thrombosis (HATT) is a well-established risk of heparin therapy.

  d. Thrombolytic therapy:

     1) Thrombolytic therapy is reserved for patients who are extremely symptomatic, who have large, (>two lobes) emboli, who have mild to moderate hemodynamic stability, and in whom anticoagulation is not contraindicated.

     2) Thombolytic therapy is contraindicated in immediate postoperative period.

     3) Use of thrombolytic therapy for PE has become standardized:

       a) Streptokinase IV as a loading dose of 250,000
units followed by 100,000 units/hr for 12–24
hours.

       b) Urokinase locally or systemically. For sys-
temic use 300,000 units as a loading dose followed by 300,000 units/hr for 12–24 hours.
If used locally 1 million units are infused over
10 hours.

  e. Alternative therapy:

    1) If anticoagulation is contraindicated or if a des-
perate situation with significant hemodynamic
compromise is present, emergent pulmonary embolectomy may be indicated.

    2) Procedures can be performed either to prevent re-
current emboli or to treat the embolic episode itself.

    3) Techniques to prevent recurrent emboli include
placement of a Greenfield filter (IVC filters) and
IVC interruption.

    4) Thrombi can be retrieved directly from the pul-
monary circulation either by aspiration or by manual extraction.

    5) Neither of these approaches can be compared rig-
orously with anticoagulation therapy and operation to remove the embolus is recommended only
in those in whom anticoagulation has failed or
cannot be used.

IV. MECHANICAL VENTILATION.
A. Indications for Intubation.

  1. Ventilatory support is indicated when PaO_2 is inadequate
or excessive $PaCO_2$ results in acidosis (see Table 7–2).

    a. Level of consciousness inadequate to protect airway or
adequately ventilate.

    b. Volume of secretions in excess of patient's capacity to
clear.

    c. Inadequate muscle strength.

    d. Excessive work of breathing.

    e. Airway obstruction.

    f. Atelectasis or consolidation unresponsive to more con-
servative therapy.

2. Intubation is indicated where airway adjuncts fail, CPAP is inadequate to reverse abnormal FRC, bag-mask-valve ventilation is ineffective, or prolonged ventilatory support is required.

3. While supplemental O_2 and other ventilatory adjuncts (airways, CPAP, positioning, reversing sedation) are appropriate immediate therapies, **elective intubation under controlled circumstances is preferable to waiting for respiratory failure requiring emergent intubation.**

4. Patients with compromised airways also require intubation.
   a. Maxillofacial fractures.
   b. Massive hemoptysis.
   c. Fatigue.
   d. Supraglottic obstruction.
   e. Protect airway in patient at high risk for aspiration.

B. Indications for Tracheostomy.

1. Upper respiratory obstruction.

2. Inability to control secretions from upper respiratory tract.
   a. Intracranial trauma.
   b. Intracranial neoplasms.
   c. CVA.

3. Inability to control secretions from lower respiratory tract, although otherwise able to ventilate.

4. Inadequate strength or VC (neurologic or COPD).

5. Mechanical ventilatory support expected to exceed 3 weeks.

6. Advantages of tracheostomy over translaryngeal intubation:
   a. Upper airway obstruction is bypassed.
   b. Greater reduction of V_D.
   c. Reduced airway resistance and work of breathing.
   d. Improved access to lower respiratory tract for pulmonary toilet.
   e. More secure airway with lower risk of kinking.
   f. Lower incidence of long-term laryngeal damage. Tracheal stenosis that does occur is relatively easy to repair.
   g. Patients can eat and talk.

7. Disadvantages of tracheostomy compared to translaryngeal intubation:
   a. Requires operative procedure.

    b. ET intubation is appropriate for up to 3 weeks.

    c. Increased exposure of lower respiratory tract to pathologic organisms with subsequent colonization. This is a particular hazard in patients with burns.

    d. Higher risk of massive hemorrhage.

  8. Complications of tracheostomy:

    a. Mortality of 1.5%, morbidity of 5.9%.

    b. Morbid events include procedure-related hemorrhage, pneumothorax, subcutaneous or mediastinal emphysema. Early events include displaced tube, infection, obstruction. Late complications include dysphagia, tracheal stenosis, tracheoesophageal fistula, and hemorrhage from erosion into mediastinal vessels.

  9. Tracheostomy is an elective procedure, performed in the OR, where proper lighting, equipment, and assistance is available.

    a. Emergent airway access should be a cricothyrotomy.

    b. Patients who are status post–median sternotomy may require cricothyrotomy to maintain isolation from sternotomy incision.

    c. Nasopharyngeal humidification or filtering is lost.

    d. Effective cough is precluded.

C. Ventilator Types.

  1. Partial ventilatory support is appropriate in most situations where spontaneous ventilations are present. Partial ventilatory support has advantages over controlled mechanical ventilation (CMV) or total ventilatory support.

    a. Periodic normalization of pleural pressure improves venous return and cardiac performance.

    b. Limits disuse atrophy and muscular dyscoordination.

    c. Allows ventilatory support with less pharmacologic restraint.

    d. Improved gas distribution to dependent portions of the lung.

    e. All ventilator circuits increase the work of spontaneous breathing so that partial support may be needed to compensate for the resistance of the machine.

  2. **Volume-cycled ventilation:**

    a. Ventilator attempts to deliver a preset constant TV.

    b. Pressure limits are set to avoid excessive inspiratory pressures.

    c. Provides more constant ventilation under conditions of changing total lung compliance.

    d. Part of TV is lost to the compliance of the breathing circuit (usually 3–4 mL/cm H_2O). This loss is a larger proportion of TV at smaller TV and higher inspiratory pressures.

    e. Difficult to compensate for delivered volume lost to air leaks.

3. **Pressure-cycled ventilation:**

    a. Inspiration is terminated when airway pressure reaches preset peak value.

    b. TV is dependent on the applied pressure and the compliance of the lung and chest wall.

    c. Incomplete exhalation limits TV and respiratory rate increases to compensate, creating a situation similar to breath stacking where mean airway pressure may reach pathologic levels.

    d. Compensation is good for airway leaks.

    e. This mode is primarily used in infants and small children where compliance is more constant and appropriate ET tube size selection mandates a small leak.

4. **Time-cycled pressure-limited ventilation:**

    a. Identical to pressure-cycled ventilation with the addition of inspiratory pause that maintains airway pressure at the preset maximum for a predetermined time.

    b. If airway-alveolar pressure equilibration does not occur, TV will vary. Where compliance is decreased and ventilation time constants for some ventilatory units are markedly increased or airway resistance is elevated, the inspiratory pause provided by this mode allows gas equilibration with all ventilation units.

    c. This is a common mode in infant ventilators.

D. Ventilator Modes.

1. **CMV:**

    a. The ventilator mode delivers a minute ventilation, determined by the preset rate and TV, independent of patient's breathing.

    b. CMV is appropriate where patient is unable to initiate breaths because of paralyzing agents, anaesthesia, or neurologic disease.

    c. Patients who require hyperventilation, inverse I/E ventilation, or differential ventilation generally also require controlled ventilation with deep sedation and perhaps muscle relaxation.

    d. Patients who cannot synchronize with the ventilator must be paralyzed or ventilated with an alternate mode.

    e. No air flow is provided between breaths so sedation may be required to abolish respiratory drive.

2. **Assist/control ventilation (AC):**

    a. Ventilator cycles through preset TV when patient initiates a breath by creating negative airway pressure.

    b. A full breath is delivered each cycle; no partial breaths are possible.

    c. Total support cannot be provided as this mode only assists spontaneous ventilations.

    d. Anxious or hyperpneic patients are at risk for hyperventilation.

    e. This mode requires meticulous attention to triggering sensitivity to prevent respiratory alkalosis (too sensitive) or wasted effort that fails to initiate a breath (excessive threshold).

    f. Respiratory muscles are at risk for atrophy and discoordination.

3. **IMV, synchronized IMV (SIMV):**

    a. Machine-delivered respiratory rate and TV are set. Level of ventilatory support may be varied from 0%–100% by varying TV or minimal breath frequency. The actual level of support is easily quantified in this mode.

    b. Air flow is provided so that patient may breath spontaneously, although unassisted, between ventilator breaths. Patients who have muscular strength that is inadequate for spontaneous breaths either need controlled ventilation, the breath-to-breath assistance of pressure support, or AC.

    c. In SIMV, ventilator breaths are synchronized by inspiratory effort. This synchronization has no physiologic effect on ventilation or patient safety.

    d. In absence of spontaneous respiratory activity, ventilation is the same as CMV.

    e. As a partial ventilatory support, this mode requires less sedation and causes less disuse atrophy of respiratory muscles than CMV or AC modes.

4. **Pressure support (PS) ventilation:**

    a. The ventilator provides a constant pressure during patient-triggered inspiration, augmenting the patient's own inspiratory effort.

b. May be used alone or in conjunction with other ventilator modes.

c. When used alone, PS is synchronized and requires spontaneous respiratory effort but does not guarantee a minimum minute ventilation.

d. Advantageous in weaning from mechanical ventilation as inspiratory support can be weaned independently from IMV rate.

e. PS allows the patient to gradually take over the work of ventilation and may help prevent disease disuse atrophy.

5. **High frequency jet ventilation (HFJV):**

a. Minute ventilation is accomplished with TV (3–4 mL/kg) $<V_D$, at high rates (50–300/min).

b. May be accomplished as high frequency oscillation (HFO), high frequency positive pressure ventilation (HFPPV), or high frequency jet ventilation (HFJV), which is most common in the United States.

c. Theoretically can provide ventilation at reduced mean airway pressures, and hence reduced incidence of pulmonary barotrauma, diminished CO, and elevated ICP.

d. Established indications: bronchopleural fistula (BPF), bronchoscopy, laryngoscopy.

e. Possible indications: excessive peak inspiratory pressure (PIP >70–80 cm H_2O) on standard ventilator modes.

f. TV may be adjusted by altering duty cycle (% inspiratory time) or drive pressure.

g. Methods include jet injector–lumen ET tube, 14-gauge needle injector, and sliding Venturi tube, which provides greatest the TV. The 14-gauge needle injector or injector-lumen ET tube provide a smaller TV.

h. Position tip of ET tube 5–10 cm from carina to prevent preferential ventilation of one lung.

i. If indication is BPF, PIP must be less than opening pressure of BPF to avoid continued air leak and allow healing.

j. Setup of ventilator includes frequency (100–150/min), duty cycle (20%–30%), drive pressure (5–50 psig).

k. Complications: inadequate $\dot{V}_E$, inadequate humidification, tracheal mucosal injury secondary to high shear forces, inspissation of secretions on ET tube.

E. Ventilator Settings.

1. **Rate** frequency of respiratory cycle must be adjusted in tandem with inspiratory flow rate (IFR) to provide for appropriate I/E. As rate is increased at a constant IFR, total and percentage exhalation times drop (normally 10–15/min).

2. **TV** is set directly on volume-cycled ventilators. TV is a function of inspiratory pressure, rate, and IFR in pressure-cycled ventilators. TV is usually set at 10–15 mL/kg for volume ventilators. For HFJV TV is usually 3–5 mL/kg.

3. **Inspiratory flow rate (IFR)** lungs with normal compliance are relatively insensitive to IFR, but when compliance is diminished, high IFR results in excessive **peak inspiratory pressure (PIP)**. A higher IFR accomplishes inspiration in a shorter period of time, providing a longer period for exhalation. A high IFR is particularly useful in diseases where exhalation is prolonged (emphysema). Normally the I/E is set at 1:2–1:3.

4. **PIP** is the point at which pressure-cycled ventilators terminate inspiration. If an inspiratory pause is combined with this setting, airway pressure will plateau at PIP, producing pressure-limited time-cycled ventilation. An adequate PIP produces good breath sounds bilaterally, visual chest movement, and delivers a TV sufficient to maintain a normal $PaCO_2$.

5. Start at **FiO_2** of 1.0 and adjust to provide for PaO_2 of 60–90 mm Hg (SaO_2 of 90%). Prolonged use of FiO_2 >0.5 subjects patient to risks of O_2 toxicity.

6. **PEEP** maintains positive airway pressure at end expiration. PEEP of 5 cm H_2O is comparable to physiologic PEEP provided by glottic closure.

   a. PEEP counterbalances airway closing forces, maintaining small airway patency at end expiration. This is particularly critical when FRC approaches closing volume.

   b. The purpose of PEEP is to improve PaO_2, ostensibly by reversing regions of low $\dot{V}/Q$, so that FiO_2 can be reduced from potentially toxic levels.

   c. RV performance is limited by PEEP, which secondarily affects LV performance by preload limitation.

      1) Airway pressure transmitted to PAs increases pulmonary vascular resistance, shifts capacitance

volume out of thorax, and limits preload to RV. Thus the RV which must pump against a higher afterload with a limited preload. Increased intravascular volume may compensate for these adverse effects.

2) Use of PEEP above 10 cm H_2O mandates invasive monitoring of intravascular volume.

d. In time-cycled, pressure-limited ventilation, high levels of PEEP narrow the delivered pressure amplitude, limiting TV.

e. PEEP redistributes extravascular lung water, improving diffusion by thinning the air-blood interface.

1) PEEP may actually increase extravascular lung water.

2) Patients on high levels of PEEP cannot have ventilator disconnections, even for ET suctioning.

3) Suctioning of these patients must be performed using a closed system.

f. PEEP may be critical to adequate ventilation and oxygenation.

1) Since high levels adversely affect cardiovascular performance and predispose to increased barotrauma, levels should be optimized.

2) Optimal PEEP is dependent on delivered TV.

3) Total lung compliance, minimal shunt, total DO_2, or minimal FiO_2 are all potential criteria.

4) Although the goal of PEEP is to reach a minimal FiO_2, maximizing total lung compliance more directly measures physiologic action of PEEP.

5) **The ultimate goal for optimization of PEEP is maximum DO_2 at an acceptable FiO_2.**

7. **Sensitivity is the level of negative inspiratory force (NIFM)** generated by the patient that is required to initiate a respiratory cycle.

a. If sensitivity is set too high, patient may have insufficient strength to initiate breaths and waste energy trying to generate sufficient NIFM to trigger ventilation.

b. If too low, i.e., more sensitive, breaths may be triggered too easily and result in hyperventilation.

8. **PS ventilation** may be combined with other ventilator modes to allow inspiratory support of patient-initiated breaths. Progressive reduction of PS allows gradual

strengthening of respiratory muscles in difficult-to-wean patients.

9. **CPAP** is physiologically equivalent to PEEP + PS and maintains airway patency by improving FRC.

   a. CPAP enhances inspiration by improving compliance, decreasing work of breathing, and improving gas exchange.

   b. Administration of CPAP to patients with a normal FRC may result in overexpansion, decreased compliance, increased work of breathing, and diminished gas exchange.

   c. Administration of CPAP to patients postoperatively hastens return to normal FRC.

F. **Alarms and Troubleshooting.**

   1. **Hypercarbia.**

      a. Mechanical problems:

         1) Correct ventilator malfunction (disconnection, inadequate TV because of circuit capacitance or air leak) by reconnecting patient, reviewing alarm settings, and eliminating air leaks.

         2) Correct inadequate TV (bronchospasm, mucus plugging, atelectasis, tension pneumothorax, incorrect ventilator settings, inadequate compensation for V_D) by treating bronchospasm and plugging. Exclude pneumothorax. Increase TV or PEEP to improve compliance and recruit alveoli.

         3) Correct increased physiologic dead space (PE, diminished CO with inadequate perfusion) by excluding or treating PE and improving cardiovascular dynamics.

      b. Increased CO_2 production:

         1) Caused by fever, shivering, rewarming, hypermetabolic state, sepsis, excessive carbohydrate calories.

         2) Treat and correct underlying problem.

         3) Muscle paralysis may be essential to control shivering.

   2. **Hypoxia and sudden respiratory decompensation:**

      a. Disconnect patient from ventilator. Hand-ventilate with 100% O_2.

      b. Perform physical examination.

    c. Obtain stat ABG, CXR, mixed venous blood gas if available.
- 1) Evaluate for adequate bilateral ventilation.
- 2) Evaluate hemodynamic status.
- 3) CXR: Check tube position, exclude pneumothorax, assess lung fields for edema, consolidation, or Westermark's sign.
- 4) Evaluate pH, PaO_2, and PCO_2.

    d. **If ventilation is easy manually:**
- 1) In hemodynamically stable patients exclude ventilator malfunction, consider PE, subjective dyspnea, shortness of breath. Correct subjective dyspnea by increasing TV. **Exclude pathologic processes before increasing sedation.**
- 2) In hemodynamically unstable patients exclude pneumothorax. Consider PE, sepsis, relative hypovolemia.

    e. **If ventilation is difficult manually:**
- 1) Exclude obstructed ET tube by performing ET suctioning to differentiate between kinked tube and mucus or thrombus plug obstructing tube.
- 2) If no obstruction, consider malpositioned tube (exclude by breath sounds bilaterally), mucus or thrombus plugging distal to tube (correct with deep ET suctioning and lavage with 5 mL NS), bronchospasm, or pulmonary edema (indistinguishable by physical examination; administer bronchodilators as diagnostic and therapeutic maneuver, consider aspiration, PE, or cardiac dysrhythmias).
- 3) **Consider reintubation or emergent cricothyroidotomy if adequate ventilation is not reestablished.**

3. **Alarms** (Table 7–8):
    a. **Low pressure (disconnect alarm):** Senses absence of positive pressure in circuit. Excellent monitoring of disconnections. **Most common failure of this alarm is failure to reactivate after ET suctioning.**
    b. **Low exhaled volume:** If exhaled TV does not match inhaled TV, an air leak or disconnection exists. Alarm may be set at 90%–100% of TV as part of delivered volume is lost to circuit capacitance.

TABLE 7–8.

Complications Attributable to
Ventilator Operation

Mechanical failure of ventilator	5.9%
Alarm failure	3.7%
Overheating of inspired air	6.8%
Alarm disabled without supervision	9.0%
Inadequate humidification	43.7%

    c. **Maximum peak inspiratory pressure:** Alarm should be set 15% above peak inspiratory pressure. This alarm signals increased risk of barotrauma and may be triggered by lack of synchronization with patient's breathing, inadequate exhalation time resulting in breath-stacking, kinked or malpositioned ET tube.

    d. **O_2 concentration of inspired gases** should be set within narrow range about set F_IO_2. Alarm signals ventilator failure or failure of O_2 source.

    e. End-tidal CO_2 ($ETCO_2$) is frequently measured in OR and is the gold standard in verifying tracheal intubation.

       1) Low $ETCO_2$ signals disconnection.

       2) Measurement gives an on-line assessment that is usually 4–6 mm Hg lower than $PaCO_2$, but may be 10–12 mm Hg lower in patients with increased V_D.

G. Weaning from Mechanical Ventilation.

  1. Correct underlying pathologic processes.

  2. Methodology:

    a. Most patients are ventilated in IMV. Weaning usually consists of progressive decreases in IMV rate, allowing increasing fraction of ventilation to be provided by patient.

    b. Patients who have difficulty overcoming resistance of the ventilator often benefit from small amounts of PS to assist spontaneous breaths. This can be started at a level that allows TV of spontaneous breaths to equal TV of ventilator breaths and weaned as the patient's strength increases. PS may be weaned independently of IMV rate.

   c. Decrease sedation as weaning progresses so that patient will have adequate respiratory drive to ventilate adequately.

3. Criteria (Table 7–9).

   a. Mechanics: Assess patient's capability to adequately ventilate. These parameters reflect strength and respiratory drive for extubation.

   b. Oxygenation Ventilation: Patient is able to maintain a PaO_2 >60–80 mm Hg on FiO_2 <0.5. $P(A-a)O_2$ <350 mm Hg on FiO_2 of 1.0.

   c. Ventilation: Maintain $PaCO_2$ <42 mm Hg and pH <7.43 with spontaneous respiratory rate <25/min.

   d. Physical examination: Assess patient's muscular strength and mental status for adequate alertness and ability to maintain and protect airway:

     1) Responds to commands.

     2) Sustained head lift (>5 seconds).

     3) Bilateral breath sounds.

     4) Bilateral hand grip.

     5) Assess ability to cough.

   e. Ventilator support from which the patient may be extubated:

     1) IMV <4 min.

     2) PEEP <5 mm Hg.

     3) PS <8 cm H_2O.

     4) FiO_2 <0.50.

TABLE 7–9.
Pulmonary Mechanics
for Extubation

Negative inspiratory force (NIFM)	>−25 cm H_2O
VT	>6 mL/kg
Respiratory rate	<25/min, >8–10/min
VC	>10–15 mL/kg

4. Difficult-to-wean patients.
   a. Patient factors:
   1) Correct or treat pulmonary edema, broncho-spasm, infection, oversedation, malnutrition, hy-pophosphatemia, excessive secretions.
   2) A degree of acidosis (pH near 7.3) may be required to effect adequate respiratory drive.
   3) Reduce excessive ventilation demands by holding carbohydrates to <33% of calories.
   4) Theophylline increases diaphragmatic contractility.
   5) CPAP may be helpful in maintaining FRC without ventilator support.
   6) Reduce FiO_2, keep PaO_2 about 60 mm Hg.
   7) Respiratory rates >30 /min indicate fatigue and require that ventilatory support be increased.
   b. Ventilator factors:
   1) Partial ventilatory support is not possible on some ventilators owing to excessive resistance of circuit and valves.
   2) PEEP of 5 cm H_2O and PS of 3–5 cm H_2O may be required during mechanical ventilation to overcome ventilator impedance.
   c. Airway factors:
   1) ET tube size may be inadequate to allow spontaneous ventilation without excessive work.
   2) ET tube may be partially obstructed, limiting its internal diameter.
   3) V_D may be too large, particularly in patients with underlying COPD or asthma. Tracheostomy in these patients reduces V_D by 100–150 mL and favorably improves V_D/TV.
5. Extubation:
   a. **Perform expeditiously with all equipment for reintubation immediately available.**
   b. Explain process to patient to minimize anxiety.
   c. Review again respiratory mechanics, last ABG, and physical examination to insure that extubation is appropriate.
   d. ET suctioning
   e. Suction oropharynx, trachea above ET tube cuff, and NG tube (if present)

     f. Deflate balloon. If patient can ventilate around ET tube, laryngeal edema is not critical.

     g. Give large breath and remove ET tube on exhalation, encouraging patient to cough.

     h. Apply supplemental O_2 via face mask at FiO_2 that is $>0.10-0.15$ above preextubation value.

     i. Encourage coughing.

     j. Check ABG after 10–15 minutes. Monitor respiratory rate and hemodynamics for decompensation.

H. Complications of Mechanical Ventilation.

  1. Disconnection is the most frequent complication of mechanical ventilation. It is easily diagnosed by appropriate alarms and settings **if they have not been disabled.**

  2. Infection.

    a. Intubation predisposes patients to infectious complications.

      1) Colonization of oropharynx and normally sterile trachea with gram-negative rods proceeds rapidly after intubation (<72 hours).

      2) Normal defenses such as the mucociliary elevator, macrophage killing, and nasotracheal filtering and humidification are circumvented by intubation or impeded by hypoxia or hyperoxia and acidosis of critical illness.

    b. Sinusitis occurs in 2%–5% of patients with nasotracheal intubation.

      1) Diagnosis is based on sinus films, fever, and purulent exudate.

      2) CT may be required.

      3) Treatment is changing intubation route to oropharyngeal or tracheostomy, administering antibiotics based on culture and sensitivity, and if no resolution, sinus drainage.

    c. Mechanical ventilation increases risk of pneumonia by 20-fold.

      1) Organisms are most likely enteric gram-negatives, arising from oropharyngeal colonization, covert aspiration, inhalation from contaminated ventilator circuitry, or hematogenous spread.

      2) Diagnosis is based on pulmonary consolidation, purulent sputum, and fever.

3. Barotrauma:
   a. As alveoli rupture at their bases, air follows perivascular tissue planes and dissects to the mediastinum, neck, or subcutaneous space, and, if the parietal pleura ruptures, results in a pneumothorax.
   b. Barotrauma is a function of PIP, and is more likely when high PIP occurs in conjunction with distended alveoli. Ventilation at a high TV and ventilation of regions of normal tissue when large areas of low compliance are present (atelectasis, contusion, pneumonia) carries an increased risk of barotrauma.
   c. Barotrauma may be limited by utilizing ventilatory modes that permit spontaneous assisted ventilation (SIMV, PS, CPAP).
      1) Spontaneous ventilation lowers mean airway pressure and improves patient-ventilator synchronization.
      2) Pressure limit alarm should be set 15% above PIP.
   d. Patients with COPD, asthma, or other causes of mucus plugging or air trapping, and patients undergoing bronchoscopy or CPR are at increased risk for barotrauma.
4. Tracheal and laryngeal stenosis:
   a. Placement of an ET tube causes mucosal ulceration and chronic inflammation that extends to involve tracheal cartilages and eventually results in fibrosis, tracheomalacia, and stenosis. Tracheoesophageal fistula may also develop.
   b. Although thin-walled, low pressure, high volume cuffs improve outcome, damage still occurs readily.
   c. Maintaining the lowest effective cuff pressure (preferably <20–25 mm Hg) is the most effective prevention.
5. Disuse atrophy and respiratory muscle discoordination:
   a. Minimized by using partial ventilatory support and allowing spontaneous ventilatory effort.
   b. In patients who have been on total ventilatory support for prolonged periods, gradual reductions in support over the course of several days may be necessary.
   c. It is important to maintain good nutritional balance to avoid catabolism of the respiratory muscles.

V. NONCARDIAC THORACIC SURGERY.

A. Preoperative Pulmonary Evaluation (see Table 7–1).

1. Clinical:

   a. A complete history including concomitant diseases, environmental exposure, tobacco use, and functional limitation.

   b. Physical examination with special attention to depth and pattern of respiration, chest physiognomy, and pathologic changes consistent with pulmonary insufficiency.

   c. A time-honored and useful test of pulmonary reserve is to walk the patient up two flights of stairs. Patients able to tolerate the climb will most likely be able to tolerate major pulmonary resection or major abdominal or vascular surgery.

   d. Further testing is warranted for all patients undergoing pulmonary resection, and for any patient having major abdominal or vascular surgery who is suspected to have a limited pulmonary reserve on the basis of history and physical examination.

2. Laboratory examination:

   a. CBC (chronic anemia, polycythemia, leukocytosis suggesting infection).

   b. Blood chemistries.

   c. Sputum for bacterial, fungal, AFB, and cytologic examination (as indicated).

   d. ECG (ischemia, arrhythmia).

   e. PA and lateral CXR. Comparison with previous films may be extremely useful to assess progression of disease.

   f. A room air ABG should be obtained on all patients. Moderate hypoxemia (PaO_2 50–65 mm Hg) or hypercarbia ($PaCO_2$ >40–45 mm Hg) are associated with an increased risk of perioperative pulmonary complications. Prohibitive operative risk is associated with severe hypoxemia (PaO_2 <50 mm Hg) or hypercarbia ($PaCO_2$ >45 mm Hg).

B. Pulmonary Function Testing.

   a. For patients undergoing procedures other than pulmonary resection, an Fev_1 > 2 L carries minimal risk; 1–2 L, moderate risk; and 0.8–1 L, high risk. Fev_1 <0.8 L contraindicates major abdominal or vascular surgery.

b. For patients being evaluated for pulmonary resection, assessment should include both preoperative PFTs and an estimate of postoperative PFTs based on percentage of pulmonary parenchyma to be removed (right lung 45%–50%, left lung 35%–40%)

    1) Postoperative F_{EV_1} should be > 0.8 L to allow existence independent of a ventilator.

    2) Postoperative MBC should be $>40\%$ of predicted.

    3) Postoperative FVC should be >1.5 L (see Table 7–1).

c. Determination of operability for a patient with a pulmonary lesion is based on many factors, including adequate pulmonary function reserve, no evidence of distant metastatic spread, associated medical problems, general condition, and biologic nature of the primary lesion. An individualized analysis of risk vs. benefit should then be applied in each patient (see Table 7–1).

C. **Perioperative Management of Common Thoracic Procedures.**

1. Pulmonary resection:

  a. Preoperative preparation should include:

    1) Cessation of smoking.

    2) Maximization of pulmonary reserve by institution of bronchodilators or treatment of infection, as warranted.

    3) Teaching of pulmonary physiotherapy techniques, including coughing.

  b. Postoperative ventilatory support:

    1) Most patients can be extubated in the OR at the end of the procedure, with only selected patients requiring a ventilator.

    2) Supplemental O_2 should be provided to keep the PaO_2 between 60–100 mm Hg, being careful to maintain the $PaCO_2$ <50 mm Hg. Patients who retain CO_2 preoperatively may require a lower PaO_2 to maintain their adaptive hypoxic drive for ventilation.

    3) Pulmonary physiotherapy to include turning, coughing, and deep breathing q. 1 h., and percussion q. 4 h. Careful nasotracheal suctioning may be necessary in patients with a poor cough. Bron-

choscopy should be employed for refractory pulmonary collapse or secretions.

4) ET suctioning should be avoided in postpneumonectomy patients to prevent disruption of staple lines.

c. Chest tube management depends on the extent of the procedure, and postoperative chest tube drainage.

1) The purpose of pleural drainage is to reexpand the remaining pulmonary parenchyma by removing air and fluid from the pleural space.

2) Anterior (apical) chest tubes are generally placed to drain air, and posterior (dependent) tubes are placed to drain fluid.

a) Large wedge resections, segmentectomies, and lobectomies usually warrant both an anterior and a posterior tube.

b) Small wedge resections and lung biopsies are often drained with a single pleural tube.

3) Chest tubes are usually removed beginning on postoperative day 2, provided certain criteria are satisfied.

a) No air leak (anterior tube).

b) Drainage <100 mL/day (posterior tube).

c) Both of the above (single tube).

d) Patients with two tubes usually have them removed on successive days.

d. The empty hemithorax following a pneumonectomy is a special case.

1) It fills in by mediastinal shift toward the side of resection, gradual collection of serous fluid, and eventual organization and fibrosis of fluid to form a fibrothorax. Therefore, most surgeons employ no pleural tubes in these patients.

2) At the time of repositioning the patient from lateral to supine in the OR, the pressure in the closed hemithorax must be equalized with the unoperated thorax to prevent cardiorespiratory embarrassment from mediastinal shift towards the operated hemithorax.

a) One method is to aspirate air via the second intercostal space anteriorly using a large syringe, a stopcock, and a needle until sufficient negative pressure exists in the empty hemithorax to shift the mediastinum and trachea to a midline position. Adequacy of this maneuver must be checked initially and at intervals during the first 24 hours postoperatively by assessing tracheal position and obtaining serial CXR.

b) A second method is to leave a small chest tube in the empty hemithorax and connect it to a balanced suction device, which allows adjustment of the pressure in the cavity to a preselected value. The chest tube is then removed on postoperative day 1.

e. Fluid therapy is designed to minimize overload, which might interfere with pulmonary function and result in pulmonary edema.

1) IV fluids at 1 mL/kg/hr.

2) NPO overnight.

3) A urinary output of 20–25 mL/hr is acceptable.

f. Perioperative antibiotics:

1) Established infections are treated with a preoperative course of sensitivity-directed antibiotics which are continued during surgery and for 3–5 days postoperatively.

2) Otherwise, prophylactic antibiotics are given immediately before, and for 24 hours after surgery.

2. Esophageal resection.

a. Preoperative considerations:

1) Nutritional status is of primary importance, as patients for esophageal resection are often severely malnourished. Preoperative alimentation via feeding tube or TPN will improve wound healing and immune defenses.

2) Cessation of smoking and optimization of pulmonary reserve.

b. Types of operation:

1) The Ivor-Lewis approach involves a right thoracotomy and an upper midline abdominal incision. Postoperatively, the patient will have an NG tube and a right chest tube.

2) The left thoracic approach (sweet) to distal esophageal lesions involves a left thoracotomy and par-

tial division of the left diaphragm. Postoperatively, the patient will have an NG tube and a left
chest tube.

    3) Blunt transhiatal esophagectomy (Orringer proce-
dure) involves upper midline abdominal and cervical incisions. The patient will have an NG tube.

  c. Postoperative management:

    1) NG tube may be removed on postoperative days
2–3 if bowel function has returned and drainage
has diminished.

    2) The patient is kept NPO until a contrast esophago-
gram is obtained demonstrating no leak at the
anastomosis. This is usually done on day 5–7.

    3) The chest tube, if present, remains until after the
first oral intake, in case of a leak.

    4) TPN, if used preoperatively, is restarted on day 1
and continued until oral alimentation is resumed.

  d. Prophylactic antibiotics should be given preoperatively
and for 24 hours postoperatively.

SELECTED REFERENCES

American Heart Association Cardiopulmonary Council: Manual
for evaluation of lung function by spirometry. *Circulation*
1982; 65:644A.

Bone RC, Jacobs ER, Balk RA. Adult respiratory distress syndrome, in Bone RC, George RB, Hudson LD: *Acute Respiratory Failure.* New York, Churchill Livingstone Inc., 1987.

Chew JY, Cantrell RW: Tracheostomy: Complications and their
management. *Arch Otolaryngol* 1972; 96:538–545.

Corey R, Hla KM: Major and massive hemoptysis: Reassessment
of conservative management. *Am J Med Sci* 1987; 294:301.

Comroe JH: *Physiology of Respiration,* ed 2. Chicago, Year
Book Medical Publishers, Inc, 1974.

Credle WF Jr, Smiddy JF, Elliott RC: Complications of fiberoptic bronchoscopy. *Am Rev Respir Dis* 1974; 109:67–72.

Fahey PJ: Management of the chronic obstructive pulmonary
disease patient in the intensive care unit, in MacDonnell KF,
Fahey PJ, Segal MS (eds): *Respiratory Intensive Care.* Boston, Little, Brown & Co, 1987.

Kirby RR, Banner MJ, Downs JB (eds): *Clinical Applications of
Ventilatory Support.* New York, Churchill Livingstone Inc,
1990.

Mecca RS: Respiratory failure in the postoperative period, in Kirby RR, Taylor RW (eds): *Respiratory Failure*. Chicago, Year Book Medical Publishers, Inc, 1986.

Pepe PE: Acute post-traumatic respiratory physiology and insufficiency. *Surg Clin North Am* 1989; 69(1):157–173.

Richardson JD, Adams L, Flind LM: Selective management of flail chest and pulmonary contusion. *Ann Surg* 1982; 196:481–487.

Sabiston DC, Spencer FC (eds): *Surgery of the Chest,* ed 5. Philadelphia, WB Saunders Co, 1990.

Tisi GM: Preoperative evaluation of pulmonary function: Validity, indications and benefits. *Am Rev Respir Dis* 1979; 119:293.

West JB: Ventilation-perfusion relationships. *Am Rev Respir Dis* 1977; 116:919.

West, JB: *Ventilation/Blood Flow and Gas Exchange,* ed 4., Oxford, England, Blackwell Scientific Publications, Inc, 1985.

West JB: *Respiratory Physiology—the Essentials,* ed 4., Baltimore, Williams & Wilkins Co, 1990.

THE VASCULAR SYSTEM

8

I. VASCULAR ANATOMY AND PHYSIOLOGY.

A. The Lower Extremity

1. The vascular supply begins at the bifurcation of the aorta into the common iliac arteries at the level of the umbilicus (Fig 8–1).

   a. On each side, the common iliac artery branches into the external iliac artery (lower extremity) and the internal iliac or hypogastric artery (pelvis). The external iliac artery passes beneath the inguinal ligament and becomes the common femoral artery.

   b. The common femoral divides into the profunda femoris artery (thigh musculature) and the superficial femoral artery (lower leg musculature). As the superficial femoral artery emerges from the adductor canal in the lower thigh, it becomes the popliteal artery.

2. Below the knee, the popliteal artery gives rise to the anterior tibial artery (anterior compartment musculature) and the tibioperoneal trunk. The latter divides into the peroneal artery (lateral compartment musculature) and the posterior tibial artery (posterior compartment musculature).

3. The foot is supplied by both the dorsalis pedis artery (continuation of the anterior tibial artery) and by the plantar arch (continuation of the posterior tibial artery)

   a. The plantar arch is usually the more important of the two systems.

   b. The pulses of the foot include the dorsalis pedis (continuation of the anterior tibial artery on the dor-

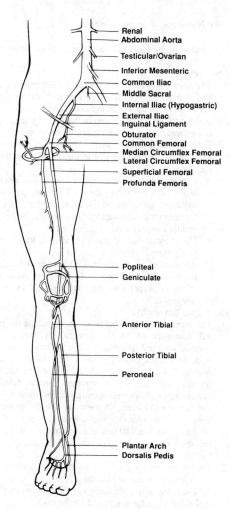

Renal
Abdominal Aorta

Testicular/Ovarian

Inferior Mesenteric
Common Iliac
Middle Sacral
Internal Iliac (Hypogastric)
External Iliac
Inguinal Ligament
Obturator
Common Femoral
Median Circumflex Femoral
Lateral Circumflex Femoral
Superficial Femoral
Profunda Femoris

Popliteal
Geniculate

Anterior Tibial

Posterior Tibial

Peroneal

Plantar Arch
Dorsalis Pedis

FIG 8–1.
Arterial circulation of the lower extremity.

sum of the foot) and the posterior tibial (posterior to the medial malleolus).

B.   The Neck.

1. The neck and brain are supplied by the paired carotid and vertebral systems. The common carotid artery arises from either the innominate artery (right) or the aortic arch (left) and ascends the neck in the carotid sheath underlying the sternocleidomastoid muscle.

2. Each common carotid artery divides into the internal and external carotid arteries at the level of the thyroid cartilage.

   a. The internal carotid artery has no named branches in the neck but enters the skull through the carotid canal and gives rise to the ophthalmic artery (eye), the anterior cerebral artery (anteromedial brain), and middle cerebral artery (lateral brain).

   b. The external carotid has eight named branches: superior thyroid (thyroid), lingual (hyoglossus), facial (muscles of facial expression), occipital (occiput), posterior auricular (auricle), ascending pharyngeal (pharynx), superficial temporal (temple), and maxillary (maxilla).

C.   The Upper Extremity.

1. The branches of the subclavian artery include the internal mammary or internal thoracic (pericardium and breast), vertebral (brainstem), thyrocervical trunk (thyroid, neck musculature), costocervical trunk (shoulder musculature), axillary (continuation of subclavian after the first rib), superior or supreme thoracic (shoulder musculature), thoracoacromial trunk (pectoral muscles and acromion), lateral thoracic (pectoralis minor and breast), subscapular (scapula), circumflex humeral (upper humerus), brachial (continuation of the axillary after the teres major), and profunda brachii (triceps) (Fig 8–2).

2. The brachial artery bifurcates into the radial and ulnar arteries just below the bend of the elbow.

   a. The radial artery terminates at the deep palmar arch below the flexor tendons of the fingers.

   b. The ulnar artery terminates at the superficial palmar arch just below the palmar fascia

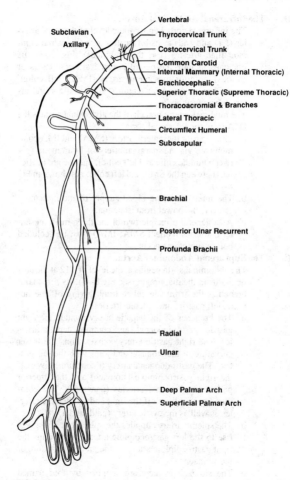

Subclavian
Axillary

Vertebral
Thyrocervical Trunk
Costocervical Trunk
Common Carotid
Internal Mammary (Internal Thoracic)
Brachiocephalic
Superior Thoracic (Supreme Thoracic)
Thoracoacromial & Branches
Lateral Thoracic
Circumflex Humeral
Subscapular

Brachial

Posterior Ulnar Recurrent

Profunda Brachii

Radial
Ulnar

Deep Palmar Arch
Superficial Palmar Arch

FIG 8–2.
Arterial circulation of the upper extremity.

D. The Infrarenal Abdominal Aorta.

1. The infrarenal aorta begins at the level of the renal arteries (L1) and ends at its bifurcation into the paired common iliac arteries (L4, the umbilicus) (Fig 8–3). Its branches include the paired gonadal arteries (testes or ovaries), inferior mesenteric artery (IMA) (left colon, sigmoid colon, superior rectum), and middle sacral artery (coccygeal body).

2. The final mesenteric branch of the abdominal aorta is the IMA from the infrarenal aorta.

   a. The superior mesenteric artery (SMA) and IMA communicate via the marginal artery of Drummond (between middle colic and left colic), and the arc of Riolan (between the SMA and left colic, not shown in Fig 8–3).

   b. The interconnecting blood supply of the mesentery protects the bowel from ischemia.

   c. As a general principle two of the three main mesenteric arteries (celiac, SMA, IMA) must be occluded before symptoms occur.

E. The Suprarenal Abdominal Aorta.

1. The abdominal aorta begins at the level of T12 at the aortic hiatus in the diaphragm (see Fig 8–3). Its first major branch is the trifurcate celiac trunk giving off the hepatic, left gastric, and splenic arteries.

   a. The branches of the hepatic artery include the right gastric, gastroduodenal, and common hepatic arteries. The right gastric artery courses along the lesser curvature of the stomach and joins with the left gastric. The gastroduodenal artery (duodenum) gives off the right gastroepiploic (stomach) and the superior pancreaticoduodenal arteries (pancreas). The common hepatic gives off the right and left hepatic arteries as well as the cystic artery (gallbladder).

   b. The splenic artery supplies the spleen but also gives rise to the left gastroepiploic artery which joins the right gastroepiploic artery on the greater curvature of the stomach.

   c. The stomach is therefore supplied by four named branches: the right gastric, left gastric, right gastroepiploic, and left gastroepiploic. Because of the stom-

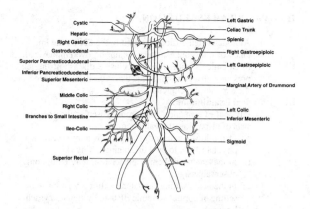

FIG 8–3.
The suprarenal abdominal aorta and the mesenteric circulation.

ach's rich collateral network, only one of the four branches is usually necessary for its viability.

2. The next aortic branch is the SMA.
   a. The SMA immediately gives off the inferior pancreaticoduodenal artery followed by multiple jejunal and ileal arteries (small intestine), the right colic artery (right colon), middle colic artery (transverse colon), and ileocolic artery (terminal ileum, cecum, and appendix).
   b. The celiac trunk and SMA interconnect via the superior and inferior pancreaticoduodenal arteries in the pancreas.
   c. The most common variation in the mesenteric circulation is the origin of the right hepatic artery from the SMA instead of the common hepatic artery (approximately 12% of cases).
3. The next branches of the aorta are the right and left renal arteries. One or more accessory renal artery may be present.

II. **VASCULAR EVALUATION.**

A. **History.**

    1. Although often difficult to elicit in the SICU, the importance of a thorough history cannot be overemphasized. Most patients with chronic occlusive disease of the leg present with a pain syndrome that is easily recognized by the experienced clinician.

B. **Physical Examination.**

    1. Physical examination for chronic vascular disease consists of inspection and palpation.

        a. In the lower extremity, inspection may reveal atrophy, hair loss, toenail thickening, shiny skin.

        b. In mesenteric ischemia, emaciation may be the only observable sign.

        c. In the acute setting, unilateral extremity pallor in the setting of normal systemic BP usually signals a vascular insult.

    2. **While palpation of pulses has been considered the hallmark of the vascular evaluation, it should be noted that pulses are solely dependent on pulse pressure and not on the true culprit in vascular disease — poor perfusion.** Serial examinations of carotid, brachial, femoral, popliteal, dorsalis pedis, and posterior tibial pulses as well as assessment of perfusion (color, capillary refill, temperature, symptomatology) are necessary.

C. **Doppler Ultrasound.**

    1. The Doppler ultrasonic probe is particularly useful in the SICU where serial examinations are required in patients who are often noncommunicative.

        a. It should be remembered that the Doppler probe generates only velocity signals and not flow signals. Assessment of blood flow should be performed clinically.

        b. The minimum velocity necessary for Doppler detection is about 5 cm/sec.

    2. The character of the Doppler waveform is indicative of the degree of stenosis in a vascular bed.

        a. In a normal peripheral artery, the Doppler signal is triphasic. There is a large forward flow signal, followed by a reverse flow signal, followed by a smaller second forward signal (Fig 8–4). With compromised

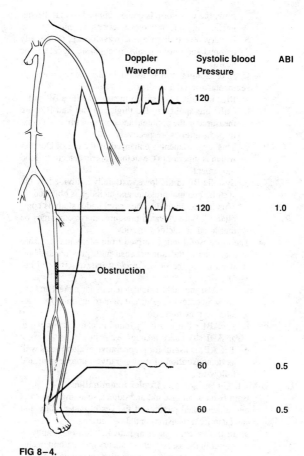

	Doppler Waveform	Systolic blood Pressure	ABI
		120	
		120	1.0
Obstruction			
		60	0.5
		60	0.5

FIG 8–4.
Doppler examination of the lower extremity proximal to the obstruction. The Doppler waveform is triphasic. Distal to the obstruction the waveform is monophasic.

flow, the waveform becomes damped so that the signal has only one or two distinct components.

b. In very severe disease, the waveform is profoundly damped and only a weak, monophasic signal can be heard.

3. Doppler examination is useful in the measurement of segmental arterial pressures.

a. Brachial artery pressure is measured with a BP cuff.

b. Cuffs are applied to the thigh and calf and BPs are measured in the popliteal and posterior tibial or dorsalis pedis arteries, respectively.

c. This measurement is enhanced by the use of Doppler which is superior to the stethoscope in detecting blood movement.

d. Systolic BP in the lower extremity is divided by the systolic brachial pressure and an index is obtained.

e. This test assumes that the vessel under study is compliant; falsely elevated pressures may sometimes be measured in calcified arteries.

4. The most useful index derived from segmental pressure measurement is the ratio between ankle pressure and brachial pressure (the *ankle-brachial index*, ABI; see Fig 8–4).

a. The ABI should be calculated both during rest and exercise in order to evaluate the contribution of fixed lesions to flow limitation.

b. An ABI <0.6 is usually found in claudication while an ABI <0.2 accompanies rest pain.

c. The ABI is useful for preoperative evaluation as well as demonstration of postoperative improvement and follow-up.

D. B-Mode Ultrasound and Duplex Examinations.

1. Both B-mode ultrasound and duplex scanning construct two-dimensional pictures of the vessel under study and can quantify dimensions and flow patterns.

a. In the vascular surgical patient, ultrasonography is useful in the assessment of aneurysms, carotid occlusive disease, and in postoperative surveillance of vascular grafts.

b. Color-flow imaging has further enhanced the quantitative capabilities of ultrasound examinations and provides information on individual vessel flow pat-

terns and aids in the diagnosis of arteriovenous fistulas.
2. Ultrasound has become the diagnostic modality of choice
in the initial survey and monitoring of AAAs.
   a. This simple examination is highly accurate with
   nearly 100% diagnostic sensitivity and ±3 mm resolution.
   b. Ultrasound is noninvasive, reproducible, and allows
   for serial measurements of aneurysm size.
E. Computed Tomography (CT).
1. CT scanning can be helpful in visualization of AAA, and
can define the extent of adjacent organ and artery involvement. Images through the aneurysm can outline arterial wall integrity, true and false lumens, and intraluminal thrombus.
2. CT is extremely useful in patients with known AAAs and
abdominal pain.
3. CT scanning may aid in the evaluation of anastomotic
leaks, pseudoaneurysmal formation, and possible graft
infection.
4. CT evaluation should only be considered in the hemodynamically stable patient.
F. Arteriography.
1. Arteriography is not employed as a diagnostic tool but
rather as a guide for the surgeon in patients who require
revascularization, and is considered the gold standard for
delineating vascular anatomy.
2. Complications occur in approximately 5% of cases and
include allergic dye reactions, renal dysfunction, CVA,
hemorrhage, thrombosis, pseudoaneurysm formation,
embolization, and cardiac arrest.
3. Contrast reactions generally occur following use of an
ionic agent. If a true allergy has been documented in the
past, it is best to avoid all contrast agents if possible.
   a. Elective arteriography:
      1) Select a nonionic contrast agent.
      2) Pretreat with prednisone 20 mg po (or equiva-
      lent) q. 6 h. for four doses.
      3) Cimetidine (Tagamet) 300 mg po and diphenhy-
      dramine (Benadryl) 25–50 mg po or IV should
      be given on call.

      b. Emergent arteriography.
         1) No definite protocol has proved to be effective.
         2) Nonionic contrast agents should be utilized.
         3) Cimetidine and diphenhydramine may be given.
         4) A bolus injection of steroids may be given but the efficacy is unproven.
    4. Renal dysfunction: careful attention to prearteriogram and postarteriogram hydration may diminish the risk of renal dysfunction. The incidence is lower with nonionic contrast agents.

G. Magnetic Resonance Imaging.
    1. MRI can be used to create high resolution cross-sectional images analogous to CT cuts or to image selected blood vessels and their flow patterns (MRI angiography).
    2. MRI is particularly useful for evaluation of areas such as the portal system where catheter access is limited.

III. PERIOPERATIVE MANAGEMENT.
A. General Considerations.
    1. In the majority of patients with vascular disease requiring an operation, the process at issue is **atherosclerosis, a systemic disease usually involving multiple organ systems.**
    2. The risk factors associated with the development of atherosclerosis include family history, male gender, increased age, history of hypertension, diabetes mellitus, and tobacco abuse (Table 8–1).
    3. The presence of these factors can have additional injurious effects on organ system function.
      a. Tobacco is a short- and long-term pulmonary toxin.
      b. Diabetes mellitus and hypertension often have deleterious effects on renal function.
      c. Elderly patients are more likely to have coexisting medical problems, in addition to decreased organ reserve.
    4. The perioperative care of the patient undergoing a vascular operation must include consideration of the common presence of coexisting cardiac, pulmonary, and renal disease.

TABLE 8–1.

Criteria for High-Risk Vascular Surgery*

Age	>85 yr
Cardiac	Class III, IV angina
	Resting LVEF >30%
	Recent CHF (<30 days)
	Complex ventricular ectopy
	Large LV aneurysm
	Severe valvular disease
	Recurrent CHF or angina after CABG
	Severe coronary artery disease (not revascularized)
Renal	Serum creatinine >3 mg/dL
Pulmonary	On O_2 at home
	PO_2 < 50 mm Hg (room air)
	$FEF_{25\%-75\%}$ <25% of predicted value
	PCO_2 >50 mm Hg
Hepatic	Biopsy-proven cirrhosis with ascites
Abdominal	Diffuse retroperitoneal fibrosis

*Modified from Rutherford RB (ed): *Vascular Surgery*, ed 3. Philadelphia, WB Saunders, 1989, p 915.

B. Preoperative Evaluation.

  1. Routine laboratory assessment:

   a. Serum electrolytes, CBC, BUN, creatinine, PT, PTT, urinalysis, PA and lateral CXR, ECG.

   b. Serum levels should be obtained of any antiarrhythmic agent that the patient is receiving.

   c. A history of significant bleeding diathesis or thromboembolic events requires a hematologic assessment.

   d. Crossmatching for blood:

    1) Carotid endarterectomy—2–4 units.

    2) Aortic dissection or aneurysm—6 units.

    3) Aortoiliac occlusive disease—4 units.

    4) Infrainguinal arterial procedures—2–4 units.

    5) Renal and visceral artery procedures—4 units.

    6) Arch vessel procedures—4–6 units.

   e. Bowel preparation using cathartics and enemas may be performed in patients undergoing transperitoneal procedures on the abdominal aorta.

  2. Cardiac evaluation (Table 8–1).

   a. Coronary artery disease: **The majority of patients with cerebrovascular disease, peripheral vascular**

disease, or aneurysmal disease have coronary artery disease.

   1) Ten percent to 25% of patients without cardiac symptoms undergoing vascular operations will have severe, correctable coronary artery disease.
   2) MI occurring in association with a vascular operation has a mortality of 30%–70%.
   3) Because of the high incidence of coronary artery disease, the threshold for preoperative evaluation with a MUGA scan, exercise tolerance testing, or cardiac catheterization must be low.

b. Valvular heart disease: Clinically important valvular heart disease is associated with a 20% incidence of either new onset CHF or exacerbation of preexisting failure.

c. Arrhythmias:

   1) The presence of a non–sinus rhythm was associated with a 10% mortality in Goldman's series (see Chapter 5).
   2) The presence of >five PVCs per minute carried an associated 14% mortality.

d. Preoperative invasive cardiac monitoring (see Table 8–1):

   1) In patients with LV dysfunction, history of recent MI, significant coronary artery disease, or moderately to severely impaired renal function, preoperative admission to the SICU for invasive monitoring may lessen postoperative complications.
   2) Intraarterial and Swan-Ganz catheter placement is performed.
      a) A baseline room air blood gas is obtained.
      b) Measurements of PCWP, CO, arterial pressure, and mixed venous O_2 are performed at baseline and following position changes (Trendelenburg and reverse Trendelenburg)[1] and after volume loading with a rapid infusion of 250 mL and 500 mL of lactated Ringers' solution.
      c) From these measurements a modified Starling curve can be formulated (CO vs. PCWP) to determine optimal preload.

    d) SVR and C(a−v)O$_2$ are calculated.

    e) Institution of inotropic agents or afterload reduction therapy can be instituted.

3. Pulmonary (see Table 8–1).

  a. The patient's smoking history, symptoms of dyspnea, and other pulmonary symptoms must be evaluated.

  b. A routine CXR is obtained.

  c. Pulmonary function testing:

    1) Hypercapnea, hypoxia, decreased FVC and FEV$_1$ indicate an increased risk of pulmonary complications.

    2) Preoperative institution of bronchodilators, cessation of smoking, antibiotic therapy for chronic bronchitis, and the use of aminophylline and occasionally steroids for the reversible component of obstructive disease decrease postoperative complications.

4. Renal.

  a. Patients with elevated serum creatinine or those undergoing revascularization procedures involving the renal arteries should have a C$_{CR}$ determined.

  b. Hypertension is present in the majority of patients with vascular disease.

    1) Poorly controlled hypertension is associated with hemodynamic instability in the perioperative period.

    2) In patients with diastolic pressures >110 mm Hg, elective operative procedures should be postponed until better control can be obtained.

    3) Antihypertensive regimens should be continued until surgery.

5. Cerebrovascular disease.

  a. The incidence of concomitant cerebrovascular disease and peripheral vascular disease is approximately 15%–20%.

  b. The risk of a CVA appears to be increased in patients with neurologic symptoms and an associated carotid artery lesion.

  c. Patients with significant carotid artery lesions who are asymptomatic do not appear to have an increased incidence of CVAs unless they are undergoing procedures on the ascending aorta or aortic arch.

6. Nutritional assessment.

    a. In high-risk patients, including those with advanced age, alcoholism, prosthetic graft infections, short-gut syndrome, chronic ischemic rest pain, chronic intestinal ischemia, or with a history of extensive weight loss (>25%–30%), preoperative nutritional evaluation and supplementation may be necessary.

    b. Determination of serum levels of total protein, albumin, transferrin, absolute lymphocyte count, and skin testing of recall antigens are performed.

    c. Patients with severe visceral protein abnormalities will benefit from preoperative nutritional support via an enteral or parenteral route as indicated (see Chapter 12).

C. **Extracranial Cerebrovascular Disease.**

1. Increased incidence of CVA is associated with increasing age, male gender, history of hypertension, transient ischemic attacks (TIAs), prior stroke, and cardiac disease.

    a. Cerebral infarction.

       1) The mortality rate with initial stroke approaches 40%.

       2) Over two-thirds of survivors will have residual neurologic deficits.

       3) The recurrent stroke rate is approximately 10%/yr.

    b. Transient ischemic attacks.

       1) The annual stroke rate averages 7%/year in patients who have experienced TIAs.

       2) Approximately one-third of patients with TIAs will suffer a stroke within 5 years from onset of symptoms.

    c. Asymptomatic lesions.

       1) Carotid artery stenosis:

          a) In patients with carotid artery stenosis >75% of lumen, the neurologic event rate is 18%/yr, with a stroke rate of 5%/yr.

          b) Development of stroke without antecedent symptoms is 2%–3%/yr.

2) Ulcerative plaques:
   a) Patients with medium or large ulcerative plaques have a stroke rate of 5%–8%/yr.
   b) A fifth of these strokes will occur in patients without antecedent symptoms.
d. Pathogenesis.
   1) Atherosclerosis accounts for 90% of lesions.
   2) Other causes include fibromuscular dysplasia, arterial kinking, extrinsic compression, traumatic occlusion, intimal dissection, radiation injury, inflammatory angiopathies, Wegener's granulomatosis, granulomatous angiitis, giant cell arteritis, infectious arteritis, and migraine.

2. **Surgical treatment.**
   a. Indications:
      1) TIAs.
      2) Reversible ischemic neurologic deficit (RIND).
      3) Stroke with recovery.
      4) Stroke in evolution.
      5) Subclavian steal syndrome.
      6) Global ischemia.
      7) Asymptomatic carotid stenosis or ulcerative plaque (controversial).
   b. Contraindications:
      1) In patients with an acute stroke there is a prohibitive risk of converting an ischemic cerebral infarct into a hemorrhagic infarct or exacerbating the existing neurologic deficit. A higher mortality and morbidity follow surgery when compared with medical treatment.
      2) The presence of a coexisting medical condition that would shorten the expected life span so that any purported benefit from a prophylactic operation could not be realized.
      3) Severe nonreversible neurologic deficit already present.
   c. **Preoperative evaluation:**
      1) Evaluate for the presence of **significant concurrent disease, particularly coronary artery disease.**
         a) **The majority of postoperative deaths are due to cardiac events.** The treatment of pa-

tients with both carotid occlusive disease and coronary artery disease requiring operative intervention remains controversial.

b) A policy of treating the more unstable disease process first, whether neurologic or cardiac, with a delayed staged revascularization of the more stable system appears warranted.

c) In patients undergoing carotid endarterectomy as the initial procedure, the ability to place an IABP should the patient become unstable is advantageous.

d) Patients with unstable angina and unstable neurologic symptoms can undergo simultaneous CABG and carotid artery endarterectomy. These patients have a higher complication rate regardless of the timing of operations.

2) Document preoperative neurologic function including hand dominance to enable an accurate comparison with the postoperative examination.

d. **Postoperative care.**

1) Wound care:

a) The neck dressing should be placed longitudinally.

b) Circumferential dressings may cause compression of the airway and other neck structures.

c) Serial examinations are performed specifically looking for evidence of excessive drainage or hematoma.

d) Hematoma formation or an increase in wound drainage often follow Valsalva maneuvers, as occur with extubation or ET suctioning, and after periods of significantly elevated BP.

2) Monitoring:

a) Following carotid endarterectomy or other vascular procedures performed on the cranial arteries, the patient is observed in an intensive nursing area for monitoring and frequent neurologic examinations.

b) Patients should have an intraarterial catheter and ECG leads for continuous arterial BP and rhythm monitoring.

c) The patient should be kept NPO until the following day to allow urgent reoperation should complications develop.

d) A thorough neurologic examination including level of consciousness, cranial nerve function, language function, motor and sensory function in the four extremities, and reflex evaluation is mandatory in the early postoperative period and should be repeated serially through the day of surgery.

e) Any changes in the neurologic examination should be communicated to the operating surgeon immediately.

3) Periods of hypertension or hypotension occur in over a third of patients undergoing carotid endarterectomy.

a) **The incidence of postoperative neurologic deficits and myocardial events is significantly higher in this subset of patients.**

b) The risk of bleeding complications is increased in patients with postoperative hypertension.

c) The etiology of this hemodynamic instability may be related to carotid sinus nerve dysfunction associated with the surgical exposure.

d) Relative hypovolemia, which may occur in patients receiving chronic diuretic therapy, increases the incidence of postoperative hypotension.

e) Inadequate medical control of hypertension preoperatively is associated with a significantly higher incidence of postoperative BP lability.

f) Correction of deficits in the intravascular volume, and achieving medical control of hypertension preoperatively is imperative,

g) Pharmacologic control of BP is warranted whenever the BP differs significantly from the preoperative norm.
  i) The patient should be restarted on pre-operative antihypertensive medications as soon as feasible.
  ii) Generally, if the systolic BP is >180 mm Hg or <100 mm Hg, or if the diastolic BP is >100 mm Hg, treatment should be initiated.
  iii) Sodium nitroprusside and nitroglycerin are the most frequently used antihypertensive agents.
h) Treatment of hypotension should start with correction of any intravascular volume deficits with an IV fluid bolus and subsequent initiation of appropriate pharmacologic therapy.

4) Any change from preoperative rhythm, usually sinus, requires investigation and therapy if unstable. Sinus tachycardia and bradycardia occur more frequently owing to carotid sinus dysfunction (see Chapter 5).

5) Antithrombotic agents are commonly utilized in the perioperative period.
a) Almost all patients are on a preoperative antiplatelet regimen, usually aspirin and occasionally dipyridamole.
b) In addition, patients are heparinized during the procedure. Often the heparin is not reversed with protamine following completion of the endarterectomy.
c) The use of aspirin on the night prior to surgery and postoperatively has been shown to decrease the risk of perioperative stroke and carotid thrombosis. The usual dose is 325 mg daily. Dipyridamole has not been shown to offer any additional benefit.
d) Patients undergoing reoperation for carotid thrombosis should not have their heparin reversed. Continuation of heparin postoperatively is common in these patients.

6) A preoperative dose and two postoperative doses of a first-generation cephalosporin are usually given as prophylaxis.

7) Obtain an ECG in patients with cardiac disease, or who have hemodynamic instability perioperatively.

   a) ECG evidence of myocardial ischemia, significant hypotension, or rhythm alterations are indications for ruling out an MI.

   b) Patients with known or suspected coronary artery disease are usually maintained on IV nitroglycerin perioperatively.

8) Laboratory examination:

   a) CBC, baseline Hct and hemoglobin, platelet count.

   b) Serum electrolytes, particularly K^+ to minimize cardiac dysrrhthmias

   c) PT and PTT to assess effect of residual heparin, dilutional coagulopathy.

   d) ABG is necessary in patients with significant pulmonary dysfunction, and intubated patients.

e. **Complications.**

1) A cervical hematoma can compress the trachea and cause airway compromise. A suture removal kit and tracheostomy tray must be available at the bedside.

   a) ET intubation may not be successful in these circumstances.

   b) The wound should be opened under sterile conditions at the bedside as expeditiously as possible.

   c) The patient should be returned to the OR for a formal exploration to identify and correct the cause of bleeding and reclosure under optimal conditions.

   d) Emergency tracheostomy may be necessary.

   e) Patients with cervical hematomas or excessive drainage from the wound should be returned to the OR for exploration and evacuation of blood.

2) The incidence of CVA in most large series is
1%–3%. The incidence in community hospitals
is 3%–13%.

   a) CVAs in patients undergoing endarterectomy occur more commonly in patients who
   have sustained a previous stroke, as compared to those with asymptomatic stenosis or
   TIAs.

   b) Occlusion of the contralateral carotid artery
   also increases the risk of perioperative CVA.

   c) CVAs may be due to emboli released during
   the operation, platelet or atheromatous emboli, ischemia during clamping, thrombosis
   of the carotid artery, or cerebral hemorrhage.

   d) In the majority of cases, CVAs develop after
   a lucid interval.

   e) **Differentiating carotid thrombosis from
   other etiologies is mandatory. Carotid
   thrombosis requires emergency reoperation.** Patients with dense hemispheric neurologic deficits or alteration in level of consciousness should be returned to the OR immediately to rule out carotid thrombosis.

   f) Although exploration should be undertaken
   as quickly as possible, similar improvement
   in neurologic deficit has been reported in
   those patients operated upon up to 4 hours after onset of neurologic symptoms due to carotid thrombosis.

   g) Approximately two-thirds of patients will
   have improvement in their neurologic deficit
   and a third will have complete recovery.
   The reported mortality is approximately
   15%–20%.

3) **Cerebral hemorrhage** is a rare condition without effective treatment.

   a) Cerebral hemorrhage causes severe neurologic deficits and is frequently fatal.

   b) The proposed mechanism is the introduction
   of normal systemic pressures to capillary net-
   works previously poorly perfused.

  c) The relative fragility of the capillary systems results in rupture with subsequent extravasation of blood.

4) Prospective studies identify **cranial nerve dysfunction** in 13%–20% of patients undergoing carotid endarterectomy. A third of these patients may be asymptomatic. Over 80% of patients will have full recovery of function, usually within 3 months.

  a) Injury of the vagus or recurrent laryngeal nerve (incidence 7%–15%) causes ipsilateral vocal cord paralysis in the paramedian position with resulting hoarseness and impaired cough mechanism. If paralysis persists beyond 6–12 months, the cord can be injected with Teflon to restore function.

  b) Hypoglossal nerve injury (incidence 4%–6%) causes ipsilateral deviation of the tongue with resulting inarticulate speech and clumsy mastication.

  c) Superior laryngeal nerve injury (incidence 1%–2%) causes voice fatigue and loss of high-pitch phonation.

  d) Marginal mandibular nerve injury (incidence 1%–2%) causes drooping of the mouth on the ipsilateral side.

  e) Glossopharyngeal nerve injury causes paralysis of the middle pharyngeal constrictor and the tensor muscle of the soft palate. Difficulty swallowing solid foods, and if associated with recurrent nerve injury, recurrent aspiration of liquids may result. Enteric alimentation via a feeding tube may be necessary until recovery of function.

  f) Horner's syndrome may be seen following carotid endarterectomy secondary to damage to the superior cervical ganglion.

D. Thoracic Aortic Dissection.
Thoracic aortic dissection is the most common catastrophic event involving the aorta and results from an intimal tear in the aorta with dissection of blood in the aortic wall (media) separating the inner layer from the outer layer resulting in true and false lumens (Fig 8–5).

TYPE A   TYPE B

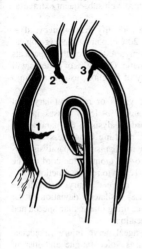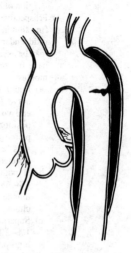

FIG 8–5.
Type A aortic dissections involve the ascending aorta and may extend to the descending aorta. The intimal tear may be in the ascending aorta *(1)*, aortic arch *(2)*, or descending aorta *(3)*. This group includes DeBakey type I (ascending and descending aorta) and DeBakey type II (ascending aorta only). Type B aortic dissections begin distal to the left subclavian artery and involve only the descending aorta (DeBakey type III). (From Miller DL, Stinson EB, Oyer PE, et al: Operative Treatment of Aortic Dissections. *JTCVS* 1979; 78:365—382.)

1. **Pathogenesis:**
   a. Aortic dissections usually occur in the presence of uncontrolled hypertension and especially in patients with an abnormal aortic wall (atherosclerosis, cystic medial necrosis, Marfan's syndrome, coarctation of the aorta, etc.).
   b. Extension of the dissection is dependent upon the rate of rise of aortic pressure dp/dt, the rate and rise of aor-

tic recoil pressure, mean aortic pressure, and the cohesive strength of the aortic wall.

    c. Reentry points (fenestrations) with communications between the true and false lumens may be present.

    d. Occlusion of the aortic branches may result from extrinsic compression (Fig 8–6). Perfusion may be from the true lumen, the false lumen, or both. Retrograde dissection with occlusion of a coronary artery or aortic insufficiency may occur. Rupture into the pericardium may cause cardiac tamponade. Free rupture may also occur.

2. **Classification** (see Fig 8–5).

    a. Type A aortic dissection (DeBakey type I and II) occurs in approximately 67% of patients, and is defined as involvement of the ascending aorta.

    b. Type B aortic dissection (DeBakey type III) is defined as involvement limited to the descending thoracic and abdominal aorta (beginning distal to the left subclavian artery).

3. **Clinical presentation:**

    a. Patients usually experience severe chest pain that is described as stabbing, cutting, or tearing. Classi-

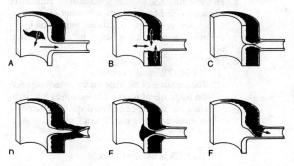

FIG 8–6.
Aortic dissection and branch vessel perfusion. **A,** branch not involved. **B,** branch involved but partial. **C,** Branch occlusion at orifice. **D,** Dissection involving branch with distal occlusion. **E,** thrombosis of branch. **F,** Reentry of dissection into branch. (From Doroghazi RM, Slater EE: *Aortic Dissections.* New York, McGraw–Hill, 1983, p. 198.)

   cally, chest pain is associated with ascending aortic
   involvement, while midscapular back pain is associated with descending aortic involvement. However,
   pain may be reported in the neck, abdomen, flank, or
   any extremity.
   b. Hypotension or cardiac arrest may follow rupture or
   tamponade.
   c. Pulmonary edema with CHF is caused by aortic insufficiency or pump failure secondary to MI.
   d. Approximately 25% of patients present with symptoms of arterial insufficiency such as stroke, visceral
   or renal ischemia or infarction, or a cold pulseless extremity.
4. **Differential diagnosis:**
   a. Acute MI.
   b. Rupture of sinus of Valsalva
   c. CVA.
   d. Acute surgical abdomen.
   e. PE.
   f. Aortoiliac occlusion (acute—embolus or thrombosis).
5. **Diagnosis:**
   a. Physical findings include hypotension, pulmonary
   edema, muffled heart sounds, a murmur of aortic insufficiency, neurologic deficits due to cerebral hypoperfusion, and unequal pulses or BP in the extremities.
   b. ECG:
      1) The ECG is usually normal.
      2) The presence of an acute injury pattern supports
      the diagnosis of myocardial ischemia, but, isch-
      emia can also be caused by dissection extending
      to involve the coronary arteries with subsequent
      occlusion.
   c. CXR.
      1) The CXR is usually abnormal.
      2) Common findings include widened mediastinum
      either superiorly or to the left of the cardiac sil-
      houette, cardiomegaly, aortic arch hump, dispar-
      ity of size between ascending and descending
      thoracic aorta, and displacement of intimal calci-
      fication.

    d. Aortography:
       1) This study is the gold standard and should be obtained as quickly as possible in patients with a characteristic history, physical examination, CXRs, and ECG for an aortic dissection.
       2) Accuracy is approximately 95%.
       3) The study establishes the diagnosis, identifies the site of the intimal tear, delineates the proximal and distal aortic involvement and evaluates for the presence of AI or branch occlusion.
    e. CT and MRI scanning:
       1) These techniques both can establish the diagnosis of aortic dissection in approximately 90% of cases.
       2) CT is used most frequently to differentiate dissection from myocardial ischemia prior to aortography in patients in whom the diagnosis of dissection is thought to be unlikely.
    f. Echocardiography:
       1) Two-dimensional (2-D) echocardiography can establish the presence of pericardial fluid and provide an estimate ventricular function.
       2) Color-flow Doppler can quantitatively assess the degree of aortic insufficiency and can help guide the decision as to whether the aortic valve requires repair or replacement.
       3) Transesophageal echocardiography (TEE) can provide a rapid diagnosis of aortic dissection and may become the imaging modality of choice.

6. Perioperative management.
    a. Monitoring:
       1) A Foley catheter, an intraarterial catheter placed into the extremity with the highest BP, ECG leads, and a CVP or PA catheter are placed.
       2) PA catheters are used liberally in many centers, and is indicated in the patient with LV dysfunction, aortic insufficiency, coronary artery disease, or renal impairment.
    b. Antihypertensive management:
       1) Immediate medical therapy is desired to decrease aortic wall tension and decrease shear forces (dp/dt), preventing extension of the dissection.

2) Treatment with IV sodium nitroprusside and IV β-blockers such as labetalol infusion (200 mg/200 mL D5W; usual starting dose is 1–2 mg/min), or metoprolol (repeated 5-mg doses).

3) Trimethaphan camsylate may be useful in the treatment of refractory hypertension or when thiocyanate toxicity limits the use of nitroprusside.

    a) It is administered as an infusion (500 mg/500 mL D5W; starting dose of 2–3 mg/min).

    b) The head of the bed must be elevated on blocks for trimethaphan to be effective.

4) BP is titrated to the lowest possible pressure that allows continued normal function of the CNS, cardiac, and renal systems.

  c. The IV administration of narcotics and short-acting agents such as midazolam are used to alleviate pain and anxiety.

7. **Treatment.**

  a. Type A aortic dissection:

    1) Surgery is undertaken in almost all patients unless severe neurologic deficit, concurrent malignancy, or other systemic disease is present that would preclude meaningful rehabilitation. In such patients medical therapy is indicated.

    2) Otherwise, patients undergo surgical repair of the ascending aorta with placement of a prosthetic graft via a median sternotomy utilizing CPB. The aortic valve may require resuspension, repair, or replacement.

  b. Type B aortic dissection:

    1) Although controversy exists, the majority of patients are treated medically using an aggressive antihypertensive regimen. Indications for urgent surgical therapy include:

      a) Rupture.

      b) Renal, visceral, or extremity ischemia or infarction.

      c) Persistent pain.

      d) Medically refractory hypertension.

    2) Surgical repair is performed through a posterolateral thoracotomy replacing the most severely affected portion of the aorta with proximal and dis-

TABLE 8–2.

Mortality Following Aortic Surgery

Thoracic aneurysms	
Ascending aorta	5%–15%
Aortic arch	10%–30%
Descending aorta	5%–15%
Thoracoabdominal	10%–40%
Aortic dissection	
Type A	5%–20%
Type B	10%–20%
Abdominal aortic aneurysms	
Elective repair	2%–5% in non–high-risk patients
	5%–20% in high-risk patients
Ruptured AAA	20%–40% with contained leak
	60%–80% with free rupture and renal failure
Aortoiliac occlusive disease	1%–3%

tal obliteration of the false lumen. Mortality following aortic dissection is shown in Table 8–2.

   3) To prevent spinal ischemia during aortic cross-clamping, a shunt (heparin-bonded shunt [Gott], Bio-Medicus pump, or partial CPB) is frequently utilized.

E.   Thoracic and Thoracoabdominal Aneurysms.

The majority of thoracic and thoracoabdominal aneurysms are secondary to atherosclerosis. Other etiologies include trauma, syphilis associated with annuloaortic ectasia, Marfan's syndrome, cystic medial necrosis, and infection (mycotic).

The natural history of thoracic aneurysms parallels that of AAAs. Aneurysms >6 cm and symptomatic aneurysms are more likely to rupture. Five-year survival in patients with thoracic aneurysms is 19%–58%. Rupture is the cause of death in 33%–74% of patients.

   1. **Diagnosis.**
      a. CXR:
          1) Aneurysms are often visualized on routine films. However, a normal CXR does not eliminate the possibility of the presence of an aneurysm.
          2) By plain film, an aneurysm may resemble a mediastinal neoplasm.

    b. CT scanning is useful in diagnosing and following patients with descending thoracic aortic aneurysms, but is less useful in visualizing ascending aortic aneurysms.

    c. MRI scanning is expensive, not widely available, and not readily applicable for emergency evaluations. MRI provides equivalent information to CT with regard to descending aneurysms, and better demonstration of ascending and transverse arch anatomy.

    d. **Aortography remains the gold standard** and can accurately demonstrate the extent of aneurysmal involvement and define the anatomic relationship to major branches.

    e. Echocardiography with Doppler is useful to evaluate degree of aortic insufficiency.

2. **Indications for operation:**

    a. Patients with symptoms due to the aneurysm or an aneurysm >6 cm unless coexisting medical conditions limit the patient's longevity (such as end-stage heart failure or metastatic carcinoma) or increase the operative risks prohibitively.

    b. Evidence of expansion is an indication for repair even in the asymptomatic patient.

3. **Operative treatment:**

    a. Operative therapy is designed to replace the aneurysmal segment with a prosthetic graft. Usually an endoaneurysmal technique is utilized and the vessel wall is wrapped around the graft.

    b. Ascending aneurysms are approached through a median sternotomy, utilizing CPB with RA and femoral artery cannulation. Aortic valve replacement and coronary reimplantation may be necessary.

    c. Arch aneurysms are approached through a median sternotomy or high posterolateral thoracotomy using CPB, and a period of deep hypothermia with either circulatory arrest or very low CPB flow. The arch vessels are reimplanted as a single arterial patch.

    d. Descending thoracic aneurysms are approached via a posterolateral thoracotomy, employing one-lung ventilation (double-lumen ET tube). Shunts or partial (femorofemoral) bypass may be utilized to maintain spinal cord perfusion.

    e. Thoracoabdominal aneurysms are approached through a posterior thoracoabdominal incision, with the abdominal portion performed through a retroperitoneal exposure. Major visceral and intercostal arteries are reimplanted using arterial (Carrel) patches.

F. Abdominal Aortic Aneurysm (AAA).

AAA is defined as a dilatation of the abdominal aorta that is twice its normal size. Over 90% of AAAs are degenerative and related to atherosclerotic changes. Other causes include trauma, syphilis, acute or chronic infections, and anastomotic pseudoaneurysms. Approximately 98% of AAAs are infrarenal. The iliac arteries have aneurysmal involvement in 70% of patients.

1. **Clinical presentation:**
   a. **The majority of patients with an AAA are asymptomatic.**
   b. Symptoms can be due to a leak causing severe back, flank, or abdominal pain.
      1) Back pain can result from retroperitoneal hemorrhage or vertebral body erosion.
      2) Partial small bowel obstructive symptoms can occur owing to the duodenum being stretched over the aneurysm.
      3) GI bleeding can occur as a result of mucosal ulceration or erosion of the aneurysm into the duodenum (rare without previous grafting).
      4) Ureteral obstruction can occur, particularly with inflammatory aneurysms.
      5) Emboli from the mural thrombus can cause extremity ischemia (trash foot).
   c. Rupture of an aneurysm into the vena cava creates an aortocaval fistula manifested by lower extremity edema, CHF, widened pulse pressure, and a continuous abdominal bruit.
2. The **risk of rupture** best correlates with aneurysm size and significantly increases with AAA >6 cm. The 5-year risk of rupture is approximately 10% for a 4-cm aneurysm and 75% for an 8-cm aneurysm.
3. **Preoperative evaluation:**
   a. Radiographic assessment is usually by serial ultrasonography or CT scans. Both techniques reliably estimate aneurysm size as well as proximal and distal

extent. CT scanning is more accurate. Both techniques can identify the presence of an abnormally located kidney.

    b. Aortography is obtained for specific indications:

       1) Renovascular hypertension.

       2) Renal insufficiency.

       3) Significant peripheral vascular disease by history and noninvasive examination.

       4) History of visceral angina.

       5) Suprarenal involvement indicated by prior radiographic studies.

       6) Horseshoe or ectopic kidney to identify accessory renal arteries.

       7) Suspected aneurysmal or occlusive disease involving other vessels such as the femoral or popliteal arteries.

4. Elective repair:

    a. Patients with symptoms or AAA >6 cm should be repaired.

    b. Coexisting life-limiting disease or severe comorbidity factors that make the operative risk prohibitive are relative contraindications (see Table 8–1).

5. Ruptured AAA.

    a. Clinical presentation.

       1) Patients usually present with severe abdominal or flank pain.

       2) Signs and symptoms of blood loss and usually hypotension and shock if free intraperitoneal rupture has occurred.

       3) Rarely, a ruptured aneurysm will manifest GI bleeding or a continuous abdominal bruit indicative of an aortocaval fistula.

    b. Preoperative evaluation:

       1) **Patients with a known AAA or a palpable pulsatile epigastric abdominal mass who present with severe abdominal or flank pain and hypotension should be taken immediately to the OR without waiting for additional studies or resuscitative efforts.**

       2) Patients who have a clinical presentation consistent with contained rupture but who are hemodynamically stable should undergo emergency CT

scanning to establish the presence or absence of extravasation of blood from the aorta. If extravasation is present the patient is taken immediately to the OR.

3) Patients without extravasation of blood and who are without another etiology to explain the abdominal or flank pain are considered to have a symptomatic aneurysm. These have a high rate of rupture and are therefore repaired on an urgent but semielective basis. While being prepared for surgery the patient is admitted to an SICU or well-monitored ward.

G. **Aortoiliac Occlusive Disease.**

 1. **Pathologic considerations:**

   a. Atherosclerosis is usually a generalized disease.

   b. Disease restricted to the terminal aorta and common iliac arteries occurs in approximately 10% of patients with aortoiliac occlusive disease.

   c. Twenty-five percent of patients have disease limited to the aorta and iliacs but not extending below the inguinal ligaments.

   d. Sixty percent to 70% of patients have disease above and below the inguinal ligaments.

   e. Symptoms referable to the aortoiliac component include claudication, usually of the buttocks and thighs, and vasogenic impotence in men (Leriché syndrome).

   f. The presence of ischemic rest pain or tissue gangrene usually indicates concurrent disease below the inguinal ligament.

 2. **Evaluation:**

   a. Physical findings include diminished femoral pulses, bruits over the femoral vessels or lower quadrants of the abdomen, as well as stigmata of tissue ischemia distally.

   b. In the presence of significant disease, the segmental upper thigh Doppler pulse will be low.

   c. The most accurate assessment of hemodynamically significant disease is direct femoral arterial pressure measurement. A pressure gradient compared with central aortic or brachial artery pressure of 5 mm Hg at rest or 15 mm Hg with flow augmentation (papaverine administration, reactive hyperemia, after exercise) is clinically important.

d. Aortobifemoral arteriography with runoff is obtained in patients in whom revascularization is planned.

3. **Indication for surgical intervention:**
   a. Ischemic rest pain, gangrene, nonhealing ulcers.
   b. Claudication that prevents employment or interferes with lifestyle.
   c. Patients with peripheral thromboemboli originating from the atherosclerotic plaques undergo bypass and exclusion of the involved segment.

4. **Operative procedures:** Long-term patency is most dependent on extent of outflow disease, particularly with regard to patency of the SFA.
   a. Aortobifemoral bypass is the most common, most durable reconstruction method and provides the best physiologic results. Five-year patency is approximately 80%–90%.
   b. Axillobifemoral or axillofemoral bypass is useful in high-risk patients (see Table 8–1). Long-term patency is much higher with bifemoral bypass. Patency at 5 years is approximately 75% if the SFA is patent, and 35%–50% if it is occluded.
   c. Femorofemoral bypass is applicable in patients with unilateral iliac disease.

H. **Postoperative Care After Aortic Surgery.**
   1. **Monitoring:**
      a. Invasive monitoring using continuous measurement of arterial BP, ECG, CVP, or PA pressure is continued in the SICU.
      b. In patients with coronary artery disease, impaired LV function, renal insufficiency, moderate to severe impairment of pulmonary function, or postoperative hypotension not readily responsive to volume loading, a PA catheter is used.
      c. Pulse oximetry, mixed-venous oximetric recordings from the PA catheter, end-tidal CO_2 (intubated patients) are also useful.
   2. SICU admission studies include CBC, electrolytes, BUN, creatinine, ABG, ECG, PT, PTT, and CXR (line placement, ET tube placement, and rule out pneumothorax).

3. Patients returning to the SICU are frequently hypothermic ($<35°$ C) and require aggressive rewarming using heating circuits on the ventilator, warming blankets, overbed heaters, higher room temperature, and warmed IV fluids.

4. **Vascular status:**

   a. Upon arrival in the SICU, the patient's lower extremities should be evaluated. Particularly in the reconstructed limb, color, capillary refill, motor, sensation, and pulses should be checked every 1–2 hours during the first 24 hours after surgery.

   b. Measurement of Doppler pressures and comparison to preoperative values is useful. If femoral or tibial disease is present, hemodynamic improvement may be delayed 12–24 hours. Patency of bifurcated aortic grafts is determined by palpation of femoral pulses. Patency of extraanatomic grafts is evaluated by direct palpation or, in obese individuals, by Doppler study.

   c. Patients who are hypothermic or who have a low CO may have extremities that appear ischemic (appearance of extremities is usually symmetric) not requiring operative intervention. Aggressive correction of the hypothermia and augmentation of CO is essential.

   d. Persistence of the circulatory abnormalities requires evaluation using either arteriography or reoperation.

5. **Renal function:**

   a. It is imperative to maintain a urinary output (UO) of at least 0.5–1.0 mL/kg/hr to protect renal function. **The most common cause of low UO is hypovolemia.**

   b. Full utilization of invasive monitoring to optimize the determinants of CO, particularly preload, is essential.

   c. In patients with renal insufficiency, care must be taken to avoid nephrotoxic insults of which prolonged hypotension is the most common and severe. The postoperative use of low-dose dopamine (1–3 μg/kg/min) may be helpful.

6. **Hemorrhage:**

   a. A hematologic and coagulation profile should be obtained immediately postoperatively.

b. With any evidence of bleeding, abnormal coagulation parameters are corrected by appropriate administration of platelets, FFP, or cryoprecipitate.

c. An elevated PTT may reflect heparinization which can be reversed using protamine after determining ACT.

d. It is useful to monitor abdominal girth when bleeding is suspected.

7. **Analgesia:**

a. Postoperative pain relief can be obtained using bolus administration of narcotics, PCA, epidural administration of either narcotics or local anesthetic using bolus therapy or continuous infusion, or a continuous infusion of narcotic (see Chapter 21).

b. The IV route for bolus administration of narcotics is preferred in the SICU because of better titration of pain relief, more reliable volumes of distributions, and fewer overdosing side effects.

8. **Cardiac:**

a. In patients with important cardiac disease, the Swan-Ganz catheter is used to optimize cardiac performance by assisting in determining optimal preload and afterload (see Chapter 2, pp 20–26).

b. In patients with inadequate CO or hypotension, the Swan-Ganz catheter can aid in determining whether the etiology is hypovolemia (volume infusion), vasogenic (vasoconstrictors such as phenylephrine or norepinephrine), or myocardial failure (inotropic agents).

c. Patients with coronary artery disease are usually maintained on IV nitroglycerin (0.5–3.0 µg/kg/min).

9. Pulmonary:

a. Vigorous pulmonary toilet is important following aortic procedures, particularly in obese patients or those with pulmonary disease. Early mobilization improves pulmonary toilet.

b. Patients with pulmonary insufficiency receiving β-agonist agents and aminophylline preoperatively should be maintained on them postoperatively. These agents should be considered in patients with postoperative pulmonary dysfunction.

    c. Careful attention to fluid management using cardiac filling pressures provided by a PA catheter minimizes postoperative respiratory difficulties.

    d. Postoperative ventilation:

        1) Most patients undergoing procedures on the intrathoracic aorta are maintained on mechanical ventilation the first postoperative night.

        2) Most patients undergoing procedures on the abdominal aorta can be extubated either in the OR or in the early postoperative period, particularly if an epidural catheter is in place.

    e. **Contraindications to early extubation:**

        1) Hypothermia (body temperature $<35°$ C).

        2) Continued hemorrhage, large intraoperative blood loss, or large volume of fluid administration.

        3) Hemodynamic instability.

        4) Inadequate pulmonary mechanics.

        5) Inadequate oxygenation or ventilation.

10. Hypertension:

    a. Systolic BP is maintained <170 mm Hg to reduce stress on suture lines and limit bleeding.

    b. BP can be controlled in the immediate postoperative period with either IV sodium nitroprusside or nitroglycerin titrated to the desired BP.

11. Antibiotics:

    a. Infections following vascular procedures cause grave complications. They can lead to generalized sepsis, anastomotic dehiscence, anastomotic aneurysm, or prosthetic graft infection.

    b. Infected grafts must be removed, frequently necessitating extraanatomic bypass or amputation.

    c. Prophylactic antibiotics are routinely used following vascular procedures; prospective randomized trials have demonstrated that cefazolin is useful in decreasing wound and prosthetic infections in vascular reconstructive operations.

        1) The benefit of prophylactic cefazolin extends 24–48 hours postoperatively.

        2) It is prudent to continue prophylaxis longer in patients with indwelling lines and catheters which pose an additional risk of bacteremia. Generally

these lines and antibiotics are discontinued 3–5 days postoperatively.

d. Surgical incisions may become infected from exogenous sources up to 3 or 4 days postoperatively; incisions should be covered with sterile gauze dressings until this time.

e. Any incisional drainage should be cultured and catheter tips should be routinely cultured at time of removal.

f. Staphylococcus is the organism most frequently cultured from vascular incisions and its source is usually the skin. Axillary and groin incisions are the most frequently infected sites owing to the proximity of the axillary and femoral vessels to the skin.

I. **Postoperative Complications of Aortic Surgery.**

Morbidity and mortality may be high following aortic surgery (see Table 8–2). Complications are greatest following emergency procedures and in high-risk patients (see Table 8–1).

1. Hemorrhage.

a. Thoracic aorta procedures:

1) Bleeding may occur from suture lines, porous graft material, raw surface areas, pulmonary parenchyma, and a variety of vessels present within the operative field.

2) Aggressive and rapid correction of coagulation defects is essential.

3) Prevention of significant hypertension is important in minimizing blood loss and suture line disruption.

4) Patients with excessive blood loss, chest tube output >500 mL in the first hour or >1,000 mL over 4 hours after correction of clotting deficiencies should undergo reoperation.

b. Abdominal aortic or iliac artery procedures:

1) Significant bleeding is rare following abdominal aortic procedures and hemostasis should be assured prior to closing the abdomen.

2) In the immediate postoperative period if there is a rapid fall in Hct, progressive abdominal distention or flank discoloration, or unexplained shock, bleeding must be considered as a cause.

       3) Blood replacement should be instituted immediately and the patient's coagulation profile evaluated. Platelet or coagulation defects should be corrected, but if hemorrhage persists, it may be necessary to return to the OR.

2. **Hypotension:**

   a. Hypotension not due to hemorrhage or inadequate blood replacement may occur following prolonged aortic cross-clamping.

   b. Etiologic factors include inadequate preoperative or intraoperative hydration, dilation of the distal arterial tree during cross-clamping due to ischemia, with release of lactic acid and toxic metabolites from the lower extremities following unclamping, and transfusion or drug reaction.

   c. Hypotension is relatively rare and can be prevented by good preoperative and intraoperative fluid management and expeditious aortic surgery.

   d. Treatment consists of fluid replacement and correction of acidosis and hyperkalemia.

   e. MI with low CO may also be a cause of postoperative hypotension. Invasive monitoring must be instituted if hypotension fails to respond to initial resuscitative efforts.

3. **Renal failure:**

   a. Owing to the high incidence of diabetes mellitus, hypertension, and renal artery occlusive disease in this patient population, postoperative renal failure is a recognized complication of aortic surgery. The risk of renal dysfunction increases if suprarenal aortic cross-clamping is required.

   b. Perioperative management should aim for prophylaxis of renal failure by preventing prerenal azotemia through appropriate fluid management aided by invasive monitoring.

   c. Patients with a prolonged cross-clamp time, suspected blood transfusion reaction, or with severely ischemic extremities are at risk for muscle necrosis with release of myoglobin following reperfusion.

       1) Some patients may require fasciotomy to release a compartment compression syndrome.

2) These patients are at risk of ATN secondary to myoglobinuria and should be treated with mannitol 25 g IV and bicarbonate to alkalinize the urine and prevent precipitation of myoglobin in the renal tubules.

d. Low-dose infusion of dopamine $(1-3\mu g/kg/min)$ may improve renal perfusion and function in the perioperative period.

e. Ureteral obstruction in the early postoperative period can be caused by edema, ischemia due to interruption of blood supply, direct surgical trauma, or compression of the ureter between the graft and the iliac artery.

f. Localized fibrosis or compression by the graft are the primary causes of late ureteral obstruction.

1) Identification of hydronephrosis can be made by ultrasound, CT, or IVP.

2) The exact level of the obstruction is determined by retrograde pyelography.

3) Progressive ureteral dilation, recurrent pyelonephritis, and renal deterioration are indications for operative intervention.

4. **Peripheral vascular complications:**

a. **Peripheral vascular insufficiency:**

1) Distal thrombosis or embolization may cause arterial occlusion which should be recognized and treated in the OR.

2) Occasionally this is diagnosed in the SICU by the loss of previously present pulses or the absence of flow by Doppler examination.

3) Such patients need to return to the OR for Fogarty thrombectomy or embolectomy or repair of an intimal flap. Delay in diagnosis or treatment risks myonecrosis, limb loss, and renal failure.

b. **Distal emboli:**

1) Microembolization of the foot (trash foot) is manifest by cutaneous ischemia despite the presence of palpable pulses.

2) The skin is partly discolored or a mottled blue color with associated sluggish refill.

3) Frequently, the involved area is very painful and tender.

    4) If collateral flow is adequate, healing will occur; otherwise, progression to gangrene ensues. The feet should be observed for several weeks prior to amputation to allow all potential tissue recovery.

    5) Treatment with heparin or dextran has been advocated, although its efficacy has not been documented.

    6) In patients with diffuse emboli and loss of pedal pulses, exploration of the tibial vessels with embolectomy may be beneficial.

    7) Owing to the importance of collateral circulation on healing, avoidance of low CO or hypotension is crucial.

  c. **Compartment syndrome:**

    1) Following reperfusion of a severely ischemic extremity, muscle edema and swelling can occur.

    2) In the fascial compartments of the lower legs muscle edema can lead to elevated pressure and venous or arterial obstruction.

    3) Distal ischemia and myonecrosis with release of myoglobin can occur.

    4) Physical signs include tense painful swelling of the lower leg, absent pedal pulses, and neurologic dysfunction.

    5) If the compartment syndrome is suspected, compartmental pressure should be measured. A compartment pressure >30 mm Hg is an indication for fasciotomy.

    6) Elective fasciotomy may also be considered following reperfusion of severely threatened extremities.

5. GI complications.

  a. Ileus or diarrhea:

    1) Prolonged intestinal ileus in not uncommon in patients undergoing abdominal aortic procedures.

    2) Often diarrhea occurs prior to recovery of complete intestinal function. Attention to the possibility of gastric distention despite continued diarrhea is important to prevent aspirations, and NG decompression may be necessary.

  b. Ischemic colitis:

    1) Ischemic colitis occurs in approximately 2% of patients, although prospective studies examining

all patients with sigmoidoscopy report an incidence of 4%–8%.

    a) The incidence is twice as great for procedures done for aneurysmal disease as compared to occlusive disease.

    b) The incidence is >10% following repair of a ruptured AAA.

2) Ischemia of the sigmoid colon may occur following ligation of the IMA if inadequate collaterals are present.

    a) If recognized intraoperatively, the IMA should be reimplanted onto the graft.

    b) If colonic ischemia persists, the bowel should be exteriorized (Mikulicz procedure). Resection must be avoided to prevent contamination of the graft.

3) Clinical presentation:

    a) The most common symptom is diarrhea usually within 24–48 hours of surgery.

    b) Bloody diarrhea is an ominous sign.

    c) Other manifestations include left-sided abdominal pain out of proportion to the usual postoperative pain, unexplained leukocytosis, refractory metabolic acidosis, falling platelet count, fevers, progressive abdominal distention, and/or marked fluid sequestration.

4) Evaluation:

    a) Supine and right lateral decubitus films are obtained to evaluate for pneumatosis or increasing intraperitoneal air.

    b) Emergency endoscopy is performed. The involved segment is usually within 40 cm of the anal verge. Once the diagnosis is established the endoscopy is terminated.

    c) Ischemia may be limited to the mucosa, which usually heals without sequelae; partial thickness, which heals with fibrosis; or transmural, which leads to gangrene and perforation. The time to resolution of reversible lesions is 1–2 weeks.

d) The patient is followed carefully with close monitoring of vital signs, abdominal symptoms and signs, serial ABG, WBC count, platelet count, serial KUBs, and repeat endoscopy.

e) Broad-spectrum antibiotics and bowel rest with NG decompression are instituted.

f) Progressive clinical deterioration requires removal of all involved bowel, and if graft contamination has occurred, removal of the graft and extraanatomic bypass.

6. **Neurologic complications.**

a. Stroke:

1) Embolization of air or particulate matter may occur during any procedure on the ascending aorta or aortic arch.

2) Inadequate CNS protection during procedures on the aortic arch may result in cerebral injury.

a) Most procedures are performed during hypothermic circulatory arrest at core temperatures of 15–18° C.

b) The safe time period for circulatory arrest in adults is 20–40 minutes.

b. Paraplegia:

1) Paraplegia due to spinal cord injury occurs in 3%–12% of patients undergoing procedures on the descending aorta, but in <1% of patients undergoing infrarenal AAA repairs.

2) Procedures for extensive thoracoabdominal lesions and dissections have a higher incidence of paraplegia. The onset of paraplegia can occur during the postoperative period, usually following a period of hypotension.

3) The incidence is higher in patients operated upon as an emergency.

4) Although half of patients make some neurologic recovery, full recovery is unusual.

7. **Pulmonary insufficiency:**

a. Acute respiratory insufficiency develops in 3%–5% of patients undergoing procedures on the thoracic aorta (Chapter 7).

b. Etiologies include blood product utilization, adverse effects of CPB, hemodilution, protamine reaction, contusion, and hemorrhage of the lung due to retraction.

8. **Aortic injury** may occur secondary to occlusive clamp injury, at the site of vent or cannula placement, cardioplegia needle site, and at suture lines, and can result in a variety of complications including hemorrhage, dissection due to separation of layers of the aortic wall, and pseudoaneurysm.

9. The **mortality for aortic surgery** depends on multiple factors including specific operations performed, emergent or nonemergent nature, and patient characteristics (see Table 8–2).

J.   **Infrainguinal Vascular Occlusive Disease.**

1. **Acute arterial insufficiency.**

a. Acute arterial occlusion is most commonly due to intrinsic obstruction secondary to emboli or thrombosis. Early diagnosis and treatment is imperative to prevent limb loss and the systemic effects of tissue ischemia. Nerve and muscle tolerate ischemia poorly, and permanent damage may result with as little as 8 hours of ischemia.

1) **Emboli are the most common cause of acute vascular occlusion in the lower extremity.**

a) In 80%–90% of cases, the heart is the source of emboli. Atrial fibrillation is the most common cause, but cardiac emboli can also be seen with a recent MI, LV aneurysm, valvular disease, or atrial myxoma.

b) Noncardiac sources are less common but include proximal large vessel disease (aneurysm, atherosclerotic plaques) and paradoxical embolism.

c) The most common sites of occlusion in the lower extremity are at the femoral and popliteal artery bifurcations.

2) **Thrombosis usually occurs in atherosclerotic vessels at sites of severe stenosis.**

a) Low flow states (CHF, shock, dehydration), intimal damage (intraplaque hemorrhage, trauma), and hypercoagulable states (polycythemia) predispose these areas to thrombosis.

   b) The signs and symptoms of acute occlusion may not be as severe as seen with emboli because of the previous development of collateral circulation around these stenotic areas.

b. Preoperative evaluation: The signs and symptoms are characterized by the "five P's" of vascular occlusion: pain, pallor, pulselessness, paresthesia, paralysis.

   1) History:
      a) Acute vs. chronic lower extremity symptoms.
      b) Preexisting cardiac disease.
      c) Atherosclerotic vascular disease (claudication, aneurysm).

   2) Physical examination:
      a) Presence of pulses, bruits, aneurysm.
      b) The temperature and any color change of the skin should be noted. Waxy and white skin implies patent arterioles, while cyanotic, blotchy skin implies occluded arterioles and skin necrosis.
      c) Neurologic examination to assess sensory and motor function.
      d) Doppler flow signals and pressures.

   3) Laboratory, CXR, ECG:
      a) CXR to assess heart size.
      b) ECG to assess rhythm and presence of ischemic changes.
      c) CBC, electrolytes, BUN, creatinine, PT, PTT.
      d) Urinalysis and urine myoglobin.
      e) If hypercoagulability is suspected, blood for protein C and S levels, a DIC screen, and a thrombosis panel should be obtained prior to anticoagulation.

   4) Special studies:
      a) **If acute occlusive disease is suspected, the most important aspect of management is early intervention to prevent tissue and limb loss.**

b) Often, an arteriogram will only delay necessary operative intervention. However, if there is a question of diagnosis, an arteriogram can help define the area of occlusion.

c) Peripheral arteriogram can be performed in the OR to facilitate early intervention and to evaluate results.

c. Management (Table 8–3):

1) The key is prompt intervention. Surgical options include thrombectomy or embolectomy, fasciotomy (to prevent compartment syndrome), and amputation. Nonoperative management includes heparinization and thrombolytic therapy.

2) Thrombolytic therapy (streptokinase, urokinase, tPA, either as a primary modality or as an adjunct to catheter embolectomy (intraoperative, intraarterial infusion), is increasing in popularity.

a) Indications: documented diagnosis of recent thrombosis (<7 days)

b) Contraindications.

i) Absolute: active internal bleeding, recent (<2 months) CVA or intracranial

TABLE 8–3.

Heparin and Thrombolytic Therapy in Acute Vascular Occlusion

Drug	Dosage	Monitoring
Heparin sodium*	Load: 5,000 units IV Infusion: 800–1,500 units/hr IV	PTT (1.5–2.5 × normal) Hct, platelet count
Streptokinase*	Load: 250,000 IU/30 min Infusion: 100,000 IU/hr × 24–72 hr	TT (2–5 × normal) PTT, PT, FDP‡ Fibrinogen Hct, platelet count
Urokinase*†	Load: 300,000 IU/10 min Infusion: 300,000 IU/hr × 12 hr	Same as for streptokinase
Tissue plasminogen activator†	Infusion: 0.5–0.1 mg/kg/hr × 1–8 hr (intraarterial)	No specific recommendation

*Recommendations for 68-kg adult.
†Not FDA-approved for this indication.
‡Fibrin degradation products.

bleed, recent (<10 days) major surgery, obstetric procedure, organ biopsy, GI bleed, trauma, severe hypertension.

 ii) Relative: minor trauma, high likelihood of left heart thrombus, endocarditis, pregnancy, age >75 years, diabetic hemorrhagic retinopathy, hemostatic defects, recent CPR.

 c) Complications: bleeding (superficial or internal).

 d) Management (see Table 8–3):

  i) Monitor thrombin time (TT), PTT, PT, platelet count, fibrinogen, and Hct pre-infusion, 3 hours after thrombolytics are administered and as appropriate thereafter.

  ii) Begin heparin infusion (without a loading dose) 3–4 hours after thrombolytics are discontinued.

  iii) Monitor vital signs during and after the infusion.

  iv) Avoid IM injections or arterial punctures. Patients usually require SICU monitoring.

2. **Chronic arterial insufficiency:**

 a. Chronic insufficiency is usually secondary to atherosclerotic vascular disease, which predisposes to thrombosis and may become manifest as limb ischemia during low flow or hypercoaguable states.

 b. Evaluation:

  1) The preoperative evaluation is most often performed outside of the SICU. A careful history and physical examination should be performed to determine the severity of the disease.

  2) Noninvasive Doppler studies complement physical examination.

  3) ABIs help to assess the severity of the vascular insufficiency: <0.6—claudication; <0.2—rest pain; absent—impending gangrene

  4) An absolute ankle systolic pressure <40 mm Hg is consistent with limb-threatening ischemia and poor wound healing.

3. **Postoperative management:**
   a. Following revascularization patients are monitored in an SICU where frequent observation of the limb and evaluation of hemodynamic status is possible.
   b. **Coronary artery disease is the leading cause of postoperative morbidity and mortality.** Hemodynamic monitoring and optimization of cardiac function is imperative in the immediate postoperative period.
   c. Limb perfusion should be assessed frequently in the first 24 hours postoperatively. Evaluate for the five P's.
   d. Doppler ultrasound can be used to evaluate distal perfusion.
   e. Graft infections carry an extremely high morbidity and mortality and antibiotic prophylaxis should be begun preoperatively and continued postoperatively until sources of bacteremia (i.e., indwelling catheters) are removed.
   f. IV fluids are administered to maintain renal perfusion. Fluid management should be guided by urinary output, BP, HR, and invasive monitoring techniques (arterial line, CVP, or PA catheters).
   g. Antiplatelet agents are started in the early postoperative period to maintain graft patency. Heparin is not routinely used following revascularization because of the risk of bleeding and wound hematoma.

4. **Complications:**
   a. Graft occlusion: Intensive monitoring postoperatively is important. A loss of a previously palpable pulse, change in the Doppler signal, or severe pain not relieved with narcotics should raise the suspicion of graft occlusion and warrant reexploration.
   b. Wound hematoma is a potential source of infection as well as extrinsic compression of the graft and may require evacuation.
   c. Graft infection:
      1) The most common organism is *Staphylococcus aureus* followed by *Staphylococcus epidermidis* and *Escherichia coli*.
      2) The risk of infection is lowered by the use of perioperative antibiotics, careful operative tech-

nique, good hemostasis, and antibiotic prophylaxis during episodes of suspected bacteremia.

   d. Compartment syndrome:

     1) Increased capillary permeability and tissue hyperemia following revascularization of the severely ischemic limb can lead to tissue edema and subsequent compartment syndrome. The edema within the fascial compartments can lead to elevated compartmental pressures with subsequent vascular, neural, and muscular injury.

     2) This entity presents as severe lower extremity pain followed by loss of motor and sensory function in the foot. The fascial compartments are tense and compartment pressures are elevated.

     3) Compartment pressures over 30 mm Hg impair tissue perfusion and may lead to muscle necrosis and nerve injury. Muscle necrosis can cause myoglobinuria and ARF. Patients must be kept well hydrated and the urine alkalinized to prevent renal tubular injury.

     4) Four-compartment fasciotomy should be performed as soon as compartment syndrome is suspected. Impaired perfusion can lead to permanent nerve and muscle injury within 8 hours.

     5) Patients with compartment syndrome and muscle necrosis are at risk for acidosis, hyperkalemia, and renal failure. Management should include hemodynamic monitoring, hydration, maintenance of UO >50 mL/hr, treatment of acidosis and hyperkalemia, and alkalinization of urine.

K. Other Vascular Problems.

   1. Peripheral aneurysms:

     a. Ninety percent of peripheral aneurysms are of the popliteal or femoral arteries. Popliteal artery aneurysms are the most common. Subclavian and upper extremity aneurysms are relatively rare.

     b. Atherosclerotic vascular disease is the most common cause of peripheral aneurysms. Traumatic, mycotic, syphilitic, anastomotic, and pseudoaneurysms occur much less frequently.

     c. There is a high incidence (60%–85%) of multiple aneurysms (including AAAs) in patients with femoral and popliteal aneurysms. Bilateral aneurysms can be demonstrated in 50%–75% of cases.

d. Complications of untreated peripheral aneurysms include thrombosis, distal embolization, expansion with compression of adjacent nerves or veins, and rupture. Thromboembolic complications predominate and can be limb-threatening.

e. The diagnosis can be made by careful history and physical examination. Ultrasound is an effective screening test. Aortic, iliac, femoral, and distal arteriograms are required preoperatively to define the anatomy and to rule out associated aneurysms.

f. Preoperative evaluation should also focus on diffuse atherosclerotic disease, including coronary artery disease, cerebrovascular disease, and peripheral vascular disease.

g. Aneurysmectomy and arterial reconstruction is the treatment of choice for arterial aneurysms.

h. Postoperative care usually involves management in the SICU:
   1) Evaluate distal perfusion hourly.
   2) Examine wound for evidence of hematoma formation.
   3) Hemodynamic monitoring in patients with associated atherosclerotic disease.
   4) Prophylactic antibiotic coverage.

2. **Arteriovenous fistula:**
   a. These may be congenital or acquired. Acquired fistulas are most often secondary to injury of adjacent arteries and veins, but can also be a result of neoplasm, infection, or degenerative changes in atherosclerotic aneurysms. The most common cause is surgical creation for hemodialysis assess.
   b. Local effects include a bruit or thrill, aneurysmal dilation, venous hypertension with pulsating veins, and edema formation.
   c. Systemic effects include increased pulse rate, increased CO, increased blood volume, enlarged cardiac size, and increased pulse pressure.
   d. Diagnosis is made by history and physical examination, Doppler flow and pulsed Doppler studies, plethysmography, and arteriography.

e. Complications include CHF, venous hypertension, ischemia distal to the fistula, and local degenerative changes.

f. Arteriovenous fistulas rarely close spontaneously and therefore surgical intervention is employed to prevent potential complications. Direct closure with restoration of arterial and venous continuity is the procedure of choice. Selective intraarterial embolization may also be useful.

g. Postoperative management includes elevation of the limb to promote venous return and frequent evaluation for signs of distal ischemia.

IV. MESENTERIC OCCLUSIVE DISEASE.
A. Pathophysiology.

1. Compromise of the blood supply to the bowel occurs through stenosis or occlusion of the celiac axis, SMA, or IMA.

2. Owing to the abundant collateral circulation of the bowel, vascular compromise occurs only when two of the three major vessels are affected.

3. The most common causes of acute mesenteric ischemia are embolism and thrombosis; less common causes include low CO syndrome, shock, vasopressor administration, aortic dissection, and digitalis administration (controversial).

4. The most common cause of chronic mesenteric ischemia is atherosclerosis; less common causes are celiac artery entrapment syndrome and radiation arteritis.

5. As with atherosclerosis in other anatomic locations, lesions of the celiac axis, SMA, and IMA tend to occur in the ostia or main channels of the vessels.

6. Inadequate perfusion of small bowel produces pain via the splanchnic sensory nerves.

7. Because O_2 consumption of the bowel increases following meals, the abdominal pain is often postprandial producing "intestinal angina" and "food fear."

8. Chronic food fear results in weight loss in the majority of patients.

B. Diagnosis.

1. Acute mesenteric ischemia.
   a. **Acute mesenteric ischemia is a surgical emergency.**

    b. **Diagnosis is difficult and requires a high index of suspicion.**

    c. It occurs almost exclusively in the elderly or infirm. A significant number of cases are seen in the intensive care population.

    d. Risk factors include previous MI, cardiac surgery, other evidence of generalized atherosclerosis, dysrhythmia, cardiac failure, and history of intestinal angina. The syndrome should be suspected in all patients with low CO syndrome and abdominal pain.

    e. All patients have abdominal pain, often crampy and sudden in onset, which may be associated with sudden bowel evacuation (often bloody and massive) or vomiting, or both.

    f. **The classic physical sign is abdominal pain out of proportion to physical examination.** Other signs are late and include distention, rigidity, and hypotension.

    g. Laboratory values are nonspecific and include hemoconcentration, hyperamylasemia, metabolic acidosis, and hyperphosphatemia.

    h. Plain radiographs are of little value. The classic finding is pneumatosis intestinalis (gas in the bowel wall) but it occurs late and usually indicates nonsalvageability.

    i. Angiography confirms the diagnosis but should not delay therapy and should be reserved for stable patients in whom the diagnosis is in question.

2. Chronic mesenteric ischemia:

    a. Risk factors include advanced age and generalized atherosclerosis. Virtually all patients with chronic mesenteric ischemia will have evidence of atherosclerotic disease elsewhere.

    b. Abdominal pain is a *sine qua non*. Pain is dull and achy, located in the midabdomen or epigastrium, frequently radiating to the back. Pain rarely lasts more than 1 hour following meals and often correlates with the amount of food ingested (intestinal angina).

    c. Weight loss is a common sign produced by the patient's food fear. Intestinal malabsorption may produce diarrhea.

    d. Laboratory tests are unrewarding.

    e. Angiography is essential for diagnosis and allows for the planning of revascularization. However, it must be noted that many patients have asymptomatic atherosclerotic involvement of the mesenteric circulation.

C.   Preoperative Preparation.

    1. Preparation of patients undergoing revascularization for chronic mesenteric ischemia should follow guidelines for generalized aortic surgery. The major source of morbidity and mortality is cardiac; a low threshold for MUGA scanning and catheterization is warranted.

    2. A suspected diagnosis of acute mesenteric ischemia in an unstable patient should be followed by immediate operative exploration. Further diagnostic evaluation delays definitive therapy and compromises outcome.

    3. The stable patient in whom the diagnosis is entertained may undergo preoperative arteriography for confirmation and to expedite revascularization.

D.   Operative Procedures.

    1. Acute mesenteric ischemia:

        a. Treatment should be individualized depending on the integrity of the bowel and anatomy of the lesions.

        b. Nonviable bowel should be resected.

        c. Viable bowel should be revascularzied with a combination of thromboembolectomy, endarterectomy, and autogenous vein bypass grafting.

        d. Bowel continuity can be established by reanastomosis or creation of enterostomies. Creation of temporary enterostomies has the advantage of allowing inspection of the mucosal ends of the resection. A second procedure is required for takedown.

        e. Some advocate reexploration after 24 hours to assess the quality of the revascularization and the integrity of the remaining bowel.

    2. Chronic mesenteric ischemia:

        a. Revascularization of all stenotic or occluded arteries (when feasible) produces the best results.

        b. The preferred conduit is autogenous vein although synthetic prostheses are also acceptable.

E.   Postoperative Management.

    1. Postoperative management is similar to care following other procedures on the abdominal aorta

2. If ischemic or threatened bowel is present after revascularization a second-look procedure should be planned at 24 hours to determine viability of the involved segments.
3. If small areas of bowel become necrotic, perforation with formation on an intraabdominal abscess or enterocutaneous fistula may occur.

V.   PERCUTANEOUS TRANSLUMINAL ANGIOPLASTY (PTA).

A.   Therapeutic Applications.

PTA is most successful treating single stenotic lesions that are short in length. Multiple lesions, occlusions, and long stenoses are associated with poorer patency rates. Indications for PTA are the same as for surgical revascularization: ischemic rest pain, gangrene, nonhealing ulcers, lifestyle-limiting claudication.

1. Iliac artery:
   a. The best results have been obtained with PTA of iliac stenoses.
   b. Technical success is achieved in 85%–95% of patients, with 3-year patency of 78%–89%.
   c. PTA of iliac occlusions appears to have a high rate of embolic complications.
2. Femoral and popliteal arteries: Technical success is achieved in 70%–95% of patients with 3-year patency rates of 43%–84%.
3. Infrapopliteal arteries:
   a. Because vasospasm is more likely, and thrombosis can result in limb loss, PTA of infrapopliteal vessels is limited to threatened extremities.
   b. Clinical success at 2–3 years is usually 50%–60%; however, recent series report success in 70%–80% of patients.
4. Renal artery:
   a. PTA of fibrodysplastic lesions is technically successful in 85%–95% of patients, with a clinical benefit achieved in over 80%.
   b. Technical success treating atherosclerotic lesions is more variable and less favorable (37%–90%).
   c. Ostial lesions are not amenable to PTA.
   d. Clinical benefit occurs in ~60% of patients.

     5. Coarctation of the aorta:

       a. Early success is achievable in almost all patients. However, late complications of restenosis and especially aneurysm formation limit the efficacy of PTA for the treatment of native aortic coarctation.

       b. Balloon dilatation of recurrent coarctation following surgical repair is more successful and may be the procedure of choice.

     6. Hemodialysis access fistula:

       a. Early technical success is 80%–90%.

       b. Six-month and 1-year patency rates are 40%–60% and 30%–45%, respectively.

     7. Subclavian artery: Technical success is achievable in 80%–90% of patients with 4-year patency rates of 80%.

     8. Vein grafts: success has been limited.

B.   **Pre-PTA Patient Management.**

All patients undergoing PTA should be prepared for possible general anesthesia which may be required to treat complications.

     1. Obtain CBC, electrolytes, PT, PTT, ECG, CXR, BUN, creatinine, urinalysis.

     2. Patients with a contrast dye allergy require a course of corticosteroids prior to the procedure.

     3. IV hydration is important to minimize adverse renal effects.

     4. Examine vessels of the affected extremity with measurement of segmental Doppler pressures (see section II).

C.   **Post-PTA Patient Management.**

     1. Serial vascular examinations of the extremity treated with PTA are performed.

       a. Evidence of extremity ischemia or change in the distal pulses indicates the need for reevaluation of the extremity with arteriography or operative exploration.

       b. Early intervention using vasodilators to treat spasm, and thrombolytics in conjunction with repeat PTA is frequently successful.

     2. Examination of the femoral artery access site:

       a. Serial examinations are performed with attention to the size of the hematoma, auscultation for bruits indicative of a pseudoaneurysm or arteriovenous fistula, presence of a pulse in the femoral artery, and adequacy of circulation in the distal extremity.

      b. Ultrasound can be useful to evaluate for pseudoaneurysm or arteriovenous fistulas.

    3. Renal:

      a. Ensure adequate urine output (>0.5–1.0 mL/kg/hr) by administration of IV fluids with continuation until the urine specific gravity is <1.025 to limit renal injury.

      b. A post-PTA measurement of serum BUN and creatinine is obtained.

    4. Bleeding:

      a. A post-PTA Hct is obtained. If there is evidence of continued blood loss, serial Hcts are obtained.

      b. Transfusion and operative control of bleeding may be necessary.

      c. **Suprainguinal arterial punctures may bleed into the retroperitoneum. These are difficult to control by applying pressure, and are more likely to require operative hemostasis.**

D. Complications.

    1. PTA is associated with a complication rate averaging 5%–10%. Mortality occurs in 0%–2% of patients and usually reflects the extent of atherosclerosis in other vascular beds, particularly the coronary circulation. Diffuse thromboemboli with mesenteric and renal artery occlusion can complicate PTA leading to death. Complications of PTA can be categorized to those occurring at the puncture site, at the angioplasty site, distal to the angioplasty site, and systemic.

    2. Puncture site:

      a. Puncture site complications include hematoma, thrombosis, false aneurysm, infection, and arteriovenous fistula.

      b. The most common complication, hematoma formation, occurs most frequently in association with obesity, hypertension, and anticoagulation use.

      c. Femoral artery punctures above the inguinal ligament may lead to retroperitoneal hematomas; the diagnosis of this complication requires a high index of suspicion.

      d. Hematomas occurring after axillary artery access can cause brachial nerve injury and require early evacuation.

3. Angioplasty site:
   a. Angioplasty site complications include subintimal dissection, perforation, rupture, occlusion of adjacent or branch vessels, spasm, and thrombosis.
   b. Vasospasm most frequently complicates PTA of renal, brachiocephalic, popliteal, and infrapopliteal vessels, predisposing these vessels to occlusion.
   c. Pharmacologic treatment with calcium channel blockers, lidocaine, and nitroglycerin is useful in the prevention and treatment of vasospasm.
   d. Treatment of vessel thrombosis is dependent on the amount of collateral blood flow present.
      1) If adequate collaterals exist, elective surgical repair is usually possible.
      2) However, sudden occlusion of vessels supplying tissue that tolerates ischemia poorly, such as the kidney and heart, requires emergency treatment using thrombolytic agents and surgical revascularization.
4. Distal:
   a. Complications distal to the site of dilation include embolization and spasm and occur in 1%–5% of angioplasties, although PTA of iliac occlusions has been associated with embolic rates as high as 40%.
   b. Diffuse emboli, typically from patients with severe atherosclerosis of the aorta undergoing percutaneous renal transluminal angioplasty (PRTA), may lead to bowel infarction and can be fatal.
   c. Most embolic events can be managed conservatively, but many require surgical embolectomy or revascularization to prevent permanent tissue damage.
5. Systemic:
   a. Renal insufficiency can occur in up to 26% of patients undergoing PRTA for renovascular hypertension, with 13% requiring dialysis. This complication can be minimized by maintaining adequate hydration. In patients without renovascular disease, renal insufficiency occurs in <5%.
   b. Contrast dye allergy.
   c. Bleeding causing hypotension or anemia.
6. Restenosis rates range from 10% with iliac artery angioplasties to 40% with coronary artery angioplasties.

VI. DEEP VENOUS THROMBOSIS.

A. Incidence.

The incidence of subclinical DVT after high-risk surgical procedures is estimated at >50%. Acute DVT may lead to fatal PE; chronic DVT may lead to severe disability owing to the consequences of venous stasis.

B. Pathogenesis.

1. Virchow's triad of hypercoagulability, intimal damage, and stasis is required. Hypercoagulability and stasis predominate as etiologic factors in most postsurgical patients.

2. Maximal stasis occurs in the cusps of the venous valves where a thrombus composed primarily of RBCs and fibrin develops. Complete occlusion of the lumen precedes retrograde propagation of the thrombus and promotes anterograde propagation.

3. While 90% of venous thrombi occur in the veins of the calves, it is propagation of these thrombi into the popliteal veins and above that confers the greatest risk of PE. Propagating thrombi are poorly adherent to normal intima and are dislodged easily by relatively minor mechanical disruption.

4. DVT in patients undergoing total hip replacement tend to arise de novo in the femoral veins, possibly due to vascular trauma from manipulation of the extremity.

5. Common risk factors are listed in Table 8–4. Additional risk factors include prolonged immobilization, varicose veins, pregnancy, oral contraceptives, chronic ulcerative colitis, sepsis, nephrotic syndrome, AT-III deficiency, protein C and S deficiency, paroxysmal nocturnal hemoglobinuria, polycythemia, and the presence of the lupus anticoagulant.

C. Diagnosis.

1. Physical examination.

    a. **Clinical signs and symptoms are highly unreliable.**

       1) At least one-half of documented cases are asymptomatic.

       2) Clinical signs in order of decreasing frequency are induration of calf muscles, unilateral edema, limb hyperthermia, and pain.

      3) Homan's sign (resistance to dorsiflexion of the foot) is unreliable.

      4) Any suspicion of DVT warrants objective testing.

2. Objective tests:

  a. Radiocontrast venography:

    1) Venography is the standard against which others are compared and can assess site and extent of occlusion as well as the presence of collateral vessels.

    2) Sensitivity is 90% when thrombi are below the internal iliac, 30% above.

    3) Postvenographic DVT averages <5%, but may be as high as 30%.

  b. ^{111}In-platelet uptake:

    1) Labeled platelet studies are nearly 100% sensitive for detecting thrombosis in calf veins but less sensitive for detecting thigh and pelvic thrombi.

    2) Radiolabeled autologous blood (50 mL) is required and imaging of the lower extremities 24 and 48 hours after injection.

    3) It is the best screening test for research purposes. Clinical utility is hampered by poor specificity, the requirement for ongoing thrombosis, and the prolonged time course of the test. It is not useful in detecting thrombi in the vicinity of a wound.

  c. Venous plethysmography:

    1) All plethysmographic tests attempt to detect venous outflow obstruction noninvasively using various methods to measure changes in calf muscle volume.

    2) These tests are accurate in detecting >80% of proximal thromboses, but incapable of detecting thrombus in calf veins and are usually combined with ^{111}In-platelet testing.

    3) Equivocal results warrant definitive testing.

  d. Ultrasonography:

    1) The detection of flow from the popliteal to common femoral veins by 2-D color Doppler ultrasonography effectively rules out thrombi, but failure to detect flow may be related to technique rather than thrombosis.

TABLE 8–4.
Risk of Deep Venous Thrombosis and Prophylactic Regimens

Type of Surgery	Risk of DVT (%)	Risk of Pulmonary Embolus (%)	Factors Conferring High Risk*	Prophylactic Regimen for High-Risk Patients
General	10–40	1–6	Age >40 yrs, obesity, previous DVT or PE, malignancy, lengthy procedure (>1 hr)	Lower extremity (LE) elevation, pneumatic compression stockings, low-dose heparin
Orthopedic	25–70	1–3	Hip and knee procedures	LE elevation, warfarin or dextran
Urologic	10–40	1–3	Transvesical prostatectomy	LE elevation, pneumatic compression stockings, low-dose heparin
Gynecologic	7–45	1–5	Malignancy	LE elevation, pneumatic compression stockings, early ambulation, low-dose heparin or dextran

Neurosurgical	9–50	1.5–3.0	Spinal cord surgery, laminectomy	Extracranial: pneumatic compression stockings, low-dose heparin Intracranial: pneumatic compression stockings
Trauma	20–40	>1	Hip fracture, severe musculoskeletal trauma	Without head injury: pneumatic compression stockings, dextran or warfarin With head injury: pneumatic compression stockings

*Risk factors listed for general surgery apply equally to other surgical specialties.

341

2) Visualization of the iliac and saphenous veins is poor.
3) Ultrasound is most useful in quickly confirming a strong clinical diagnosis and is considered by many the test of first choice.
4) Two-dimensional ultrasonography is superior to handheld, audible output, Doppler blood velocity detectors.

e. MRI:
1) Clinical experience is limited, but early studies indicate 90% contrast specificity and 100% sensitivity compared to venography.
2) MRI is noninvasive, but expensive, and is an excellent test for patients in whom ionizing radiation is contraindicated.

D. Treatment.

1. Prior to any pharmacologic therapy, baseline CBC, PT, PTT, TT, fibrinogen level, and FDP levels should be obtained. Bed rest must be enforced with ankles elevated above knees, and knees elevated above heart (Fig 8–7). If compression stockings are employed, care must be taken to avoid the tourniquet effect of stocking cuff roll-over.

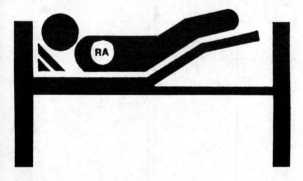

FIG 8–7.
Proper patient positioning for prophylaxis of DVT. The legs should be positioned above the right atrium *(RA)* to avoid venous stasis.

2. In most cases, initiation of medical therapy should be preceded by definitive diagnosis.
   a. Anticoagulation:
      1) Heparin 5,000 units IV immediately upon diagnosis, then approximately 500 units/kg/day as a continuous infusion (PTT 1.5–2.0 × control) for 7–14 days (usually 800–1,200 units/hr).
      2) Begin oral warfarin sodium 10 mg/day on day 3 with dosage adjustment to maintain PT 1.5–2.0 × control.
      3) Discontinue heparin when stable oral anticoagulation is achieved.
      4) Continue warfarin 3–6 months.
   b. Thrombolytic therapy:
      1) 20%–70% of thrombi <5 days old will undergo lysis with streptokinase (SK) or urokinase (UK).
      2) A loading dose of SK 250,000 IU over 30 minutes will neutralize streptococcal antibodies. The maintenance dose is 100,000 IU/hr IV.
      3) Corresponding doses for UK are 4,400 IU/kg loading, followed by 4,400 IU/kg/hr maintenance.
      4) Maintain TT or PTT two to four times control (first measurement 2–4 hours after loading) and continue therapy for 72 hours.
      5) Begin full-dose heparin 6 hours after discontinuing lytic therapy (PT <2 times control), and follow by routine conversion to warfarin.
      6) Indications for early discontinuation of lytic therapy are a TT or PTT >5 times control (temporary), a TT or PTT that is initially elevated but returns to baseline, or a body temperature >39° C after initiating therapy.
3. Surgical.
   a. Acute DVT: Venous thrombectomy in acute DVT is reserved for patients with threatened extremities due to phlegmasia cerula dolens (tense edema, tenderness, and cyanosis).
   b. Chronic DVT:
      1) Saphenous vein bypass of discrete obstructions in major veins should be considered only after fail-

ure of medical therapy (compression stockings, elevation).
2) Venous valvuloplasty and valvular transposition are promising new techniques.

E. **Prophylaxis.**
1. **Proper elevation of the lower extremities** (see above) **cannot be overemphasized, and should be enforced routinely** (see Fig 8–7). Care must be taken not to allow ankles to become dependent as this promotes infrapopliteal stasis. In some high-risk patients, low-dose heparin, warfarin, dextran, and pneumatic compression stockings have been shown to be effective (see Table 8–4).
2. Low-dose heparin 5,000 units preoperatively, then 5,000 units q. 8–12 h. for 7 days is advocated by some clinicians. Low-dose heparin in patients undergoing total hip replacement is controversial.
3. Dextran 40 or 70 5–10 mL/kg IV of 10% solution intraoperatively, followed by 4–7 mL/kg/day for 7 days. Dextran may cause osmotic nephrosis and, possibly, ATN at high doses.
4. Warfarin sodium 2.5–7.0 mg/day (PT 1.5–2.0 × control) until 7 days after ambulation begins (contraindicated in pregnancy).

VII. **UPPER EXTREMITY REPLANTATION.**
A. **Care of the Amputated Part and Transport.**
1. Immerse the amputated part in a plastic bag or sterile specimen cup containing lactated Ringer's solution.
2. Place the plastic bag or specimen cup on ice.
3. Do not put the amputated part in direct contact with ice in order to prevent frostbite.
4. Apply a compressive dressing to amputation stump.
5. Do not ligate or clamp exposed vessels.
6. If the patient's condition is stable, patient and part are transported to a replantation center as rapidly as possible.

B. **Patient Selection.**
1. The ability to restore circulation is not in itself an absolute indication for replantation. The decision must be individualized with restoration of painless function as the primary goal of treatment. Various factors (occupation,

age, underlying disease states) influence the decision to perform replantation.

2. Priorities for upper extremity replantation:
   a. Thumb.
   b. Multiple digits.
   c. Amputation through the palm, wrist, or forearm.
   d. Isolated individual digits if the laceration is distal to the superficialis tendon insertion at the middle phalanx.
   e. Any part in a child.

3. Relative contraindications for upper extremity replantation:
   a. Severely avulsed, crushed, or mangled parts.
   b. Multiple level amputations.
   c. Isolated border digits in the index or the little finger if the injury is proximal to the superficialis tendon insertion at the middle phalanx.
   d. Presence of severe arteriosclerosis or nicotine addiction.
   e. Patients who are mentally unstable or who have systemic diseases such as diabetes or coronary artery disease.
   f. Prolonged ischemia of the amputated part.
   g. These contraindications are not absolute but must be considered when making the final assessment. Often a final decision cannot be made until the status of the damaged vessels has been determined under the operating microscope. This should be explained to the patient so that his expectations are not unreasonable.

C. **Preoperative Evaluation.**
   1. Pertinent history:
      a. Patient's age, sex, occupation, hand dominance.
      b. Mechanism and extent of injury.
      c. Ischemia time from injury to arrival at the hospital. Irreversible changes occur in muscle after 4 hours of warm ischemia, but cooling does prolong the safe time for replantation. Since digits have essentially no muscle, they may be replanted successfully up to 24 hours after amputation if they have been cooled appropriately.
      d. Associated injuries.

      e. Past medical history (alcohol and tobacco usage).

      f. Psychological profile.

  2. Physical examination:

      a. General physical examination.

      b. Examination of the injured extremity and amputated part.

         1) Bone injury.

         2) Skin injury.

         3) Tendon injury.

         4) Evidence of avulsion of nerve, artery, or other soft tissues.

         5) In cases of incomplete amputation check capillary refill, turgor, color, and two-point discrimination with calipers or paper clip.

  3. Laboratory workup:

      a. CBC, electrolytes, PT, PTT, ECG, CXR.

      b. Blood type and crossmatch.

      c. Radiograph of amputated part and injured extremity.

      d. Wound culture in instances of forearm or above-elbow amputation.

  4. Patient preparation for the OR:

      a. Resuscitation, stabilization as indicated by patient's condition.

      b. Appropriate antibiotics:

         1) First-generation cephalosporin.

         2) Add an aminoglycoside in highly contaminated wounds.

         3) Add penicillin in farm injuries.

      c. Tetanus prophylaxis.

D. Postoperative Care.

  1. Patients should remain in a quiet environment for several days following operation to avoid wide shifts in vasomotor tone.

  2. A bulky dressing is applied in the operating room.

  3. Patients are kept NPO for 24 hours in the event that reoperation is necessary.

  4. A bedside chart recording the color, capillary refill, and turgor of the digit is maintained. The patient is kept well hydrated.

  5. Replanted parts may be monitored with surface temperature probes. A sustained digital pulp temperature of $<30°$ C is diagnostic of inadequate perfusion which, if

uncorrected, will cause loss of the digit. If the temperature of a digit drops suddenly, the following steps should be taken:

    a. Notify the operating surgeon.

    b. Release constricting dressings.

    c. Elevate or lower the involved extremity depending on whether arterial or venous flow is compromised.

    d. Raise the room temperature.

    e. Administer an analgesic or sedative to diminish anxiety.

    f. Administer IV heparin bolus (5,000 units).

    g. Obtain an axillary or stellate block using bupivacaine to relieve vasospasm.

    h. Consider reexploration of vascular anastomoses if there is no improvement after the above steps are taken.

6. Postoperative medications (Table 8–5):

    a. Aspirin 325 mg po b.i.d., and dipyridamole 25 mg po t.i.d.

    b. Antibiotics for 3 days.

    c. Dextran −40 at 20–30 mL/hr IV.

    d. Heparin 1,000 units/hr IV in the case of severe trauma to vessels or difficult anastomoses.

    e. Chlorpromazine 25 mg po t.i.d. for sedation and peripheral vasodilation.

    f. Modify drug doses in children.

TABLE 8–5.

Postoperative Management of Extremity Replantation

1. Elevation of operated part
2. Immobilization
3. Adequate volume resuscitation
4. Adequate pain relief
5. NPO for 24 hr
6. Low-molecular-weight dextran at 20–30 mL/hr
7. Aspirin 325 mg/day
8. Dipyridamole 25–50 mg t.i.d.
9. Chlorpromazine 25 mg t.i.d.
10. Heparin or pneumatic compression stockings for DVT prophylaxis
11. No smoking, caffeine, or chocolate (to avoid vasoconstriction)

    7. No smoking, chocolates, or caffeine as these may cause vasoconstriction.

    8. Room temperature >72° F (22° C) at all times.

    9. Overhead heater.

    10. Patients are usually discharged from the hospital 3–10 days after replantation depending on the magnitude of injury.

        a. Discharge medications include aspirin and dipyridamole for several days.

        b. Patients should be told to keep warm and avoid smoking.

        c. Patients are discharged in the bulky hand dressing that was applied at operation unless this becomes soiled or there is a problem with a "blood cast" causing vascular compromise to the part.

        d. Patients return 2–3 weeks postoperatively for initiation of physical therapy and splinting.

        e. No motion of the part is encouraged during the immediate perioperative period.

VIII. COMPOSITE TISSUE TRANSFER.

Various tissues may be transferred via local rotation as a pedicled transfer or by microsurgical free tissue transfer. These tissues include bone, muscle, musculocutaneous, fascial, fasciocutaneous, omentum, or enteric tissues. The advantage of such transfer is that these tissues bring in their own blood supply and do not necessarily rely upon the recipient wound bed. Composite tissue transfer may actually augment the blood supply to the recipient bed, as well as provide bulk and stable yet pliable wound coverage.

A.   **Preoperative Evaluation.**

    1. As with any clinical problem a complete history and physical examination are required including an assessment of mechanism of injury, associated medical problems (coronary artery disease, diabetes, renal failure), medications, allergies, chronicity of the wound, attempts at previous closure, presence of peripheral vascular disease, and previous surgery which may influence treatment options.

    2. Preoperative preparation of the wound may include multiple debridements, repeated dressing changes, and possibly hyperbaric O_2 therapy preceding composite tissue surgery.

B. **Laboratory Assessment.**
1. Routine evaluation:
   a. CBC.
   b. PT, PTT.
   c. Blood type and crossmatch.
   d. Wound culture (qualitative, quantitative).
   e. ECG (where indicated).
   f. CXR.
2. Specific studies:
   a. In extremity reconstruction, preoperative angiography for the donor or recipient site, or both, may be indicated.
   b. With exposed bone or potential areas of osteomyelitis, preoperative radiographs and nuclear scans are indicated.
   c. Duplex scanning may be indicated where venous anatomy is important (e.g., femoral-distal bypass with free tissue transfer).

C. **Preoperative Medications.**
1. Routine medications should be continued as necessary.
2. Aspirin for its antiplatelet effect (325 mg q. d.), chlorpromazine for its smooth muscle relaxant properties (25 mg b.i.d.), and dipyridamole for its vasodilator properties (25 mg t.i.d.) may be started on the day preceding operation if not contraindicated.
3. Heparin or pneumatic compression boots should be utilized for DVT prophylaxis as most surgeries are performed under general anesthesia and may be prolonged in length.
4. Antibiotics are utilized for treatment (based on culture results) or prophylaxis.

D. **Postoperative Management:**
1. Postoperatively, the flap should be closely monitored by trained personnel for any evidence of vascular insufficiency. Flap color, temperature, turgor, and assessment of capillary bleeding in response to needle stick are important indicators of flap viability.
2. Flap monitoring can be accomplished by any number of different techniques. Each method has advantages and drawbacks.
   a. Laser Doppler:
      1) The unit is reliable in the early detection of vascular insufficiency.

2) The instrument shows trends in blood flow. "Normal values" have been determined for a large number of free tissue transfers. These are of less importance than the trends, although absolute flow <0.4 mL/min/100 g of tissue correlates with poor flap survival.

3) Using the laser Doppler, the success rate with flaps is >95% and the salvage of failing flaps >85%.

4) Various probe designs are available to allow assessment of surface or deep tissue blood flow.

5) The monitor and fiberoptic probes are expensive and relatively fragile.

b. Photoplethysmography detects flow by detecting the phase shift in light from moving RBC mass. This monitor is somewhat more tedious to use and interpret than the laser Doppler.

c. Temperature probes provide an inexpensive means to monitor flap viability. Temperatures <30° C usually indicate vascular insufficiency but must be considered in comparison to adjacent tissue temperature.

d. Transcutaneous PO_2 monitors measure the transcutaneous delivery of O_2 via a heated probe. There is individual and systemic variation depending upon the physiologic condition of the patient. Preoperative and control tissue values are required. The usual indication of vascular insufficiency is a O_2 <25 mm Hg.

E. **Complications.**

1. Vascular insufficiency (Table 8–6):

a. The laser Doppler has been useful in conjunction with clinical observation in the early detection of vascular insufficiency. Prompt recognition and treatment is important for optimal flap survival.

b. Treatment of vascular insufficiency:

1) Prompt inspection of patient, flap, and monitoring device.

2) Release of constricting dressing.

3) Check for tight flap closure, hematoma, etc.

4) If a vascular problem is diagnosed a low threshold for prompt reexploration in the OR is warranted.

5) Since most venous or arterial problems are encountered during the first 24 hours, it is reason-

TABLE 8-6.

Vascular Insufficiency Following Composite Tissue Transfer

Venous thrombosis (flap characteristics)
Flap appears blue and engorged
Flap is cool
Brisk capillary refill (<2 sec)
Dark venous blood with needle stick
Arterial thrombosis (flap characteristics)
Flap is white or pale
Decreased flap turgor
Absent or delayed capillary refill

able to maintain the patient NPO during this time.
6) Heparin as a bolus may be given in preparation
for reexploration unless a hematoma is suspected
or contraindicated by other conditions.
2. Hematoma:
a. Hematoma may be manifested by swelling beneath
the flap with signs of vascular embarassment to all or
a portion of the flap.
b. Hematoma may cause a fall in laser Doppler flow
numbers. Prompt recognition and treatment are important for flap survival.
c. Hematoma may be seen with increased frequency if
low-molecular-weight dextran is continued beyond
postoperative day 5.
3. Infection:
a. Infection may be seen as with any surgical wound.
b. Muscle and musculocutaneous flaps have been demonstrated to have an elevated tolerance to bacterial
loads.
c. These flaps are not a substitute for proper wound management and thorough debridement.
4. DVT:
a. DVT and PE may be seen with reconstructive micro-
surgery as the procedures are lengthy and patients
tend to be immobilized postoperatively.
b. Many patients have preexisting trauma or other risk
factors for DVT and PE.
c. Heparin or pneumatic compression stockings should
be utilized where possible (see Table 8-4).

SELECTED REFERENCES

Comorota AJ: *Thrombolytic Therapy.* Orlando, Fla, Grune & Stratton, Inc, 1988.

Glaget GP, Reisch JS: Prevention of venous thromboembolism in general surgical patients: Results of meta-analysis. *Ann Surg* 1988; 208:227.

Mathes SJ, Nahai F: *Clinical Atlas of Muscle and Musculocutaneous Flaps.* St Louis, CV Mosby Co, 1979.

National Institutes of Health: Consensus development conference statement, prevention of venous thrombosis and pulmonary embolism. March 24–26, 1986 *JAMA* 1986; 256:744.

Rutherford RB (ed): *Vascular Surgery,* ed 3. Philadelphia, WB Saunders Co, 1989.

Sabiston DC (ed): *Textbook of Surgery,* ed 13. Philadelphia, WB Saunders Co, 1987.

Serafin D, Buncke HJ: *Microsurgical Composite Tissue Transplantation.* St Louis, CV Mosby Co, 1979.

Urbaniak JR: Replantation, in Green DP (ed): *Operative Hand Surgery,* ed 2. New York, Churchill Livingstone, Inc, 1988.

THE RENAL SYSTEM

9

I. **FUNCTIONS OF THE NORMAL KIDNEY.**
A. **Regulation of Water and Electrolyte Balance.**
B. **Excretion of Metabolic Wastes and Foreign Chemicals.**
C. **Regulation of Arterial Blood Pressure.**
  1. The renin-angiotensin system.
     Renin, produced by the juxtaglomerular apparatus, cata-
     lyzes the splitting of *angiotensin I* from *angiotensinogen*
     (secreted in the liver). Upon contact with *angiotensin-
     converting enzyme* (usually in the lungs or kidneys), an-
     giotensin I is converted into *angiotensin II.*
  2. Other vasoactive substances. The kidneys produce other
     substances, such as prostaglandins and kinins, that cause
     vasoconstriction and vasodilation.
  3. Regulation of erythrocyte production. The kidneys se-
     crete *erythropoietin* which induces the production of
     RBCs in the bone marrow.
D. **Regulation of vitamin D activity.**
  1. Production of the active form of vitamin D (1,25-dihy-
     droxyvitamin D_3) occurs in the kidneys.

II. **BASIC RENAL PROCESSES.**
A. **Glomerular Filtration.**
  The *glomerular filtration rate* (GFR) is the amount of ultrafiltrate generated by the glomerulus per unit time and is
  approximately 180 L/day in a 70-kg male. The typical concentrations of solutes after the various renal processes are
  listed in Table 9.1.
  1. **Determinants of GFR.** Whereas the permeability and
     surface area of the glomerular filter are relatively fixed,
     the most significant determinant of GFR is the glomerular
     capillary hydraulic pressure and is directly proportional

TABLE 9–1.

Daily Renal Solute Exchange

	Filtered	Reabsorbed	Secreted	Urine
Sodium (mEq)	25,200	25,050	—	150 (100 mEq/L)
Potassium (mEq)	720	720	100	100 (67 mEq/L)
Chloride (mEq)	18,000	17,870	—	130 (87 mEq/L)
Bicarbonate (mEq)	4,000	4,000	—	0
Urea (mM)	900	500	—	400 (267 mM)
Creatinine (mM)	15	—	—	15 (10 mM)
Glucose (mM)	900	900	—	0
Total solutes (mOsm)	49,735	49,040	140	910 (607 mOsm/L)
Water (mL)	180,000	178,500		1,500

to renal perfusion pressure (RPP). RPP can be regulated by changing systemic mean arterial pressure (MAP), renal vascular resistance (RVR), or renal venous pressure (RVP) according to the formula:

$$RPP = \frac{MAP - RVP}{RVR}$$

Therefore, GFR will increase with increased MAP or decrease with RVP or RVR. Factors which increase RVR include adrenergic stimulation and ADH. Factors which decrease RVR are dopaminergic receptor stimulation and prostaglandins.

2. **Composition of ultrafiltrate.** The composition of ultrafiltrate is determined by the combined semipermeable membranes of the glomerular capillaries and Bowman's capsule. Water and solutes <7,000 mol wt pass freely into Bowman's capsule, while most proteins and cells continue through the renal circulation and out the renal veins. Hence, the glomerular ultrafiltrate is a protein-free crystalloid solution with an electrolyte concentration nearly identical to that of the circulating plasma.

3. **Tubular reabsorption.** Many of the filtered plasma solutes are either completely absent from the urine or present in substantially smaller quantities than were present in the initial ultrafiltrate (see Table 9–1). The reabsorption capabilities of the renal tubules are further

demonstrated by the fact that 99% of the 180 L/day of ultrafiltrate produced by the glomerulus is reabsorbed. Reabsorption is accomplished by several mechanisms, including simple diffusion (concentration gradient), facilitated diffusion, active transport, and endocytosis.

4. **Tubular secretion.** An alternative pathway to glomerular filtration for excretion of solutes into the urine is through *tubular secretion*. This process begins with simple diffusion of the substance out of the peritubular capillaries and into the interstitium. Transport into the tubule may be active or passive depending on the gradients of the particular solute. Tubular secretion plays a major role in H^+ and K^+ excretion.

III. CLINICAL ASSESSMENT OF RENAL FUNCTION.

A. History and Physical.

1. A history of uremia, hypertension, hematuria or proteinuria, and review of all medications is sought.
2. Signs suggestive of renal insufficiency include hypertension, alopecia, peripheral neuropathy, conjunctival calcification, band keratopathy, gynecomastia or testicular atrophy, peripheral edema, pericardial rub, and CHF.

B. Urinalysis.

1. Urine output (UO).
   a. Under conditions of normal hydration, UO should be within the range of 0.5–1.0 mL/kg/hr.
   b. *Polyuria* may indicate diuretic use, diabetes mellitus, diabetes insipidus, nervous diseases, ARF, or certain types of chronic nephritis.
   c. *Oliguria* (UO <400 mL/day in an adult) or *anuria* (absence of UO) may result from dehydration, cardiogenic shock, renal failure, or urinary outflow obstruction.
2. Urine pH.
   a. Normal urine pH is 4.6–8.0.
   b. Acidic urine may be due to ketoacidosis, high protein diet, COPD, or various medications.
   c. Basic urine indicates urinary tract infection (UTI), renal tubular acidosis, diet, or bicarbonate therapy.
3. Urine specific gravity (SG).
   a. SG is normally 1.003–1.030.

    b. Elevated SG indicates dehydration, CHF, adrenal insufficiency, or SIADH.

    c. Decreased SG reflects overhydration, diabetes insipidus, pyelonephritis, or glomerulonephritis.

    d. SG is an unreliable indicator of volume status or renal function in the presence of glycosuria, following use of IV radiographic contrast agents, or in patients receiving diuretics.

    e. Following a night of fluid restriction, SG >1.018 indicates appropriate tubular function and a requirement for increased intravascular volume.

4. Urine dipstick.

    a. Glucose.

      1) Glucose is normally absent from urine.

      2) Glucosuria reflects hyperglycemia due to diabetes mellitus, pancreatitis, shock, sepsis, steroids, hyperthyroidism, renal tubular dysfunction, or iatrogenic causes.

    b. Protein.

      1) Urine protein is normally 0.0–0.1 g/24 hr.

      2) Proteinuria, if detected by dipstick, should be quantified in a 24-hour urine collection prior to elective operation. Excretion in excess of 150 mg/24 hr indicates significant renal parenchymal disease and warrants a more detailed evaluation.

    c. Ketones.

      1) Ketones are normally absent from urine.

      2) Ketonuria is due to DKA, starvation, hyperthyroidism, fever, or pregnancy.

    d. Nitrite.

      1) Positive urine nitrite indicates UTI.

      2) Microscopic analysis and urine culture and sensitivity are indicated.

    e. Bilirubin and urobilinogen.

      1) Bilirubin and urobilinogen are normally absent from urine.

      2) Positive urine bilirubin or urobilinogen indicates obstructive jaundice, hepatitis, cirrhosis, cholangitis, hemolysis, or suppression of intestinal flora by antibiotics.

    f. RBCs and WBCs.

      1) Neither RBCs nor WBCs are normally present in urine.

       2) Positive dipstick indicating hematuria or pyuria is an absolute requirement for microscopic analysis.

5. Microscopic analysis (sediment).

   a. Hematuria.

     Microscopic hematuria may be due to trauma, pyelonephritis, cystitis, prostatitis, nephrolithiasis, urinary tract cancer, coagulopathy, menses, polycystic kidneys, hemolytic anemia, transfusion reaction, or interstitial nephritis (see p. 381–382).

   b. Pyuria.

     1) The presence of >10 WBCs per HPF is strong evidence of urinary tract infection. A clean-catch or straight catheter urine sample should be obtained for urine culture and sensitivity. Elective operation is usually postponed if pyuria is documented.

     2) Pyuria also occurs with acute glomerular nephritis, urinary tract cancer, renal tuberculosis, or interstitial nephritis.

   c. Epithelial cells. Identification of epithelial cells in urine occurs with acute tubular necrosis (ATN) and necrotizing papillitis.

   d. Casts.

     1) Urinary casts are cylindric masses of cellular elements derived directly from the kidney.

     2) The presence of RBC casts suggests an acute glomerular nephritis, while the presence of WBC casts suggests nephritis or pyelonephritis.

     3) Identification of fatty casts with proteinuria is diagnostic of the nephrotic syndrome.

   e. Crystals.

     1) In acidic urine, calcium oxalate and urate crystals may be normally present.

     2) In alkaline urine, calcium carbonate and phosphate crystals may be normally present.

     3) Cystine, sulfonamide, leucine, tyrosine, and cholesterol crystals in urine are abnormal.

6. Urine electrolytes and fractional excretion of sodium.

   a. Normal urine electrolytes are listed in Table 9–1.

   b. A spot determination of urine electrolytes may be useful for assessment of intravascular volume status and aids in potassium supplementation. However, concentrations of electrolytes in urine may vary considerably with salt intake.

1) Urine Na^+ <20 mEq/L suggests hypovolemia, shock, or hyponatremia.

2) Urine K^+ <10 mEq/L indicates hypokalemia or renal failure.

c. **Fractional excretion of sodium** (FE_{Na}) is a more reliable indicator of volume status and etiology of ARF and is calculated by the formula:

$$FE_{Na} \ (\%) = \frac{U/P \ sodium}{U/P \ creatinine} \times 100$$

where U/P sodium is the ratio of urine and plasma sodium concentrations and U/P creatinine is the ratio of urine and plasma creatinine concentrations.

1) In the presence of hypovolemia and hypoperfusion, the renin-angiotensin system is activated and the subsequent release of aldosterone will induce the kidney to reabsorb sodium. Therefore, a FE_{Na} <1% is indicative of volume depletion.

2) An elevated FE_{Na} >3% is consistent with tubular injury or obstruction.

d. *Note:* Assessment of renal function or volume status by urine electrolytes is unreliable in the presence of a preexisting prerenal state (e.g., CHF, cirrhosis), with diuretic therapy, or following the use of contrast dye.

C. **Plasma Creatinine and Creatinine Clearance (C_{Cr}).**

1. Creatinine is a metabolic end product of high-energy phosphates in muscle. It is removed from the plasma mostly by glomerular filtration with only minor secretion by the proximal tubule. Therefore, it is an accurate reflection of GFR.

2. Plasma creatinine is determined by the rate of production (related to muscle mass) and the rate of excretion (related to GFR).

3. As renal failure progresses, creatinine is a less reliable indicator of GFR owing to increasing tubular secretion of creatinine. In these circumstances, other nonsecreted molecules, such as inulin, should be used to determine GFR.

4. A gradual rise in plasma creatinine does not necessarily

reflect continuing renal injury. A steady-state level will take several days to develop and creatinine will rise continually until a new plateau is reached.

5. In patients with decreased muscle mass, creatinine can remain within normal limits despite significant impairment to renal function.

6. **Creatinine clearance** (C_{Cr}).

   a. GFR can be accurately assessed by measuring C_{Cr}. **Predicted C_{Cr}** is usually 90–150 mL/min, but can be estimated from age (yr), body weight (kg) and plasma creatinine, P_{Cr} (mg/dL), by the formula:

   $$C_{Cr} \text{ (mL/min)} = \frac{(140 - \text{age}) \times \text{wt}}{72 \times P_{Cr}}$$

   b. **Actual C_{Cr}** can be determined after a timed urine collection by the formula:

   $$C_{Cr} \text{ (mL/min)} = \frac{U_{Cr} \times U_{vol} \times 1.73}{P_{Cr} \times \text{time} \times \text{BSA}}$$

   where U_{Cr} is urinary creatinine (mg/dL), U_{vol} is urine volume (mL), P_{Cr} is plasma creatinine (mg/dL), time is minutes of urine collected; and BSA is body surface area (m^2).

   c. Many therapeutic agents require adjustment of dosage for patients with renal insufficiency. This adjustment is based on the ratio between the actual vs. predicted C_{Cr}. Section VII lists some of these drugs and their respective dosing adjustments for renal failure.

D. **Blood Urea Nitrogen (BUN).**

   1. BUN (normal range 10–20 mg/dL) is the end product of protein degradation via the urea cycle. It is freely filterable, but approximately 50% of filtered urea is reabsorbed. This reabsorption occurs passively and is dependent on water reabsorption to establish the diffusion gradient for urea. Therefore, BUN reflects both renal function and volume status.

   2. Since urea generation is directly dependent on protein intake and degradation, BUN may be unreliable as an indicator of renal dysfunction in malnourished patients.

   3. The relationship between BUN and renal function (GFR)

is essentially loglinear. Therefore, assuming constant fluid and nutritional balance, if a patient has a BUN of 10 mg/dL, a reduction in GFR of 50% is required before BUN becomes >20 mg/dL.

E. **Urine and Plasma Osmolarity (U_{osm}, P_{osm}).**

1. Healthy kidneys excrete an osmolar load while retaining free water. If damage to renal tubules occurs, this ability to excrete becomes impaired, and U_{osm} and P_{osm} approach equal values.

2. The maximal concentration of urine by the normal kidney is 1,400 mOsm/L. Because approximately 910 mOsm/day of metabolic wastes are produced, if urine volume is inadequate (<30 mL/hr or <500 mL/day), these waste products will accumulate in the circulation owing to impaired excretion.

3. Normal P_{osm} is 285 ± 15 mOsm/L.

4. U_{osm} (normal 40–700 mOsm/L) indicates the amount of solute in a given volume of urine.

5. The concentrating ability of the kidney, indicating renal tubular function, correlates with the U_{osm}/P_{osm} ratio. **Osmolar clearance** (C_{osm}) is represented by the formula:

$$C_{osm} \text{ (osm/min)} = \frac{U_{osm}}{P_{osm}} \times V \text{ (mL/min)}$$

where V = urine volume (mL/min).

6. **Free water clearance** (C_{H_2O}) is calculated using the following formula:

$$C_{H_2O} = V - \frac{U_{osm} \times V}{P_{osm}}$$

a. C_{H_2O} is usually negative (<−20) and becomes increasingly negative as renal concentration increases.

b. As renal tubular function decreases, concentrating ability falls and C_{H_2O} approximates 0 (±10). C_{H_2O} may become positive (>+20) in diabetes insipidus or water intoxication.

7. P_{osm} may be falsely elevated owing to osmotically active molecules present in excess amounts. These usually are glucose, urea, or alcohol. In the presence of hyperglyce-

mia or elevated BUN, P_{osm} may be corrected by the formula:

$$P_{osm} = 2 \times [Na^+] + \frac{BUN \ (mg/dL)}{2.8}$$
$$+ \frac{glucose \ (mg/dL)}{18}$$

IV. PERIOPERATIVE MANAGEMENT.

A. Established (Chronic) Renal Failure.

1. *Chronic renal failure* (CRF) results from the irreversible impairment or destruction of nephrons and is assigned when renal insufficiency persists >3 months. Conditions encountered with this syndrome include impaired fluid and electrolyte regulation, suppressed erythropoiesis and immune function, atherosclerosis, hypertension, pericarditis, encephalitis, and distal neuropathy.
2. Perioperative considerations for patients with CRF.
   a. For elective procedures, dialyze pre- and postoperatively.
   b. Owing to suppressed immune function, prophylactic antibiotics and careful wound management are essential.
   c. FFP and vitamin K should be administered for correction of renal failure–associated coagulopathy.
   d. **Desmopressin acetate** (DDAVP) is administered to correct platelet dysfunction.
3. Aggressive application of renal replacement therapy (usually hemodialysis or peritoneal dialysis) is essential to minimize complications of CRF patients in the perioperative setting.

B. Prevention of Acute Renal Failure.

1. Maintenance of renal perfusion by aggressive management of hypovolemia, hypoxemia, and low CO are obvious goals.
2. Contrast agents and nephrotoxic drugs should be used only when the benefits outweigh the risk.
3. In posttraumatic cases where severe rhabdomyolysis may exist, diuretics, haptoglobin therapy, and alkaline solute diuresis may be protective from myoglobin-induced ARF.

4. Diuretics such as furosemide or mannitol afford renal protection through saluretic effects which clear the tubule of obstruction and prevent backleakage of filtrate.

   a. **Mannitol** produces an osmotic diuresis and increases renal blood flow to cortical areas. In the setting of adequate intravascular volume, mannitol infusion affords protection from ARF in several experimental and clinical settings, particularly prior to renal ischemia in open heart and aortic resection procedures.

   b. Loop diuretics such as **furosemide** and **ethacrynic acid** have also been tested, although evidence of protection from ARF is inconsistent. Furosemide may convert oliguric ARF to nonoliguric ARF in combination with dopamine infusion.

C. **Preoperative Measures.**

   1. Preoperative assessment of renal function includes a careful history and physical, urinalysis, plasma electrolytes, BUN, and creatinine, as well as urine volume. An accurate weight should be obtained the night before operation.

   2. Administer IV fluids the night prior to operation to maintain normal hydration while restricted by NPO orders.

D. **Intraoperative Measures.**

   1. Neuromuscular blocking agents such as pancuronium and tubocurarine may cause acidosis and hyperkalemia, and should be avoided in CRF patients and in those at risk for ARF.

   2. Aggressive measures should be taken to avoid hypotensive episodes. This includes close monitoring of hemodynamic status (HR, BP, CVP) during induction and throughout the procedure.

   3. Maintain an accurate record of fluid balance throughout the operation, including UO, blood loss, and fluid replacement. Use of vasoactive, inotropic, and diuretic agents should be noted for dose and corresponding response.

E. **Postoperative Measures.**

   1. Initial postoperative assessment should begin with careful review of intraoperative fluid balance (UO, blood loss, fluid replacement) and hemodynamic course.

   2. VS and UO should be monitored immediately and throughout the postoperative period.

      a. Intravascular volume status must be assessed, including breath sounds (rales), neck veins (JVD), and peripheral perfusion (pulses, capillary refill, extremity temperature).

      b. Invasive monitoring of CVP, PCWP, and CO must be instituted for patients at risk for ARF, with major cardiac, vascular, or intraabdominal operations, and in patients whose volume status is difficult to determine.

      c. Daily weights are also essential.

3. Hourly UO should be $\geq 0.5 - 1.0$ mL/kg/hr. The quality of the urine should also be determined by urinalysis.

4. The presence of glucosuria must be identified and monitored at least q. 4h.

      a. Glucosuria reflects the metabolic control of serum glucose and surgical stress may lead to glucosuria in up to 50% of surgical patients.

      b. Glucose acts as an osmotic diuretic and elevates urine output even if the patient has inadequate preload and renal perfusion.

5. Note deteriorating renal function and correct early. Identify and correct any postrenal etiologies (see pp 376–380). Then eliminate prerenal etiologies of oliguria (see section V. A, pp 363–376).

V. SPECIFIC CONDITIONS.
A. Acute Renal Failure.

1. ARF, by definition, is an abrupt decrease in kidney function that results in accumulation of nitrogenous solutes.

2. UO in ARF may be oliguric (<400 mL/day) or nonoliguric, in which UO is normal or increased while solute clearance is markedly decreased. Mortality from nonoliguric ARF is significantly less than from oliguric, although many cases progress to oliguria and its poor outcome.

3. Regardless of urine output, the sequela of ARF results from retention of metabolic wastes and is indicated by a progressive rise in BUN and serum creatinine concentrations. Hypervolemia and electrolyte imbalances further complicate management of oliguric ARF.

4. ARF is commonly classified as prerenal, postrenal, or intrinsic parenchymal.

a. Prenatal ARF.
   1) ARF caused by hypoperfusion of the kidneys is classified as prenatal.
   2) Surgical patients are at risk for hypovolemia and hypoperfusion. Therefore, any patient with oliguria should be assumed to be hypovolemic until proved otherwise. Causes of prenatal ARF are listed in Table 9–2.
   3) Evaluation of prenatal etiology of ARF includes:
      a) Review of recent (past hours and days) fluid balances. Fluid output significantly greater than input suggests a prenatal etiology of oliguria.
      b) Review of weight change over the past days. Weight loss in the acute setting is most likely secondary to fluid loss.
      c) Determine the extent of insensitive losses from diarrhea, sweat, ascites, pleural effusions, third-space sequestration due to small bowel obstruction. Fluid loss also occurs with large open wounds or burns. Large amounts of intravascular volume may be lost via these routes.
      d) Assessment of renal perfusion according to MAP and O_2 delivery ($CO \times CaO_2$).
      e) Identify factors that may increase renal vein pressure and decrease renal perfusion including mean airway pressure, RV failure and increased intraabdominal pressure.
   4) Results of urinalysis are often helpful in discerning prenatal vs. parenchymal ARF (Table 9–3).
      a) In the presence of tubular injury, U_{osm} is close to that of plasma owing to lack of tubu-

TABLE 9–2.

Causes of Prerenal Acute Renal Failure in Surgical Patients

Volume Changes	Hemodynamic Changes	Vascular Changes
Dehydration	Septic shock	Renal artery stenosis
Blood loss	Cardiogenic shock	Renal vein thrombosis
Third-space sequestration	Neurogenic hypotension	Operative vessel occlusion

TABLE 9–3.

Diagnostic Urine Chemistry

Test	Prerenal	Parenchymal
Urine osmolarity (mOsm/L)	>500	250–350
U/P osmolarity	>1.5	<1.1
U/P urea	>8	<3
U/P creatinine	>20	<10
Urine sodium (mEq/L)	<20	>40
FE_{Na}	<1%	>3%

lar concentrating ability. Conversely, U_{osm} >500 mOsm/L demonstrates excellent concentrating function and suggests prerenal etiology.

b) In the presence of hypovolemia and hypoperfusion, the renin-angiotensin system is activated and the subsequent release of aldosterone will induce the kidney to reabsorb sodium. Therefore, a FE_{Na} <1 indicates volume depletion while an elevated FE_{Na} is more consistent with tubular injury or obstruction.

c) Caution must be taken in interpreting any of these parameters in the presence of a preexisting prerenal state (e.g. CHF, cirrhosis), diuretics, or following the use of contrast dye.

5) With established oliguria, monitoring of CVP, PCWP, and CO is essential.

6) Administration of a fluid challenge (250–500 mL in an adult) and restoration of normal renal perfusion will usually result in increased UO when oliguria is due to prerenal causes.

b. Postrenal ARF.

1) Obstructive uropathy must always be ruled out in the oliguric patient.

2) Patients may complain of flank pain due to acute distention of the renal capsule or suprapubic discomfort caused by bladder distention.

3) Renal ultrasonography is a quick and simple procedure to evaluate the urinary outflow tract and

      detect the presence of calculi, tumor, or blood clot.

  4) Removal of the obstruction should return renal function to normal. However, oliguria and uremia are unlikely to result from a unilateral obstruction without disease in the contralateral kidney (see pp 376–379).

c. Parenchymal ARF.

After excluding pre- and postrenal causes of oliguria, parenchymal etiologies must be considered. These include ATN, pigment nephropathy (due to circulating myoglobin and hemoglobin), and nephrotoxic agents (various drugs and contrast material). Other causes of parenchymal renal disease such as acute glomerular nephritis and vasculitis are not typically responsible for ARF in the surgical patient.

  1) Acute tubular necrosis.

    a) ATN results from ischemia to the renal parenchyma and is the most common cause of ARF.

    b) Under conditions of diminishing renal blood flow, perfusion of the kidneys is first maintained by vasomotor responses which dilate the afferent arteriole and constrict the efferent arteriole.

    c) As continued hypotension is detected by the juxtaglomerular apparatus, the renin-angiotensin system is activated in concert with sympathetic release of other vasoactive hormones. These substances produce vasoconstriction of the afferent arteriole and further exacerbate cortical hypoperfusion.

    d) As a result, GFR is sharply reduced, and the tubules experience profound ischemia.

    e) With damage to the tubular system, casts of cellular debris obstruct the lumen and cellular edema occurs. As tubular cells necrose and slough off, glomerular ultrafiltrate leaks back across the proximal tubular membrane into the interstitium. This back-leakage causes vascular congestion within the renal parenchyma and may prolong ARF.

2) Pigment nephropathy (myoglobinuria and hemoglobinuria).

   a) Pigment nephropathy due to hemolysis or rhabdomyolysis is a common cause of ARF and may occur after trauma, burn, operation, cardiopulmonary bypass (CPB), seizures, alcohol or drug intoxication, prolonged ischemia to muscle groups, or extended coma.

   b) With ischemia or blunt injury to large muscle masses, myoglobin is released to the circulation. In the kidney, it is filtered from blood and reabsorbed by the tubule. Although myoglobin is not a direct nephrotoxin, in the presence of aciduria, myoglobin is converted to ferrihemate which is toxic to renal cells.

   c) Diagnosis can be made with elevated CPK, serum hemoglobin or myoglobin, and a urine microscopy that shows prominent heme pigment without RBCs in the urine sediment. Hyperkalemia and elevated serum creatinine are also consistent with injury to muscle masses.

   d) Prevention of myoglobin-induced ARF include:

      i) Generous hydration.

      ii) Use of diuretics to keep VOP > 100 cc/h.

      iii) Alkalinization of urine to pH >6.0 by administration of sodium biocarbonate.

3) Nephrotoxic agents.

   a) Contrast media.

      i) Radiographic contrast dye has been documented to cause ARF. The incidence of contrast nephropathy is approximately 1%–10% and may be predicted according to a number of risk factors, including contrast load, age, preexisting renal insufficiency, diabetes.

      ii) The incidence in patients with normal renal function is significantly lower at 1%–2%.

      iii) Contrast nephropathy is usually experi-

   enced as an asymptomatic, transient rise
   in creatinine, but may progress to oliguric renal failure requiring hemodialysis.

   iv) Induced diuresis with fluids and diuretics
   prior to contrast injection may decrease
   the incidence and severity of ARF in
   high-risk patients.

b) Nephrotoxic drugs.

   i) Drug-induced ARF (DI-ARF) is responsible for approximately 5% of all cases.

   ii) The pathophysiology of DI-ARF differs
   according to the offending agent. The
   site of damage of several well-docu-
   mented nephrotoxic drugs is listed in Table 9-4. Through normal reabsorption
   and secretion, the kidney is exposed to
   high concentrations of drugs and solutes
   which may be toxic. This is compounded
   by hypovolemia, which causes increased
   reabsorption of water and solutes and ex-
   poses the lumen to even higher concentrations of toxins.

   iii) While the damage to tubular function can
   be significant, much of DI-ARF remains
   nonoliguric owing to sparing of glomerular function.

5. General care of ARF patients.

In surgical patients, ARF rarely occurs in an isolated
fashion. Rather, ARF is only one component of a MOFS
often accompanied by infection. Management of these
patients should therefore be focused on treatment of the
underlying disease process(es). Development of ARF
complicates the care of surgical patients by introducing
difficulties to fluid, electrolyte, and nutritional management. The adverse effects of renal replacement therapies
further compound these problems. Aggressive intervention is necessary. This includes surgical drainage of septic foci, excision of necrotic tissue, early implementation
of effective renal replacement therapy, and full nutritional support.

a. Nonoliguric ARF.

   1) With nonoliguric ARF, treatment may differ little

TABLE 9-4.
Nephrotoxic Drugs

Glomerulus	Renal Arterioles	Proximal Tubule	Distal Tubule	Interstitium
Heroin	Allopurinol	Aminoglycosides	Amphotericin B	Acetaminophen
Hydralazine	Penicillin G	Amphotericin B	Lithium	Aspirin
Penicillamine	Propylthiouracil	Cephaloridine	Vitamin D intoxication	Methicillin
Probenecid	Sulfonamides	Polymixin B		Penicillin G
Procainamide	Thiazides			Phenacetin

  from that required for identical patients with normal renal function.

 2) Except for an elevated BUN, management of fluids, solutes, and nutrition is usually unaffected by
  nonoliguric ARF.

 3) The extent of renal dysfunction is limited and almost always reversible. Use of renal replacement
  therapies is rarely necessary.

b. Oliguric and anuric ARF.

 1) Problems of fluid overload can lead to anasarca,
  pulmonary edema, and CHF.

 2) The pharmacokinetics of drugs become difficult to
  predict as a result of decreased elimination and increased volume of distribution. For adjustments of
  dosages, see pp 394-399.

 3) The volume status of patients with ARF must
  therefore be carefully monitored. Fluid intake and
  output must be tabulated precisely and weight
  measured daily. PA catheterization may be necessary to more closely monitor fluid status.

 4) Treatment options for hypervolemia consist of
  fluid restriction or fluid removal, or both, with artificial kidney techniques. Nutrition and other critical medications are essential to postoperative recovery and should not be limited. Renal replacement should be selected and conducted to allow
  full nutrition without restriction.

 5) "Renal dose" dopamine.

  a) The renal circulation contains specific vasodilating dopaminergic receptors that respond to
   dopamine in low doses of $1-3$ µg/kg/min.

  b) This low-dose (renal-dose) dopamine has
   been shown to increase renal blood flow,
   GFR, and UO.

  c) In addition, renal-dose dopamine and furosemide have shown synergism in successfully converting oliguric to nonoliguric ARF.

  d) For these reasons, renal-dose dopamine is accepted as effective in the treatment of established ARF.

  e) However, its usefulness in preventing ARF is
   doubtful. It is also important to note that do-

pamine will cause renal vasoconstriction when administered in doses >5–10 µg/kg/min.

c. Electrolyte derangements in ARF.
  1) Perform serum electrolyte measurements daily.
  2) Hyperkalemia (serum K^+ >6.5 mEq/L associated with ECG changes) is a medical emergency and a frequent electrolyte disorder with ARF (see pp 420–421).
      a) Under the conditions of hypercatabolism and tissue necrosis, large amounts of K^+ may be generated and accumulate over a short period of time.
      b) Acute hyperkalemia decreases cardiac excitability, which may ultimately result in asystole. These events are usually preceded by changes in the ECG that indicate hyperkalemia. These include loss of P waves, widening of the QRS complex, and peaked T waves.
      c) Immediate treatment of hyperkalemia.
          i) See p 421.
          ii) Hemodialysis is the preferred method of renal replacement.
  3) Hyponatremia, hyperphosphatemia, hypocalcemia, and metabolic acidosis are also common with ARF and must be monitored closely. Treatment consists of appropriate additions or restrictions to IV solutions, and effective use of the artificial kidney.

d. Hematologic derangements in ARF.
  1) Anemia.
      a) In addition to blood loss due to hemorrhage or operation, erythropoietin production has been shown to decrease in direct proportion with decreasing renal function.
      b) In the surgical patient with ARF, PRBCs should be transfused to maintain a Hct >30%.
  2) Platelets.
      a) Although poorly understood, platelet dysfunction and coagulopathy are often associated with ARF. A reproducible platelet defect can

               be demonstrated experimentally with a BUN of 100 mg/dL. The cause of this defect is unidentified.

    b) Desmopressin is used to improve uremic platelet function. (0.3 μg/kg in NS IV over 15–30 min).

    c) Platelets should be transfused to maintain a platelet count >100,000/mm³ in the presence of bleeding.

6. Nutrition and ARF.

  a. The goal is to provide optimal amounts of caloric and protein substrates to minimize autocatabolism and allow tissue anabolism, wound healing, and sustained immune function.

  b. Nutrition for ARF vs. CRF patients.

    1) In CRF, patients are generally healthy with energy requirements that differ little from normal individuals. Protein intake is required only for metabolic turnover and is restricted to minimize urea generation and other products of protein metabolism.

    2) By contrast, the metabolic requirements of ARF patients are those of a critically ill hospitalized patient. Actual measurement of resting energy expenditure has shown that caloric requirements of MOFS patients with ARF average 50% above normal, healthy individuals. Measured protein requirements are also increased to as much as 2 g/kg in order to provide for anabolic wound healing and sustained immune function. For these patients, protein restriction is counterproductive and potentially detrimental. Urea generation is best minimized by providing enough energy substrates (carbohydrates and lipids) to prevent cannibalization of endogenous protein as an energy source. Recent investigations emphasizing energy and protein balance have demonstrated improvement of outcome from ARF.

  c. Guidelines for nutrition in surgical ARF.

    1) Glucose and lipids should be supplied to maintain positive energy balance to reduce protein catabolism, urea generation, and hyperkalemia.

2) Protein should be administered with the goal of achieving positive nitrogen balance. In the absence of conclusive evidence supporting the use of specialized formulations (i.e., essential or branched chain solutions), use of mixed amino acids is recommended.

7. Special considerations in surgical patients.

   a. The mortality of ARF in surgical patients is significantly greater than in medical patients. ARF in nonsurgical patients is usually the primary disease in an otherwise healthy patient. By contrast, surgical patients with ARF are more severely ill and experience ARF secondary to some other primary disease such as burns, trauma, or operative or postoperative complications. These etiologies of ARF are specific to surgical patients and require special consideration.

   b. Burns.

      1) The burn patient is at risk for developing ARF owing to hypovolemia, sepsis, and myoglobinuria.

      2) Effective fluid and electrolyte resuscitation should prevent hypovolemia, and renal failure is rare in burn injury.

      3) When burn or trauma produces muscle necrosis and myoglobinuria, renal failure is common.

      4) The use of daily hemodialysis in massively burned patients does not improve survival, suggesting that neither nitrogenous wastes nor soluble toxins play a role in burn mortality.

   c. Cardiopulmonary bypass.

      1) The incidence of ARF after cardiac operation is ~1%–2%.

      2) Blood flow is nonpulsatile during CPB and this may exacerbate renal ischemia, but only if total body O_2 delivery is inadequate.

      3) Some hemolysis always occurs during CPB which may cause ARF if it becomes excessive.

      4) Perioperative low CO is the most important consideration in the development of ARF.

   d. Renal transplantation.

      1) The most common pathophysiology of ARF in the posttransplant patient is ATN.

   2) Factors which may contribute to posttransplant ATN include donor hypotension, prolonged "warm ischemia," poor perfusate flow, reduced allograft blood flow, cold lymphocytotoxins, and the use of nephrotoxic drugs.

   3) Less common causes of ARF in transplant grafts are hyperacute rejection, ureteral obstruction or leakage, and vascular occlusion.

   4) Cyclosporine.

      a) Although cyclosporine has become the drug of choice in blunting the rejection of transplanted organs, it is also a direct nephrotoxin to renal cortical cells and may also cause ARF through impairment of renal blood flow. These effects are potentiated when combined with other nephrotoxic drugs such as aminoglycosides.

      b) Daily levels and careful dosing of cyclosporine are critical to preventing ATN in the transplant graft.

 e. Liver failure.

   1) The development of ARF secondary to liver dysfunction is referred to as the *hepatorenal syndrome* (HRS).

   2) Clinically, HRS is slowly progressive and characterized by intense NaCl retention with absence of NaCl in urine.

   3) The ensuing renal dysfunction is unresponsive to volume or hemodynamic maneuvers.

   4) HRS commonly occurs in alcoholic cirrhosis but is also reported in patients with cholestatic jaundice, acute hepatitis, and hepatic malignancy.

   5) Regardless of etiology, patients with HRS are characterized by portal hypertension and tense ascites, although the degree of jaundice may be variable.

   6) Management should focus on the state of the intravascular volume in light of ascites and hypoproteinemia. Sodium and fluid intake is carefully restricted.

   7) In severe cases, a peritoneovenous (LeVeen)

shunt may correct the maldistribution of extracellular fluid in HRS and aid management of ARF.

f. Sepsis.

1) Infection is the major cause of death in surgical patients who develop ARF.

2) Sepsis can also cause ARF through direct and indirect effects which cause both renal injury (ATN) and prerenal azotemia.

   a) Direct effects include endotoxin and prostaglandin damage to the renal microvasculature.

   b) Indirect effects include hypotension, impaired regional O_2 delivery, and metabolic disturbances that may result in ATN.

   c) In addition, management of septicemia often requires the use of nephrotoxic antibiotics which may further exacerbate tubular damage.

3) Prophylactic antibiotics and aggressive wound management are required to prevent sepsis in ARF patients.

g. Trauma.

1) Like thermal injury, the development of ARF in the posttraumatic patient is multifactorial with hypovolemia being the major problem. Rapid fluid resuscitation must be instituted to avoid shock, which may lead to ARF if untreated.

2) If after stabilization and restoration of intravascular volume the patient becomes oliguric, the possibility of traumatic injury to the ureter, bladder, or urethra must be ruled out.

3) With blunt trauma to large muscle masses, rhabdomyolysis-induced ARF is a significant concern. Microscopic urinalysis for myoglobin and serum CPK measurements will define the extent of muscle injury and risk. Prevention of ARF in this circumstance may be accomplished by prompt induction of an alkaline solute diuresis using IV mannitol and $NaCO_3$.

h. Vascular surgery.

1) The incidence of ARF in vascular surgery is di-

rectly related to the position and duration of cross-clamping the aorta or renal vessels as well as preexisting renal disease.

2) Resection of a thoracic aortic aneurysm (TAA) requires clamping of the aorta proximal to the renal arteries. ARF has been reported to occur in as many as 50% of patients undergoing TAA repair. However, the rate of ARF after resection of AAAs (in which renal blood flow is usually maintained) is ~7%.

8. Prognosis.

a. Survival of patients with ARF is a function of the successful treatment of the primary disease(s). The mortality of ischemic ATN without other organ failure is 6%. By contrast, mortality of multiple organ failure complicated by ARF ranges from 40%–80%.

b. Outcome of ARF is related to the number of organ systems failed, the interval from onset of ARF to first dialysis, the maximum serum creatinine prior to dialysis, and the presence of cardiac failure. In patients with ARF, 90% of deaths can be attributed to sepsis or multiple organ failure.

c. Both survival and recovery of renal function is better in patients with nonoliguric vs. oliguric ARF.

d. In patients who survive the acute phase of illness, recovery of renal function after ARF is dependent on the type and extent of injury to the renal parenchyma.

1) Renal replacement therapy may be required for several weeks until urine output and solute excretion return to acceptable levels.

2) If renal function has not returned after 6 weeks, recovery is unlikely, and provisions should be made for long-term renal substitution therapy.

B. Urinary Obstruction.

1. Upper tract obstruction.

a. Pathophysiology.

1) Complete unilateral ureteral obstruction with normal contralateral kidney results in elevation of pressure in pyelocaliceal system, diminution of renal blood flow, progressive impairment of renal function, and atrophy of obstructed kidney.

2) Recovery of function after relief of obstruction is

dependent on duration of obstruction, morphology of renal pelvis, and presence or absence of infection.

3) Compensatory hypertrophy of contralateral kidney occurs and is most marked in neonates.

  b. Etiology.

    1) Intrinsic.

      a) Stones—85% radiopaque.

      b) Tumor—95% transitional cell carcinoma.

      c) Sloughed papilla—primarily seen in diabetes, sickle cell disease, analgesic nephropathy.

      d) Clot—important to find source of bleeding. Consider renal cell carcinoma, urothelial carcinoma, vascular anomalies.

      e) Stricture.

        i) Primary (congenital UPJ, obstructed megaureter).

        ii) Secondary (stones, infection, TB, iatrogenic or traumatic).

    2) Extrinsic.

      a) Retroperitoneal tumor—lymphoma, sarcoma, metastatic carcinoma.

      b) Inflammatory processes—retroperitoneal fibrosis, abscess.

      c) Endometriosis.

  c. Diagnosis.

    1) IVP.

      a) Preferred initial study in suspected obstruction in patient with normal renal function.

      b) Delayed nephrogram, delayed excretion.

    2) Renal ultrasonography.

      a) Pelvocaliectasis suggestive of obstruction.

      b) May have obstruction without pelvocaliectasis or pelvocaliectasis without obstruction.

      c) Useful as screening modality, particularly in acute azotemia.

    3) Diuretic radionuclide renography.

      a) ^{99}Tc DTPA scan is to assess whether upper tract obstruction exists by monitoring washout of radionuclide from renal pelvis after administration of loop diuretic.

      b) Utility declines in presence of marked azotemia (creatinine >5 mg/dL).

4) Retrograde pyelography.
  a) "Gold standard"—excellent anatomic detail.
  b) Invasive—cystoscopy required, possibly anesthesia.
5) CT.
  a) Particularly useful in assessing extrinsic upper tract obstruction.
  b) Also useful in distinguishing radiolucent stone from tumor, clot, papilla (must have unenhanced as well as enhanced study).
d. Treatment.
  1) Varies with etiology of obstruction.
  2) Goal is to relieve obstruction expeditiously to salvage renal function.
  3) When obstruction is complicated by infection or azotemia, intervention is urgent.
  4) When possible, retrograde ureteral stenting (double-J stent or ureteral catheter) is preferable.
e. Indications for percutaneous nephrostomy.
  1) Failed retrograde attempt at relief of obstruction.
  2) High-grade obstruction with inability to achieve retrograde decompression owing to anatomic factors such as inaccessible ureteral orifices, presence of urinary diversion (ileal loop, Kock pouch, etc.).
  3) Urosepsis due to upper tract obstruction in patients with prohibitive anesthesia risk.
  4) Pylonephrosis—need larger-bore catheter for drainage than can be placed cystoscopically.
2. Lower tract obstruction.
  a. Pathophysiology.
    1) Anatomic or functional obstruction at or distal to bladder neck.
    2) Efficiency of bladder emptying is a result of strength of detrusor contraction relative to bladder neck or urethral resistance.
    3) Micturition in the neurologically intact patient is a result of detrusor contraction with coordinated sphincter relaxation.
    4) Chronically elevated bladder neck or urethral resistance results in detrusor hypertrophy, elevated micturitional detrusor pressure with ultimate de-

compensation resulting in elevated postvoid residual urine or urinary retention.

- a) Predisposes to UTI, bladder calculi, bladder diverticula.
- b) Elevated bladder pressures result in impairment of upper tract drainage with hydronephrosis.
- c) In severe cases, may lead to ARF with attendant metabolic abnormalities (usually resolve with relief of obstruction).

b. Etiology.

1) Anatomic obstruction.
   - a) Most common cause is BPH.
   - b) Prostatic carcinoma.
     - i) Present in 50%–75% of men over age 70.
     - ii) May also cause upper tract obstruction by local extension into bladder trigone.
   - c) Bladder neck hypertrophy.
   - d) Urethral stricture.
     - i) Most common cause is iatrogenic.
     - ii) Postgonoccocal.
   - e) Miscellaneous causes include bladder or urethral stone, bladder tumor, clot in bladder, fecal impaction, foreign body, meatal stenosis, phimosis.

2) Functional obstruction.
   - a) Hypocontractile neuropathic bladder is frequently seen in diabetes, sacral cord injury, spinal shock.
   - b) Detrusor or sphincter dyssynergia.
     - i) Detrusor contraction is associated with simultaneous sphincter contraction.
     - ii) Seen in spinal cord lesions above sacral reflex arch, multiple sclerosis.
     - iii) Results in incomplete emptying, elevated voiding pressure, and upper tract deterioration.

3) Pharmacologic retention.
   - a) Anticholinergics, cold preparations, antidepressants.
   - b) Narcotics.

c) Spinal or general anesthesia.

d) Ethanol.

c. Diagnosis.

1) Evaluation often prompted by obstructive voiding symptoms (hesitancy, decreased force of stream, postvoid dribbling, double voiding, intermittency, nocturia). May have mild urgency component.

2) Occasionally urinary retention or "anuria" is presenting sign—often postoperatively or after taking medications with anticholinergic effects.

3) Initial diagnostic test should be rectal examination and postvoid residual urine determination.

a) Urine for analysis and culture.

b) Check medications.

4) Other helpful diagnostic aids include cystourethroscopy, urodynamics, retrograde urethrography.

d. Treatment.

1) Dependent on cause and severity of obstruction, and presence or absence of infection or azotemia.

2) Anatomic obstruction generally at bladder neck resolved by insertion of Foley catheter.

a) Larger catheter (18F–22F) with coudé tip is generally more effective if obstruction is at prostatic level.

b) Smaller catheters (12F–14F) are more effective in urethral stricture disease.

c) Filling urethra with 10–15 mL of lubricant via catheter tip syringe is often helpful in difficult catheterization.

3) Prior to manipulation of the infected lower urinary tract, broad-spectrum antibiotics should be administered and the patient should be observed closely following manipulation for sign of sepsis.

4) The hypocontractile neuropathic bladder is best served by intermittent clean catheterization.

5) Watch closely for **postobstructive diuresis** in the postrenally azotemic patient who has undergone relief of lower urinary tract (or bilateral upper tract) obstruction. UO should be replaced ½ mL/mL with D5 ½ NS while monitoring serum electrolytes until resolution of the diuresis.

6) Impassable stricture or difficult or traumatic catheterization should prompt urologic consultation. Filiform and followers or suprapubic cystostomy may be required.

C.   Hematuria.

1. Microhematuria.

    a. Accompanied by proteinuria or pyuria.

        1) Evaluate with urine culture (catheter specimen preferable).

        2) If culture negative, consider TB, fastidious organisms, chlamydia, medical renal disease, papillary necrosis.

        3) If hematuria persists after appropriate therapy, proceed as in gross hematuria (see section V. C. 2).

    b. Unaccompanied by proteinuria.

        1) Rule out urolithiasis, urothelial malignancy, renal cell carcinoma with IVP (or renal ultrasonography and retrograde pyelography in the presence of azotemia), urine cytology, cystoscopy.

        2) Exclude trauma, coagulopathy, sickle cell trait, foreign body, or pseudohematuria.

        3) "Benign" hematuria is a diagnosis of exclusion.

2. Gross hematuria.

    a. Upper tract.

        1) Posttraumatic:

            a) High index of suspicion with penetrating trauma, lower rib fracture, lumbar transverse process fracture, or hemodynamic instability.

            b) Assess bilateral function with IVP or CT scan—urgent renal arteriography if no perfusion documented to renal unit.

            c) Conservative management unless penetrating trauma with associated visceral injury, renal pedicle injury, expanding retroperitoneal hematoma with hemodynamic instability, or extensive urinary extravasation.

        2) Nontraumatic: exclude malignancy, nephrolithiasis, arterial venous malformation, etc.

    b. Lower tract.

        1) Urethral.

            a) High index of suspicion with pelvic fracture,

blood at the external meatus, prostatic displacement on digital rectal examination, penetrating pelvic trauma, or "anuria."
   b) Evaluate with retrograde urethrography. Suprapubic cystostomy for partial or complete urethral disruption with delayed primary repair.
   c) High index of suspicion for associated injury (rectal, vascular) after pelvic trauma.
   2) Bladder.
      a) Cystography with drainage film.
      b) Immediate repair for free intraperitoneal extravasation.
      c) Extraperitoneal extravasation managed with Foley catheter drainage alone in the absence of other lower tract disorder.
   c. **Intractable vesical hemorrhage.**
      1) Multiple blood transfusions are required to declare vesical hemorrhage as intractable. It is usually the result of advanced pelvic malignancy, radiation, or cyclophosphamide-induced **hemorrhagic cystitis.**
      2) The mainstay of therapy is correction of contributing or exacerbating factors (coagulopathy, thrombocytopenia, etc.) and thorough clot evacuation with fulguration of any discrete bleeding points. If bleeding persists, continuous bladder irrigation via large-bore three-way Foley catheter is indicated.
         a) Irrigate initially with NS followed by 1% alum or 1% silver nitrate solution.
         b) In recalcitrant cases the addition of systemic ϵ-aminocaproic acid may be beneficial (1 g IV q. 1 h. $\times$ 4 followed by 1 g IV q. 4 h.).
      3) Intravesical formalin (2%–10% solution) is reserved for unresponsive cases. It is potentially morbid and requires general anesthesia. Perform a cystogram immediately prior to instillation of the formalin to assure absence of vesicoureteral reflux.
      4) Hyperbaric O_2 (in radiation cystitis) and external

beam radiotherapy (in locally advanced malignancy) may be efficacious in selected cases.

5) Embolization or ligation of hypogastric arteries has been advocated.

6) Cystectomy with urinary diversion is occasionally required when conservative measures fail.

VI. RENAL REPLACEMENT THERAPIES.

A. General Guidelines.

1. Indications for use of renal replacement therapy include fluid overload (pulmonary edema, CHF), hyperkalemia, metabolic acidosis, uremic encephalopathy, coagulopathy, acute poisoning. Recent data indicate that initiation of renal replacement early in the course of ARF correlates with improved outcome.

2. Volume (IV fluids, TPN, etc.) should be given as needed, independent of method of renal replacement. Priority must be placed on treatment of underlying disease processes and renal replacement selected and performed to allow usual treatment of the critically ill surgical patient.

3. Renal replacement therapy should be instituted early in the course of ARF, before hypervolemia, azotemia, or hyperkalemia occur.

4. Currently, renal replacement modalities available for treatment of ARF in the critically ill patient are hemodialysis (HD), peritoneal dialysis, and continuous arteriovenous hemofiltration. These therapies are described below and contrasted in Table 9–5.

B. Hemodialysis.

1. Description of technique.

a. The patient's blood is pumped via an extracorporeal circuit through a porous hollow-fiber membrane (artificial kidney) which is permeable to solutes of <2,000 daltons. An isotonic solution surrounds the membrane that provides a concentration gradient for the selective removal of solutes such as K^+, urea, and creatinine, while maintaining plasma concentrations of Na^+, Cl^-, and HCO_3^-.

b. Vascular access consists of an arteriovenous shunt or a double-lumen venovenous access.

1) Percutaneous venovenous catheters are usually

TABLE 9–5.

Comparison of Renal Replacement Therapies

Description	Hemodialysis	Peritoneal Dialysis	CAVH/CAVHD
Assessment	Rapid-intermittent	Slow-intermittent	Slow-continuous
Vascular access	Arteriovenous/venovenous	Abdominal catheter	Arteriovenous
Anticoagulation	Required	None required	Required
Solute removal	Excellent	Excellent	Good (CAVH) Excellent (CAVHD)
Fluid removal	Good-excellent	Good	Excellent
Hemodynamic instability	Potentially significant	None	None
Risks of procedure	Hypotension Hemorrhage Dysequilibrium syndrome	Infection/peritonitis Intrabdominal adhesions Respiratory distress	Dehydration Hemorrhage Electrolyte imbalance
Overall appraisal	Useful for urgent removal of solutes or poisons Hemodynamic instability may limit use in SICU patients	Contraindicated with abdominal operation Useful in burn patients and patients with poor vascular access	Broad flexibility with fluid-electrolyte balance Solute removal and fluid management enhanced with CAVHD

placed in the SICU at the bedside for initial therapy. The catheter and access site should be changed frequently to prevent sepsis.

   2) Placement of permanent access (SC arteriovenous shunt) is indicated if renal replacement is required for >2 weeks with no signs of renal recovery.

  c. Systemic anticoagulation is usually required for this procedure, although less heparin may be used on patients with a baseline coagulopathy.

  d. HD is typically performed q.o.d. for a 3–4-hour period but is required more frequently in catabolic patients with a high urea generation rate.

  e. Solute and volume removal is considered very efficient with HD relative to other methods of renal replacement.

2. Advantages.

  a. HD is the method of choice for rapid removal of large amounts of fluid, life-threatening electrolyte imbalances, toxins, and poisons.

  b. HD may also be applied to hemodynamically stable surgical patients with isolated ARF where contraindication for peritoneal dialysis exists (i.e., postoperative laparotomy).

3. Disadvantages.

  a. In critically ill surgical patients with ARF, HD can cause hypotension, hypoxemia, hemolysis, and precipitate cardiac arrhythmias. These events limit the application of dialysis in unstable patients.

  b. Hypotension may be managed by:

   1) Decreasing transmembrane pressure and sodium gradient during dialysis.

   2) Transfusion to maintain Hct > 20%.

   3) Keeping patient npo prior to HD to avoid splanchnic pooling of blood.

   4) Trendelenburg position during HD.

   5) Substitution of **bicarbonate for acetate** during HD. Acetate in dialysate may act as a vasodilator. It is used because it is more stable than bicarbonate, hence has a longer shelf life.

   6) α-Agonist use during HD (phenylephrine).

  c. Anticoagulation is also required and may be undesirable in the immediate postoperative or posttrauma setting.

    d. Acute CNS disturbances ranging from mild stupor to coma can occur with hemodialysis ("disequilibrium syndrome"). They are attributed to rapid intracellular and extracellular fluid and electrolyte movement across the brain.

    e. Muscle cramping may occur due to rapid fall in serum osmolarity. This may be decreased by increasing the dialysate sodium to 132–140 mEq/L or the use of mannitol to increase osmolarity.

C. Peritoneal Dialysis (PD).

1. Description of technique.

    a. PD is performed by infusion of several liters of a sterile electrolyte solution with hypertonic dextrose into the abdominal space. Using the peritoneal membrane as a selective barrier, the dialysate solution creates an osmotic pressure gradient that extracts extracellular fluid and solutes out of the mesenteric circulation and into the peritoneal cavity. This fluid is then drained after an equilibration period of 1–2 hours.

    b. Dialysate composition:

       1) Lactate or acetate 0–45 mEq/L (replaces bicarbonate).

       2) Electrolytes: Na^+ 131–141 mEq/L, K^+ 0–4 mEq/L, Ca^{2+} 3.5–4.0 mEq/L, Mg^{2+} 0.5–1.5 mEq/L, Cl^- 96–107 mEq/L.

       3) Dextrose 1.5%–4.5%. Concentrations of dextrose >4.25% irritate the peritoneum.

       4) Osmolarity is 345–510 mOsm/L depending on the dextrose concentration.

    c. Fluid removal usually ranges 0.5–2.0 L/hr although greater fluid and solute clearance can be accomplished by:

       1) Using larger volumes of dialysate.

       2) Increasing the frequency of exchange cycles.

       3) Using a higher dextrose concentration in the dialysate.

    d. Placement of intraperitoneal (Tenckhoff) catheter can be performed in the SICU or OR.

2. Technique:

    a. The dialysis fluid (500–1000 mL) is allowed to flow freely into the peritoneal cavity through the Tenckhoff catheter.

b. After a dwell time of 15–60 minutes, the fluid is emptied by lowering the original bag below the patient.

c. Determination of cycle frequency and dialysate composition depends on assessment of fluid and electrolyte balance. Usually start with a 500-mL volume and a short dwell time. A smaller volume reduces the leakage around a new catheter.

3. Advantages of PD:

a. PD does not require vascular access or systemic anticoagulation, making it useful in patients with peripheral vascular disease or risk of hemorrhage. It is the treatment of choice for the postcardiothoracic surgical patient with ARF.

b. The slow rate of equilibration and fluid extraction minimizes the problems of disequilibrium and hemodynamic compromise experienced with conventional HD.

4. Disadvantages of PD:

a. Catheter infection and peritonitis.

1) Rigid peritoneal catheters inserted percutaneously in the acute setting become predictably colonized after 48–72 hours.

2) Silastic catheters placed SC are associated with a lower incidence of peritonitis (1.6 episodes per patient-year) and should be implanted with prolonged use of PD.

3) Other access-related complications include visceral injury at time of catheter placement and formation of intraabdominal adhesions.

4) In light of these risks, PD is generally the last-choice method of renal replacement after abdominal operation or trauma.

b. Hyperglycemia can occur due to the hypertonic glucose of the dialysate. Insulin therapy may be required.

c. Respiratory distress may develop from reduced diaphragmatic compliance and increased intraabdominal pressure.

d. Repeated lavage of the peritoneal cavity causes protein loss of ≥ 10 g/day and may exacerbate malnutrition in catabolic ARF patients. Hypovitaminosis can occur.

e. Catheter misplacement may require water-soluble contrast studies to document location of catheter in the peritoneal cavity.

D. Continuous Arteriovenous Hemofiltration (CAVH) and Continuous Arteriovenous Hemodiafiltration (CAVHD).

1. Description of techniques.

   a. CAVH and CAVHD are extracorporeal ultrafiltration techniques that remove extracellular fluid (ECF) across a synthetic membrane via the hydrostatic pressure gradient created between indwelling arterial and venous catheters.

   b. With a systolic BP of ≥80 mm Hg, blood flows through the porous hollow-fiber capillary membrane at a rate of 50–150 mL/min thus driving plasma water and solutes of up to 10,000 daltons (ultrafiltrate) out of the hemofilter at 500–700 mL/hr.

   c. Arteriovenous access is accomplished by percutaneous cannulation of the femoral artery and vein with a low incidence of complications.

   d. Heparinization of the extracorporeal circuit is required, usually at a rate of 500 units/hr.

   e. With CAVH, a substitution solution formulated to resemble ECF without toxic solutes is simultaneously infused into the venous access of the circuit at a rate to achieve a desired hourly fluid balance.

   f. This exchange transfusion of 12–17 L/day of ECF provides clearance of approximately 10–14 g/day of urea (assuming a BUN of 80 mg/dL) (see Fig 9–1).

   g. With CAVHD, a dialysate solution is circulated in the extracapillary space countercurrent to blood flow. This creates a concentration gradient for selective removal of large amounts of solute. The ultrafiltration rate is regulated to achieve desired net fluid balance and no substitution fluid is necessary (see Fig 9–2).

   h. CAVH and CAVHD are run continuously for as many days as renal replacement is required. Hemofilter performance (as monitored by the ultrafiltration rate) decreases over time, requiring replacement with a new hemofilter approximately every 2 days.

2. Advantages of CAVH and CAVHD.

   a. Little or no incidence of hemodynamic instability is encountered with treatment of unstable critically ill

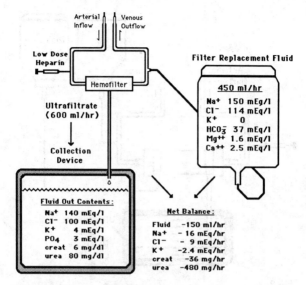

FIG 9–1.
Principles of continuous arteriovenous hemofiltration (CAVH). Arteriovenous access provides blood flow through the hemofilter. Hydrostatic pressure creates an isoelectric ultrafiltrate at a rate of 600 mL/hr. A replacement fluid is reinfused to maintain normal electrolytes and achieve a desired net fluid balance. Low-dose heparin is also required with this therapy. (From Mault JR, Dirkes SM, Swartz RD, et al: *Continuous Hemofiltration: A Reference Guide for SCUF, CAVH, and CAVHD.* Ann Arbor, University of Michigan Printing, 1990. Used by permission.)

ARF patients. This is attributed to slow and continuous fluid and solute removal in addition to the low blood activating properties of the hemofilter membrane.

b. Both CAVH and CAVHD permit generous flexibility with volume management and eliminate the need for fluid restriction in oliguric ARF. Fluid balance and serum electrolyte concentrations can be titrated to any

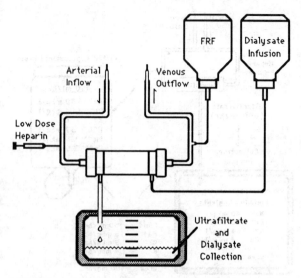

FIG 9–2.
Continuous arteriovenous hemodialysis (CAVHD). CAVHD combines the
advantages of continuous hemofiltration with the selective properties and
clearance capabilities of hemodialysis. A sterile dialysate solution is infused
countercurrent to hemofilter blood flow and provides a concentration gradient for selective removal of large amounts of uremic solutes. FRF = filter
replacement fluid. (From Mault JR, Dirkes SM, Swartz RD, et al: *Continuous Hemofiltration: A Reference Guide for SCUF, CAVH, and CAVHD*.
Ann Arbor, University of Michigan Printing, 1990. Used by permission.)

           value and optimum amounts of nutrition can be pro-
           vided.
      c. Solute clearance with CAVHD is approximately equal
           to that achievable with standard HD.
   3. Disadvantages of CAVH and CAVHD:
      a. Owing to continuous fluid and electrolyte removal,
           dehydration and electrolyte imbalance may occur.
      b. Hemorrhage may occur as a result of systemic antico-
           agulation.

4. Management considerations of CAVH and CAVHD.
   a. Ultrafiltration rate (UFR).
      1) UFR is dependent on patient's BP, the blood flow through the hemofilter, the available free water, and distance between the collection container and the hemofilter.
      2) In order to prevent excess hemoconcentration of blood at the venous end of the hemofilter (which decreases hemofilter performance and longevity), the maximum ultrafiltration rate (UFR$_{max}$) should be calculated. First, the hemofilter blood flow rate (BF) is calculated from the circuit time (recorded upon unclamping the hemofilter blood tubing) and the hemofilter circuit volume as follows:

$$BF \ (mL/min) = \frac{circuit \ volume \ (mL)}{circuit \ time \ (sec)} \times \frac{60 \ sec}{min}$$

Next, determine the plasma flow (PF) and UFR$_{max}$:

$$PF \ (mL/min) = BF \times \frac{(100\% - Hct)}{100}$$

$$UFR_{max} \ (mL/min) = 0.2^* \times PF$$

7*For Hct <40%, use 0.3 instead.

      3) With CAVH, the UFR should be maintained below UFR$_{max}$ and is usually regulated to 400–600 mL/hr with a Hoffman clamp or volumetric control pump on the ultrafiltrate line.
      4) With CAVHD, both the dialysate and the ultrafiltrate fluids will drain through the ultrafiltrate line into the collection container. To determine the actual UFR, subtract the dialysate infusion rate (DI) from the total fluid collected (TFC) as follows:

$$UFR_{CAVHD} \ (mL/min) = TFC \ (mL/min) - DI \ (mL/min)$$

      5) As described earlier, the clearance capabilities of CAVHD eliminate the need for replacement fluid and limit the use of ultrafiltration to maintenance

of a desired fluid balance (DFB). Therefore, by using a Hoffman clamp or volumetric control pump on the ultrafiltrate line, the TFC is limited to the sum of the DI plus total IV fluids (TIV) minus all other fluid output (OFO) (i.e., UO, chest tube and NG drainage), plus or minus DFB (for a net negative fluid balance, add DFB; for net positive fluid balance, subtract DFB) as follows (units in mL/hr):

$$\text{TFC} = \text{DI} + \text{TIV} - \text{OFO} + \text{DFB}$$

    a) The minimum TFC allowed equals the rate of dialysate infusion (DI) and must not be restricted below that rate.

    b) If the calculated TFC is less than the DI rate, then a filter replacement fluid (FRF) should be infused to make up the difference.

6) Clotting of the hemofilter will result in a decrease in blood flow and a subsequent decrease in UFR. If the systolic BP is ≥80 mm Hg, and the unrestricted UFR is ≤100 mL/hr, the hemofilter should be discontinued to prevent thrombosis of the vascular access. Increasing the heparin infusion will not reverse clotting that has occurred in the hemofilter and should not be attempted as a means of "saving the filter."

b. Anticoagulation.

1) The objective of heparinization in continuous hemofiltration is to prevent thrombosis of blood in the hemofilter without necessarily effecting systemic anticoagulation. This objective may or may not be achieved with an individual patient. In most cases, a continuous heparin infusion of ~7–10 units/kg/hr is administered to patients with normal clotting times, and hemofilter longevity averages 48 hours. However, a single hemofilter may last several days with little or no heparin in a patient with a coagulopathy.

2) In order to monitor anticoagulation status, the activated clotting time ACT, normal range 100–120 seconds, should be checked frequently. The ACT

is a measure of whole blood clotting and is the preferred method for monitoring heparin therapy (if the ACT is unavailable, TCT or PTT can be substituted effectively).

c. Fluid and electrolyte balance.
   1) Strict records of all fluids in and out are essential!
   2) In CAVH, approximately 8–14 L/day of ultrafiltrate are removed according to patient conditions. This ultrafiltrate contains uremic solutes (urea and creatinine) but also essential solutes (Na^+, Cl^-, HCO_3^-, etc.) which must be replaced. The concentration of these solutes in the ultrafiltrate is identical to that in the patient's plasma. Solute losses can be calculated by multiplying the plasma concentration by the UFR.
   3) Filter replacement fluid (FRF) is a premixed IV solution formulated to replace water, electrolytes, and other solutes removed by ultrafiltration. The exact composition of the FRF is determined by the requirements of the individual patient. FRF rate is calculated as follows (units in mL/hr):

$$FRF = UFR + OFO - TIV + DFB$$

d. Drug clearance.
   1) All nonprotein-bound drugs will be cleared with the ultrafiltrate. These losses should be compensated by increasing dosages to maintain therapeutic levels.
   2) The amount of drug clearance (DC) can be estimated from the plasma concentration of the drug ($[D]_p$), the percent of drug-protein binding (%PB), and the UFR as follows:

$$DC \ (amount/min) = [D]_P \times UFR \times (100\% - \%PB)$$

e. Complications.
   1) For severe hypotension, clamp the ultrafiltrate line but allow the blood flow to continue through the hemofilter. The heparin infusion must also be maintained. With CAVH, the FRF infusion may

TABLE 9-6.
Medication Adjustments for Renal Failure*†

	Dosage Interval (hr) for Creatinine Clearance (mL/min)			Supplement After Dialysis	Monitor Serum Levels
	>50	10–50	<10		
Aminoglycosides					
Amikacin	12	12	>24	H,P	Yes
Gentamycin	8	12	>24	H,P	Yes
Kanamycin	24	24–72	72–96	H,P	Yes
Streptomycin	24	24–72	72–96	H	Yes
Tobramycin	8	12	>24	H,P	Yes
Netilmicin	8–12	12	>24	H,P	Yes
Cephalosporins					
Cefamandole	4–6	6–8	8–12	H	
Cefazolin	8	12	24–48	H	
Cefoperazone	N	N	N	H	
Cefotaxime	6–8	8–12	12–24	H	
Cefoxitin	8	8–12	24–48	H,P	
Ceftazidime	6–8	12–24	24–36	H	
Ceftizoxime	6–8	8–12	12–24	H	
Cephalothin	6	6	6–12	H,P	
Moxalactam	8	12	12–24	H	

Penicillins					
Azlocillin	4	4–8	8–12	H	
Ampicillin	6	6–12	12–16	H	
Carbenicillin	4–6	8–12	12–24	H,P	
Mezlocillin	4	4–8	8–12	H	
Methicillin	4	4	8–12	H,P	
Nafcillin	6	6	6	H	
Penicillin G	4–6	6–12	12	H	
Piperacillin	4–6	6–8	8	H	
Ticarcillin	4–6	8–12	12–24	H,P	
Miscellaneous antimicrobials					
Acyclovir	8	24	48	H	
Amantadine	12–24	24–72	72–168	N	
Amphotericin B	24	24	24–36	?	
Chloramphenicol	N	N	N	H	
Clindamycin	N	N	N	N	
Ethambutol	24	24–36	48	H,P	
Flucytosine	6	24	24–48	H,P	Yes
Imipenem	6–8	8–12	12	H	
Isoniazid	N	N	75%	H,P	
Ketoconazole	N	N	N	N	
Metronidazole	8	8–12	12–24	H	Yes

(Continued.)

TABLE 9-6 (cont.).
Medication Adjustments for Renal Failure*†

	Dosage Interval (hr) for Creatinine Clearance (mL/min)			Supplement After Dialysis	Monitor Serum Levels
	>50	10–50	<10		
Miconazole	N	N	N	N	
Rifampin	N	N	N	?	
Sulfamethoxazole	12	18	24	H	
Sulfisoxazole	6	8–12	12–24	H,P	
Tetracycline	12	12–18	18–24	N	
Timentin	4–6	8	12–24	H	
Trimethoprim	12	18	24	H	
Vancomycin	24–72	72–240	240	N	Yes
Diuretics					
Acetazolamide	6	12	Avoid		
Ethacrynic acid	6	6	Avoid		
Furosemide	N	N	N		
Mercurials	24	Avoid	Avoid		
Metolazone	N	N	N		
Spironolactone	6–12	6–24	Avoid		
Thiazides	N	N	Avoid		
Antihypertensives					
Captopril	N	N	50%	H	
Clonidine	N	N	N	N	
Hydralazine	8	8	8–16	N	

Drug					
Methyldopa	6	9–18	12–24	H,P	
Minoxidil	N	N	N	H	
Nitroprusside	N	N	N	H	
Prazosin	N	N	N		
Miscellaneous medications					
Cimetidine	6	8	12	N	
Metoclopramide	75%	75%	50%	?	
Terbutaline	N	50%	Avoid	?	
Theophylline	N	N	N	H,P	
Nonnarcotic analgesics					
Acetaminophen	4	6	8	H	
Acetylsalicylic acid	4	4–6	Avoid	H	
Narcotics					
Codeine	N	N	N	N	
Meperidine	N	N	N	N	
Morphine	N	N	Avoid	N	
Antiarrhythmics					
Amiodarone	N	N	N	?	
Bretylium	N	25%–50%	Avoid	?	
Disopyramide	75%	25%–50%	10%–25%	H	Yes
Flecainide	N	25%–50%	Avoid	?	Yes
Lidocaine	N	N	N	N	Yes
Procainamide	4	6–12	12–24	H	Yes
Quinidine	N	N	N	H,P	Yes
Tocainide	N	N	N	H	Yes
Verapamil	N	N	N	?	

(Continued.)

TABLE 9–6 (cont.).
Medication Adjustments for Renal Failure*†

	Dosage Interval (hr) for Creatinine Clearance (mL/min)			Supplement After Dialysis	Monitor Serum Levels
	>50	10–50	<10		
Miscellaneous cardiac drugs					
Atenolol	N	50%	25%	H	
Digoxin	24	36	48	N	Yes
Diltiazem	N	N	N	N	
Esmolol	N	N	N	N	
Nifedipine	N	N	N	N	
Nitrates	N	N	N	N	
Metoprolol	N	N	N	H	
Nadolol	N	50%	25%	H	
Pindolol	N	N	N	?	
Propranolol	N	N	N	N	
Timolol	N	N	N	N	
Psychoactive drugs					
Amitriptyline	N	N	N	N	
Chlordiazepoxide	N	N	N	N	
Chlorpromazine	N	N	N	N	
Diazepam	N	N	N	N	
Flurazepam	N	N	N	N	
Haloperidol	N	N	N	N	
Imipramine	N	N	N	N	
Lithium	N	50%–75%	25%–50%	H,P	
Medazolam	N	N	N	N	

Anticoagulants					
Heparin	4	4	4	H	Yes
Warfarin	24	24	24	?	Yes
Anticonvulsants					
Carbamazepine	N	N	75%	N	
Phenobarbital	N	N	12–16	H,P	
Phenytoin	N	N	N		
Corticosteroids					
Cortisone	8	8	8	H	
Dexamethasone	6	6	6	?	
Hydrocortisone	8	8	8	?	
Methylprednisolone	24	24	24	H	
Prednisone	8	8	8	?	
Hypoglycemic agents					
Chlorpropamide	24–36	Avoid	Avoid	P	
Insulin (regular)	N	N	N	?	
Tolbutamide	8	8	8	H	

*Adapted from Bennett WM: *Clin Pharmacokinet* 1988; 15:326–354.
†H = hemodialysis; P = peritoneal dialysis.

be continued if required to expand intravascular volume. With CAVHD, the dialysate infusion must be discontinued when clamping the ultrafiltrate line.

2) If any portion of the extracorporeal circuit becomes disconnected, immediately occlude the arterial and venous cannulas and disconnect the hemofilter circuit.

3) Any change in ultrafiltrate color to pink or red indicates rupture of a hemofilter capillary and requires immediate removal and replacement.

f. Discontinue hemofiltration:

1) If the maximum unrestricted UFR is ≤100 mL/hr.

2) If the ultrafiltrate color changes to pink or red, indicating hollow fiber rupture.

3) If renal function recovers sufficiently (UO, decreasing BUN and creatinine) so that all IV lines and nutrition can be maintained without fluid restriction.

4) If renal function is not recovered when all other organ failure(s) have resolved, the patient should be treated with HD or PD.

I. MEDICATION ADJUSTMENTS FOR RENAL FAILURE (see Table 9–6).

SELECTED REFERENCES

Abel RM, Beck CH, Abbott WM, et al: Improved survival from acute renal failure after treatment with intravenous essential I-amino acids and glucose: Results of a prospective double-blind study. *N Engl J Med* 1973; 288:645–699.

Bartlett RH, Mault JR, Dechert RE, et al: Continuous arteriovenous hemofiltration: Improved survival in surgical acute renal failure? *Surgery* 1986; 100:400–408.

Bennett WM: Guide to drug dosage in renal failure. *Clin Pharmacokinet* 1988; 15:326–354.

Bywaters EGL, Beall D: Crush injuries with impairment of renal function. *Br Med J* 1941; 1:427–434.

Cioffi WG, Taka A, Gamelli RL: Probability of surviving postoperative acute renal failure. *Ann Surg* 1984; 200:205–211.

Graziani G, Cantaluppi A, Casati S, et al.: Dopamine and furosemide in oliguric acute renal failure. *Nephron* 1984; 37:39–42.

Kramer P, Wigger W, Rieger J, et al: Arteriovenous hemofiltration: A new and simple method for treatment of overhydrated patients resistant to diuretics. *Klin Wochenschr* 1977; 55:1121–1122.

Kolff WJ, Berk HTJ: Artificial kidney: Dialyzer with great area. *Acta Med Scand* 1944; 117:121–134.

Mault JR, Dirkes SM, Swartz RD, et al: *Continuous Hemofiltration: A Reference Guide for SCUF, CAVH, and CAVHD.* Ann Arbor, University of Michigan Print, 1990.

Martin PV, Dixon SM, Baker JD, et al: Risk of renal failure after major angiography. *Arch Surg* 1983; 118:1417–1420.

McDonald RH, Goldberg LI, McNay JL, et al: Effect of dopamine in man: Augmentation of sodium excretion, glomerular filtration rate, and renal plasma flow. *J Clin Invest* 1964; 43:1116–1124.

Schetz M, Lauwers PM, Ferdinande P: Extracorporeal treatment of acute renal failure in the intensive care unit: A critical review. *Intensive Care Med* 1989; 15:349–357.

Vander AJ: *Renal Physiology*, ed 4. New York, McGraw-Hill Book Co, 1991.

FLUID AND ELECTROLYTES/ ACID-BASE REGULATION

10

I. NORMAL DISTRIBUTION OF BODY FLUIDS.

A. Total Body Water (TBW).

The TBW is distributed between two main compartments (Fig 10–1).

1. **Intracellular water** (ICW) consists of $\sim$ 30%–50% of TBW.

2. Extracellular water (ECW) is distributed among interstitial, plasma, and transcellular compartments which make up 16%, 4%, and 2% of TBW, respectively.

B. Compartment Composition.

The protein and electrolyte composition of the various compartments is shown in Figure 10–2. The integrity of these compartments is maintained by the vascular endothelium and the cell membranes that surround the compartments.

C. Water Movement Between Compartments.

1. Osmolality: The amount of water in a compartment is determined by the number of osmotically active particles present within that compartment. Because cell membranes and endothelium are freely permeable to water, osmotic equilibrium between the various compartments is usually maintained.

2. Fluid shifts.

   a. Nonisotonic fluid shifts: When the osmolality of either the intracellular or extracellular compartment changes, water moves along the osmotic gradient from the hypotonic compartment to the hypertonic compartment until a new osmotic equilibrium is reached. At this

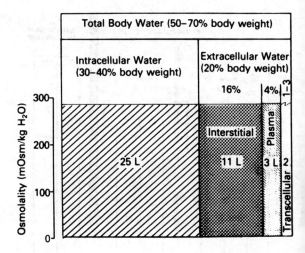

FIG 10–1.
Approximate sizes of body fluid compartments.

new equilibrium, each compartment has a new volume and osmolality (Table 10–1), thus minimizing the magnitude of the initial change.

b. Isotonic fluid shifts: Isosmotic fluid gains or losses are distributed only within the ECW compartment because without a change in osmolality, water will not shift between the intracellular and extracellular compartments.

c. Starling forces: Some fluid movement between the plasma and the interstitium is governed by the balance between intracapillary hydrostatic pressure (IHP) and interstitial oncotic pressure (IOP) on one side and plasma oncotic pressure (POP) and tissue turgor pressure (TTP) on the other. When IHP plus IOP are greater than POP and TTP, ultrafiltration across the capillary membrane occurs. When TTP and POP are greater than IHP and IOP, there is a net fluid reabsorption into the capillary.

3. Calculation of osmolality: Plasma osmolality can be mea-

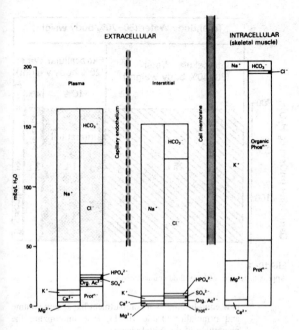

FIG 10–2.
Solute constituents of major body fluid compartments.

sured directly or estimated. The main osmotically active particles within plasma are Na^+ and Cl^-. Glucose and urea usually account for approximately 5 mOsm/L. However, if either is markedly elevated, as in diabetes or renal failure, their effect on plasma osmolality can be pronounced. The following formula for approximating **plasma osmolality** (P_{osm}) shows the relative contribution of each.

$$P_{osm} \cong 2[Na^+] + \frac{glucose\ (mg/L)}{18} + \frac{BUN}{2.8}$$

TABLE 10–1.

Classification of Imbalances of Body Fluids and Associated Changes in Volume and Composition

	Changes in					
	Volume*			Concentration		
Extracellular Type of Imbalance	ECF	ICF	Na+	Protein	Osmality	Hct
Isosmotic contraction	↓	0	0	↑	0	↑
Hyperosmotic contraction	↓	↓	↑	↑	↑	0
Hyposmotic contraction	↓	↑	↓	↑	↓	↑
Isosmotic expansion	↑	0	0	↓	0	↓
Hyperosmotic expansion	↑	↓	↑	↓	↑	0
Hyposmotic expansion	↑	↑	↓	↓	↓	0

*ECF = extracellular fluid; ICF = intracellular fluid.

II. NORMAL FLUID AND ELECTROLYTE BALANCE.

Neuroendocrine controls maintain the fluid and electrolyte composition of the intracellular and extracellular compartments. In the steady state, fluid and electrolyte intake equals fluid and electrolyte output. For the healthy individual, fluid intake comes from liquids, solids, and oxidative metabolism. Fluid output is from sensible and insensible losses (Table 10–2).

TABLE 10–2.

Water, Sodium, and Potassium Balance in Normal Patient

	Water (mL/day)	Sodium (mEq/day)	Potassium (mEq/day)
Intake			
Liquids	800–1,500	50–150	50–80
Solids	500–1,000		
Oxidation	150–300		
Output			
Sensible			
Urine	800–1,500	10–150	50–80
Intensive	0–250	0–20	Trace
Sweat	0–100	10–60	0–10
Insensible			
Lungs	250–450	0	0
Skin	250–450	0	0

III. INTRAVENOUS FLUID THERAPY.

Intravenous fluid therapy is required when patients are unable to maintain fluid and electrolyte balance by oral intake. Fluid and electrolyte therapy can be divided into three categories: maintenance, replacement of previous losses, and replacement of ongoing losses.

A. Maintenance Therapy.

1. **Water:** In calculating maintenance fluid requirements, several factors must be considered. For a 70-kg patient, daily obligatory losses that must be replaced include insensible losses (800 mL), fecal losses (200 mL), and sweat (100 mL) (see Table 10–2). In addition, enough urine must be produced to excrete a solute load of 600 mOsm produced each day by the body. Surgical patients, injured patients, and severely ill patients have decreased urine-concentrating abilities. These patients have a minimum obligatory UO of ~900 mL. In total, the 70-kg patient requires from 2,000–2,500 mL/day of H_2O to maintain fluid balance. From this information 24-hour IV fluid requirements have been formulated based on weight for adults and children:

Weight (kg)	IV Fluid Requirements
0–10	100 mL/kg
10–20	1,000 mL + 50 mL/kg for every kilogram >10
>20	1,500 mL + 20 mL/kg for every kilogram >20 until adult level is reached
Adults	30–35 mL/kg

2. **Sodium:** Sodium losses amount to about 30 mEq/day from stool and sweat with a variable amount lost in the urine. In times of severe water deprivation, the kidneys can reabsorb most of the filtered sodium in response to increased aldosterone secretion. When this occurs, large amounts of potassium can be lost. Therefore, administration of approximately 1–2 mEq/kg/day of sodium in adults or 1 mEq/kg/day in children will not only replace obligatory sodium losses but will also suppress aldosterone secretion enough to help prevent potassium wasting. If NaCl is used, the body's daily requirement for chloride will also be met.

3. **Potassium:** Daily losses of potassium in urine and sweat amount to 40–60 mEq. Replacement with 0.5–1.0 mEq/

kg/day is usually enough to maintain potassium balance in a patient with normal kidneys.

4. **Standard IV therapy solutions:** The electrolyte composition of various commercially available IV solutions is listed in Table 10–3. Daily maintenance requirements can be met by using a D5W ¼ NS + 20 mEq KCl/L solution at a rate calculated in section III.A.1.

B. **Replacement of Previous Losses**

1. **Hemodynamically unstable patient:** Initial treatment of patients who are hypovolemic is geared toward preventing or correcting shock. Rapid volume expansion is usually required. Isotonic crystalloid or colloid can be used. Although there is some controversy as to which type of solution is preferred, both are efficacious.

   a. **Crystalloid**—electrolyte solutions with or without dextrose.

      1) **Distribution:** To expand the intravascular space, isosmotic solutions must be used. Since the crystalloids equilibrate across the extracellular space, only about **one fourth** of any volume of isotonic crystalloid will stay within the intravascular compartment.

      2) **Complications:** Large volumes of crystalloids usually lead to peripheral and potentially pulmonary edema. Large amounts of dextrose may cause hyperglycemia. Large amounts of normal saline may lead to hyperchloremic metabolic acidosis and lactated Ringer's solution given in the setting of hypovolemia, and metabolic alkalosis (e.g., NG drainage, vomiting) may exacerbate the alkalosis when the lactate is metabolized.

      3) **Indications:** In most situations, except as mentioned below, crystalloid volume expansion should be the initial therapy with consideration of concurrent colloid administration if a shock state persists or returns after rapid infusion of 2 L of crystalloid.

   b. **Colloid:** The use of colloid solutions is directed toward augmenting the body's own response of releasing albumin from the liver (up to 50 g or 40% of the normal intravascular pool) into the intravascular space within 3 hours of the onset of the hypovolemia.

      1) **Distribution:** Colloid solutions stay mainly within the intravascular space. However, to remain within

TABLE 10–3.

Electrolyte Composition of Commercially Available Intravenous Solutions

	Electrolytes (mEq/L)							
	Na⁺	Cl⁻	K⁺	HCO₃⁻	Ca²⁺	Osmality	pH	Calories/L
Crystalloid								
0.9% NaCl (NS)	154	154				292	5	
0.9% NaCl + 5% dextrose (D5W NS)	154	154				565	5	200
0.45% NaCl (½ NS)	77	77				146		
0.45% NaCl + 5% dextrose (D5W ½ NS)	77	77				420		200
0.2% NaCl + 5% dextrose (D5W ¼ NS)	34	34				330		200
D5W						274	4	200
D10W						548	6.5	400
Ringer's lactate	130	109	4	(28)	3	277		
3% NaCl	513	513				960		
Colloid								
Hetastarch	154	154				310	5.5	
5% plasma protein factor	145	100	.25				6–7	

this space and be effective, colloids require intact capillary membranes across which they can exert oncotic pressure.

2) Complications: Although controversial, some authorities believe that colloid administration is associated with an increased incidence of PE and respiratory failure requiring mechanical ventilation if given to patients with leaky capillary syndrome. Colloid solutions are also more expensive than crystalloids.

3) **Indications:**

    a)   If the hypovolemic state persists or returns after rapid infusion of 2 L of crystalloid.

    b)   Patients with low effective circulating volumes but total body excess of sodium and water: This group includes patients with ascites, CHF, and postcardiac bypass patients. The exogenous colloid may help mobilize fluid reserves as seen by infusion of 100 mL of 25% albumin which increases plasma volume by $\sim 450 \pm 50$ mL compared to infusion of 1,000 mL of LR which increases plasma volume only 200 ± 20 mL.

    c)   Patients unable to synthesize adequate amounts of albumin include those having liver transplants, hepatic resections, malnutrition, and liver disease. These patients may not have or make enough protein to exert significant amounts of oncotic pressure.

    d)   Severe hemorrhage or coagulopathy: In this setting, blood product replacement such as PRBCs and FFP may help increase the Hct and correct the coagulopathy while the underlying problem is being addressed.

2. **Hemodynamically stable patients:** Once circulating volume has been restored or in patients who are dehydrated but not in shock, volume deficits can be corrected at a slower rate. These volume deficits are best **corrected over a 24–36-hour period** with half of the estimated volume deficit replaced within the first 8 hours and the remaining half being replaced over the ensuing 16–24 hours. Calculation of the volume loss requires a careful history and physical examination, attempting to document weight loss, as well as

laboratory data consisting of electrolytes and plasma osmolality. Isotonic volume losses must be determined by the degree of weight loss or estimation of the degree of dehydration as plasma sodium and osmolality are normal. Hypertonic or hypotonic volume losses can be estimated by formulas based on plasma sodium and osmolality (see section IV, pp 412-413).

C. **Ongoing Volume Losses.**

Critically ill patients often have additional volume losses that must be quantitated and completely replaced to prevent severe fluid and electrolyte derangements. The source of these fluids and their electrolyte composition determine the nature of the replacement fluid. The composition of many of these fluids is shown in Table 10–4.

1. **Fever:** Each degree centigrade above 37°C adds 2.0–2.5 mL/kg/day of insensible water loss. D5W ¼ NS plus 5 mEq KCl/L is the best replacement fluid to approximate sweat.

2. **Loss of body fluids.**

   a. **Gastric:** D5W ½ NS plus 30 mEq KCl/L is the best approximation of gastric contents for replacement secondary to losses from vomiting, NG drainage, or fistulas. If a metabolic alkalosis is present, D5W NS plus 40 mEq

TABLE 10–4.

Electrolyte Composition of Various Body Fluids

| | Electrolytes (mEq/L) | | | | |
	Na^+	K^+	Cl^-	HCO_3^-	Volume (L/day)
Saliva	30	20	35	15	1.0–1.5
Gastric juice, pH<4	60	10	90		2.5
Gastric juice, pH >4	100	10	100		2
Bile	145	5	110	40	1.5
Duodenum	140	5	80	50	
Pancreas	140	5	75	90	0.7–1.0
Ileum	130	10	110	30	3.5
Cecum	80	20	50	20	
Colon	60	30	40	20	
Sweat	50	5	55		0–3
New ileostomy	130	20	110	30	0.5–2.0
Adapted ileostomy	50	5	30	25	0.4
Colostomy	50	10	40	20	0.3

KCl/L should be used to provide enough chloride to help correct the alkalosis. Lactated Ringer's should not be used in this setting as metabolism of lactate to HCO_3 may exacerbate the alkalosis.

b. **Biliary and pancreatic losses:** Lactated Ringer's is the replacement fluid of choice. Extra HCO_3 may be needed when replacing pancreatic fluid losses.

c. **Small bowel and colon:** Lactated Ringer's is used for small bowel loses. LR or ½ NS plus 20 mEq KCl/L plus 25 mEq $NaHCO_3$/L may be used for colon losses or diarrhea.

3. **Third-space losses:** Third-space fluid is similar in composition to extracellular interstitial fluid. Volume losses may be difficult to estimate. **In adults, there is approximately 1 L of third-space fluid intraabdominally for each quadrant of the abdomen that is traumatized, inflamed, or operated upon.** In children, approximately one fourth of the calculated maintenance rate per 24-hour period is sequestered for each quadrant of the abdomen that is traumatized, inflamed, or operated upon. Lactated Ringer's is the appropriate replacement solution.

4. **Burns:** Many standard formulas exist for estimating volume losses in burn patients (see pp 751-753).

5. **Osmotic diuresis** (secondary to urea, mannitol, or glucose): Urine electrolytes should be checked to help determine the composition of a replacement fluid, if one is necessary.

D. **Goals of Fluid Therapy.**

The goals of fluid therapy are to maintain an adequate state of hydration and tissue perfusion with electrolyte balance. The physical examination and appropriate laboratory data must be reviewed frequently and carefully.

1. **Vital signs:** Tachycardia, decreased pulse pressure, and orthostatic BP are all early signs of hypovolemia. BP is not persistently lowered until 20%–30% of the circulating volume is lost.

2. **Physical examination:**

a. Neck veins provide "poor man's CVP." Low CVP implies hypovolemia.

b. Lungs: Rales suggest volume overload or CHF.

c. Heart: Presence of S_3 suggests volume overload or CHF.

    d. **Periphery:** Signs of edema suggest volume overload or CHF. Poor tissue turgor, dry mucous membranes, and cool extremities all suggest hypovolemia.

3. **Input, output, weights:** Daily weights provide one of the more accurate methods for assessing volume status, especially when followed serially. Day-to-day changes reflect acute volume losses or gains. Careful measurements of inputs and outputs are helpful in planning appropriate fluid replacement and following UO.

4. **UO:** Normal UO ranges between 30–125 mL/hr. Lower rates imply renal failure, low flow states, or hypovolemia. Rates above this imply overhydration or pathologic states such as DI, osmotic diuresis, or postobstructive diuresis.

5. **Laboratory data:** Serum electrolytes should be determined frequently in SICU patients on IV fluid to not only make sure that any preexisting electrolyte abnormality is resolving with current treatment but also to prevent iatrogenic electrolyte abnormalities from developing. Serum electrolytes can also shed light on the volume status. BUN-creatinine ratios are a marker of hydration: ratios <15 imply adequate hydration whereas ratios >20 imply low intravascular volume. Urine electrolytes and urine osmolality, if obtained before or at least 12 hours after the last diuretic use, can also be useful in oliguric patients to differentiate prerenal etiologies that are usually related to hypovolemia or low flow states from ARF (see p 364–365).

6. **Invasive monitoring:** Frequently patients in the SICU have multiple complex problems involving multiple organ systems which can make clinical assessment of their volume status very difficult. In these cases, a Swan-Ganz catheter should be used to follow CVP, PCWP, and CO. These measurements help guide fluid management.

IV. ELECTROLYTE DISTURBANCES: DIAGNOSIS AND TREATMENT.

A. **Hyponatremia (Na^+ <136 mEq/L).**

    1. **Evaluation and differential diagnosis:** Initial workup consists of obtaining a serum osmolality. From this, the hyponatremic patient can be put into one of three groups:

        a. **Hypertonic hyponatremia** (P_{osm} >280 mOsm/kg H_2O) usually secondary to hyperglycemia or hypertonic infusions (mannitol, glucose, glycine). Serum Na^+ falls 1.6 mEq/L for every 100-mg/dL increase in glucose or mannitol.

b. **Isotonic hyponatremia** (P_{osm}=280–285mOsm/kg H_2O) is usually secondary to hyperlipidemia, hyperproteinemia, or isotonic infusions of glucose, mannitol, or glycine.

c. **Hypotonic hyponatremia** (P_{osm}<280 mOsm/kg H_2O) can be divided into three categories based on an assessment of extracellular volume status: hypovolemic, hypervolemic, or isovolemic. The differential diagnosis of each of these categories is seen in Fig 10–3. History, physical examination, urine osmolality, urine sodium, BUN, serum creatinine, and serum electrolytes are used to determine the diagnosis.

2. Symptoms include confusion, anorexia, lethargy, nausea, vomiting, coma, and seizures. Their severity depends on the rate of fall of serum Na^+ as well as the degree of hyponatremia. Symptoms usually do not occur until serum Na^+ concentration has fallen to 120–125 mEq/L.

3. **Treatment.**

a. **Asymptomatic hyponatremia:** Treatment depends on etiology.

1) Hypertonic or isotonic hyponatremia: Correct underlying disorder. Insulin may be required if increased Na^+ is secondary to hyperglycemia.

2) Hypovolemic hypotonic hyponatremia: isotonic saline.

3) Hypervolemic hypotonic hyponatremia: water restriction; consider diuresis.

4) Isovolemic hypotonic hyponatremia: water restriction of <500 mL/day.

b. **Symptomatic hyponatremia** requires more aggressive treatment: 3% NaCl to correct the sodium deficit no faster than 2 mEq/L/hr or 20 mEq/L/day. The rate of 3% NaCl administration to raise serum sodium 2 mEq/L/hr can be approximated by the following formula:

$$\frac{(2 \text{ mEq/L})(0.6 \text{ body weight [kg]}) \times 1{,}000}{513 \text{ mEq/L}}$$

$$= 3\% \text{ NaCl/hr (mL)}$$

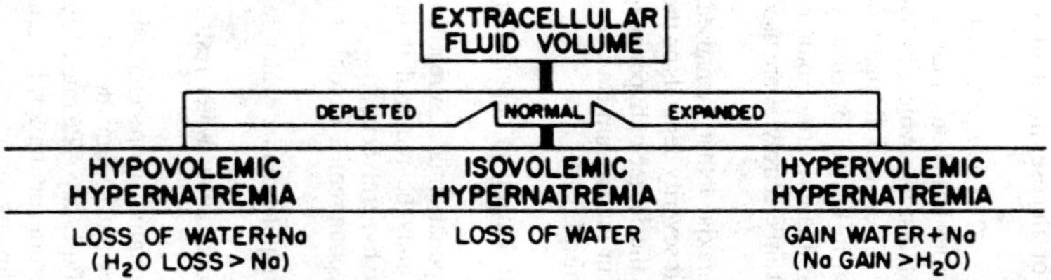
EXTRACELLULAR FLUID VOLUME
DEPLETED
NORMAL
EXPANDED
HYPOVOLEMIC HYPERNATREMIA
ISOVOLEMIC HYPERNATREMIA
HYPERVOLEMIC HYPERNATREMIA
LOSS OF WATER+Na (H_2O LOSS > Na)
LOSS OF WATER
GAIN WATER+Na (Na GAIN > H_2O)

CAUSES	BUN/Cr.	URINARY (Na)	URINARY Osm	CAUSES	BUN/Cr.	URINARY (Na)	URINARY Osm	CAUSES	BUN/Cr.	URINARY (Na)	URINARY Osm
RENAL:				DIABET. INSIP.*				IATROGENIC	V	↑↓(V)	V
DIURETICS	↑↑/↑	↑	↓	CENTRAL	↑/N	N	↓	MINERALOCORT.			
GLYCOSURIA	↑/N,↑	↑	↓	NEPHROG.	↑/N	N	↓	EXCESS			
UREA DIURESIS	↑↑/N,↑	↑	↓	RESET				1° ALDO	N	N	V
ACUTE/CHRONIC	↑↑/↑↑	↑	↓	OSMOSTAT	N/N	N	V	CUSHING'S	N	N	V
RENAL FAIL.				SKIN LOSS	↑/N	↓	↑	CONG. ADR.			
PARTIAL OBST.	↑↑/↑↑	↑	↓	IATROGENIC	N/N	V	↑	HYPERPLAS.	N	N	V
ADRENAL:								EXOGENOUS	N	N	V
CONG./ACQ.	↑↑/↑	↑	±↑								
DEFICIENCIES											
GI LOSSES	↑↑/↑	↓	↑								
RESPIRATORY	↑↑/↑	↓	↑								
LOSSES											
SKIN LOSSES	↑↑/↑	↓	↑								

FIG 10–3.
Differential diagnosis of hyponatremia.

Concurrently, the underlying cause of the hyponatremia should be determined and aggressively treated. When the symptoms resolve, usually when serum Na^+ rises to 120–125 mEq/L, the 3% NaCl can be stopped. Continued correction of the hyponatremia based upon its etiology can be continued at a slower rate as described above. Overzealous correction of the hyponatremia can cause seizures, central pontine myelinolysis, and permanent brain damage.

B. Hypernatremia (Na+>144 mEq/L).

1. **Evaluation and differential diagnosis:** Because hypernatremia is always associated with hypertonicity, it is not necessary to measure serum osmolality. Evaluation begins by clinically assessing extracellular volume status. From this information, one can put the hypernatremic patient into one of three categories: hypovolemic hypernatremia, hypervolemic hypernatremia, and isovolemic hypernatremia. The differential diagnosis for each of these categories can be seen in Fig 10–4. A careful history, physical examination, electrolytes, BUN, serum creatinine, urine Na^+ and U_{osm} will help make the diagnosis. In the SICU, iatrogenic hypernatremia and diabetes insipidus (DI) are the two most common causes.

2. Signs and symptoms depend on the rate of development and the extent of the hypernatremia as well as the accompanying volume status. **Neurologic abnormalities** are most frequently seen and include restlessness, lethargy, twitching, tremulousness, ataxia, seizures, dementia, delirium, and strokes, secondary to subarachnoid and subcortical hemorrhages. Cellular dehydration and shrinkage of brain cells that causes tearing of cerebral blood vessels is thought to be the mechanism of the most severe neurologic changes.

3. Treatment of hypernatremia depends upon extracellular volume status and the rate of development of the hypernatremia.

   a. **Extracellular volume status:**

      1) **Volume depletion:** In hypovolemic hypernatremia, the first goal of therapy is restoration of extracellular volume. Isotonic saline is used initially until euvolemia is achieved. Then, hypotonic saline or D5W can be used to correct the hyperna-

TACHYCARDIA, HYPOTENSION POOR SKIN TURGOR — EDEMA — NORMAL PULSE, BLOOD PRESSURE, SKIN TURGOR, NO EDEMA

HYPOVOLEMIC HYPOTONIC HYPONATREMIA

CAUSES	BUN/Cr.	URIC ACID	URINARY Osm.	(Na)
1. GI LOSSES	↑↑/↑	↑	↑↑	↓↓
2. SKIN LOSSES	↑↑/↑	↑	↑↑	↓↓
3. LUNG LOSSES	↑↑/↑	↑	↑↑	↓↓
4. 3rd. SPACE	↑↑/↑	↑	↑↑	↓↓
5. RENAL LOSSES				
a. DIURETICS	↑↑/↑	↑	ISO	↑
b. RENAL DAMAGE	↑↑/↑↑	↑	ISO	↑
c. PARTIAL URINARY TRACT OBSTRUCT.	↑↑/↑	↑	ISO (↑)	↑
6. ADRENAL INSUFFICIENCY	↑↑/↑	↑	↑	↑

HYPERVOLEMIC HYPOTONIC HYPONATREMIA

CAUSES	BUN/Cr.	URIC ACID	URINARY Osm.	(Na)
1. CHF	↑↑/↑	↑	↑	↓
2. LIVER DAMAGE	↑↑/↑	↑	↑	↓
3. NEPHROSIS	↑↑/↑ (↑↑/↑↑)*	↑	↑ (ISO	↓ ↑)*

ISOVOLEMIC HYPOTONIC HYPONATREMIA

CAUSES	BUN/Cr.	URIC ACID	URINARY Osm.	(Na)
1. H_2O INTOX.	↓/↓	↓	↓,(↑)*	↓
2. RENAL FAIL.	↑↑/↑↑	↑	ISO	↑
3. K^+ LOSS	↓/↓(N)*	↓	↑	↑
4. SIADH	↓/↓	↓↓	↑	↑
5. RESET OSMOSTAT	N	N	V	V

FIG 10–4.
Differential diagnosis of hypernatremia.

tremia. The **H$_2$O deficit** can be calculated with the following formula:

$$0.6 \, (BW)\frac{(current \; P_{Na^+})}{140} - 1 = H_2O \; deficit$$

$$BW = Body \; weight \; (kg)$$
$$H_2O \; deficit \; (L)$$

In cases secondary to DI, aqueous vasopressin 5 units SC q. 4–6 h. or IV drip may be necessary (25 units in 250 mL at a rate of 1 unit/hr, titrated to maintain UO between 100–200 mL/hr).

2) **Volume expansion:** In the hypervolemic hypernatremic patient, a loop diuretic (furosemide), in conjunction with D5W or D5¼ NS is the treatment of choice. In the setting of renal failure, dialysis may be required to remove the excess volume.

3) **Euvolemia:** In the euvolemic hypernatremic patient, the hypernatremia can be treated with water replacement orally or D5W parenterally.

b. **Rate of correction.**

1) **Acute hypernatremia:** When accompanied by neurologic signs and symptoms, acute hypernatremia should be corrected rapidly over a few hours. Patients without neurologic symptoms should be treated like patients that develop hypernatremia slowly.

2) **Chronic hypernatremia:** Because the brain can compensate during chronic hypernatremia by creating idiogenic osmoles to prevent cell shrinking, a rapid correction of a hypernatremia that developed slowly would lead to cerebral swelling and edema. Therefore, slowly developing hypernatremias should be corrected slowly over at least 48 hours and no faster than 2 mOsm/hr.

C. **Hypokalemia.**

1. **Evaluation:** Although only a small amount of the total body potassium is present in the serum (65 mEq in serum vs. 4,000 mEq intracellularly), hypokalemia is defined as a serum K$^+$ <3.5 mEq/L. A delicate equilibrium exists between extracellular and intracellular potassium (Fig

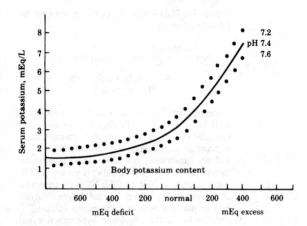

FIG 10-5.
Relationship between serum and tissue potassium.

10-5). Because of the way potassium is distributed within the body, hypokalemia can result from:

a. Altered transcellular distribution of potassium.
b. Total body depletion of potassium.
c. Combination of the above.

The presence of hypokalemia can be suggested by flattened T waves and a U wave on an ECG (Fig 10-6).

2. **Differential diagnosis:** History, physical examination, acid-base status, and urinary electrolytes are useful in working up the hypokalemic patient. Four general mechanisms lead to hypokalemia:

a. **Hypokalemia secondary to redistribution:** Several factors lead to altered transcellular distribution of potassium: respiratory and metabolic alkalosis, exogenous HCO_3, insulin and glucose administration. The effect of decreased pH on serum K^+ can be estimated. For every 0.1-unit change in pH, there is a 0.6-mEq/L change in serum K^+.

b. **GI losses:** urine K^+ <20 mEq/day; etiologies include diarrhea, intestinal or biliary fistulas, villous adeno-

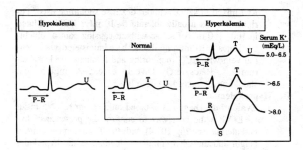

FIG 10–6.
ECG abnormalities seen in hypokalemia and hyperkalemia.

mas, laxative abuse, vomiting, NG suction. Urine K^+
in the last two disorders may be >20 mEq/day owing
to increased urine K^+ excretion that occurs with alkalosis.

   c. **Renal losses:** urine K^+ >20 mEq/day; etiologies include renal tubular acidosis, diuretic phase of ATN,
postobstructive diuresis, osmotic diuresis, diuretics,
corticosteroids, hyperaldosteronism, or Cushing's syndrome.

   d. Poor intake of potassium.

3. **Signs and symptoms.**

   a. Cardiac: increased incidence of arrhythmias, especially
PACs, PVCs, and predisposition to digoxin toxicity.

   b. Neuromuscular: intestinal ileus, constipation, rhabdomyolysis, skeletal muscle weakness, paralysis. Respiratory arrest may occur with K^+ <2 mEq/L.

   c. Renal: decreased GFR, increased ammonium production, metabolic alkalosis.

   d. Endocrine: decreased aldosterone and insulin release,
increased renin release.

4. **Treatment:** Serum K^+ should be confirmed in addition to
adequate renal function and urine output. If the GI tract is
functional, then oral supplementation is preferred. Total
body deficits can be calculated from Figure 10–3 and replaced at a rate of 80–120 mEq/day. If the patient's GI
tract is not functional or the hypokalemia is severe, IV

KCl mixed in saline without dextrose should be used. Peripheral veins usually tolerate 5–10 mEq KCl/hr diluted in 100–150 mL of saline without causing pain or phlebitis. Rates >10 mEq/hr should be administered via a central vein with ECG monitoring and frequent checks of serum K^+. Rates rarely have to exceed 20 mEq/hr and should never exceed 40 mEq/hr.

D. Hyperkalemia.

1. **Evaluation:** Diagnosis is based on a serum K^+ >5 mEq/L. **ECG** is the best way to confirm the presence of hyperkalemia (see Fig 10–4) with the T wave increasing in height and the QRS complex widening as the hyperkalemia worsens.

2. **Differential diagnosis:** A careful history and physical examination, ECG, blood chemistry, and ABG are helpful.

   a. **Redistribution** is usually seen in the setting of acidosis where a 0.1-unit decrease in pH causes a 0.6-mEq/L increase in serum K^+.

   b. **Decreased K^+ excretion** is most commonly seen with ARF and adrenal insufficiency, less commonly in CRF unless the patient is challenged with a potassium load.

   c. **Increased K^+ load** may be endogenous secondary to increased tissue breakdown such as major surgery, crush injury, rhabdomyolysis, massive hemolysis, or GI bleeding. Exogenous sources include oversupplementation, blood transfusions, especially when blood has been stored for extended periods, and high doses of penicillin (potassium salts).

   d. **Pseudohyperkalemia** usually occurs secondary to a hemolyzed blood sample. It may also be seen in patients with a leukocytosis $>5 \times 10^5/mm^3$ or thrombocytosis $>7.5 \times 10^5/mm^3$ because of potassium released by these cells during clotting. The diagnosis of pseudohyperkalemia is confirmed by a normal ECG and a normal repeated potassium performed on **heparinized** blood.

3. **Signs and symptoms.**

   a. Cardiac: Alterations in cardiac conduction (see Fig 10–4) secondary to hyperkalemia may lead to cardiac arrest. Although ECG changes do not correlate exactly with a given potassium level, it is rare to see ECG changes other than peaked T waves with a serum K^+ <6.5 mEq/L.

   b. **Neuromuscular:** tingling, malaise, weakness, pares-
      thesias, paralysis.
   c. **Endocrine:** increased aldosterone and insulin.
4. Treatment of hyperkalemia depends on the level of potassium and ECG changes.
   a. For K^+ **<6.5 mEq/L with no ECG changes,** all sup-
      plemental KCl should be stopped. Repeat a stat serum
      K^+ on heparinized blood.
   b. For K^+ **<6.5 mEq/L with ECG changes** consisting
      only of peaked T waves, stop supplemental KCl. Give
      sodium polystyrene sulfonate (either po or per rectum)
      or furosemide (Table 10–5) in an attempt to eliminate
      excess K^+. Search for underlying cause of hyperkale-
      mia that can be corrected.
   c. For K^+ **>6.5 mEq/L or any level of K^+ with ECG
      changes more extensive than peaked T waves,** ag-
      gressive therapy aimed at lowering serum and total
      body potassium should be undertaken (see Table
      10–7).
E. **Hypocalcemia.**
   1. **Evaluation:** Calcium exists in plasma in various forms:
      50% is free or ionized, 40% is bound to proteins, and
      10%–15% is bound to ions such as citrate or phosphate.
      Although free Ca^{2+} is the only form that is physiologi-
      cally active, most laboratories measure total serum Ca^{2+}
      (8.8–10.4 mg/dL normal in men, 8.5–10.1 mg/dL nor-
      mal in women). When interpreting this value, the serum
      albumin should also be checked because the **total serum
      Ca^{2+} will fall 0.8 mg/dL for every 1-g/dL decrease in
      serum albumin.** Hypocalcemia secondary to hypoalbu-
      minemia is called pseudohypocalcemia and is asympto-
      matic because ionized Ca^{2+} is not lowered. If possible,
      the diagnosis of hypocalcemia should be based on **ionized
      Ca^{2+} levels,** the normal range for which is **1.12–1.23
      mmol/L.**
   2. Differential diagnosis: Pseudohypocalcemia should be ex-
      cluded by documenting hypocalcemia with either a low
      ionized Ca^{2+} or a low adjusted total serum Ca^{2+}. The
      most common causes of hypocalcemia include:
      a. Hypoparathyroidism—surgical, neoplastic or infiltra-
         tive.
      b. Pancreatitis.

TABLE 10–5.
Treatment of Hyperkalemia

Drug	Rationale	Dose	Onset	Duration
Calcium gluconate*	Antagonizes membrane effects of ↑ K^+	10 mL of 10% solution slowly over 2–3 min; may repeat × 1	Minutes	1 hr
Glucose and insulin*	Redistribution of K^+ into cells	1 ampule D50 + insulin 10 units regular IV	15–30 min	2–4 hr
$NaHCO_3$†	Redistribution of K^+ into cells	50–100 mEq IV	15–30 min	1–2 hr
Sodium polystyrene sulfonate‡	Removes K^+ by anion exchange in GI tract	Enema: 50–100 g mixed in sorbitol as retention enema for 45 min; repeat q.h.	60 min	4 hr
		Oral: 40 g mixed in sorbitol q. 2–4 h.	120 min	
Furosemide§	Removes K^+ by increased renal excretion	20–40 mg IV	15–30 min	4 hr
Dialysis‖	Removes K^+ directly; redistributes K^+ into cells	Hemodialysis, peritoneal dialysis	Minutes Minutes	

*Should be done immediately. Use Ca^{2+} cautiously in patients on digoxin as it may precipitate digoxin toxicity.
†Depends on arterial pH.
‡May cause hypernatremia. Oral administration removes 1 mEq K^+/g. Per rectum, removes 0.5 mEq K^+/g.
§May not be effective in patients with ARF or may require larger doe.
‖Usually only necessary in severe ARF or massive crush injuries. Hemodialysis can remove 20–30 mEq K^+/hr. Peritoneal dialysis can remove 10–15 mEq K^+/hr.

    c. Hypomagnesemia.

    d. Hyperphosphatemia—renal failure, rhabdomyolysis.

    e. Hypovitaminosis D—CRF, malabsorption.

    f. Drugs or toxins—transfusions with citrated blood, gentamicin, protamine, mithramycin, phenytoin, phenobarbital.

3. **Signs and symptoms:**

    a. CNS—mental status changes, seizures, extrapyramidal movement disorders.

    b. Neuromuscular—circumoral and acral paresthesias, tetany, myopathy.

    c. Cardiovascular—hypotension, increased QT interval, occasionally ventricular dysrhythmias.

4. **Treatment.**

    a. **Acute:** Patients with neuromuscular symptoms may be at risk for developing seizures and laryngospasm. Therefore, they should be given 200–300 mg of elemental calcium. This amount is present in 20–30 mL of 10% calcium gluconate (90 mg/10 mL ampule) or 5–10 mL of 10% calcium chloride (273 mg/10 mL ampule). The IV calcium should be given slowly over several minutes because it can potentiate hypertension and digoxin toxicity. It should never be given in the same line as $NaHCO_3$ as it will precipitate into the calcium salt. With any type (acute or chronic) of hypocalcemia, concomitant hypomagnesemia and hyperphosphatemia should be corrected.

    b. **Chronic:** Asymptomatic hypocalcemia can be treated by adding calcium to a liter of maintenance IV fluid to run in over several hours or with po calcium (1,500–3,000 mg/day) plus vitamin D.

F. **Hypercalcemia.**

1. Hypercalcemia is defined as **total serum Ca^{2+} >10.4 mg/dL** in men and **>10.1 mg/dL** in women or an **ionized Ca^{2+} >1.23 mEq/L.** Hyperalbuminemia or conditions such as multiple myeloma where total serum protein is increased may elevate total serum Ca^{2+} by 0.8 mEq/dL for each gram increase in serum protein.

2. **Differential diagnosis:** Malignancy, hyperparathyroidism, and granulomatous disease account for almost 90% of all cases. More than two thirds of the cases seen in the SICU are secondary to a known malignancy. When no known malig-

nancy exists, a serum PTH level should be obtained. If the serum PTH is elevated, hyperparathyroidism is usually the cause. If the serum PTH is low, then a workup for occult malignancy should be undertaken. Other causes of hypercalcemia that should be considered if there is no evidence of malignancy and the serum PTH is not elevated include:

a. Thyrotoxicosis.
b. Paget's disease.
c. Sarcoidosis.
d. Tuberculosis.
e. Addison's disease.
f. Immobilization.
g. Thiazide diuretics.
h. Milk-alkali syndrome.
i. Vitamin D intoxication.
j. Vitamin A intoxication.
k. Hypophosphatemia.

3. **Signs and symptoms:**
   a. General—malaise, fatigue, weakness.
   b. Neuropsychiatric—lethargy, confusion, polydipsia, headache, decreased concentration and memory.
   c. GI—anorexia, nausea, vomiting, constipation.
   d. Renal—polyuria, nephrocalcinosis, nephrolithiasis, ARF, CRF.
   e. Cardiovascular—bradycardia, heart block.

4. **Treatment** of hypercalcemia is supportive until the underlying causes can be corrected. Supportive measures include:
   a. **Saline and furosemide:** Hydration accompanied by diuretics which inhibit renal calcium reabsorption are effective in decreasing serum Ca^{2+}. **One to 2 L NS over 1–2 hours followed by 200–400 mL/hr given in conjunction with furosemide 20–80 mg IV q. 2–3 h.** is usually effective in lowering total serum Ca^{2+} 1–3 mg/dL within the first 24 hours. The serum K^+ and Mg^{2+} levels must be followed closely, especially if the patient has any degree of renal failure. The rate of IV fluid administration must be slowed if signs of overhydration develop.
   b. **Etidronate disodium (EHDP)** is a synthetic diphosphate analogue of the naturally occurring inhibitor of bone metabolism, pyrophosphate. As such, EHDP acts

primarily to reduce normal and abnormal bone resorption which in turn leads to diminished bone formation and turnover. The drug is most effective in treating hypercalcemia secondary to neoplastic disease. EHDP does not have any direct antineoplastic activity and is not effective in treating hypercalcemia secondary to hyperparathyroidism. EHDP should only be used after adequate UO has been achieved with hydration and furosemide. **The IV dosage given over 2 hours is 7.5 mg/ kg/day × 3 days.** A second IV course may be tried after 7 days. Maintenance of normocalcemia can be achieved with a po dosage of EHDP 20 mg/kg/day for 30 days.

c. **Phosphate** causes calcium to be removed from the blood and deposited in the extravascular tissues. **Phosphate should be given to any hypercalcemic patient with a serum PO_4^{2-} <3 mg/dL until the PO_4^{2-} increases to 5 mg/dL.** Effects are immediate with IV administration. However, oral administration is the route of preference (phosphosoda 5 mL po t.i.d. or q.i.d. = 1,800–2,400 mg PO_4^{2-}). IV PO_4^{2-} should be used if calcium is ≥15 mg/dL. The usual IV dose is 0.16 mmol/kg or 5 mg/kg of PO_4^{2-} administered over a 6-hour period until the serum PO_4^{2-} is 5–6 mg/dL.

d. **Mithramycin** inhibits bone resorption. Usual dose is **10–25 μg/kg IV** repeated as necessary for severe hypercalcemia (Ca^{2+} ≥15). Serum Ca^{2+} should begin to fall within 12–24 hours. Repeated doses may be associated with thrombocytopenia, platelet dysfunction, or liver damage, so liver function tests, WBC, and platelet counts should be followed daily.

e. **Steroids** help to decrease intestinal Ca^{2+} absorption and in malignancies may not only inhibit bone resorption but also be tumoricidal. **Prednisone 5–15 mg po q. 6 h.** or its steroid equivalent can be used. Steroids exert their effect in 2–3 days.

f. **Calcitonin** reduces bone resorption. However, even at doses of **4 units/kg IV followed by 4 units/kg SQ q. 12 h.,** 25% of patients do not respond. In general, calcitonin is less effective than PO_4^{2-} or mithromycin.

g. **Dialysis** is usually necessary if hypercalcemia is accompanied by ARF.

G. Hypophosphatemia.

1. **Evaluation:** Normal serum PO_4^{2-} levels range from **2.7–4.5 mg/dL,** with the majority of the total body store being intracellular (3,000 mg/dL). Hyperphosphatemia can occur secondary to excess external losses of PO_4^{2-} or secondary to its redistribution from extracellular to intracellular pools.

2. **Differential diagnosis:** The history and physical examination are important. Urine PO_4^{2-} excretion may also be useful as <100 mg/day implies GI losses or redistribution and >100 mg/day implies renal losses.

   a. **GI losses:** inadequate intake, malabsorption, alcoholism, aluminum containing antacids, chronic diarrhea.

   b. **Primary renal losses:** primary hyperparathyroidism, diuretics, burns, alcoholism.

   c. **Redistribution into cells:** The most common causes of hypophosphatemia seen in the sick are usually secondary to glucose infusion, insulin administration, TPN, or food administration after periods of starvation, malnutrition, respiratory alkalosis, or catecholamine administration.

3. **Signs and symptoms:**

   a. CNS—obtundation, coma, seizures.

   b. Muscle—rhabdomyolysis, myopathy, weakness, cardiomyopathy, respiratory arrest.

   c. Hematopoietic—anemia.

   d. Bone—osteomalacia.

   e. General—weakness, fatigue.

4. **Treatment** (1 mmol PO_4^{2-} = 31 mg elemental PO_4^{2-}).

   a. **Severe life-threatening hypophosphatemia (PO_4^{2-} <1 mg/dL):** Administer 0.16 mmol/kg (5 mg/kg) of elemental phosphorous over 6 hours.

   b. **Hypophosphatemia with PO_4^{2-} between 1–2 mg/dL:** Administer 0.08 mmol/kg (2.5 mg/kg) over 6 hours.

   c. For the above two situations, increase dose by 25%–50% if patient symptomatic and decrease dose by 25%–50% if patient hypercalcemic. Recheck PO_4^{2-} after infusion and base further treatment on new PO_4^{2-} level obtained.

   d. For mild asymptomatic hypophosphatemia, po supplementation may be used such as phosphosoda 5 mL t.i.d. (4.2 mmol/mL). Diarrhea is an occasional side effect.

   e. Correct concurrent hypocalcemia.

H. Hyperphosphatemia.

1. **Evaluation and differential diagnosis:** Hyperphosphatemia is defined as a **serum PO_4^{2-} >5 mg/dL.** In patients with normal renal function, hyperphosphatemia is unusual. The three settings in which renal excretion is insufficient to prevent hyperphosphatemia are:

   a. **Massive phosphate infusion:**
      1) Endogenous—cytotoxic therapy, rhabdomyolysis.
      2) Exogenous—phosphate enemas, laxative abuse.

   b. **Decreased GFR:**
      1) ARF.
      2) CRF.

   c. **Increased tubular reabsorption:**
      1) Hypoparathyroidism.
      2) Thyrotoxicosis.
      3) Hypovolemia.
      4) Excess growth hormone.
      5) Tumoral calcinosis.

2. **Signs and symptoms** are usually related to hypocalcemia that develops when high serum PO_4^{2-} levels form insoluble calcium-phosphate complexes.

3. **Treatment:**

   a. Acute hyperphosphatemia resolves in ~12 hours if renal function normal and source of PO_4^{2-} controlled. If symptoms of hypocalcemia are present, **acetazolamide 15 mg/kg q.3–4h.** may help by increasing PO_4^{2-} excretion, but usually dialysis is required.

   b. **Mild or chronic** hyperphosphatemia is usually seen in CRF or neoplastic calcinosis and is treated with a low phosphate diet and aluminum-binding antacids such as $Al(OH)_3$.

I. Hypomagnesemia.

1. **Evaluation:** Magnesium deficiency is often accompanied by disturbances in calcium and potassium balance because magnesium is not only required for proper function of cell membrane ATPase-dependent Na^+, K^+ pumps but also for proper PTH secretion. Therefore, conditions in which hypomagnesemia should be considered include hypokalemia, hypocalcemia, alcoholism, postchemotherapy, intractable ventricular arrhythmias, and in chronically ill or malnourished patients. The **normal serum Mg^{2+} level is 1.3–2.1 mEq/L.**

2. **Differential diagnosis** requires a careful history and physical examination as well as appropriate laboratory data. Most often Mg^{2+} deficiencies arise from abnormal losses from the urinary or GI tract.
   a. Malabsorption.
   b. Chronic diarrhea: inflammatory bowel disease, laxative abuse, intestinal infections.
   c. Alcoholism: secondary to malnutrition and alcohol's effects on the kidney.
   d. Low intake of Mg^{2+}: malnutrition, prolonged IV therapy.
   e. Large GI fluid losses: fistulas, NG tubes, prolonged vomiting.
   f. Increased urinary Mg^{2+} losses secondary to drugs such as cisplatin, digoxin, aminoglycosides, amphotericin B, diuretics.
3. **Signs and symptoms:**
   a. Neuromuscular—paresthesias, tremors, weakness, vertigo, ataxia, nystagmus, seizures, coma.
   b. Psychiatric—mood alterations, psychosis.
   c. Cardiovascular—ventricular arrhythmias resistant to conventional treatment, predisposition to digoxin toxicity.
   d. GI—anorexia, vomiting, dysphagia.
   e. Hematopoietic—anemia.
4. **Treatment.**
   a. **Acute hypomagnesemia:** If symptomatic hypomagnesemia is present, **2 g of $MgSO_4$ (8 mEq/g) as a 20% solution can be given IV over 2–5 minutes** followed by up to 10 g during the next 24 hours if normal renal function is present. Then, 4–6 g/day for 4–5 days should restore depleted magnesium stores. If kidneys are not functioning normally, supplementation must be given slowly with frequent monitoring of serum levels. IV magnesium can cause hypotension, and BP should be followed closely.
   b. **Chronic hypomagnesemia:** In symptomatic patients, 3–6 g/day $MgSO_4$ for 3 days should help correct the deficiency. Oral magnesium salts are available. In high doses, these agents may serve as cathartics but in the replacement dose range of 10–160 mEq/day, they are usu-

ally well tolerated (i.e., 10 mL of milk of magnesia = 28 mEq Mg^{2+}, 600 mg MgO = 28 mEq Mg^{2+}).

c. **Prophylactic:** $1-2$ g/day $MgSO_4$ in IV fluid can help prevent hypomagnesemia in ill patients with normal renal function.

J. Hypermagnesemia.

1. **Evaluation and differential diagnosis:** Hypermagnesemia is defined as **serum Mg^{2+} >2.2 mEq/L.** Minor elevations (usually <4 mEq/L) have been reported with lithium therapy, metastatic neoplasms to bone, hypothyroidism, viral hepatitis, and acute acidotic states. Most instances of hypermagnesemia follow a combination of impaired renal function and the administration of magnesium-containing drugs (mainly antacids).

2. **Symptoms** of hypermagnesemia usually do not occur until the magnesium level exceeds 4 mEq/L. One of the earliest signs of magnesium intoxication is loss of deep tendon reflexes which occurs at Mg^{2+} levels ≥ 6 mEq/L. Other symptoms include hypotension, nausea, vomiting, cutaneous flushing, bradycardia. Muscle paralysis can occur with Mg^{2+} levels >10 mEq/L, with respiratory depression occurring at Mg^{2+} levels of $12-14$ mg/L and asystolic cardiac arrest at levels exceeding 15 mg/L.

3. **Treatment.**

a. Calcium: $100-200$ mg IV as calcium gluconate or CaCl over $5-10$ minutes will immediately but only transiently reverse the effects of Mg^{2+} toxicity.

b. Dialysis: Peritoneal or hemodialysis may be necessary if renal function is poor.

c. Removal of Mg^{2+} source.

d. Avoid Mg^{2+}-containing compounds in patients with renal failure.

V. ACID-BASE REGULATION.

Acid-base disturbances are extremely common in the SICU. The body is usually able to maintain the blood pH within a range of $7.37-7.42$, which is necessary for optimal function of clotting factors, enzymes, and contractile proteins. To appropriately diagnose and treat acid-base disorders, an understanding of normal acid-base physiology is necessary.

A. Acid Production.

1. **Volatile acids:** Healthy humans produce $13,000-20,000$ mEq/day of CO_2 via oxidative metabolism. When the CO_2

produced is hydrated, the H_2CO_3 is formed by the following reaction:

$$CO_2 + H_2O \leftrightharpoons H_2CO_3 \leftrightharpoons H^+ + HCO_3^-$$

H_2CO_3 is referred to as a *volatile acid* because the CO_2 with which it is in equilibrium can be removed by ventilation.

2. **Nonvolatile acids:** Another 50–100 mEq/day of mainly H_2SO_4 and H_3PO_4 are produced through protein catabolism and the incomplete oxidation of fat and carbohydrates. These acids are not in equilibrium with CO_2 and thus are referred to as *nonvolatile acids*.

B. **Calculation of pH.**

1. **Henderson-Hasselbach (HH) equation:** Because CO_2 represents a much larger acid load than the nonvolatile acids, the major determinant of blood pH is the equilibrium between CO_2, HCO_3^-, and H^+. This equilibrium is represented by the HH equation:

$$pH = 6.1 + \frac{\log [HCO_3^-]}{0.03 \times PaCO_2}$$

where 6.1 is the pH of the bicarbonate system, and 0.03 is the solubility constant of CO_2 in arterial blood. Primary derangements affecting the numerator are usually metabolic in origin, whereas those affecting primarily the denominator are usually respiratory in nature.

2. The Henderson equation is more useful clinically:

$$[H^+] \text{ mEq/L} = \frac{24 \times PaCO_2}{[HCO_3^-]\text{mEq/L}}$$

$[H^+]$ can be approximated by knowing the arterial pH. At a pH of 7.4, the $[H^+] = 40$ mEq/L. Changes of 0.01 in the pH correspond inversely with 1-mEq/L changes in the $[H^+]$. Approximations of $[H^+]$ based on pH are close to actually measured values in the pH range of 7.1–7.5 (Table 10–6). By knowing any of the two variables in the Henderson equation, the third variable can be calculated. Most ABGs obtained in the SICU measure pH and $PaCO_2$, then calculate the HCO_3^- concentration using the HH equation.

TABLE 10-6.
Estimated vs. Actual H⁺ Concentrations for Given pH

pH	Estimated H^+ (mEq/L)	Actual H^+ (mEq/L)	
7.00	80	100	
7.10	70	79	Range within which
7.20	60	63	estimation of H^+
7.30	50	50	concentration is useful
7.35	45	45	
7.40	40	40	
7.45	35	35	
7.50	30	32	
7.60	20	25	

C. Lines of Defense.

The body has three lines of defense (buffers, respiratory compensation, renal compensation) to help preserve the blood's slightly alkaline pH in the presence of large daily acid loads.

1. **Buffers** are a mixture of a weak acid and its conjugate base or a weak base and its conjugate acid. Buffers are located intracellularly and extracellularly. They usually have pKa's (the point where the amount of acid and conjugate base or base and conjugate acid are equal) in the physiologic range. Within 1 pH unit on either side of their pKa, buffers show the least amount of change in pH for a given amount of H^+ or OH^- added to the system. Thus, while buffers do not prevent a pH change in response to an acid or base load, they help minimize it.

   a. The **extracellular buffers** consist mainly of the bicarbonate system.

      1) **Nonvolatile acids:** ~45% of nonvolatile acids are buffered by extracellular HCO_3. As the buffering occurs, CO_2 is rapidly generated by the following reactions:

$$H_2SO_4 + 2\ NaHCO_3 \rightarrow Na_2SO_4 + 2\ H_2CO_3$$
$$\rightarrow 2\ CO_2 + 2\ H_2O$$

$$H_3PO_4 + 2\ NaHCO_3 \rightarrow Na_2HPO_4 + 2\ H_2CO_3$$
$$\rightarrow 2\ CO_2 + 2\ H_2O$$

The CO_2 generated by this buffering action is released by the lungs.

2) **Volatile acids:** H_2CO_3 generated by oxidative metabolism cannot be buffered by the H_2CO_3 system because the addition of H^+ and HCO_3^- regenerates H_2CO_3.

$$H_2CO_3 + HCO_3^- \rightarrow HCO_3^- + H_2CO_3$$

b. The **intracellular buffers** consist of hemoglobin, organic phosphates, proteins, and bone.

1) **Nonvolatile acids:** About 50% of the H^+ generated by nonvolatile acids is not buffered by the extracellular buffers. Over the course of minutes to hours the unbuffered H^+ moves intracellularly where it is buffered by bone, organic phosphates, and proteins.

2) **Volatile acid:** Because H_2CO_3 cannot be buffered extracellularly by the HCO_3 system, it is buffered predominantly (97%) intracellularly. The majority of H_2CO_3 is buffered by deoxygenated hemoglobin within RBCs.

2. **Respiratory compensation:** The lungs help maintain the body's pH by regulating CO_2 exchange. The rapidity with which the lungs can respond to acid or base loads increases the efficiency of the HCO_3 system manyfold. Chemosensitive areas in the brainstem responsive to changes in $PaCO_2$ and chemoreceptors in the carotid body responsive to changes in PaO_2 mediate this compensatory response. Hypercarbia and hypoxemia stimulate increased ventilation. Hypocarbia leads to decreased ventilation.

3. **Renal compensation:** The kidneys provide the final line of defense via reabsorption of filtered HCO_3 and excretion of the 50–100 mEq of H^+ generated by nonvolatile acids.

a. **HCO_3 reabsorption:** HCO_3^- is freely filtered at the glomerulus. Below plasma HCO_3^- concentrations of 26 mEq/L, virtually all HCO_3^- must be reabsorbed as a HCO_3^- molecule lost in the urine is equivalent to the addition of a H^+ molecule to the blood. Reabsorption is mediated by carbonic anhydrase. Above a plasma HCO_3^- concentration of 26 mEq/L, increasing amounts of HCO_3^- are lost in the urine.

b. **H^+ secretion:** In addition to reabsorbing HCO_3^-, the kidney must also excrete the daily nonvolatile acid load. Excretion of free H^+ in the urine does not occur because the lowest urine pH that can be achieved by humans is 4.5 which corresponds to a free H^+ concentration of only 0.04 mEq/L. Therefore, H^+ is secreted in the urine in two forms: titratable acid and ammonium ion.

1) **Titratable acid:** Approximately 10–40 mEq/day of H^+ can be excreted in the urine as titratable acid. $Na_2H(PO_4)_2$ is the main titratable acid in urine because of its relatively high urine concentration and favorable pK for buffering.

2) **Ammonium ion:** The remainder of the H^+ generated each day is secreted by the renal tubular cell along with NH_3. The NH_3 is generated by the renal tubular cell from glutamine metabolism. Because the pK of the NH_3/NH_4 system is 9.3, the acidic pH of the urine favors the association of H^+ with NH_3, forming NH_4^+. The NH_4^+ is trapped in the tubular lumen and excreted in the urine. Although only 30–50 mEq/day of H^+ is normally excreted as NH_4^+, H^+ excretion can increase to >250 mEq/day in the presence of a metabolic acidosis. This is in contrast to titratable acid which can only increase slightly in acidotic patients. The mechanism of increased glutamine metabolism and generation of NH_3 in metabolic acidosis is poorly understood but takes several days to reach its maximum, thus accounting for some of the delay in renal compensation of acid-base disorders.

D. Evaluation of Acid-Base Status.

1. **Normal values:** The above-described mechanisms allow the body to maintain normal acid-base values (Table 10–7).

2. In the SICU, acid-base disturbances are frequently diagnosed by routinely obtained arterial blood samples. Knowledge of various artifacts that may affect the reading of blood gases is important for proper interpretation of these values.

a. **Temperature:** Metabolism within uncooled blood gas samples will decrease the PaO_2 and increase the

TABLE 10–7.

Normal Acid-Base Values

	pH	H^+ (mEq/L)	PCO_2 (mm Hg)	HCO_3^- (mEq/L)
Arterial	7.37–7.43	37–43	36–44	22–26
Venous	7.32–7.38	42–48	42–50	23–27

$PaCO_2$ by as much as 3 mm Hg/min. Samples should be cooled on ice as soon as they are obtained and read within 1 hour.

b. **Air bubbles:** The presence of air bubbles within the syringe will cause the blood gas sample to equilibrate with room air (the PaO_2 will drift toward 150 mm Hg and the $PaCO_2$ will drift toward 0). Therefore, air bubbles should be removed from the syringe immediately after the sample is obtained.

c. **Heparin:** Because aqueous heparin is acidic (pH 5), it may artificially lower the sample's pH if an excess is present in the syringe or if it is not mixed well within the sample. Therefore, only enough heparin to coat the edges of the tubing and syringe should be used and the sample should be agitated gently after it is obtained.

d. **Venous blood gases:** In certain situations (difficult arterial punctures, children), acid-base determinations may be made on venous blood as pH, $PaCO_2$, and HCO_3^- values are relatively similar to arterial values (see Table 10–2). **An important exception to this rule occurs during cardiopulmonary arrest.** In this setting, although studies have shown the HCO_3^- concentrations of arterial and venous blood to be similar, the mixed venous pH is generally lower and the $P\overline{v}CO_2$ as much as 40 mm Hg higher than simultaneously obtained arterial values. Mixed venous values may reflect a more accurate guide to acid-base derangement.

VI. ACID-BASE DISORDERS.

A. Definitions and Compensatory Responses.

1. **Definitions:** Changes in extracellular pH are seen when renal or respiratory function is abnormal or when an acid or base load overwhelms the normal excretory capacity of

the body. **Acidemia is a decrease in blood pH <7.36 and alkalemia is an increase in blood pH >7.44. Acidosis and alkalosis refer to the processes that tend to cause the change in pH.** There are four basic categories of acid-base disturbances. Primary abnormal changes in $PaCO_2$ are referred to as **respiratory acidosis** (increased $PaCO_2$) and **respiratory alkalosis** (decreased $PaCO_2$), because ventilation controls the $PaCO_2$ level. Primary changes in plasma HCO_3^- concentration are referred to as **metabolic acidosis** (decreased plasma HCO_3^-) and **metabolic alkalosis** (increased plasma HCO_3^-).

2. **Compensatory responses:** The kidneys and lungs respond to primary acid-base derangements with compensatory responses that attempt to minimize the change in H^+ concentration by minimizing the change in the $PaCO_2/HCO_3^-$ ratio (see Henderson equation, section V.B.2). Therefore, the kidneys compensate for respiratory disorders and the lungs compensate for metabolic disorders. The compensatory response is always in the opposite direction to the primary disturbance and tends to minimize the change in pH but never return it to normal. Figure 10–7 is a nomogram outlining the evaluation of acid-base disturbances. The degree of compensation in the various acid-base disorders is shown in Table 10–8.

3. **Mixed acid-base disorders** may occur when more than one primary disorder is present in a patient. They are diagnosed clinically and by recognizing discrepancies between the calculated compensatory responses to primary disturbances and actually obtained values. Since these processes may have either additive or nullifying effects, the deviation in H^+ concentration and thus pH from normal may be marked or minimal.

B. **Metabolic Alkalosis.**

1. **Definition and compensatory response:** A metabolic alkalosis is caused by a primary elevation in plasma HCO_3^- concentration >27 mEq/L leading to a pH >7.44. The increased pH stimulates a decrease in ventilation. Decreased ventilation leads to an increase in $PaCO_2$, thereby minimizing the deviation in blood pH. The appropriate compensatory response is a 5–7-mm Hg increase in $PaCO_2$ for each 10-mEq/L increase in HCO_3^-. Elevation of $PaCO_2$ much above this range implies the presence of a

TABLE 10–8.
Acid-Base Disorders and Appropriate Compensatory Responses

Disturbance	pH	H⁺	Primary Disturbance	Compensatory Response
Metabolic acidosis	$\downarrow$	$\uparrow$	$\downarrow HCO_3^-$	$PaCO_2 \downarrow$ by 1.0–1.3 mm Hg for each mEq/L $\downarrow$ in HCO_3^-; $PaCO_2$ rarely $\downarrow$ below 10 mm Hg
Metabolic alkalosis	$\uparrow$	$\downarrow$	$\uparrow HCO_3^-$	$PaCO_2 \uparrow$ by 5–7 mm Hg for each 10 mEq/L $\uparrow$ in HCO_3^-; $PaCO_2$ rarely $\uparrow$ over 55 mm Hg
Respiratory acidosis				
Acute	$\downarrow$	$\uparrow$	$\uparrow PaCO_2$	$HCO_3^- \uparrow$ by 1 mEq/L for each 10 mm Hg $\uparrow$ in $PaCO_2$; HCO_3^- rarely $\uparrow$ over 30 mEq/L
Chronic	$\downarrow$	$\uparrow$	$\uparrow PaCO_2$	$HCO_3^- \uparrow$ by 3–4 mEq/L for each 10 mm Hg $\uparrow$ in $PaCO_2$; HCO_3^- rarely $\uparrow$ over 45 mEq/L
Respiratory alkalosis				
Acute	$\uparrow$	$\downarrow$	$\downarrow PaCO_2$	$HCO_3^- \downarrow$ by 2 mEq/L for each 10 mm Hg $\downarrow$ in $PaCO_2$; HCO_3^- rarely $\downarrow$ below 18 mEq/L
Chronic	$\uparrow$	$\downarrow$	$\downarrow PaCO_2$	$HCO_3^- \downarrow$ by 5 mEq/L for each 10 mm Hg $\downarrow$ in $PaCO_2$; HCO_3^- rarely $\downarrow$ below 12 mEq/L

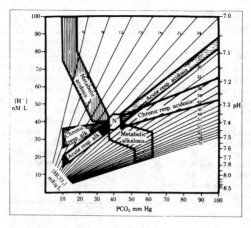

FIG 10–7.
Nomogram for acid-base disorders. (From Goldberg *JAMA* 1973; 223:269. Used by permission.)

superimposed respiratory acidosis. A $PaCO_2$ level much below the calculated compensatory response implies a concurrent respiratory alkalosis.

2. **Pathophysiology:** Because the kidney has the ability to correct a metabolic alkalosis by not reabsorbing excess HCO_3^- in the urine, the perpetuation of a metabolic alkalosis requires an impairment in renal HCO_3^- excretion. This impairment can result from either decreased HCO_3^- filtration, enhanced HCO_3^- reabsorption, or both. Situations in which HCO_3^- reabsorption is enhanced include hypovolemia, hypochloremia, acidemia, hypokalemia, hypercapnea, and mineralocorticoid excess. Decreased HCO_3^- filtration occurs in low flow states and hypovolemia. These underlying states must be corrected.

3. **Differential diagnosis:** The causes of a metabolic alkalosis can be divided into **saline-responsive** and **saline-unresponsive** depending on whether the alkalosis can be corrected by volume restoration with NaCl (Table 10–9). Physical examination, history, urinary Cl^-, and selected

TABLE 10-9.

Differential Diagnosis of a Metabolic Alkalosis

Saline-Responsive (Urine Cl⁻ <10 mEq/L)	Saline-Unresponsive (Urine Cl⁻ >10 mEq/L)
Vomiting	Excess mineralocorticoid
Gastric drainage: NG tube, gastrostomy	Cushing's syndrome
Diuretic therapy: contraction alkalosis	Hyperaldosteronism
Relief from prolonged hypercapnea	ACTH-secreting tumors
Congenital chloridorrhea	Licorice ingestion
Bicarbonate therapy of organic acidosis	Renal artery stenosis
Administration of organic salts which, when	Exogenous steroids
metabolized, make HCO₃⁻	Bartter's syndrome
Lactate	Severe potassium deficiency
Citrate (transfusions)	Magnesium deficiency
Acetate	
Renal failure + alkali therapy	
Milk-alkali syndrome	

electrolytes can also be important in classifying patients with metabolic alkalosis. Chloride-responsive patients show signs of hypovolemia and have urine Cl⁻ <10 mEq/L. Patients with chloride-unresponsive metabolic alkalosis usually have urine Cl⁻ >10 mEq/L and are euvolemic.

4. **Symptoms:** Patients may be asymptomatic or show signs of hypovolemia. Alkalosis may also produce signs and symptoms secondary to electrolyte disturbances such as hypokalemia, hypocalcemia, or hypophosphatemia. The alkalosis may also impair oxygen delivery to tissues by shifting the oxyhemoglobin curve to the left.

5. **Treatment.**
   a. **Saline-responsive:** Correct volume deficits with NaCl and give potassium supplementation simultaneously to achieve serum K^+ levels of 4.5–5.5 mEq/L. H_2 receptor antagonists (ranitidine, cimetidine) can also help diminish H^+ secretion.
   b. **Saline-unresponsive:** Correct electrolyte deficiencies and remove the mineralocorticoid source. If the source cannot be removed, then the mineralocorticoid action can be blocked with either spironolactone or amiloride.

    c. **Severe alkalosis:** A rapid renal loss of HCO_3^- can be achieved with **acetazolamide 250–500 mg IV** in addition to the above treatments. In severe renal failure or life-threatening metabolic alkalosis (pH>7.6, HCO_3^- >40), HCl can be given via a central vein to correct the alkalosis. The amount of 0.1N HCl to be given is based on calculation of the chloride deficit by the following formula:

$$\text{Chloride deficit} = 0.2 \text{ L/kg} \times \text{wt (kg)} \times (103 - \text{observed Cl})$$

    Replacement is carried out with 100 mEq HCL/L at a rate no faster than 125 mL or 2 mEq/kg/hr. If the situation permits, a slower infusion is better tolerated. Frequent monitoring of ABGs to follow the efficacy of HCl treatment is mandatory. Complications of HCl administration include hemolysis and tissue necrosis.

C. Metabolic Acidosis.

1. **Definition and compensatory response:** A metabolic acidosis is characterized by a arterial pH <7.36 secondary to a reduction in plasma HCO_3^- < 22 mEq/L. This reduction in pH leads to a compensatory hyperventilation that decreases the $PaCO_2$ and minimizes the change in arterial pH. The appropriate compensatory response is a 1.0–1.3-mm Hg fall in $PaCO_2$ for 1 mEq/L fall in HCO_3^-. A fall in $PaCO_2$ greater than calculated implies a concurrent respiratory alkalosis. A change in $PaCO_2$ less than calculated implies a superimposed respiratory acidosis.

2. **Pathophysiology:** The reduction in plasma HCO_3^- can occur by either a loss of HCO_3^- or by addition of a non-volatile acid load, both of which lead to an increase in H^+ concentration. The body responds to the H^+ load initially with intracellular and extracellular buffers followed by respiratory compensation. These mechanisms help minimize the increase in H^+ concentration until the kidneys can excrete the excess H^+ by generation of ammonium ion and titratable acid.

3. **Differential diagnosis.**

    a. **Anion gap:** Evaluation of a metabolic acidosis begins with a careful history and physical examination as well as measurement of serum electrolytes. From the electrolytes, the anion gap (AG) can be calculated:

$$AG = Na^+ - [Cl^- + HCO_3^-]$$

The normal AG = 8–12 mmol/L.

b. When an acid load is presented to the body, it is rapidly buffered extracellularly by the bicarbonate system. If the acid is HCl, the net buffering effect is a milliequivalent-for-milliequivalent exchange of extracellular HCO_3^- for Cl^-. Since the sum of these two anions remains the same, the anion gap does not increase. If, however, H^+ accumulates with another anion besides Cl^-, then the extracellular HCO_3^- will be replaced by an unmeasured anion resulting in an increase in the anion gap as the sum of HCO_3^- and Cl^- decreases. The anion gap is useful in determining the etiology of the acidosis (Table 10–10).

TABLE 10–10.

Etiology of Metabolic Acidosis Based on Anion Gap

Increased Organic Acids With Increased Anion Gap	Increased Inorganic Acids With Normal Anion Gap and Hyperchloremia
Renal failure	Inability to excrete acid
Lactic acidosis	Distal renal tubular acidosis
Ketoacidosis	Addison's disease
Diabetes	Hypoaldosteronism
Starvation	Excessive loss of HCO_3^-
Drugs or ingestions	GI fistula
Ethylene glycol	Pancreatic
Salicylates	Biliary
Methanol	Diarrhea
Paraldehyde	Proximal renal tubular acidosis
	Ureterosigmoidostomy
	Early renal failure
	Carbonic anhydrase inhibitors (acetazolamide)
	Administration of acid
	Blood transfusions (citrate)
	Ammonium chloride
	Arginine hydrochloride
	Hyperalimentation

c. With review of history and physical examination, other useful tests in assessing acidosis include lactate, ketone, ETOH, methanol, and ethylene glycol levels, and serum osmolality.

d. **Lactic acidosis** is extremely common in the SICU.

1) **Pathophysiology:** Lactate is derived by the metabolism of pyruvate (Fig 10–8). Healthy individuals produce 15–20 mmol/kg/day of lactic acid generated from the metabolism of glucose and alanine. This lactic acid load is buffered by the extracellular bicarbonate system until the liver or kidney can convert it into either $CO_2 + H_2O$ (80%) or glucose (20%). Both reactions regenerate the HCO_3^- used to buffer the acid as seen below:

$$Lactate + 3\ O_2 \rightarrow HCO_3^- + 2\ CO_2 + 2H_2O$$

$$2\ Lactate + 2\ H_2O + 2\ CO_2 \rightarrow 2\ HCO_3^- + glucose$$

The normal lactic acid level in humans is **0.5–1.5 mEq/L**. Accumulation of lactate occurs in a variety of settings due to derangements in lactate pro-

PYRUVATE METABOLISM

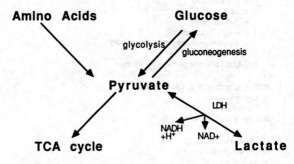

FIG 10–8.
Pyruvate metabolism. *TCA* = tricarboxylic acid.

duction or metabolism (Table 10–11). If the lactate level is >4 mEq/L, mortality rates may be 60%–80%. If >15 mEq/L, patients rarely survive.

2) **Diagnosis:** Although the diagnosis of lactic acidosis is made by obtaining elevated serum lactate

TABLE 10–11.

Differential Diagnosis of Lactate Acidosis Based on Etiology

I. Increased lactate production
   A. Increased pyruvate production
      1. Enzymatic defects in glycogenolysis or gluconeogenesis
      2. Respiratory alkalosis
   B. Impaired pyruvate utilization
      1. Decreased activity of pyruvate dehydrogenase of pyruvate carboxylase
        a. Congenital
        b. ? Role of diabetes mellitus, Reye's syndrome
   C. Altered redox state favoring pyruvate conversion to lactate
      1. Enhanced metabolic rate
        a. Grand mal seizure
        b. Severe exercise
        c. Hypothermic shivering
      2. Decreased O_2 delivery
        a. Shock (cardiogenic, septic, hypovolemic)
        b. Asphyxia (PaO_2 <30 mm Hg)
        c. CO poisoning
        d. CHF
        e. Cardiac arrest
      3. Reduced O_2 utilization
        a. Cyanide intoxication (high-dose SNP)
        b. ? Phenformin
      4. D-Lactic acidosis (abnormal gut flora)

II. Primary decreases in lactate utilization
   A. Liver disease
   B. Alcoholism
   C. Severe acidemia (pH < 7.1)

III. Mechanism uncertain
   A. Diabetes mellitus
   B. Malignancy
   C. Hypoglycemia
   D. Idiopathic

levels, its presence can be suggested by history, physical examination, and an increased anion gap metabolic acidosis.

3) **Treatment:** Attempts to reverse lactic acidosis must be aggressive as soon as the diagnosis is made. Treatment is directed toward correction of the underlying problems that are suspected of causing the acidosis. In the intensive care setting, these problems are most often hypovolemia, hypoxemia, sepsis, or heart failure as well as any end organ damage that may have occurred secondarily such as ischemic bowel or extremities. The use of $NaHCO_3$ is discussed below.

4) **Symptoms** can be varied depending on the underlying etiology of the acidosis, the rapidity with which the acidosis develops, and its magnitude. Symptoms and signs include lethargy, confusion, decreased myocardial contractility, increased arrhythmias, hyperkalemia, increased PVR, and a shift of the oxyhemoglobin curve to the right.

5) **Treatment:** Most clinicians feel that $NaHCO_3$ should be given when the arterial pH is <7.2 to help prevent cardiac arrhythmias, improve cardiac contractility, and improve the body's responsiveness to catecholamines. Above a pH of 7.2, whether or not to treat an acidosis becomes an individual decision as correction of the underlying process may obviate the need for $NaHCO_3$. In using $NaHCO_3$, one must remember many of its unwanted side effects. **$NaHCO_3$ can induce hyperosmolarity, hypokalemia, hypernatremia, and fluid overload.** $NaHCO_3$ may also produce a paradoxical acidosis if ventilation is not adequate, secondary to the accumulation of CO_2 generated when the H^+ is buffered. Thus, CO_2 may diffuse freely into myocardial and cerebral cells, depressing the function of both. Finally, in cardiac arrest, $NaHCO_3$ has not been shown experimentally to improve the ability to defibrillate or improve survival, it may exacerbate a central venous acidosis, and it may inactivate simultaneously administered

catecholamines. When $NaHCO_3^-$ is used, a base deficit should be calculated:

$$\text{Base deficit} = (\text{body wt in kg})(0.4) \times (\text{desired } [HCO_3^-] \text{ in mEq/L}) - \text{actual } [HCO_3^-] \text{ (mEq/L)}$$

About one third to one half of the calculated HCO_3^- deficit should be given with subsequent dosages based on follow-up ABGs and blood chemistries. Monitor serum K^+ during bicarbonate administration to avoid hypokalemia.

D. **Respiratory Alkalosis.**

1. **Definition and compensation:** Respiratory alkalosis is characterized by a primary decrease in $PaCO_2$ secondary to increased alveolar ventilation above that necessary to eliminate the daily load of metabolically produced PCO_2.

   a. **Acute compensation:** The body compensates acutely by rapid extra- and intracellular buffering as evidenced by a 1–2 mEq/L-fall in HCO_3^- for every 10-mm Hg decrease in $PaCO_2$. The HCO_3^- rarely goes below 18 mEq/L. Decreases in HCO_3^- greater than this imply a concurrent metabolic acidosis and changes in the HCO_3^- less than this imply a superimposed metabolic alkalosis.

   b. **Chronic compensation:** If hypercapnea persists, the kidneys begin to compensate by decreasing the secretion of H^+. As a result, the serum HCO_3^- decreases 4–5 mEq/L for every 10-mm Hg decrease in $PaCO_2$. Decreases in HCO_3^- less than the calculated compensatory response for a chronic respiratory alkalosis imply a superimposed metabolic alkalosis. Decreases in HCO_3^- greater than the calculated compensatory response suggest a concurrent metabolic acidosis.

2. **Pathophysiology:** The underlying etiology of a respiratory alkalosis is related to one of three processes which can lead to an increase in ventilation.

   a. Decreased pH in the CSF sensed by the central respiratory chemoreceptors in the medulla.

   b. Hypoxemia sensed by the peripheral respiratory chemoreceptors in the carotid bodies.

   c. Nonphysiologic stimuli (e.g., pulmonary disease, direct stimulation of the respiratory chemoreceptors).

3. **Differential diagnosis:** Evaluation of a respiratory alkalosis involves first deciding if the process is acute or chronic (Table 10–12). This classification reduces the differential diagnosis. An evaluation based on history, physical examination, CXR, drug review, blood cultures, and other tests can suggest the specific diagnosis.

4. **Symptoms:** Changes secondary to decreased cerebral blood flow (e.g., altered mental status) may be seen. Patients may also complain of lightheadedness, cramps, circumoral numbness, and acral paresthesias.

5. **Treatment** usually revolves around correcting the underlying disorder, especially one that is life-threatening. In the SICU, hypoxemia and improper ventilatory settings are the most common causes. Rebreathing in a paper bag can help the patient with psychogenic hyperventilation. Treatment of the alkalosis per se is usually not necessary.

E. **Respiratory Acidosis.**

1. **Definition and compensatory response:** Respiratory acidosis is characterized by a primary increase in arterial $Paco_2$ secondary to decreased alveolar ventilation insufficient to excrete the metabolically produced CO_2. The accumulation of CO_2 leads to a decrease in arterial pH.

TABLE 10–12.

Differential Diagnosis of Respiratory Alkalosis

Acute
  Psychogenic hyperventilation
  Errors in mechanical ventilation
  Acute hypoxemia (pneumonia, pulmonary embolism, pneumothorax, atelectasis, asthma)
  Drugs (salicylates, progesterone, catecholamines, theophylline)
  Fever
  CNS (tumor, infection, trauma, CVA)
  Sepsis
Chronic
  Prolonged hypoxemia (anemia, congenital heart disease, high altitude)
  Cirrhosis
  Prolonged mechanical hyperventilation
  Sepsis
  CNS (tumor, infection, trauma, CVA)

a. **Acute compensation:** The body attempts to minimize the decrease in pH caused by CO_2 retention acutely with intracellular buffers. This buffering results in the acute compensatory response of a 1-mEq/L increase in HCO_3^- for each 10 mm Hg in $PaCO_2$. The HCO_3^- rarely rises above 30 mEq/L. If the HCO_3^- increases above 30 mEq/L, it implies a concurrent metabolic alkalosis. If the change in HCO_3^- is less than expected by the calculated compensatory response, then a superimposed metabolic acidosis is probably present.

b. **Chronic compensation:** Over the next 2–3 days, if the respiratory acidosis persists, the kidneys increase H^+ secretion leading to an elevation of serum HCO_3^- by 3–4 mEq/L for each 10-mm Hg increase in $PaCO_2$. Again, changes greater or less than the calculated compensatory response for a chronic respiratory acidosis imply a mixed acid-base disturbance.

2. **Pathophysiology:** The underlying cause of a respiratory acidosis is usually related to one of four major problems that decrease ventilation leading to CO_2 retention.

a. Inhibition of the medullary respiratory center.

b. Disorders of respiratory muscles.

c. Upper airway obstruction.

d. Disorders affecting gas exchange across pulmonary capillaries.

3. **Differential diagnosis:** Initial evaluation of respiratory acidosis involves determining if the process is acute or chronic. With the aid of a careful history and physical examination, appropriate laboratory tests (including CXR, sputum culture, electrolytes, and CBC) and careful rechecking of ventilator settings and hardware, the etiology can be determined. A complete differential diagnosis is shown in Table 10–13.

4. **Symptoms:** Sequelae of severe respiratory acidosis are similar to those discussed for metabolic acidosis. Specific symptoms are frequently related to the underlying disorder.

5. **Treatment** of respiratory acidosis is aimed at improving ventilation. Acutely, this can be done with aggressive pulmonary toilet and, if necessary, ET intubation. Once ventilation is restored, treatment of the underlying problem can be undertaken. Bicarbonate should not be given to a

TABLE 10–13.
Differential Diagnosis of Respiratory Acidosis

I. Inhibition of medullary respiratory center
   A. Acute
      1. Drugs (opiates, anesthetics, sedatives, alcohol)
      2. O_2 in chronic hypercapnea
      3. Cardiac arrest
      4. Central sleep apnea
   B. Chronic
      1. Extreme obesity
      2. CNS lesion

II. Disorders of respiratory muscles
   A. Acute
      1. Muscle weakness (crisis in myasthenia gravis, periodic paralysis, aminoglycosides, severe hypokalemia, Guillain-Barré syndrome, hypophosphatemia)
   B. Chronic
      1. Muscle weakness (poliomyelitis, amyotrophic lateral sclerosis, multiple sclerosis, myxedema)
      2. Kyphoscoliosis
      3. Extreme obesity

III. Upper airway obstruction
   A. Acute
      1. Aspiration of foreign body or vomitus
      2. Obstructive sleep apnea
      3. Laryngospasm

IV. Disorders affecting gas exchange across pulmonary capillary
   A. Acute
      1. Exacerbation of underlying lung disease
      2. ARDS
      3. Acute cardiogenic pulmonary edema
      4. Severe asthma or pneumonia
      5. Pneumothorax or hemothorax
   B. Chronic
      1. COPD (emphysema, chronic bronchitis)

V. Mechanical ventilation
   A. Acute
      1. Improper settings
      2. Defective ventilator hardware

patient with a pure respiratory acidosis because it will worsen the acidosis by increasing the CO_2 load. Oxygen should also be used with care in unintubated patients with chronic respiratory acidosis. These patients have become accustomed to high $PaCO_2$ and their ventilatory drive is stimulated by mild hypoxemia. Oxygen may suppress the hypoxic drive leading to hypoventilation with further worsening of the respiratory acidosis and possible respiratory arrest.

SELECTED REFERENCES

Friedman BS, Lumb PD: Prevention and management of metabolic acidosis. *J Intensive Care Med* 1990; 5:S22–S27.

Harrington J, Cohen J: Measurement of urinary electrolytes: Indications and limitations. *N Engl J Med* 1975; 293:1241.

Narins R: Therapy of hyponatremia: Does haste make waste? *N Engl J Med* 1986; 314:1573.

Narins R, Jones ER, Stom MC, et al: Diagnostic strategies in disorders of fluid, electrolyte and acid-base homeostasis. *Am J Med* 1982; 72:496.

Oh M, Carroll H: The anion gap. *N Engl J Med* 1977; 297:814.

Stoff J: Phosphate homeostasis and hypophosphatemia. *Am J Med* 1982; 72:489.

Symposium on acid-base disorders. *Med Clin North Am* 1983; 67(4).

Symposium on renal therapeutics. *Med Clin North Am* 1978; 62(6).

Weil MH, Rackow EC, Trevino R, et al: Difference in acid-base state between venous and arterial blood samples during cardiopulmonary resuscitation. *N Engl J Med* 1986; 315:

THE ALIMENTARY *11* TRACT

I. GENERAL CONDITIONS.

A. Gastrointestinal Hemorrhage.

1. GI hemorrhage can be a life-threatening condition that requires prompt and appropriate treatment. The management of GI bleeding involves three distinct phases (which may overlap): resuscitation, localization, and intervention.

2. The urgency in which GI bleeding is managed is dictated by the rate of bleeding.

   a. Heme-positive stool requires elective evaluation usually as an outpatient.

   b. Visible blood requires hospitalization and inpatient evaluation. Persistent bleeding or bleeding with hemodynamic instability necessitates SICU admission.

   c. Massive hemorrhage is defined as the loss of 30% of estimated blood volume or a bleed requiring blood transfusion of 6 units/24 hr.

3. **Blood loss may be estimated** by measuring the return from an NG tube or by quantitating bloody stools. In addition to the usual means of determining blood loss based on the severity of shock, an approximate estimate of blood loss can be made by the hemodynamic response to a 2-L crystalloid fluid challenge:

   a. If BP returns to normal and stabilizes, blood loss of 15%–30% has occurred.

   b. If BP rises but falls again, blood volume loss of 30%–40% has occurred.

   c. If BP continues to fall, blood volume loss of >40% has probably occurred.

4. **Resuscitation.**

   a. Monitoring in the SICU is required in the setting of hemodynamic instability or persistent visible bleeding.

It may also be advised for bleeding in an elderly or debilitated patient.

b. The basic steps of resuscitation include:

1) Establishment of two peripheral large-bore IV lines (14- or 16-gauge).

2) Continuous monitoring of VS. This requires:

   a) Indwelling urinary catheter for UO.

   b) Arterial line for continuous BP monitoring.

   c) CVP or PA catheter depending upon the stability of the patient and underlying cardiac disease.

3) Blood for hemoglobin, Hct, platelet count, PT, APTT, fibrinogen, electrolytes, and type and crossmatch for 6 units of blood are obtained. Repeat Hct determination q. 4 h. until stable. The Hct may not fall for 12–36 hours after a bleed so that a significant blood loss may occur despite a stable Hct.

4) DO_2 is optimized for the treatment of shock (see p 71). This may include blood component transfusions and pharmacologic adjustment of preload, afterload, and contractility.

5) Consider prompt blood transfusions.

   a) If the estimated blood losses are large and if the patient is hemodynamically unstable, then begin O-negative or type-specific transfusion. The risk of transfusion reaction is <1%.

   b) Because PRBCs have no clotting factors or platelets, consider transfusion of FFP after 6 units of PRBCs and platelets after 10 units.

   c) The administration of calcium is controversial (the preservative citrate in banked blood temporarily chelates calcium, a cofactor essential to coagulation) but is indicated when transfusions exceed 50 mL/min. Administer 1 ampule IV CaCl.

   d) Warming infused blood products prevents hypothermia and associated complications such as coagulopathy and arrhythmias.

6) If a coagulopathy is present, it must be treated aggressively.

    a) Prolonged PT and APTT can usually be treated with FFP, *infused rapidly*.

    b) Vitamin K 10 mg SC is usually added also.

    c) Cryoprecipitate can correct low fibrinogen levels.

    d) Platelet transfusions are administered for platelet counts below 50,000/mm^3 or in the setting of known platelet dysfunction.

    e) It is important to remember that, during rapid bleeding, coagulation factors are rapidly consumed. In the treatment of active bleeding associated with coagulopathy, aggressive surgical therapy is rarely considered until the coagulopathy is corrected.

5. **Localization.**

  a. The common causes of UGI bleeding include Mallory-Weiss tear, gastritis, duodenal ulcer, gastric ulcer, esophageal varices.

  b. Causes of significant lower GI bleeding are diverticulosis and angiodysplasia. Inflammatory bowel disease, neoplasms, hemorrhoids, Meckel's diverticulum, and aortoenteric fistula are less common.

  c. Methods of localization are described below.

    1) Obtain history and physical examination:

      a) **History** should address prior GI bleed, diverticulosis, ulcer disease; salicylate or ethanol ingestion; prior abdominal surgery (e.g., abdominal aneurysm repair).

      b) **Physical examination** should include BP and pulse measurements in both supine and sitting positions, if possible.

      c) **Rectal examination** and nature of stool may help localize the bleed (e.g., rectal cancer). A stool may be guaiac-positive for 3 weeks following a bleed. Melena (black, tarry stool) may occur with as little as 50 mL of UGI bleeding. Frankly bloody stools usually suggest lower GI bleeding but may indicate an upper GI source when the UGI bleed massive.

2) **NG intubation:** All patients with GI bleeding require NG intubation.

   a) The presence of gross blood or coffee-ground emesis suggests a source of bleeding proximal to the pylorus.

   b) If the aspirate is negative, lavage should be attempted. Bile should be detected to ensure evaluation of duodenal contents. A negative lavage in the presence of bile usually, but not always, indicates a distal source of bleeding, although it may indicate the temporary cessation of a proximal bleed.

   c) A large NG tube (Ewald tube) should be placed if a UGI bleed is suspected as this may also be used to lavage the stomach free of clots. Only UGI endoscopy can definitely exclude a UGI source.

3) **Endoscopy.**

   a) **Proctosigmoidoscopy:** Following visual inspection of the anus and manual palpation, rigid proctosigmoidoscopy should be undertaken if a lower source of bleeding is suspected. This can not only exclude a site of bleeding in the rectum and distal sigmoid but may provide information on generalized mucosal abnormalities (e.g., ischemic bowel). Careful examination of the anus directly and by anoscopy is critical. Hemorrhoidal bleeding can be massive.

   b) **UGI endoscopy:** Although endoscopy can be diagnostic (and occasionally therapeutic), the patient must be resuscitated and stabilized. While clinical trials have failed to demonstrate a decrease in mortality and morbidity with the use of early endoscopy, any patient with a UGI or unknown source of bleeding requires endoscopy to localize the source. Endoscopy can be performed at the bedside with the patient fully monitored. A specific lesion explaining the bleeding is identified in approximately 90% of patients with a complication rate <1%. In about one third of cases, two potential sources of bleeding are seen.

c) **Colonoscopy** is not usually performed during active lower GI bleeding. After a self-limited bleed, colonoscopy can be helpful in determining the *cause* of lower GI bleeding (e.g., cancer vs. angiodysplasia), but colonoscopy may not localize the precise location of bleeding unless active bleeding is directly visualized.

4) **Radionuclide scintiscanning.**

a) Scanning can be done with ^{99m}Tc sulfur colloid or, more commonly, ^{99m}Tc autologous RBCs.

b) Scintigraphy is useful in patients with low-grade or intermittent hemorrhage to help plan the timing of arteriography.

c) *Tagged RBC scans may be misleading in localizing the source of bleeding because of pooling of blood in various regions of the intestine.* **Scanning should be followed by angiography.**

d) Repeated scans can be performed after the initial injection for up to 24 hours.

e) Bleeding as little as 0.1 mL/min may be detected.

5) **Angiography.**

a) Angiography may visualize continuous bleeding as slow as 0.5–2.0 mL/min, but massive bleeding is often intermittent, making detection difficult.

b) Selective celiac or mesenteric angiography is performed after a positive tagged RBC scan and may localize the specific bleeding vessel.

c) Not only can the angiogram be diagnostic but it may also be therapeutic. The angiographer can infuse vasopressin (Pitressin) selectively or can embolize one of various substances into the bleeding vessel to induce thrombosis.

6. **Definitive therapeutic intervention.**
   a. Over 75% of all GI bleeding resolves spontaneously and requires only resuscitative care. Management depends on the source of bleeding:
   b. **Mallory-Weiss tear:**
      1) A linear gastric mucosal laceration, usually just below the esophagogastric junction, may follow forceful vomiting or alcohol ingestion.
      2) The majority cease bleeding spontaneously. Selective arterial infusion of vasopressin, endoscopic coagulation, or gastric inflation of a Sengstaken-Blakemore tube may be helpful.
      3) Surgical management is indicated only for massive bleeding unresponsive to conservative therapy. The surgical approach involves a high longitudinal gastrotomy and oversewing of the tear.
   c. **Duodenal ulcer (DU):**
      1) Bleeding ulcers are the most frequent cause of UGI bleeding.
      2) In addition to resuscitation, treat with H_2 blockers or antacids. Endoscopic electrocoagulation, Nd-YAG laser, or angiographic embolization have been used successfully.
      3) Indications for surgery include an actively bleeding ulcer, a visible vessel within an ulcer crater (seen on endoscopy), or failed medical therapy (bleeding 6–10 units/24 hr).
      4) Surgical intervention includes oversewing of the bleeding vessel followed by an acid-reducing procedure. In an unstable patient, vagotomy and pyloroplasty is performed. Antrectomy or parietal cell vagotomy may be done if the patient is more stable. Mortality rates of 5%–10% are expected and vary with age and amount of blood transfused preoperatively.
   d. **Gastric ulcer:**
      1) Indications for emergency surgery similar to DU.
      2) Surgical intervention involves resection of the ulcer without vagotomy. Oversewing of the ulcer with vagotomy and an outlet procedure has a higher incidence of rebleeding. If the ulcer is in the prepyloric region or if there are associated DUs, resection is followed by vagotomy.

e. **Esophageal varices:**

1) In the United States 90%–95% of esophageal varices are due to portal hypertension from alcoholic cirrhosis. Although only a third of patients with varices bleed, in those patients with UGI bleeding who have varices, the bleeding is from the varices. Early series, however, reported other sources of bleeding in up to 50% of these patients. The rate of rebleeding is >70% (usually within 6 weeks) with a 30%–40% mortality with each bleed.

2) Rarely is operation indicated as an emergency.

3) Resuscitative measures include restoration of blood volume and correction of coagulopathy with FFP and platelets.

4) Correct metabolic alkalosis with supplemental IV potassium.

5) Evacuate blood from the GI tract with lavage or cathartics to prevent encephalopathy.

6) **Lactulose or neomycin** is administered if encephalopathy develops (lactulose 10 mg PO or via NG tube q. 6 h., neomycin 1 g PO or via NG tube q. 6 h.).

7) **Vasopressin** is usually indicated for its vasoconstrictive effects. Systemic IV vasopressin is as effective as intraarterial infusion. Doses of 0.2–0.4 units/min are begun via a peripheral vein. With cessation of bleeding, the dose is decreased 0.1 unit/min q. 12 h. This is effective approximately 50% of the time. *Vasopressin is contraindicated in patients with coronary artery disease because of its coronary vasoconstricting effects*.

8) **Somatostatin** has fewer side effects and clinical trials suggest it may be at least as effective as vasopressin (somatostatin 100 μg SC q. 8 h.).

9) **Balloon tamponade** with a Sengstaken-Blakemore tube is effective in 50%–80%. Tamponade for 24 hours is usually required. Pressure necrosis may occur if the balloon is inflated for longer periods.

10) **Sclerotherapy** performed during endoscopy has replaced balloon tamponade for acute bleeding at

many centers. Morbidity is 2%–10%; mortality, 1%–3%. Sclerotherapy for the prevention of recurrent hemorrhage, while having a high recurrence rate (50%), has a survival advantage over distal splenorenal shunt.

11) When sclerotherapy fails, management with portocaval shunting or distal splenorenal shunt is indicated.

12) Emergency surgical procedures are reserved for patients who fail attempts at conservative therapy. **Portocaval shunting** or **esophageal transsection and reanastomosis** with the EEA stapler are the most popular emergency operations. Mortality for a class C cirrhotic undergoing emergency portocaval shunt is approximately 50%. In an elective setting, a distal splenorenal shunt with preservation of hepatic portal perfusion is indicated. Child's class may be improved medically with subsequent reduction in mortality.

13) **Propranolol** in doses to lower HR by 25% may be effective in preventing recurrent bleeding. It should not be used in the treatment of acute bleeding (propranolol 10 mg po or via NG tube q. 6 h., increasing doses until HR is lowered).

f. **Aortoenteric fistula:**

1) A patient with an intraabdominal vascular graft and GI bleed should be managed as if he has an aortoenteric fistula until proved otherwise.

2) A "herald" bleed is often followed by massive hemorrhage. Urgent endoscopy, CT scanning, and angiography have all been used to aid in the diagnosis.

a) CT scan is the diagnostic study of choice as it may demonstrate soft tissue changes proximal to the graft consistent with graft infection.

b) Angiograms usually do not demonstrate extravasation of blood. When an aortoenteric fistula is apparent enough to be diagnosed, it is often bleeding so rapidly that the patient cannot be resuscitated.

3) The failure to demonstrate another source of bleeding may support the diagnosis of aortoenteric fistula.

4) Surgical intervention requires removal of the graft, oversewing of the aorta, repair of the duodenum or jejunum, and an extraanatomic bypass. Operative mortality is >50%.

g. **Lower GI bleeding:**
1) The most common causes appear to be diverticular disease and angiodysplasia.
2) Although bleeding from diverticula reportedly occurs most often in the ascending colon, unless a site can be localized preoperatively, subtotal colectomy is warranted.
3) Preoperative localization can be accomplished with radionuclide scanning and angiography.
4) **Intraarterial vasopressin** for management of colonic bleeding is initially successful in 80% of patients, but over half rebleed with cessation of the drug. In high-risk patients, arterial embolization may be attempted.
5) **Colonoscopy** with heat probe application to angiodysplastic lesions also may be indicated in the high-risk patient.

B. Stress Erosive Gastritis.

1. Stress erosive gastritis (stress ulcer, hemorrhagic gastritis, acute mucosal ulceration, acute erosive gastritis) occurs in 80%–100% of critically ill patients when examined endoscopically. Occult UGI bleeding, while common, rarely leads to massive blood loss, primarily because of an increased awareness of the pathophysiology of the disease as well as effective prophylaxis.

2. **Definition:** Multiple gastric erosions occur superficial to the muscularis mucosa. Most begin in the proximal stomach (acid-secreting portion).

3. **Pathophysiology:** There are many important etiologic factors but all result in the inability of the stomach to protect itself against its own acid. Sepsis, shock, and burns are common settings.

4. **Clinical manifestations:** Bleeding may be massive but is more frequently minor, resulting in only slight hemody-

namic derangements. Symptoms are generally manifested 3–10 days after insult. This is a mucosal injury so perforation is rare.

5. **Curling's ulcers** occur commonly in patients with burns in whom more than one third of the body surface is involved. They occur in 12% of patients hospitalized for burns and in 40% of those with >70% burn. Almost half bleed massively. Most occur during convalescence. They may be single or multiple, in the stomach or in the duodenum.

6. **Cushing's ulcers** may be seen in the esophagus, stomach, or duodenum of neurosurgical patients or following cerebral trauma. These are true ulcers and may perforate. It is thought that these arise because of a central mechanism.

7. **Treatment:** The most important factor is prophylaxis. When bleeding occurs, the majority of patients can be treated without operation.

    a. **Prophylaxis** includes supportive care of the underlying disease (e.g., treatment of sepsis, ventilatory support, etc.) as well as alteration of the gastric milieu that may cause erosions. The drugs important in prevention and treatment are listed in Table 11–1. There are both clinical and theoretical data to recommend antacids over H_2 antagonists. Sucralfate appears to be

TABLE 11–1.

Drugs for Prophylaxis or Treatment of Upper Gastrointestinal Bleeding

Agent	Dosage	Mechanism of Action
Antacid (Mylanta II)	30–60 mL via NG tube q.1h. prn to maintain gastric pH>4	Neutralizes acid
Cimetidine (Tagamet)	300 mg IV q.6h. or 900 mg/day IV drip	H_2 antagonist
Rantidine (Zantac)	50 mg IV q.8h.	H_2 antagonist
Famotidine (Pepcid)	20 mg IV q.12h.	H_2 antagonist
Sucralfate (Carafate)	1 g in 10 mL via NG tube q.4h.	Cytoprotective: site-protective at the mucosa
Omeprazole	20 mg po q.d.	Blocks proton pump

as effective as antacids and may also decrease the risk of nosocomial pneumonias.

b. **Nonsurgical treatment:** Intensification of antacid therapy is first attempted. UGI endoscopy is helpful to exclude other causes of bleeding. Endoscopic laser photocoagulation, electrocoagulation, or local injection of epinephrine may be therapeutic. Selective left gastric artery infusion of vasopressin or angiographic Gelfoam embolization may be therapeutic.

c. When bleeding persists despite appropriate medical therapy, surgical therapy may be considered. Numerous operations have been recommended. Oversewing of the erosions with vagotomy and pyloroplasty has the widest support.

C. Acute Pancreatitis.

1. Acute pancreatitis presents in a variety of clinical settings with symptoms ranging from mild epigastric tenderness to severe pain with hemodynamic instability. Postoperative pancreatitis can be lethal because it is often unrecognized in an already compromised patient.

2. **Pathophysiology:** Several theories exist including the "common channel theory," ductal obstruction, vascular ischemia, and hyperlipidemia. Pancreatic inflammation stimulates activation of pancreatic enzymes with autodigestion and pancreatic necrosis. Morphologically, a spectrum of mild edema to hemorrhagic necrosis is seen.

3. **Etiology:** Pancreatitis is associated with a variety of clinical conditions: cholelithiasis, alcohol, trauma, postoperative state, hypercalcemia, drugs (e.g., hydrochlorothiazide, corticosteroids).

4. **Clinical manifestations:** Epigastic pain radiating to the back, nausea, vomiting, fever, a palpable mass, hypotension, jaundice, abdominal distention, Grey Turner's sign (purple discoloration of the flank), and Cullen's sign (periumbilical disoloration) are often seen.

5. **Differential diagnosis:** Perforated peptic ulcer, intestinal obstruction and strangulation, mesenteric infarction, and biliary tract disease may mimic pancreatitis clinically and have elevated serum amylase levels.

6. **Laboratory studies.**

a. **Serum amylase** is highest in gallstone pancreatitis. The test is nonspecific but elevated in 95% of patients with acute pancreatitis.

b. **Urine amylase:**

$$\frac{\text{Amylase clearance}}{\text{Creatinine clearance}} = \frac{\text{urine amylase}}{\text{serum amylase}}$$

$$\times \frac{\text{serum creatinine}}{\text{urine creatinine}}$$

A value of 1%–4% is normal. Levels >4% are seen in pancreatitis. This value identifies patients with hyperamylasemia due to impaired renal clearance of amylase.

c. **Serum lipase** levels can be obtained rapidly. The test is approximately 90%–97% specific for pancreatitis, and stays elevated longer than amylase. Elevated lipase levels occur in pancreatitis, but may also be elevated in renal failure, macrolipase syndromes, and in 5%–10% of patients with nonpancreatic abdominal pain.

d. **Metabolic aberrations:** Hypocalcemia and hyperglycemia may occur in severe pancreatitis. Both are potentially life-threatening, but easily treatable. New hyperglycemia in the setting of severe acute pancreatitis should be managed with an insulin drip.

7. **Radiologic findings:**
   a. In order of incidence, **plain films** of the abdomen and chest demonstrate segmental ileus ("sentinal loop"), colonic dilatation ("colon cutoff sign"), obscure psoas margin, increased epigastric soft tissue density, dilated duodenal loop, left pleural effusion, and pancreatic calcifications.
   b. **Ultrasound** and **abdominal CT scans** may help document enlargement of the pancreas consistent with acute pancreatitis. They may also help define the etiology of the pancreatitis (e.g., cholelithiasis) as well as the late sequelae of the disease (i.e., pseudocyst, abscess).

8. **Nonoperative treatment.**
   a. **NPO and NG suction:**
      1) Patients are kept npo while clinical and laboratory evidence of pancreatitis persist.
      2) NG suction decreases emesis but has not been proved efficacious in reducing the severity of pancreatitis. When symptoms resolve and serum

amylase returns to normal, a low fat diet may be instituted.

b. **Fluid and electrolyte replacement:**
   1) Replace third-space fluid losses with crystalloid.
   2) Blood and FFP may be indicated to correct anemia and coagulopathy in hemorrhagic pancreatitis.
   3) Total volume requirements in severe pancreatitis can be as high as 10–20 L.

c. **Prophylaxis** for stress gastritis.

d. **Respiratory support:** Hypoxemia may develop rapidly despite normal clinical and radiographic findings. Monitor ABG frequently. Intubation may be required.

e. **Analgesia:** Meperidine (Demerol) is used. It may have less effect on the ampulla of Vater than morphine.

f. **Antibiotics** are not usually indicated for alcoholic pancreatitis but are used with gallstone pancreatitis or when a pancreatic abscess or phlegmon is suspected.

g. For severe cases of pancreatitis, **parenteral nutrition** is required. Avoid fat emulsions only if hyperlipidemia is a presumed etiologic factor.

9. **Operative indication.**

a. Nonoperative treatment is generally successful in nonbiliary-associated acute pancreatitis. Operation is indicated to confirm diagnosis, manage biliary disease, or manage complications of pancreatitis.

b. Management of acute complications generally involves debridement and drainage of pancreatic abscess or phlegmon. Peritoneal lavage has not provided increased survival but there is ongoing debate about its potential role.

c. Twenty percent to 30% of patients with gallstone pancreatitis do not respond to conservative therapy. Cholecystectomy with common bile duct exploration or ERCP with papillotomy may be required.

d. Patients who recover from gallstone pancreatitis have a 30%–50% incidence of recurrence within the next several months and should undergo interval cholecystectomy, preferably when the pancreatitis has resolved to the degree that an oral diet can be tolerated.

10. **Prognosis.**

a. Three fourths of patients recover uneventfully from pancreatitis and the remainder have severe complications with a mortality of 10%. Alcohol-induced pancreatitis has the lowest mortality (<4%); postoperative pancreatitis has the highest (>40%).

b. **Ranson** has identified 11 objective signs to identify patients at risk (Table 11–2): Patients with fewer than three positive signs have a mortality of 1%; with three to four signs, 16%; with five to six signs, 40%; with seven or more signs, up to 100% mortality.

11. **Chronic sequelae:** Complications of acute pancreatitis include pseudocyst (10%), pancreatic abscess (5%), fistula, splenic vein thrombosis with gastric varices, bile duct stricture, bowel necrosis, chronic abdominal pain.

D. Intestinal Obstruction.

1. In the SICU setting, with mechanical ventilation, IV narcotics, and multisystem organ failure, the differentiation of mechanical small bowel obstruction from paralytic ileus is difficult.

2. **Small bowel obstruction (SBO).**
   a. **Pathophysiology:** Bowel obstruction leads to fluid and air accumulation with resulting bowel distention. Air swallowing accounts for 75% of the air seen in bowel obstruction. With increasing distention fluid absorption is diminished and luminal secretion increases leading to large third-space fluid losses. With strangulation obstruction, luminal distention results in tissue necrosis and subsequent bacterial proliferation.
   b. **Etiology:** Adhesions cause over half of reported cases. Hernias (external and internal) are next in frequency. In the early postoperative period, adhesions and ab-

TABLE 11–2.

Early Prognostic Signs in Acute Pancreatitis*

On Admission	During Initial 48 Hours
Age >55 yr	Fall in Hct >10 percentage points
WBC >16,000/mm³	Calcium <8.0 mg/dL
Glucose >200 mg/dL	PaO₂ <60 mm Hg
LDH >350 IU/L	Base deficit >4 mEq/L
SGOT >250 SF units	BUN increase >5 mg/dL
	Third-space loss >6,000 mL

*Data from Ranson JHC: *Am J Gastroenterol* 1982; 77:633.

dominal sepsis cause most cases. The incidence is higher following colorectal operations (especially abdominal-perineal resection), pelvic operations, and appendectomy for acute or perforated appendicitis.

c. **Clinical manifestations:** Intermittent colicky pain, feculent vomiting, abdominal distention, obstipation, fever, tachycardia, and hypotension are seen. In early postoperative obstruction, a period of normal bowel function may precede symptoms. The passage of flatus and small stools postoperatively should not deter the diagnosis if other clinical symptoms are present.

d. **Laboratory studies.** Mild leukocytosis, hyperamylasemia, and electrolyte abnormalities are seen in a number of settings including bowel obstruction. Metabolic acidosis suggests strangulation.

e. **Radiologic findings.**

1) **Plain films** demonstrate air-fluid levels in a "stepladder" pattern. Small bowel loops are centrally located and valvulae conniventes cross the entire lumen ("stack of coins"). Distended loops and lack of gas in the colon are seen. With high proximal bowel obstructions, distended loops with air-fluid levels may not be seen. Thickened bowel loops (>3 mm), thumbprinting, intramural air, free air, and air in the portal vein suggest strangulation.

2) A **barium enema**, which fills the colon, eliminates the colon as the obstructed site and reflux of barium into a collapsed terminal ileum confirms the plain film diagnosis.

3) A **UGI series** demonstrating a transition zone is helpful. The passage of barium is slow in both obstruction and ileus. **Enteroclysis** (small bowel study) is a more useful study than UGI.

f. **Management.**

1) **Fluid resuscitation:** Replace third-space losses with isotonic solution. Monitor with Foley catheter, CVP or PA catheterization, as appropriate.

2) Replace NG losses with ½ NS with 30 mEq KCL/L to prevent hypochloremic, hypokalemic metabolic alkalosis.

3) Bowel decompression is best achieved with **NG suctioning.** Occasionally, long intestinal tubes are useful but these often delay surgery and may increase morbidity. Possible indications for their use include early postoperative obstruction, recurrent partial bowel obstruction, and abdominal carcinomatosis.

4) **Surgical procedures:** Abdominal exploration following rehydration is recommended in most cases. A definite transition zone of dilated proximal bowel and collapsed distal bowel is sought. Obstruction secondary to Crohn's disease, malignancy, and recent operation may respond to conservative therapy. Reexploration in a recently operated abdomen is difficult but if obstruction has not been relieved with conservative therapy, surgery is warranted. If operation is to be delayed, nutritional support should be considered.

g. **Prognosis:** Mortality for simple obstruction is 0%–6%; for strangulation obstruction, 15%–30%; and for early postoperative obstruction, 15%.

3. **Large bowel obstruction.**
   a. Colorectal carcinoma (80%), volvulus, diverticulitis, and fecal impaction are common etiologies.
   b. **Clinical manifestations** are similar to SBO. Diarrhea may precede complete obstruction. An abdominal mass may be found.
   c. **Radiologic findings:**
      1) A dilated proximal colon with absence of gas distally is diagnostic (if no enemas are given). On plain films, haustral markings are noted in the colon.
      2) Barium enema may show a "bird beak" in volvulus or may be therapeutic in intussusception.
   d. **Treatment:** Colonic obstructions are surgical emergencies. Diverting colostomy with or without resection is required. In right-sided lesions, primary anastomosis may be attempted if soilage is minimal and the patient stable.

4. Following abdominal exploration, *paralytic ileus* may persist for 2–5 days. Return of GI motility is variable, with return in the small bowel occurring first, followed by the

stomach, and lastly the colon. NG suction and IV hydration, correction of electrolyte abnormality and minimizing narcotic use is the treatment of choice. In prolonged cases, a primary tube study (enteroclysis) may be necessary to differentiate ileus from obstruction.

5. **Colonic ileus or cecal dilation**
   a. (pseudo-obstruction, Ogilvie's syndrome, nonobstructive colonic dilation) is not uncommon postoperatively in SICU patients.
   b. May be clinically asymptomatic except for abdominal distention. Symptoms are often indistinguishable from large bowel obstruction.
   c. The diameter of the normal cecum is usually less than 9 cm on the plain film, but may approach 12 cm in extreme cases.
   d. Initial therapy is conservative, using NG decompression, IV fluid, and rectal tube decompression as tolerated. If the patient becomes symptomatic, deteriorates despite therapy, or continues to have cecal dilation at 48 hours, the treatment of choice is **colonoscopic decompression.** A 6F catheter can be placed endoscopically in the cecum and brought out through the anus for continued decompression. Colonscopy succeeds in 85% with a lower mortality and morbidity than surgical decompression. Rarely, surgery is required.

E. **Intestinal Ischemia.**
   1. Ischemia of the small or large intestine can occur acutely or chronically. The stomach has four major arteries, and gastric ischemia is exceedingly rare. Intestinal ischemia may be the result of either (a) progressive atherosclerotic occlusive disease in two or more of the three major vessels (celiac axis, SMA, IMA) or (b) acute mesenteric occlusion.
   2. **Progressive atherosclerosis.**
      a. Progressive atherosclerosis of the mesenteric arteries is compensated for by the enlargement of existing collateral vessels, but some patients are unable, despite collaterals, to achieve adequate tissue perfusion of the small and large bowel.
      b. These patients may present with recurrent postprandial pain due to chronic mesenteric ischemia.
      c. The pathophysiology parallels that of angina and claudication in that it represents pain associated with in-

creased O_2 demands of muscle. The patient usually presents with significant weight loss due to poor oral intake.

d. Oral intake is curbed because of the pain associated with eating. In selected cases, surgery may be useful.

3. **Acute mesenteric occlusion.**

a. Acute mesenteric occlusion may be the result of an embolus or an acute thrombosis. The SMA and its branches are most commonly involved.

b. The event represents a major abdominal catastrophe, and the patient classically presents with *severe abdominal pain out of proportion to physical findings*. The clinical picture is one of an acute abdomen.

c. Laboratory values confirm a metabolic **(lactic) acidosis** and leukocytosis. ECG may show atrial fibrillation.

d. **Plain films** may show air-fluid levels and dilated bowel consistent with an ileus. **Angiography** demonstrates arterial obstruction.

e. Especially in the setting of a known proximal embolic source (heart in atrial fibrillation, abdominal aortic atherosclerotic disease), the index of suspicion should be high, to permit early operative intervention.

f. In a postoperative patient, especially in the SICU, pain may not be evident, and the postoperative ileus may mask symptoms of acute mesenteric occlusion.

   1) These patients usually present with sepsis and a metabolic acidosis, resulting from gangrenous bowel.

   2) In this setting, the proper evaluation includes flat and decubitus radiographs of the abdomen and a thorough workup to rule out other sources of sepsis.

   3) The radiographs will often reveal dilated loops of bowel, air-fluid levels, thickened bowel wall, and the absence of normal haustral markings or valvulae conniventes. Extensive films are not usually helpful. Early exploration is appropriate.

F. **Malignancy.**

1. Patients with GI tract malignancy deserve special attention from an intensive care standpoint.

2. Patients admitted to the SICU with advanced malignancy often are cachectic and anergic. These patients need nutri-

tional assessment early, and if prolonged ileus is anticipated, tube feedings or TPN should be instituted early. The
only caveat is that aggressive intervention, including TPN,
in patients with metastatic cancer can have significant ethi-
cal implications. The patient's therapy in many respects
may be limited by the overall prognosis and the family's re-
quests.

3. Anergy implies immune deficits. These need to be considered when the patient has an infection or an infection-prone
wound. Also, these patients may not develop leukocytosis.

4. Metastatic cancer is a common cause of **hypercalcemia.**
Also, several paraneoplastic syndromes exist, in which hormones produced by tumors have systemic effects that complicate patient management. Islet cell tumors and related tumors may produce insulin, glucagon, gastrin, somatostatin, or other systemically active hormones with profound effects on metabolic parameters.

G. Peritonitis and Perforated Viscus.

1. A perforated viscus can lead to a localized abscess or diffuse peritonitis. A perforation usually presents with free intraperitoneal air on upright CXR or lateral decubitus abdominal film (sensitivity: 1–5 mL air). However, free air is
not present in all cases of perforation (75%).

2. In the setting of diffuse peritonitis, there is an ileus secondary to an inflammatory response. The resultant third-space
fluid accumulation can be impressive. Large-volume fluid
resuscitation (L), electrolyte management, and antibiotics
are required, almost always followed by laparotomy for definitive therapy of the cause of peritonitis.

3. A **perforated duodenal ulcer** usually presents acutely with
severe abdominal pain and peritonitis. It may occur in a person who is otherwise healthy, or it may occur in the hospitalized person in whom the stress of severe illness exacer-
bates an underlying ulcer diathesis.

   a. In this setting, diffuse peritonitis is common. The usual
   management is exploratory laparotomy, and oversewing of the ulcer with an omental patch (Graham patch).

   b. In the stable patient, a definitive ulcer operation (a
   highly selective vagotomy or vagotomy-pyloroplasty) is
   also performed.

   c. In some circumstances, especially in the poor operative
   candidate and when the perforation can be shown to

have sealed, nonoperative management and IV antibiotics have been advocated.

H. Diverticular Disease.

1. A perforated colonic diverticulum can present as a localized diverticular abscess, often managed successfully with percutaneous drainage and IV antibiotics, or as diffuse peritonitis requiring exploration and resection of the involved segment of colon. Hartmann's procedure (end colostomy and stapled distal stump of rectosigmoid) is usually performed.

2. Diverticulitis itself can present with an acute or subacute inflammatory mass, which is usually diagnosed on the clinical basis of LUQ pain and tenderness, with fever and leukocytosis. A CT scan may be useful in diagnosis, showing a thickened colon wall or an abscess. The mass usually is managed successfully with IV antibiotics and bowel rest for 7–10 days. An elective resection may be required in several weeks.

3. Diverticulitis is often chronic and may lead to few symptoms until inflammatory changes cause a sigmoid stricture, requiring resection.

4. Diverticulitis can also present as a **colovesical fistula** when a diverticulum erodes into adjacent bladder (Pneumatomia may result). Surgery is indicated to remove the diseased bowel and to excise the fistula.

I. Intraabdominal Abscess.

1. An intraabdominal abscess should be distinguished from generalized peritonitis. In the SICU, the diagnosis is difficult given the debility of the patient, sedation used, and abdominal pain from the recent operation.

2. **Etiology:** Abscesses may more commonly occur after intraabdominal trauma or following large operations in the stomach, pancreas, or liver. Incidental splenectomy is associated with left subphrenic abscesses.

3. **Location:** Pelvis, retroperitoneum, right and left subphrenic spaces, subhepatic space, lesser sac, and right and left pericolic spaces are common sites for abscess formation. Abscesses form between loops of bowel (intraloop abscess). Hematogenous seeding accounts for most solid organ abscesses (liver, spleen, kidney) except for pancreatic abscesses which result most often from pancreatitis.

4. **Clinical findings** are nonspecific and include fever, tachycardia, and leukocytosis. Tenderness and a mass may be ap-

preciated. A rectal examination may identify a pelvic abscess. The patient may also have an ileus.

5. **Plain film** findings include extraluminal gas, soft tissue mass, and ileus. Radiographs are helpful in 50% but are often nonspecific.

6. **Diagnosis.**
   a. **Ultrasound:** Ultrasound is very sensitive and very specific. Large amounts of air in the bowel, complicated wound dressings, or open wounds may limit the study. A distended gallbladder and fluid-filled loops of bowel may be confused with an abscess. Ultrasound can be performed at the bedside.
   b. **Radionuclide scan:** Indium-labeled WBCs can identify abscesses but the time delay (48 hours), need for repeat scanning, and decreased sensitivity compared to CT often precludes its use.
   c. **CT** has the highest sensitivity and specificity of any study. Abscesses may be distinguished from hematomas or phlegmon based on attenuation values. The patient must be transported to the CT scanner.

7. **Treatment:** Delay in the diagnosis of an abscess leads to multisystem organ failure and sepsis with greatly increased mortality and morbidity.
   a. **Antibiotics:** GI organisms are the majority of cultured organisms. While awaiting blood and abscess culture results, broad-spectrum antibiotics are used. An aminoglycoside, ampicillin-clindamycin, or metronidazole will cover these organisms. Synthetic penicillins and second- and third-generation cephalosporins may be useful, especially in patients with renal insufficiency.
   b. **Percutaneous drainage** via CT or ultrasound guidance should be considered with all abscesses, especially uniloculated abscesses that can be drained without traversing intestine. Intraloop abscesses, multiple abscesses, multiloculated abscesses, and abscesses that require traversing solid organs or intestine may not be amenable to percutaneous drainage. The presence of a fistula is not a contraindication to percutaneous drainage, although prolonged drainage will be necessary. Approximately 80% of intraabdominal abscesses respond to percutaneous drainage.
   c. **Surgical exploration** may be required in inaccessible abscesses, those that do not respond to percutaneous

drainage, or when the clinical suspicion of an abscess exists but cannot be identified radiographically. The success of surgical and percutaneous drainage is similar, but the morbidity from surgical reexploration appears to be greater.

8. **Prognosis:** The mortality for surgically or percutaneously drained abscesses is 10%–15%. Early diagnosis before multiorgan system failure has greatly lowered the mortality.

J. Inflammatory Bowel Disease (IBD).

1. The two forms of IBD are ulcerative colitis (UC) and Crohn's disease (CD). In CD, because the entire GI tract can be involved, attempts are made to limit surgical resection. In UC, a protocolectomy is curative, so in patients with recurrent or severe complications, this procedure or a subtotal colectomy may be indicated.

2. Patients with IBD are often chronically treated with corticosteroids. Steroids in stress doses are administered to prevent adrenal insufficiency in these patients.

3. Bowel rest, medical therapy, and TPN have been found to provide significant benefit to patients with IBD during acute exacerbations of the disease. They may allow a significant percentage of patients (~50%) to recover without surgical intervention.

4. The **acute complications** of IBD include obstruction, bleeding, perforation, abscess, and fistula.

   a. **Obstruction:** In the patient who has had no prior abdominal surgery and who has SBO in the setting of CD, it is appropriate to manage him conservatively. If such a patient has had prior surgery, then it is more likely the obstruction is due to adhesions and scarring. In the latter case, early surgical intervention is therapeutic. Bowel resection should be limited. Ninety percent to 95% of patients develop recurrent CD despite resection.

   b. **Bleeding:** Small amounts of blood in the stool are common in CD; however, massive bleeding occurs in <5% of cases. Small bowel bleeding is five times more common than colon bleeding. After one massive bleed, another occurs in about 50% of cases. It is reasonable to resect if: (1) other indications for resection exist; (2) the bleed exceeds 4–6 units of blood; (3) the bleed recurs.

   c. **Perforation:** Contained perforation and an abscess are more common than free perforation. Appropriate surgical therapy is resection of the involved segment, with primary anastomosis if soilage is minimal.

d. **Abscesses** (15%–25%) and **fistulas** (20%–50%): Abscesses can occur as a result of the inflammatory bowel disease itself or as a postoperative complication. Many are associated with fistulas. CT usually makes the diagnosis. Treatment is surgical. External drainage is adequate, but optimal therapy is excision of the involved bowel and the abscess cavity. Fistulas may be to skin, bowel, bladder, vagina, or stomach. Bowel rest, medical therapy, and TPN may result in closure in a subset of patients, but many fistulas due to IBD will require surgical division.

K. Biliary Sepsis and Cholangitis.

Sepsis within the biliary tree can constitute a diagnostic and therapeutic emergency and is becoming more common with the advent of percutaneous and endoscopic manipulation. In addition, the surgical treatment of primary and secondary biliary disorders can predispose to ascending infection of the bile ducts. The classic diagnostic signs of *cholangitis* are fever, jaundice, and RUQ pain (Charcot's triad). Advanced infection may present as Reynold's pentad of fever, jaundice, RUQ pain, hypotension, and mental status changes. The mortality rate is high in such patients, and treatment is urgent.

1. The **history** may include an indolent dull ache, low fever, and malaise that rapidly worsens. Important aspects to note are a history of gallstone disease, prior biliary surgery, alcohol abuse or pancreatitis, recent manipulation of the biliary tree (ERCP, PTC), or recent abdominal symptoms.

2. **Pathophysiology:** Bacteria may ascend the obstructed biliary tree from the intestine, from foci and infection elsewhere via the portal or systemic circulation, directly via trauma, or from surgical or other direct manipulations. Bacteria then multiply and ascend the biliary tree with eventual bilivenous and bililymphatic reflux leading to infection.

3. **Etiology:** Any condition leading to partial or complete biliary obstruction predisposes to cholangitis (Table 11–3). Approximately 90% of patients with gallstones have positive bile cultures, while <50% of patients with malignant obstruction and no stones have positive cultures.

4. The **differential diagnosis** is extensive: Acute cholecystitis; acute hepatitis; hepatic or perihepatic abscess; perforation of the stomach, duodenum, or colon; acute pancreati-

TABLE 11–3.

Conditions Associated With
Cholangitis

Iatrogenic procedures (ERCP, PTC)
Choledocholithiasis
Malignant obstruction
   (cholangiocarcinoma, pancreatic
   cancer, metastatic disease to the
   porta hepatis)
Stricture (postoperative, malignant,
   chronic pancreatitis, sclerosing
   cholangitis)
Biliary-enteric anastomosis
Foreign bodies (Ttube, indwelling biliary
   stent)

tis; appendicitis; bacterial endocarditis; and potential superinfection of malignant processes must be considered.

5. **Physical findings:** fever, RUQ tenderness to palpation, ic-
terus or jaundice, nausea and vomiting, hepatomegaly, hypotension, mental status changes.
6. **Laboratory studies:** leukocytosis with band cells, bilirubin >3 mg/dL (<10 mg/dL usually benign, >15 mg/dL
usually malignant), elevated alkaline phosphatase, moderately elevated transaminases, hyperamylasemia, positive
cultures of blood and bile.
7. **Bacteriology:** The duodenum is the most common source
of organisms. With partial obstruction infection often follows instrumentation. The most common organisms are
aerobic gram-negative rods including *Escherichia coli* and
Klebsiella sps. Enterococci are common and proteus,
pseudomonads, and *Enterobacter* are occasionally seen.
Anaerobes are relatively rare though bacteroides and *Pep-
tostreptococcus* are seen. Clostridia are common in acalculous cholecystitis but not cholangitis. Microaerophilic
streptococci are becoming more common as culture techniques improve.
8. **Diagnosis:** Ultrasonography should be performed if the
clinical diagnosis is cholangitis. Positive findings usually
include a dilated biliary tree associated with biliary stones,
an enlarged pancreatic head, aerobilia, or an abnormal gall-

bladder. Plain abdominal films may reveal aerobilia. CT of the abdomen will show dilation of the common or intrahepatic ducts, or both.

9. **Treatment.**

   a. **Prevention:** A significant percentage of cases are caused by procedural manipulation of the biliary tree, and patients undergoing ERCP, PTC or T tube cholangiogram should receive prophylactic antibiotics. Generally one dose prior to and 18–24 hours of coverage following the procedure are sufficient.

   b. **Resuscitation:** Patients with sepsis from cholangitis must be resuscitated prior to definitive treatment. Antibiotics (either conventional triple-drug therapy or broad-spectrum penicillin or cephalosporin) and IV fluids usually suffice. Patients with suppurative cholangitis and associated medical problems will need intensive care with arterial and PAP monitoring, and monitoring of UO. Large volumes of fluid and vasopressors may be required.

   c. **Decompression:** After diagnosis and resuscitation are accomplished, urgent decompression of the biliary tree must be obtained (Table 11–4). Previously, surgical drainage was necessary in all cases and mortality ranged up to 30%. Today most patients can be drained via ERCP or PTC stenting with lower mobidity and mortality (<5%). If successful, these procedures allow definitive surgical intervention in a stable patient with an established diagnosis. If urgent decompression is not deemed necessary 85% of patients are improved in 24 hours. If not, decompression should be performed.

TABLE 11–4.

Signs of Need for Urgent Biliary Decompression

Bilirubin >3.0 mg/dL
Systolic BP <90 mm Hg
Mental disorientation
Temperature >39° C
Disseminated intravascular coagulation

10. **Prognosis:** Untreated suppurative cholangitis is 100% fatal; the mortality of decompressed cholangitis is 5%.

L. Acalculous Cholecystitis.

1. Patients who are severely ill, especially with multisystem failure, are predisposed to the development of acalculous cholecystitis. Acalculous cholecystitis accounts for <5% of adult cases of acute cholecystitis in the United States, but accounts for a high proportion of cases that occur in SICU patients. The etiology is uncertain, but is presumed to be related to cholestasis, sepsis, and ischemia.

2. **Diagnosis** by ultrasound or CT may be suggested by thickening of the gallbladder wall (≥ 4 mm), pericholecystic fluid, mucosal sloughing, and intramural gas. HIDA scan is the standard for diagnosis in acute calculous cholecystitis, but may be misleading in patients suspected of acalculous cholecystitis. IV morphine during HIDA scanning may aid gallbladder filling and reduce the chance of a false-positive scan.

3. Classically, the preferred treatment has been cholecystectomy, but cholecystostomy has been performed in patients too ill to tolerate resection. Recent advances in interventional radiology have made it feasible to perform **percutaneous drainage** (PD) of the gallbladder in a large number of cases. A percutaneous cholecystostomy tube can be placed transhepatically under ultrasound guidance and left until the patient has recovered from concurrent life-threatening problems. At that time, many patients may have the tube removed without ill effect. Tube cholecystogram demonstrating cystic duct obstruction may be an indication for interval cholecystectomy.

M. Postoperative Jaundice and Hepatic Failure

1. Jaundice following major surgical procedures requiring multiple transfusions or cardiopulmonary bypass is relatively common, and usually resolves spontaneously. However, metabolic evidence of hepatic dysfunction with jaundice in critically ill patients must be investigated. Causes of jaundice fall into three broad categories: prehepatic, intrahepatic, and posthepatic.

a. Prehepatic (hemolytic) jaundice.

1) Massive transfusion of PRBCs presents the liver with an inordinate load of bilirubin. Ten percent of 2-week-old blood and 20% of 3-week-old blood is

hemolyzed within 24 hours of transfusion, doubling or tripling the normal day's bilirubin turnover (250 mg/day).

2) Large hematomas (along with the subsequent necessary transfusions) likewise result in peripheral heme absorption.

3) Hemolysis resulting from transfusion reaction causes immediate, sometimes catastrophic, reactions including hyperbilirubinemia, haptoglobinemia, fever, hemoglobinuria, and circulatory collapse.

4) Sickle cell anemia crisis or perioperative stress in sickle cell patients may lead to hemolysis and subsequent jaundice.

5) Cardiopulmonary bypass, despite advances in technology, causes jaundice from hemolysis in up to 20% of patients undergoing open heart procedures.

b. **Intrahepatic (cholestatic) jaundice.**

1) Infection by hepatitis A,B (or delta agent), C, or CMV may develop or recrudesce in postoperative patients secondary to prior exposure or infection by transfusion of blood products. Hepatic transaminases are typically markedly elevated, and specific serum tests are usually diagnostic.

2) Drugs (e.g., acetaminophen, MAOIs, tetracycline, sulfonamides, MTX) may lead to a spectrum of derangements from cholestasis to fulminant failure. Halothane, implicated in the past, is not a major cause of hepatic toxicity.

3) TPN causes intrahepatic cholestasis with mild elevations of transaminases. Recent studies showing a beneficial effect of concurrent CCK infusion are encouraging.

4) Sepsis, especially from intraabdominal sources, may cause transient jaundice.

5) Shock resulting in a low-flow hepatic state may cause hepatic ischemia or necrosis resulting in cholestasis and jaundice.

c. **Posthepatic (obstructive) jaundice:** Any source of obstruction of the biliary tree may cause jaundice.

d. **History:** The determination of preexisting hepatic conditions (hepatitis, hemolytic syndromes), previous similar episodes, and recent drug history should be obtained. Additionally, a history of gallstone disease, and a detailed operative history (shock, Pringle maneuver, transfusions) should be obtained.

  e. **Physical examination:** In addition to jaundice, hepatomegaly, RUQ tenderness, epigastic pain, clay-colored stools, cola-colored urine, or biliary fistula may be present.

  f. **Laboratory studies:** Total and fractionated bilirubin, amylase (isoamylase and lipase for differential of pancreatitis), SGOT and SGPT (indicating hepaticocellular injury), alkaline phosphatase and 5′-nucleotidase (extrahepatic obstruction), CBC (hemolysis), PT (hepatocellular metabolic dysfunction), haptoglobin, and Coombs' test (hemolysis) are useful for differential diagnosis. Viral antigen-antibody testing is necessary for the investigation of viral hepatitis.

  g. **Diagnostic studies:** In addition to the above laboratory studies, ultrasound or CT will demonstrate a dilated biliary tree (obstruction), ERCP or PTC may be useful, but attention to coagulation status is vital.

2. **Hepatic failure.**

Fulminant hepatic failure in the postoperative patient carries a mortality of 80%–90%. Patients with cirrhosis are the most common victims, and they must be approached therapeutically with extreme caution. **Child's classification** (Table 11–5) is useful in determining patients at risk. Importantly, evidence of synthetic or metabolic dysfunction (low albumin, hyperbilirubinemia) is more indicative of risk than

TABLE 11–5.

Child's Classification of Cirrhosis

Parameter	A	B	C
Serum bilirubin (mg/dL)	<2.0	2.0–3.0	>3.0
Serum albumin	>3.5	3.0–3.5	<3.0
Ascites	None	Easily controlled	Poorly controlled
Neurologic disorder	None	Minimal	Advanced; coma
Nutrition	Excellent	Good	Poor; wasting
Postoperative mortality rate (%)	0–10	10–20	20–60

transaminase elevation. Jaundice and hepatic dysfunction are extremely worrisome when found together.

a. **Clinical features:** Hepatic decompensation is manifest by mental status changes (agitation, confusion, drowsiness, coma), and may be accompanied by renal dysfunction (hepatorenal syndrome I or II) or other organ dysfunction.

b. **Laboratory investigation:** Hepatic transaminases, serum ammonia, creatinine, BUN, and arterial pH are important in guiding therapy. Albumin, bilirubin, and coagulation studies aid in determining the severity of dysfunction.

c. **Prevention:** Hepatic failure is best treated by prevention, i.e., avoiding precipitating conditions such as GI bleeding, sepsis, protein loading, excessive transfusion, and hepatotoxic drugs.

d. **Treatment:**
   1) Control GI bleeding.
   2) Reduce ammonia production by intestinal flora with lactulose (cathartic—reduces stool pH), neomycin (decreases bowel flora), and enemas (remove blood and stool from colon).
   3) Dosages: lactulose 30–45 mL q.h. until diarrhea ensues then t.i.d.-q.i.d. for two to three loose stools daily; neomycin 1 g po q. 6 h. or 1 g in 200 mL saline as a retention enema.
   4) Ensure nutrition with limited protein (20 g/day acutely and 40–60 g/day chronically) with enteral or parenteral feeding.

e. **Prognosis:** Hepatic failure with multiorgan system failure is nearly 100% fatal. Survival rates have improved because of improved supportive care but mortality in patients with Child's C cirrhosis still ranges from 20%–60% for all operative procedures. Hepatic transplantation offers some hope to victims of fulminant hepatic failure.

N. Drug Dosage in Hepatic Failure

The duration and intensity of systemic effects of drugs are determined to a large degree by their rate of elimination. The liver and kidney constitute the major routes of drug elimination, and hepatic dysfunction markedly alters the metabolism of certain drugs. General guidelines for common drugs are presented in

TABLE 11–6.
Drug Adjustment in Hepatic Failure

Drug/Class	Adjustment/Comment
Analgesics	
Ibuprofen	Avoid in severe disease
Aspirin	Avoid in severe disease
Acetaminophen	No adjustment
Morphine	Reduce dose
β-Blockers	
Atenolol	Adjustment
Propranolol	Avoid
Benzodiazapines	Drastically reduce dose
Antibiotics	
Ampicillin	No adjustment
Aminoglycosides	None, monitor levels
Mezlocillin	Reduce dose 50%
Nafcillin	Reduce
Clindamycin	No adjustment
Metronidazole	No adjustment in mild disease, reduce in severe disease
Cephalosporins	No adjustment
Vancomycin	Reduce dose 60%
H₂ blockers	
Cimetidine	None in mild disease, reduce in severe disease
Ranitidine	No adjustment
Calcium channel blockers	No adjustment
Digoxin	No adjustment
Prednisone	No adjustment
Diuretics	
Furosemide	No adjustment, may need increase
Spironolactone	No adjustment
Cyclosporine	Follow levels

Table 11–6, but for specific recommendations, consult package inserts.

II. PERIOPERATIVE CARE FOR ALIMENTARY TRACT SURGERY.
A. Hiatal Hernia Repair.
    1. Preoperative orders:
        a. NPO after midnight.
        b. Prophylactic antibiotics are unnecessary.

    c. Administer H_2 blockers or antacids and continue into postoperative period.

2. Postoperative orders:

    a. Administer IV fluids to include maintenance, NG loss, and minimal third-space loss.

    b. Secure the NG tube. The NG tube is generally removed with the demonstration of bowel function although some surgeons will remove the tube earlier.

    c. The diet is advanced after removal of the NG tube. Avoid carbonated beverages.

3. Complications:

    a. Postoperative atelectasis is common, especially if the procedure is done through the chest.

    b. Hemorrhage is uncommon and is usually a result of an unrecognized splenic injury or improper ligation of a short gastric vessel during mobilization of the fundus.

    c. The "gas bloat" syndrome is not uncommon after a Nissen fundoplication and consists of the inability to eructate and epigastric or retrosternal pain. Symptoms are generally mild and resolve within weeks. Persistent symptoms mandate a barium swallow for diagnosis and NG suction may be required.

B. Esophageal Resection.

After resection of the esophagus, several reconstructive procedures are available which involve use of the stomach, small bowel, or colon.

1. Preoperative orders:

    a. NPO after midnight.

    b. Nutritional support for an extended period preoperatively may be necessary in the severely malnourished patient. Often, this can be accomplished with placement of an enteral feeding tube distal to the obstruction.

    c. Perioperative prophylactic antibiotics are administered.

    d. If the colon is to be used as an interposition graft, a preoperative mechanical bowel preparation is begun.

2. Postoperative orders:

    a. Administer IV fluids to include maintenance, NG loss, and large third-space loss.

    b. Secure the NG tube. Emphasize to staff the critical nature of the tube remaining in place and patent.

    c. Prophylaxis for stress gastritis.

    d. A Gastrografin swallow is obtained at 5–7 days looking

for an anastomotic leak. The posterior chest tube is left in place until no leak is confirmed. Feeding may begin after the Gastrografin swallow.

3. Complications:

a. Atelectasis and pneumonia are common. Vigorous chest physiotherapy is encouraged although ET suctioning is contraindicated with an anastomosis in the neck.

b. A hematoma in the neck should be evacuated in the OR to prevent airway compromise.

c. Necrosis of the interposed viscus may manifest with fever, leukocytosis, pain, cellulitis, or wound drainage. This potentially lethal complication may not be apparent until the Gastrografin swallow is obtained.

d. An anastomotic leak is usually managed surgically with reexploration for repair of the leak. A small asymptomatic leak may occasionally be managed conservatively with prolonged chest tube drainage and nutritional support. When the drainage resolves, a Gastrografin swallow will document closure.

e. Other complications include reflux, aspiration, pneumothorax, bowel obstruction, gastric outlet obstruction, prolonged ileus, and anastomotic stricture.

C. Gastrectomy.

The choice of operation depends on several factors including cause (cancer vs. ulcer disease), indication for operation (perforation, bleeding, obstruction, intractability), and surgical preference. Parietal cell vagotomy has the lowest complication rate but the highest rate of ulcer recurrence (15%). Vagotomy and antrectomy have higher complication rates and the lowest rate of recurrence (1%).

1. Preoperative orders:

a. Replace blood losses and begin resuscitation if the patient is bleeding.

b. Massive fluid resuscitation may be required for perforation with peritonitis.

c. NG suction is instituted for bleeding, perforation, or obstruction. Prolonged NG aspiration in a grossly distended stomach from outlet obstruction may be necessary.

d. Support patients nutritionally who present with weight loss from cancer or outlet obstruction. Parenteral nutrition is necessary unless an enteral tube can be advanced past the obstruction.

e. Antibiotics are administered when the indication for surgery is obstruction, perforation, or bleeding. Although normally the stomach has few microorganisms, obstruction results in bacterial overgrowth. Patients with achlorhydria or with correction of normal gastric acidity with H_2 blockers may also have a higher concentration of bacteria in the stomach than normal. With perforation, antibiotics are continued 7–10 days postoperatively.

2. Postoperative orders:

a. Fluid replacement varies according to operative blood losses and expected third-space fluid losses. Replace NG output with appropriate fluids or send fluid for electrolytes (see Chapter 10, pp 406–412).

b. Secure NG tube. The tube is generally removed with the onset of peristalsis.

c. A Gastrografin swallow is obtained if the anastomosis was difficult or NG output remains elevated after an appropriate time of decompression.

d. Begin clear liquids with removal of NG tube and advance diet slowly. With a subtotal or total gastrectomy, a postgastrectomy diet of six small meals is appropriate.

e. H_2 blockers or antacids are generally not required if an acid-reducing operation was performed. Some surgeons continue therapy for 6 weeks postoperatively or until pathologic confirmation of a complete vagotomy.

3. Complications:

a. Prevention of atelectasis requires good chest physiotherapy.

b. The causes of postoperative hemorrhage include anastomotic bleeding, splenic injury, a recurrent ulcer, or an improperly ligated vessel. Follow the Hct, bloody NG output, and hemodynamics. Surgical reexploration may be required for intraabdominal bleeding. Anastomotic bleeding, while troublesome, generally resolves spontaneously.

c. Pancreatitis manifested by elevated serum amylase ususually resolves with medical support.

d. Postoperative jaundice is discussed on pp 474–477. Common bile duct injury may occur with suture ligation of bleeding duodenal ulcers.

e. Delayed gastric emptying should be considered when NG output remains high several days postoperatively or when the patient continually vomits after beginning a diet. The diagnosis is confirmed with a Gastrografin or barium swallow. Proposed etiologies for delayed emptying included anastomotic edema or hematoma, dysmotility, technical problems with the emptying procedure, pancreatitis, internal hernia, adhesive bands, neurogenic afferent or efferent loop obstruction, retrocolic mesenteric obstruction, gastrojejunal intussusception, and marginal ulceration. The syndrome usually resolves spontaneously, although 4–6 weeks of decompression with nutritional support may be necessary. Endoscopy may differentiate mechanical from functional obstruction but should be delayed for 4–6 weeks after surgery.

f. Late complications of ulcer procedures include dumping, diarrhea, afferent loop obstruction, blind loop syndrome, alkaline reflux gastritis, marginal ulceration.

D. Gastrostomy Tube Placement.

Gastrostomies for patients with head and neck tumors or CNS disease (e.g., dementia, stroke, tumor) may greatly facilitate feeding and decrease the risk of aspiration. Tubes may be placed by an open technique (laparotomy) or percutaneously (endoscopically or fluoroscopically). Percutaneous gastrostomy avoids the risk of anesthesia and wound complications (~10% wound infection in debilitated patients) and should be the technique of choice. Contraindications to percutaneous tubes are ascites and inability to pass the gastroscope (for PEG) or NG tube (for fluoroscopic placement). Relative contraindications are massive obesity and prior extensive gastric surgical procedures.

1. Preoperative orders:
   a. NPO after midnight.
   b. Prophylactic antibiotics are administered.
2. Postoperative orders:
   a. Place tube to gravity drainage. For percutaneous tubes, feedings can begin the following day if the procedure was uncomplicated. Open gastrostomies generally require several days for bowel motility to return.
   b. Begin feeding with dilute formulas, then advance either concentration or volume first. With the smaller percutaneous tubes, pureed diets are not recommended. For specifics on choices of formula and advancement of feedings, see Chapter 12.

3. Complications:
   a. Vomiting may be caused by obstruction of the pylorus from the tube. Gently pull back on the tube until resistance is felt.
   b. Mild peritonitis may occur after percutaneous insertion of a tube. Check that tube and stomach are snug against the anterior abdominal wall. An abdominal film is not helpful since most patients with percutaneous tubes have free air under the diaphragm. Symptoms resolve in several days with gravity drainage and IV antibiotics.
   c. Tube dislodgment within 3–4 days after laparotomy often requires reexploration and replacement. After 7 days, the tube may be replaced with a Foley catheter and the balloon inflated with water. Confirm proper placement with a contrast radiograph if dislodgment occurs within several weeks postoperatively.
   d. If the patient's condition improves such that the tube is no longer required, it can generally be removed and the site will heal spontaneously. Percutaneous tubes may require reendoscopy for removal.

E. Small Bowel Resection and Lysis of Adhesions.
   1. Preoperative and postoperative orders:
      a. IV fluid administration will include maintenance and large third-space loss replacement.
      b. The purpose of nasoenteric decompression is to suction both air and fluid from the bowel. This can usually be accomplished with an NG tube although some surgeons will use "long tubes" both pre- and postoperatively.
      c. NG tubes should have two ports: one for suctioning and the other to "sump" air so that the tube does not become lodged on the stomach wall. This allows continuous aspiration to occur (single-lumen tubes require intermittent wall suction and do not function as well). These tubes are easily passed by having the patient sit and "swallow" while the tube is passed down the pharynx. Confirm tube placement by injecting air into the suction port while auscultating over the stomach. If unsure of placement, a radiograph can document nasobronchial intubation. Although techniques have been devised for dealing with enteric contents draining from the sump port, drainage indicates nonfunctioning of the tube. Flushing the aspiration port with saline and the sump

port with air will usually correct the problem. If this fails, the tube may need to be advanced or pulled back slightly.

d. Long tubes (Miller-Abbott tube) are for nasointestinal intubation. Hg is instilled into the distal balloon and a tube is inserted into the stomach via the nose. The patient is placed in the right lateral decubitus position for 45–60 minutes with the tube untaped to the nose in hopes that the tube will pass into the duodenum. Metoclopramide (Reglan) (10 mg IV) may facilitate passage. Failing this, fluoroscopic placement is required. These tubes require intermittent suction as there is no sump port. Often a separate NG tube is required to aspirate fluid from the stomach. Proponents of these tubes argue that even if they do not effectively decompress the bowel, they act as a "stent" to prevent obstruction post-operatively.

e. In patients with massive bowel resection, a prolonged period of adaptation may be required before the intestinal tract may be used for feeding. Forty centimeters of viable small bowel is required in the adult for enteral feedings. H_2 blockers may decrease gastric acid hypersecretion and intestinal fluid output after massive resections.

2. Complications:

a. Patients often complain of a "sore throat" or dry mouth with the prolonged use of nasoenteric tubes. This is relieved with sips of water, ice chips, or topical anesthetics (e.g., viscous xylocaine, cetylpyridinium [Cepacol] anesthetic troches). Other complications include pressure necrosis to nares and middle ear infections.

b. Fluid and electrolyte abnormalities are prevented with appropriate fluid management. When in doubt, send a sample of aspirated fluid for electrolyte determination.

c. Large NG losses are often due to a tube which has slipped past the pylorus into the duodenum. A radiograph confirms proper placement. If output is still large or prolonged, consider ileus or recurrent obstruction.

d. An enterocutaneous fistula may first become manifest by drainage through the incision or drain site or as an intraabdominal abscess. First, quantify the amount of drainage by placing a collection bag over the drainage site or count the number of dressing changes required. Next, obtain a fistulogram to attempt to localize the fistula. A small bowel series or barium enema should be obtained after the fistulogram. Depending on the site and output of the enterocutaneous fistula, parenteral nutrition or an elemental diet may be tried in attempts to heal the fistula. Fistulas do not heal in the presence of distal obstruction. Include fistula output in calculating IV fluid requirements.

F. Colon and Rectal Surgery.

Nonemergent preoperative management is aimed at reducing the concentration of colonic microflora to decrease the incidence of septic wound complications and intraabdominal abscesses. The usual regimen includes a combination of mechanical cleansing oral antibiotics and IV antibiotics.

1. Preoperative orders:

   a. The duration of mechanical bowel preparation and the agents used depend on the degree of obstruction, debility of the patient, and hospital utilization. A clear liquid or elemental diet is begun several days before operation. Cathartics and enemas for 2 days preoperatively are used in one regimen. In another, NG lavage with saline is begun 24 hours preoperatively and continued until the rectal effluent is clear (generally 4–6 hours). This is contraindicated in patients with underlying renal and cardiac disease because of fluid absorption. The use of osmotic diarrheal agents containing polyethylene glycol (e.g., GoLYTELY 4 L po) circumvent fluid absorption problems and rapidly cleanse the bowel. With all mechanical preparations, attention should be directed to fluid and electrolyte imbalances (e.g., dehydration, fluid overload, hypokalemia). GoLYTELY is used increasingly in the setting of shorter preoperative hospital stays.

   b. Oral antibiotics found to be efficacious in bowel preparations are listed in Table 11–7. The appropriate use and choice of parenteral antibiotics in colonic prophylaxis continues to be controversial. As *E. coli* and *Bacteroides fragilis* are the most common aerobes and anaerobes, respectively, it would appear beneficial to at least use antibiotics to which these organisms are sensitive. Despite the drug *used*, studies show a beneficial effect only if the drug is begun *prior* to operation.

TABLE 11–7.

Oral Antibiotics Used for Colonic Bowel Preparation

Neomycin-erythromycin base	1 g each po at 1 P.M., 2 P.M. and 11 P.M. on the day preceding operation
Kanamycin	1 g po q.h. for 4 hr, then q. 6 h. for 72 hr
Metronidazole	750 mg po q. 8 h. for 72 hr

2. Postoperative orders:
   a. Administer IV fluids to include maintenance, NG losses, and moderate to large third-space losses.
   b. Secure the NG tube. This generally remains until bowel activity is noted although many remove the tube early and others do not use a tube.
   c. If an abdominal-perineal resection is performed, a Foley catheter is left in place for 5–7 days. Otherwise, it may be removed when fluid balance is normalized and when the patient is able to void spontaneously.
3. Complications: An early postoperative SBO is more likely to occur with an inflammatory process. In the setting of a low anterior anastomosis, the risk of an anastomotic leak is increased. Although leaks frequently occur, they are seldom symptomatic and rarely become a problem. Symptoms include fever, leukocytosis, and persistent ileus. Treatment may require a proximal diverting colostomy.

G. **Cholecystectomy, Common Bile Duct Exploration, Biliary Bypass Procedure.**
   1. Preoperative orders:
      a. Parenteral prophylactic antibiotics are generally indicated except perhaps in patients undergoing cholecystectomy for biliary colic or chronic cholecystitis. With active cholecystitis or cholangitis, appropriate antibiotics are mandatory. The most common microorganism is *E. coli*. Antibiotic coverage should be directed at gram-negative organisms.
      b. In patients with longstanding common duct obstruction, vitamin K (10 mg IM) may be given the day preceding operation.
      c. Several prospective studies have demonstrated no change in mortality or morbidity with preoperative de-

compression of the common bile duct in patients with serum bilirubin levels >10 mg/dL. If difficulty in identify-
ing the common bile duct is anticipated, the placement
of a stent preoperatively may be beneficial.

2. Postoperative orders:

   a. Fluid replacement is guided by the degree of inflammation and dissection required. Replace T tube drainage
   with lactated Ringer's solution.

   b. Either meperidine (preferable) or morphine may be used
   for postoperative pain.

   c. Continue therapeutic antibiotics for 5–10 days in patients with infectious processes.

   d. The diet may be rapidly advanced on the first postoperative day in the patient undergoing uncomplicated cholecystectomy.

   e. Patients undergoing **laparoscopic cholecystectomy** *are
   usually* discharged the day following surgery.

   f. For patients with acute cholecystitis or those who have a
   biliary-enteric anastomosis, feeding should be delayed
   until return of bowel function.

   g. Drainage of the gallbladder fossa is performed when
   fluid accumulation is expected (e.g., gangrenous cholecystitis) or when a biliary-enteric anastomosis has been
   performed. Both closed and open drainage systems are
   used, although closed systems are generally favored. If a
   closed drainage system (e.g., Jackson-Pratt, HemoVac)
   is used, it is removed when drainage has nearly ceased,
   usually on postoperative day 2 or 3 or after beginning a
   regular diet. Open drainage systems (e.g., Penrose
   drains) are advanced over several days, beginning on
   postoperative day 3 or later. With Penrose drains, be
   certain the drain cannot retract into the abdominal cavity. A safety pin attached to the drain will prevent this.

   h. A **T tube** is placed if the patient undergoes a common
   duct exploration. A **T tube cholangiogram** is ordered
   on postoperative day 5–7. Antibiotics are given before
   obtaining the radiograph. If no retained stones are demonstrated, the tube may be removed on postoperative
   day 10 or the patient may be discharged and the tube removed on an outpatient basis in approximately 2 weeks.
   A retained stone can be extracted by the basket technique 4–6 weeks postoperatively when the tract ma-
   tures.

3. Complications:
   a. Hemorrhage is unusual but may occur from the cystic artery.
   b. A **biliary fistula** is suspected if a large amount of biliary drainage occurs. Most biliary fistulas are due to small transected ducts in the gallbladder fossa, and they resolve spontaneously. Other causes include a retained common duct stone, bile duct injury, or a malpositioned T tube. An early cholangiogram may be indicated.
   c. **T tube dislodgment,** if it occurs within several days of operation, may require reexploration to prevent bile peritonitis. If the tube is inadvertently removed later, fluoroscopic replacement may be attempted if the tube is regarded as still being necessary.
   d. A **retained stone** can be removed at 4–6 weeks with basket extraction if a large tube (≥14F) was placed. Irrigation of the T tube with monooctanoin may occasionally dissolve a retained stone.
   e. Postoperative jaundice after a biliary tract procedure may be due to the presence of a retained stone, pancreatitis, right hepatic artery ligation with subsequent hepatic necrosis, missed or persistent tumor, or bile duct injury.

H. Gallstone Pancreatitis.

The surgical treatment of gallstone pancreatitis is cholecystectomy, intraoperative cholangiogram, and common bile duct exploration (if necessary). In poor-risk patients or in the elderly, ERCP with sphincterotomy may be the only treatment necessary.

1. Preoperative orders:
   a. Follow serum amylase closely until it returns to normal. Operation may be safely undertaken when amylase is near normal and clinical symptoms of pancreatitis have resolved. Generally, the amylase rises to several thousand IU/mL, then returns rapidly toward normal over several days. If the serum amylase does not return to normal levels and symptoms worsen, emergent exploration or emergent ERCP with sphincterotomy may be required. Patients whose symptoms resolve with conservative management may be discharged to return later for an elective cholecystectomy, although the incidence of recurrent symptoms within 6 weeks is not insignificant.

      b. Although antibiotics are not efficacious in alcoholic pancreatitis, they are generally recommended in gallstone pancreatitis.

      c. Fluid management is predicated on the severity of the pancreatitis.

  2. Postoperative care:

      a. Fluid management is predicated on the severity of the pancreatitis.

      b. Bowel function is slower to return than after a "routine" cholecystectomy.

  3. Complications: The most feared complication is worsening of the pancreatitis.

I. Radical Pancreaticoduodenectomy (Whipple Procedure).

  1. Treat as though the patient has had a combination of vagotomy, gastroenterostomy, biliary bypass, and pancreatic drainage. Considerable dissection is performed and prolonged ileus and a large amount of third-space fluid loss can be expected.

  2. Nutritional support is usually imperative.

  3. Bleeding, infection, and **pancreatic fistula** are the most frequent intraabdominal complications. Almost all pancreatic fistulas close without further operation although prolonged parenteral nutritional support is required. Skin excoriation is usually not a problem with pure pancreatic fistula because enzymes have not come in contact with an intestinal mucosa and are therefore not activated.

  4. Somatostatin should be considered for pancreatic fistula (100 μg SL q. 8h.).

J. Liver Resection.

  1. Two considerations after large liver resections are **hypoglycemia** and **hypoalbuminemia.** The liver often loses the ability to supply adequate sugar and albumin for several weeks.

      a. Hypoglycemia can be prevented by administration of a 10% dextrose solution rather than a 5% solution for several days and by continuing an IV solution for at least 1 week postoperatively.

      b. Hypoalbuminemia can also be prevented by administering albumin 50 mL IV q. 6 h. for 1–2 weeks.

  2. Hyperbilirubinemia is common following large liver resections secondary to transfusion hemolysis or transient hepatic dysfunction. Injury to the remaining hepatic ducts or liver failure must be considered if jaundice persists.

3. Drains are often left in place until GI function returns and bile leaks and collections have not been demonstrated.

K. Splenectomy.

1. Preoperative orders:
   a. PRBCs and platelets should be available prior to surgery. Preoperative platelet transfusion for thrombocytopenia is rarely necessary.
   b. Prophylactic antibiotics (cephalosporin) may be given.
   c. The patient should receive Pneumovax (polyvalent pneumococcal vaccine) 0.5 mL SC 1 week prior to surgery.
   d. If the patient has been on steroids for ITP or a similar condition, increase steroid coverage perioperatively.

2. Postoperative orders:
   a. An NG tube is used to prevent gastric distention and prevent undue tension on ligated short gastric vessels. The tube is often removed the following day.
   b. For patients with ITP, steroids may be tapered rapidly initially, then gradually over 4–6 weeks.
   c. Drainage of the LUQ is avoided because of the risk of a subphrenic abscess. However, with persistent oozing from the splenic bed or with damage to the tail of the pancreas, a closed drainage system may be used. It is removed when drainage decreases. If there is concern about possible pancreatic injury, the drain may remain until a regular diet is begun.
   d. Pneumovax 0.5 mL is given prior to discharge if not administered preoperatively.

3. Complications:
   a. Left lower lobe atelectasis is the most common complication. Postoperative hemorrhage from short gastric vessels, stomach wall necrosis, pancreatitis, and subphrenic abscess are less common.
   b. Thrombocytosis is usual after splenectomy but counts in excess of $10^6/mm^3$ are worrisome as a risk factor for thromboembolism, especially in patients with myeloproliferative disorders. Aspirin, dipyridamole (Persantine), heparin, or plateletpheresis may be effective.
   c. Postsplenectomy sepsis (overwhelming postsplenectomy infection, OPSI) is 60 times greater than normal following splenectomy and may have an annual incidence of 0.5%–1.0%. The incidence of OPSI is great-

est within the first 2 years after splenectomy. Mortality is ≥50%.

L. Portosystemic Shunts.

1. Routine postoperative care is directed at fluid and electrolyte management. The patient can be expected to develop a certain amount of ascites. Maintain adequate intravascular volume with initial liberal use of albumin and salt solutions. After 2 or 3 days the patient will respond to diuretics. Fluid administration should be decreased markedly at that time. Postoperative ascites is not uncommon, even if none was present preoperatively.

2. Treatment of the underlying coagulopathy of hepatic insufficiency may be accomplished with administration of FFP and platelets.

3. In the occasional case when the patient has had an emergency portosystemic shunt, keep the gastric balloon of the Sengstaken-Blakemore tube inflated for approximately 24 hours.

4. H₂ blockers or antacids are helpful in the postoperative period. When digestive function returns, begin a low protein diet to avoid hepatic encephalopathy. Lactulose or oral antibiotics are reserved for treatment of encephalopathy, which is more common if GI bleeding continues.

SELECTED REFERENCES

Agarwal N, Pitchumoni CS, Sivaprasad AV: Evaluating tests for acute pancreatitis. *Am J Gastroenterol* 1990; 85:356–366.

Brolin RE, Krasna MJ, Mast BA: Use of tubes and radiographs in the management of small bowel obstruction. *Ann Surg* 1987; 206:126.

Browder W, Cerise EJ, Litwin MS: Impact of emergency angiography in massive lower gastrointestinal bleeding. *Ann Surg* 1986; 204:530.

Buchman TG, Bulkley GB: Current management of patients with lower gastrointestinal bleeding. *Surg Clin North Am* 1987; 67:651.

Eggermont AM, Lameris JS, Jeekel J: Ultrasound-guided percutaneous transhepatic cholecystostomy for acute acalculous cholecystitis. *Arch Surg* 1985; 120:1354.

Garrison RN, Cryer HM, Howard DA, et al: Clarification of risk factors for abdominal operations in patients with hepatic cirrhosis. *Ann Surg* 1984; 199:648.

Henderson JM, Kutner MH, Millikan WJ Jr, et al: Endoscopic variceal sclerosis compared with distal splenorenal shunt to prevent recurrent variceal bleeding in cirrhosis. A prospective, randomized trial. *Ann Intern Med* 1990; 112:262–269.

Ihse I, Evander A, Holmberg JT, et al: Influence of peritoneal lavage on objective prognostic signs in acute pancreatitis. *Ann Surg* 1986; 204:122.

Larson DE, Farnell MB: Upper gastrointestinal hemorrhage. *Mayo Clin Proc* 1983; 58:371.

Leese T, Neoptolemos JP, Baker AR, et al: Management of acute cholangitis and the impact of endoscopic spincterotomy. *Br J Surg* 1986; 73:788.

Lurie K, Plzak L, Deveney CW: Intra-abdominal abscess in the 1980s. *Surg Clin North Am* 1987; 67:621.

Moody FG, Thompson DA: Postoperative jaundice, in Schiff L (ed): *Diseases of the Liver*, ed 6. Philadelphia, JB Lippincott Co, 1987.

Mucha P: Small intestinal obstruction. *Surg Clin North Am* 1987; 67:597.

Nunez D, Guerra JJ, Al-Sheikh WA, et al: Percutaneous biliary drainage in acute suppurative cholangitis. *Gastrointest Radiol* 1986; 11:85.

Olak J, Christon NV, Stein LA, et al: Operative vs. percutaneous drainage of intra-abdominal abscesses. *Arch Surg* 1986; 121:141.

Pessa ME, Hawkins IF, Vogel SB: The treatment of acute cholangitis: Percutaneous transhepatic biliary drainage before definitive therapy. *Ann Surg* 1987; 205:389.

Ranson JHC: Etiological and prognostic factors in human acute pancreatitis: A review. *Am J Gastroenterol* 1982; 77:633.

Rose SC, Dunnick NR: Angiographic treatment of gastrointestinal hemorrhage: Comparison of vasopressin infusion and embolization. *Invest Radiol* 1987; 22:354–356.

Shiloni E, Coronado E, Freund HR: Role of total parenteral nutrition in the treatment of Crohn's disease. *Am J Surg* 1989; 157:180–184.

Shorvon PJ, Leung JW, Cotton PB: Preliminary clinical experience with the heat probe at endoscopy in acute upper gastrointestinal bleeding. *Gastrintest Endosc* 1985; 31:364–366.

Tryba M: Risk of acute stress bleeding and nosocomial pneumonia in ventilated intensive care unit patients: sucralfate versus antacids. Am J Med, 83(supp. 38):117, 1987.

Ventrucci M, Pezzilli R, Gullo L et al. Role of serum pancreatic enzyme assays in diagnosis of pancreatic disease. Digestive Disease and Sciences, 1989, 34:39–45.

ANNOTATED REFERENCES

Moody FG, Carey LC, Jones RS, et al: *Surgical Treatment of Digestive Disease*. ed 2. Chicago, Year Book Medical Publishers, Inc., 1990.

> This excellent text discusses the surgical treatment of complex diseases of the abdomen. The chapters on stress erosive gastritis, biliary sepsis, and suppurative cholangitis, and the diagnosis and early treatment of acute pancreatitis are particularly pertinent.

Imrie CW, Moossa AR: *Gastrointestinal Emergencies*. Edinburgh, Churchill-Livingstone Ltd, 1987.

> This concise reference provides substantive discussions on gastrointestinal emergencies and is edited by respected surgeons from the United States and United Kingdom. The individual chapters are written by international experts in each aspect of GI surgery. It addresses many problems that may arise in SICUs and or that may require treatment in an SICU.

SURGICAL NUTRITION

12

I. NUTRITIONAL ASSESSMENT.

Choosing the best nutritional support method depends first on the awareness of the need for any nutritional support for a specific patient. Although it is not necessary to perform formal nutritional assessment on every patient, one must be constantly aware of factors contributing to malnutrition in the hospitalized patient in order to avoid this often unrecognized and untreated disease.

A. Risk Factors.

1. Low nutritional reserves at the time of admission.
2. Extensive preoperative evaluation required including multiple bowel preparations and pretest fasts.
3. Prolonged lack of oral intake due to disease process (bowel obstruction, pancreatitis, primary GI disease, etc.).
4. High stress (wound healing, burns, multiple surgical procedures, head injury, sepsis, etc.).

B. Indications for Formal Nutritional Assessment (Screening Tests).

1. **History of unintentional weight loss.** Unless a rapid weight loss has occurred, patients with an unintentional weight loss of <10% of their usual body weight appear to have little increase in risk of postoperative complications. As weight loss approaches 30% of usual body weight, morbidity and mortality rapidly increase and approach 95%.
2. **Serum albumin <3.4 g/dL.** Mortality risk increases by approximately 37% for each gram deficit of serum albumin if malnutrition is untreated.
3. **Anergy** to four of five standard skin test antigens.
4. **Low total lymphocyte count.** Although controversial,

counts of $1,200-2,000/mm^3$ are associated with mild nutritional depletion, while counts of $<800/mm^3$ are associated with severe deficiency.

5. **Physical signs** including fat and muscle wasting, skin rash, pallor, cheilosis, glossitis, gingival lesions, hepatomegaly, edema, neuropathy, dementia.

C. **Classification.**

Patients with protein calorie malnutrition have been divided into three groups: kwashiorkor, marasmus, and a mixed clinical picture.

1. **Kwashiorkor** is likely to be found in patients with acute, severe catabolic stress and may develop rapidly. It is characterized by hypoalbuminemia, edema, depressed cellular immune function, but patients tend to maintain normal anthropometric parameters.

2. **Marasmus,** or simple starvation, reflects a more chronic deficiency and is associated with wasting of muscle mass and SC fat. This group has markedly abnormal anthropometric measurements, but biochemical alterations are rare.

3. **Nutritional assessment** is meant to determine the patient's nutritional status and reserves as well as predict nutritional requirements (Table 12–1).

   a. **History** of weight loss (discussed above).

   b. **Anthropometric measurements** (altered by state of hydration):
      1) Triceps skin fold.
      2) Midarm muscle circumference [=arm circumference-3.14 (triceps skin fold)].

   c. **Laboratory Measurements:**
      1) Serum albumin—altered by liver disease, intravascular volume, nephrosis, acute trauma or surgery, protein-losing enteropathy.
      2) Serum transferrin [$=0.8$ (TIBC)-43]—altered by renal failure, iron deficiency anemia.
      3) Prealbumin.
      4) Retinol-binding protein—altered by trauma and surgery.
      5) Creatinine-height index [$=100(24\text{-hr urinary creatinine})/(\text{ideal height})$]—affected by strenuous exercise, diet, trauma, infection, abnormal renal function.
      6) Vitamin levels.
      7) Urinary 3-methylhistidine.

TABLE 12–1.
Nutritional Assessment

History
  Weight loss
Anthropometric measurements
  Triceps skin fold
  Midarm muscle circumference
Laboratory tests
  Serum albumin/total protein
  Serum transferrin
  Prealbumin
  Retinol-binding protein
  Creatinine-height index
  Vitamin levels
  Urinary 3-methylhistidine
Immunologic studies
  Skin testing of recall antigens
  Dinitrochlorobenzene
  Total lymphocyte count
  Lymphoblastic response

  d. **Immunologic studies:**
    1) Delayed hypersensitivity skin testing—altered by
       immunosuppressive drugs, cancer, stress, surgery.
    2) Dinitrochlorobenzene sensitization.
    3) Total lymphocyte count.
    4) Lymphoblastic response—expensive and time-
       consuming.
D. Prediction of Energy Requirements.
  1. Simple estimate: 35 kcal/kg/day.
  2. **Basal energy expenditure (BEE)** can be estimated from
     Harris-Benedict equations:

  $$BEE(<Females) = 665 + 9.6(W) + 1.7(H) - 4.7(A)$$
  $$BEE(<Males) = 66 + 13.7(W) + 5(H) - 6.8(A)$$

  where W = mass (kg), H = height (cm), A = age (yr).
  3. **Actual energy expenditure** (AEE)=BEE × MAF where
     MAF (metabolic activity factor) combines activity (AF),
     stress (SF), fever (FF), and growth (GF) factors:

$$MAF = 1 + AF + SF + FF + GF$$

    a. Activity factor (AF):
        0.2—sedentary.
        0.35—moderately active.
        0.5—active.
    b. Stress factor (SF):
        0.1–0.15—elective surgery.
        0.2–0.4—skeletal trauma.
        0.5–1.0—major burn (varies with %).
    c. Fever factor (FF): 0.13/°C.
    d. Growth factor (GF):
        0.05—moderate weight loss.
        0.1–.15—severe weight loss.
    e. Calorimetry is the most accurate method.

E. Basic Facts for Nutritional Support (Table 12–2)

    1. **Ratio of nonprotein calories to nitrogen.** Nitrogen balance depends not only on the quantity of nitrogen but also on the presence of adequate potassium, magnesium, phosphate, vitamins, and most importantly, nonprotein calories. The desirable calorie-nitrogen ratio is 135–200:1 (kcal/g nitrogen).

    2. **Protein requirements:** ~0.8–2.0 g/kg/day depending on stress level. Nitrogen = g(protein)/6.25.

    3. **Caloric sources:** General starting point is carbohydrate-fat ratio of 4:1 although stressed patients are often relatively intolerant to glucose. Excessive glucose in the stressed patient may contribute to fatty liver and abnormal liver function tests. The adverse effects of IV fat are related primarily to the individual's capacity to clear lipid from the bloodstream.

TABLE 12–2.
Important Nutritional Equations

Metabolic rate (kcal/hr) = VO_2 (mL/min) × 60 min/hr × 1 L/1,000 mL × 4.83 kcal/L

VO_2 (mL/min) = CO (L/min) × (CaO_2 [mL/L] − $C\overline{v}O_2$ [mL/L])

RQ = VCO_2/VO_2

UUN (g/day) = UUN (mg/dL) × UO (mL/day) × 1 g/1,000 mg × 1 dL/100 mL

Nitrogen loss (g/day) = UUN (g/day) × 1.2 + 2 g/day

4. **Ventilatory considerations:** Excess exogenous carbohydrate increases CO_2 production (VCO_2) and the respiratory quotient (RQ).

$$RQ = VCO_2/VO_2$$

Decreasing RQ may aid in ventilatory weaning. RQ = 0.7 with pure fat oxidation, 0.8 with pure protein oxidation, 1.0 with pure carbohydrate oxidation, 1.3 with fat synthesis.

5. Use supplemental regular **insulin** as necessary during nutritional support to maintain serum glucose at <150 mg/dL and to limit glycosuria to no more than 2+. Insulin is an anabolic hormone.

II. ENTERAL FEEDING.

This includes total enteral nutrition via a feeding tube as well as dietary supplements in the intact patient unable to take in sufficient calories to keep up with an increased metabolic rate and supplements via feeding tube. When there are no serious contraindications, enteral alimentation is preferable to parenteral feeding and capable of providing adequate nutrition.

A. Indications.

Enteral feeding is applicable to essentially all patients with intact GI function and should be the first method considered. In addition, with the availability of elemental and low residue formulas, some patients with lower GI fistulas may also be fed enterally. Patients with upper GI fistulas can often be fed enterally if a feeding tube can be placed to deliver the formula distal to the fistula site.

B. Contraindications.

1. **Absolute:** intractable vomiting, intestinal obstruction, profuse GI bleeding, hemodynamic instability.
2. **Relative:** diarrhea, intraabdominal infection, primary GI disease including malabsorption syndromes, complicated severe pancreatitis, high output enterocutaneous fistulas.

C. Benefits.

1. Maintains intestinal structure and function through the trophic effects of intraluminal nutrients.
2. Maintains normal hormonal patterns.
3. Provides normal sequence of intestinal and hepatic metabolism prior to nutrient delivery to the arterial system.

4. Augmented insulin response to enterally administered carbohydrate.
5. Approximately 1/20th the cost of TPN.
6. Avoids complications of catheter placement and line sepsis.
7. Does not require as high a level of training as TPN.

D. General Considerations.

1. **Residue content:** Reduce in treating patients with fistulas or chronic intestinal disease.
2. **Lactose content:** Deficiency of the brush border enzyme lactase is common in the adult population, especially in blacks. Secondary deficiency may develop in patients with severe stress, acute enteritis, celiac disease, inflammatory bowel disease, or short-bowel syndromes.
3. **Protein sources:** Amino acids may be supplied as intact protein from pureed meat, eggs, or milk, or isolated from casein, soybeans, or egg whites. In addition, hydrolyzed protein, oligopeptides, as well as di- or tripeptides or purified amino acids may be used.
4. **Carbohydrate sources** may be complex carbohydrates from fruits and vegetables or simple sugars such as sucrose, glucose, or oligosaccharides.
5. **Fat sources:** milk fat, corn oil, safflower oil, or medium chain triglycerides (can be directly absorbed without the requirement of hydrolysis into FFAs).
6. **Vitamin and mineral content:** Amin-Aid and Hepatic-Aid have inadequate levels and therefore require supplementation.
7. **High osmolality** formulas delivered to the small intestine may produce dumping symptoms including cramps, nausea, and severe diarrhea. Osmolarity of commercially available formulas range from 300–900 mOsm/L.
8. Formula palatability is increased with most fat sources, simple sugars, and complex proteins.

E. Specific Types of Enteral Formulas (Table 12–3).

1. **Polymeric:** may be food-based or contain combinations of intact macronutrients; contain protein, fat, and carbohydrates in HMW form; increased palatability due to large amounts of fat; milk-based formulas contain lactose.
   a. Advantages:
      1) Low osmolality.
      2) Contains required vitamins and minerals.
      3) Inexpensive.

TABLE 12–3.
Commercially Available Tube Feeding Formulas

Product	kcal/mL	mOsm/L	CHO(g/L)	Pro (g/L)	Fat (g/L)	Na (mEq/L)	K (mEq/L)
A. Blenderized							
Compleat B	1.07	405	128	43	43	55	36
Compleat B (modified)	1.07	300	140	43	37	30	36
B. Lactose-free							
Sustacal	1.0	625	140	60	23	40	53
Isocal	1.06	300	132	34	44	23	34
Isocal HCN	2.0	740	225	75	91	35	36
Ensure	1.06	450	145	37	37	32	33
Ensure Plus	1.5	600	200	55	53	46	49
Osmolite	1.06	300	145	37	38	23	27
Traumacal	1.5	490	142	82	68	52	36
C. Hydrolyzed protein							
Criticare HN	1.06	650	222	38	3	28	34
Vital HN	1.0	460	187	41	11	17	30
Travasorb	1.0	450	190	30	14	40	30
Reabilan HN	1.3	490	158	58	52	43	42

D. Crystalline amino acids							
Vivonex	1.0	550	230	21	1.5	20	30
Vivonex HN	1.0	810	207	46	1	23	30
E. Incomplete special formulas							
Travasorb (renal)	1.35	590	274	23	18	—	—
Amin-Aid	1.95	850	366	19	46	<20	<18
Hepatic-Aid	1.7	900	289	43	36	14	—
F. Fiber-containing							
Isofiber	1.18	310	160	50	38	37	32

  b. Disadvantages:
    1) Fixed nutrient composition limits use in patients with renal, liver, or cardiac disease.
2. **Chemically defined:** contain monomeric or short chain hydrolysis products of protein and carbohydrate macronutrients; calorie source is predominantly carbohydrate.
  a. Advantages:
    1) All are lactose-free.
    2) Nutritionally complete.
    3) Low residue.
    4) Contain essential fatty acids (EFAs).
  b. Disadvantages:
    1) Unpalatable.
    2) Hyperosmolar.
    3) Expensive.
    4) Poorly tolerated in the glucose-intolerant patient.
  c. Indications: inflammatory bowel disease, mild pancreatitis, short-bowel syndrome, radiation enteritis, bowel resection, lower GI fistula, severe burns.
3. **Modular formulas:** Modular products provide one or a few macronutrients only, and no micronutrients. Protein, carbohydrate, and fat modules are available.
  a. Advantage: Individual components may be altered to design a formula for a particular patient's needs and take into account the specific disease process such as liver, renal, or heart failure.
  b. Disadvantage: Complete nutrition is not provided without the addition of vitamins and minerals.
4. **Special formulas.**
  a. **Amin-Aid** (McGaw) is useful for patients with ARF or CRF and BUN >80 mg/dL. It contains essential amino acids plus histidine.
    1) Disadvantages:
      a) Lacks electrolytes, vitamins, minerals.
      b) High osmolality.
      c) Hypocaloric—must supplement with polycose for additional calories.
  b. **Hepatic-Aid** (McGaw) contains a higher content of branched chain amino acids and lower content of aromatic amino acids and is intended for use in patients with acute or chronic liver disease and impending hepatic encephalopathy.
    1) Disadvantages: As for Amin-Aid.

F. Sites of Delivery and Types of Feeding Tubes.
1. **Stomach:** NG and gastrostomy (formal or percutaneous).
   a. Advantages:
      1) Stomach acts as reservoir and tolerates high osmolar loads.
      2) Permits bolus feeding.
   b. Disadvantage: Risk of aspiration requires that the patient have an intact gag reflex, no gastric atony, and must not be debilitated, lethargic, or stuporous. Gastric residuals should be measured frequently.
   c. **Tubes:**
      1) Standard Levin or Salem sump-type NG tubes. Easy to insert (replace); large caliber allows for the delivery of viscous formulas. They have poor acceptability due to discomfort, gastroesophageal reflux, and complication of nasal cartilage erosion.
      2) Small-caliber Silastic or polyurethane tubes with weighted tips and removable guidewires (Dobbhoff, Entriflex). Increased comfort; decreased risk of aspiration; better patient compliance. Disadvantages include easy dislodgment and inability to deliver viscous or blenderized formulas.
2. **Small bowel.**
   a. Advantages:
      1) Reduced risk of aspiration.
      2) May feed distal to fistula or obstruction.
      3) Able to use in patients with gastric atony.
   b. Disadvantages:
      1) Low tolerance to high osmolar loads.
      2) Intolerance to bolus feeding requires continuous administration, usually requiring a pump.
      3) Requires frequent irrigations to maintain patency.
      4) Must use low viscosity formula.
   c. **Tubes.**
      1) Nasoduodenal (Entriflex, Dobbhoff, Vivonex tungsten tip) tube is difficult or time-consuming to replace; often requires fluoroscopic placement; must irrigate q. 8 h. with water (cranberry juice will coagulate protein within the tube); must confirm position with radiograph prior to use.
      2) Jejunostomy (needle catheter or formal) tube, once removed or dislodged, cannot be replaced; must ir-

rigate q. 4–8 h. with water; partial tube removal results in IP delivery of formula.

G. Administration.

1. **Gastric delivery.**

   a. **Intermittent feeding:** Wait at least 24 hours prior to using a new gastrostomy. Begin with 100-mL boluses of ½ strength formula (or full strength if isotonic) q. 2 h., measuring gastric residuals prior to administration of each bolus and following each bolus with water irrigation (20–50 mL). If this is well tolerated over the ensuing 8 hours, increase to ¾ strength and then full strength at 8-hour intervals. Residuals should be <100 mL. If feedings are still well tolerated, increase volume to 200 mL q. 2 h. for 24 hours and then gradually to 400 mL (or the calculated requirement) over the next 4 days. At this point, the schedule may be altered to allow for a sleep period in preparation for home or nursing home care.

   b. **Continuous flow:** Again, a 24-hour period should elapse prior to using a new gastrostomy. Start with ½ strength formula (or full strength if isotonic) at a rate of 50 mL/hr and increase rate in 25-mL/hr increments q. 8 h. until a rate of 100 mL/hr is reached. Next, increase to ¾ strength and then to full strength at 8-hour intervals. Residuals should be checked at least q. 4 h. If residual is greater than 150 mL, refeed 150 mL and discard remainder.

2. Small bowel feeding must be administered by continuous infusion. Advance as per continuous flow into the stomach as described above. Remember to irrigate the tube q. 8 h. with water. In patients with restricted fluid intake, increase strength of feeding solution to its maximum prior to increasing rate.

H. Monitoring.

1. Physical examination: chest auscultation, abdominal examination.
2. Ins and Outs: Pay particular attention to diarrhea.
3. Daily weights.
4. Laboratory studies:
   a. Potassium.
   b. Magnesium.

    c. Phosphorus.

    d. Glucose.

    e. Creatinine.

    f. Sodium.

    g. Calcium.

    h. Albumin.

    i. Urine for nitrogen excretion and glycosuria.

I. Trouble-shooting.

  1. **High residuals:** If feeding via nasoduodenal tube, check tube placement with a KUB. If feeding into the stomach, reduce the rate and increase more slowly. If residuals again become a problem, administer metoclopramide 10 mg IV q. 6 h.

  2. **Diarrhea** (defined as >300 g/day of stool or >three loose stools per day) may occur in as many as 75% of critically ill patients receiving enteral nutrition, and is usually the result of a rapid increase in the administration rate or osmolality of the solution. A high osmolar load is poorly tolerated by the small intestine. This does not mean that

TABLE 12–4.

Mechanisms of Diarrhea

Malabsorptive syndromes
  Pancreatic insufficiency
  Biliary obstruction
  Disaccharidase deficiency
  Short-bowel syndrome
  Inflammatory bowel disease
Secretory
  Gastric hypersecretion
  Dumping syndrome
  Postobstruction syndrome
Infectious
  Enterotoxins
  Enteropathogens
  Contaminated enteral formula
Iatrogenic
  Tube administration of hypertonic
    medications

the patient is permanently intolerant to tube feedings. Despite diarrhea, the patient is still absorbing some nutrients.

  a. Therapy:

    1) Check tube placement with radiograph.

    2) Reduce rate or strength, or both, and restart with a more gradual increase in rate and osmolality.

    3) Change to another lactose-free formula.

    4) Antidiarrheal agents:

      a) Paragoric 5–10 mL after each diarrheal stool up to four times daily, or 1 mL/1 dL formula.

      b) Diphenoxylate (Lomotil) 10 mL q.i.d. on the first day and 5 mL t.i.d. thereafter

    5) Consider other causes of diarrhea (Table 12–4).

III. TOTAL PARENTERAL NUTRITION.

A. Indications.

In general, the parenteral route is used in all cases requiring nutritional support where the GI tract is not available or would benefit from bowel rest.

1. **Protein-calorie malnutrition.**
   - a. Prolonged ileus or GI obstruction.
   - b. Chronic vomiting.
   - c. Chronic diarrhea.
   - d. Malabsorption syndromes.
2. **Short bowel syndrome.**
3. **Acute pancreatitis and pancreatic fistula.**
4. Inflammatory bowel disease.
5. High output enterocutaneous fistulas.
6. Hypercatabolic states.
   - a. Burns.
   - b. Trauma.
   - c. Major surgery.
   - d. Malignant disease.
7. Renal failure.
8. Hepatic failure.

B. Contraindications.

1. Lack of experienced personnel for catheter insertion, maintenance, and management.
2. Extreme fluid restriction insufficient to meet minimal caloric needs. May need dialysis to remove excess fluid.
3. Severe glucose intolerance (relative).
4. Severe hepatic failure with encephalopathy.

C. Benefits.
1. Precise and independent control of daily intake of calories, carbohydrate, fat, protein, vitamins, minerals.
2. Able to infuse high osmolar solutions and therefore minimize volume while optimizing caloric delivery.
3. Able to achieve an anabolic state.

D. Disadvantages.
1. High osmolar solutions require administration via a central venous catheter.
2. Expensive both in material costs and for required personnel (dietician, pharmacist, nurse, physician).
3. Nonphysiologic delivery of nutrients bypassing intestinal and hepatic metabolism.
4. GI mucosal atrophy with solutions containing inadequate glutamine.
5. Potential hepatic damage with long-term use.
6. Increased risk of sepsis (~4%–5%).
7. Risk of nonketotic, hyperosmolar coma.
8. Hormonal imbalances.

E. Feeding solutions.
1. **General considerations.**
   a. Amino acids: 3.5%–10% with 5–15 g N per liter.
   b. Carbohydrate: generally 50%–70% dextrose.
   c. Fatty acids: EFAs provided with twice-weekly infusions of 10% lipid solution (500 mL) or by using a 3:1 mix.
   d. Vitamins: fat- and water-soluble.
   e. Minerals: Ca, P, Mg.
   f. Trace minerals: Zn, Cu, Mn, Cr, I, Se, Mb.
2. **Commercially available amino acid solutions:**
   a. Aminosyn (Abbott): 3.5%, 5.0%, 7.0%, 8.5%, 10%.
   b. Travasol (Travenol): 5.5%, 8.5%, 10%.
   c. FreAmine (McGaw): 3.0%, 8.5%, 10%.
   d. Nephramine (McGaw), 5.4%, contains essential amino acids plus histidine for renal failure patients.
   e. Hepatamine and FreAmine HBC (McGaw), 8.0% and 6.9%, respectively, contain high levels of branched chain amino acids for use in patients with hepatic failure.
3. **Commercially available fat emulsions:**
   a. Intralipid (Kabi Vitrum): 10%, 20%.
   h Liposyn II (Abbott): 10%, 20%.
   c. Soyacal (Alpha Therapeutic): 10%, 20%.

F. Vascular Access (see Chapter 22, I).
1. Subclavian vein catheter insertion.
2. Other techniques:
   a. Internal jugular vein.
   b. External jugular vein.
   c. Supraclavicular approach to the subclavian vein.
   d. Permanent access via Hickman, Broviac, Porta-Cath, or similar catheters.

G. Writing TPN Orders.
1. Determine **daily fluid requirement** from either weight or BSA. These will underestimate the fluid requirement of TPN patients by 800–1,000 mL/day owing to the reduction of endogenous water production from orally ingested calories.
2. Determine **caloric requirements** (see pp 496–497).
3. Determine **protein requirement** (Typically 0.8–2.0 g/kg/day in the stressed patient); maintain calorie-nitrogen ratio at 135–200:1.
4. Choose appropriate **amino acid–dextrose solution** to provide necessary protein and calories in desired volume.
5. Determine amounts of **additional electrolytes** to be added (Table 12–5).
6. Add desired amount of **calcium** and **magnesium.**
7. Add **multivitamins, trace elements,** and any additional medications (regular insulin, cimetidine, albumin, etc.) (Table 12–6).

H. Complications and Side Effects.
1. Catheter complications:
   a. Pneumothorax.
   b. Malposition.

TABLE 12–5.

Electrolyte and Mineral Requirements During TPN

Sodium	1–2 mEq/kg/day
Potassium	1–2 mEq/kg/day
Chloride	Equal to Na
Calcium	0.2–0.3 mEq/kg/day
Magnesium	0.35–0.45 mEq/kg/day
Phosphorus	Extremely variable; start with 10 mmol/1,000 kcal

TABLE 12–6.
TPN Additives

Additive	Maximal Concentration
Albumin	25 g/L
Insulin	350 units/day
Heparin	20,000 units/L
Cimetidine	300 mg/L
Aminophylline	1500 mg/L
Iron dextran	100 mg/L
Antibiotics	Variable
Hydrochloric acid	100 mEq/L
Metoclopramide	20 mg/L

    c. Arterial laceration.
    d. Brachial plexus injury.
    e. Hydro- and chylothorax.
    f. Catheter sepsis.
    g. Subclavian vein thrombosis.
  2. **Metabolic complications** (Table 12–7):
    a. Deficiencies of vitamins, minerals, electrolytes, trace metals, EFAs.
    b. Hyperosmolar nonketotic coma.
    c. Hyperglycemia (Table 12–8).
    d. Hepatic dysfunction and fatty infiltration.
    e. Refeeding syndrome.
I. Monitoring.
  1. Daily weights (aim for ~400 g/day gain).
  2. I/O.
  3. Urine for sugar and ketones.
  4. Laboratory studies.
    a. Electrolytes (daily).
    b. LFTs, Ca, P, Mg, albumin (daily for 3 days, then weekly).
  5. Nitrogen balance (weekly).
  6. Repeat nutritional assessment at biweekly intervals.
J. Trouble-Shooting.
  1. **Fluid overload** (>0.5 kg/day weight gain):
    a. Check I/O daily.
    b. Check weighing technique to exclude change of scale, and assure similar conditions.

TABLE 12–7.
Metabolic Complications of TPN

Derangement	Symptoms/Signs	Etiology	Treatment
Hypoglycemia	Perioral paresthesias Headache Tachycardia Altered mental status Seizure	Excessive insulin administration Resolution of sepsis Rapid TPN wean	↓ Insulin ↓ Insulin 5% Dextrose
Hyperglycemia	Osmotic diuresis Hyperosmotic, nonketotic acidosis	Excessive glucose administration Inadequate endogenous insulin Resistance due to glucocorticoids, sepsis Chromium deficiency	Supplemental insulin Supplemental insulin Supplemental insulin; treat septic source Trace metal supplementation
Metabolic acidosis		Hyperosmolar, nonketotic acidosis Excessive chloride administration	Hydration, insulin ↓ NaCl, increase acetate
Hyperphosphatemia	Metastatic soft tissue calcifications	Excessive administration	↓ Administration
Hypophosphatemia	Muscle weakness Circumoral and peripheral paresthesias Mental obtundity Hyperventilation	Renal failure Refeeding syndrome	Phosphate binders Phosphate supplementation
Hypokalemia	Arrhythmias Muscle weakness	Refeeding syndrome Excessive losses	↑ Administration Replace losses appropriately

Condition	Signs/Symptoms	Causes	Treatment
Hyperkalemia	Hyperglycemia ileus Muscle weakness Ventricular arrhythmias	Excessive administration Ineffective excretion (renal failure)	↓ Administration Binders, dialysis
Hypocalcemia	Intestinal colic Chvostek's sign Muscle spasm, weakness, tetany Depression Arrhythmias	Inadequate administration Excessive phosphate administration	↑ Administration
Hypercalcemia	Muscle weakness CNS depression	Excessive Ca or vitamin D administration	↓ Administration
Hypomagnesemia	Digitalis toxicity Chvostek's sign Fasciculations Depression Nausea/vomiting	Refeeding syndrome	↑ Administration
Hypermagnesemia	Hypotension CNS depression	Excessive administration Renal failure	↓ Administration Convert to aluminum-based antacids
Azotemia	Nausea/vomiting Increased BUN/creatinine	Reduced renal function Excessive protein administration	
Hepatic dysfunction	Increased LFTs	Cholestasis Steatosis	↓ Administration Dialysis ↓ Carbohydrate Convert to fat fuel source Measure AEE Do not overfeed

TABLE 12–8.

Differential Diagnosis of
Hyperglycemia

Diabetes
  Type I
  Type II
  Postpancreatectomy
Pancreatitis
Infections and sepsis
Burns
Dehydration
Dialysis
  Peritoneal
  Hemodialysis
Hepatic failure
Medications
  Steroids
  Epinephrine (Dilantin)
  Phenytoin

---

   c. Concentrate TPN solution by changing to a higher amino
     acid or dextrose concentration.
2. **Hyperosmolar nonketotic dehydration:**
   a. Monitor blood glucose—assure glucose control.
   b. Check I/O—consider osmotic diuresis, dehydration.
   c. Correct hyperglycemia with insulin, dehydration with
     free water.
3. **Hypoglycemia:**
   a. Reduce insulin.
   b. Check infusion as it may be interrupted.
4. **Elevated BUN:**
   a. Assess renal function, fluid status to avoid dehydration.
   b. Reduce amino acid concentration.
   c. Increase calorie-nitrogen ratio of TPN.
5. **Catheter-related sepsis:** Be suspicious in the patient with
   frequent temperature spikes of unexplained origin or sudden onset of glucose intolerance when previously on stable
   formula.
   a. **Exclude other sources.**
     1) Completely culture patient (cultures of blood, both
       peripheral and via the TPN catheter, sputum, urine,
       and wound).
     2) CXR.

b. **Inspect insertion site** for evidence of inflammation. The majority of catheter infections track along the catheter from the skin.

c. If catheter sepsis is likely, **remove it aseptically** and send tip and subcutaneous portions separately for routine and fungal cultures. Remember to administer 5% dextrose peripherally at the same rate to avoid hypoglycemia. It is best to wait at least 24 hours before inserting another TPN catheter although some studies show no increased risk in changing catheter over a guidewire.

6. **Discontinuing TPN infusion:**

   a. **Temporary**—decrease infusion rate by one half for 2 hours, then convert to 5% dextrose solution at the same rate.

   b. **Permanent**—following the final bottle of TPN solution, change to 5% dextrose and infuse at the same rate at which TPN was infusing overnight. Remove central catheter the following morning.

7. **Obstructed TPN line:**

   a. Inspect for external catheter kinks.

   b. Irrigate catheter with normal saline using a 3-mL syringe and sterile technique.

   c. Reposition and change dressing using sterile technique.

   d. Attempt treatment with urokinase (kits available with instructions).

   e. If problem continues or is recurrent, consider changing the catheter over a guidewire.

8. **Disconnection of the TPN line:**

   a. Immediately clamp the tubing on the patient side of the disconnection to prevent blood loss or air embolism. If air embolism has occurred, place patient's head low and roll on to left side.

   b. Using sterile technique, change IV tubing to catheter hub and discard old TPN solution.

IV. **PERIPHERAL FEEDING.**

The goal of peripheral parenteral nutrition is to minimize nitrogen losses due to catabolism of somatic and visceral protein. Nitrogen losses can be reduced to $1.2-3.0$ g/m^2/day with the infusion of amino acids alone.

A. **Indications.**

   1. Mild stress and mild malnutrition.

   2. Enteral route unavailable.

    3. Central venous access not available owing to subclavian vein thrombosis.

    4. Use as temporary support following an episode of catheter sepsis prior to insertion of a new catheter.

    5. When anticipated period of starvation is <10 days.

    6. As a supplement while increasing to full enteral support.

B. Contraindications.

    1. Moderate to severe stress present.

    2. Moderate to severe malnutrition present.

    3. GI tract functional.

    4. Peripheral access not available.

    5. Anticipated need for prolonged nutritional support.

C. Benefits.

    1. Ability to supply some nutrition temporarily during periods of decreased or absent enteral intake.

    2. Less complicated than central nutrition.

    3. Avoids risks of central venous catheter insertion.

D. Disadvantages.

    1. Full nutritional support not possible.

    2. Patient remains catabolic.

    3. Not able to deliver large caloric load owing to limitations on osmolality of infused solutions.

    4. Requires frequent changes of infusion sites.

    5. High incidence of thrombophlebitis.

    6. High risk of subcutaneous infiltration.

    7. Vitamin, mineral, trace metal deficiencies can occur.

E. Different Systems.

    1. **Protein sparing:** Fluid consists of 4.25% amino acid solution infused via a peripheral vein to provide 1–2 g/kg/day of protein. No dextrose is given. This system preserves body protein mass at the expense of body fat stores, producing ketosis.

    2. **Periperipheral:** Fluid consists of 4.5% amino acids and 2.5%–10% dextrose with additional calories supplied by fat emulsion (10%–20% at 500–1,000 mL/day). This system is capable of supplying 550–2,200 kcal/day. Body protein mass is preserved although patient continues to be catabolic.

V. NUTRITIONAL SUPPORT OF THE PROBLEM PATIENT.

A. Cardiac Patients.

    1. Malnourished secondary to anorexia, unpalatable diets (low sodium), cardiac cachexia, and associated renal failure.

2. The problems of nutritional support are largely related to the requirement for severe fluid restriction.
   a. **Enteral feeding:** When advancing enteral feeding, increase the strength of the solution prior to the rate to minimize the fluid delivered. Use solutions with higher caloric density (2 kcal/mL).
   b. **Parenteral feeding:**
      1) Use central route to minimize fluid load.
      2) Increase dextrose solution to 70%.
      3) Increase amino acid solution to 10%.

B. Renal Failure Patients.
1. The optimal treatment of the patient with renal failure is to use standard nutritional support, and dialyze as indicated. Restrict potassium, sodium, and protein (20–40 g/day).
2. If dialysis is not possible, use specialized solutions containing high-biologic-value protein (essential amino acids and histidine) and hypertonic dextrose to minimize volume. These solutions are indicated when BUN >80 and creatinine >3.0.
3. **Available solutions:**
   a. **Enteral**: Amin-Aid lacks electrolytes, vitamins, minerals, and is hypocaloric.
   b. **Parenteral:** Nephramine lacks electrolytes, vitamins, minerals, and is hypocaloric.
4. **Dialysis effects** (loss or gain of nutrients).
   a. **Amino acids:**
      Hemodialysis: 6–9 g per treatment lost.
      Peritoneal: 0.3–0.5 g per exchange lost.
   b. **Protein:**
      Hemodialysis: none.
      Peritoneal: approximately 0.6 g/hr treatment lost.
   c. **Glucose:**
      Hemodialysis: 5 g/hr with a glucose-free dialysate lost.
      Peritoneal: 150–200 g/day can be absorbed depending on dialysate volume and glucose concentration. Insulin may be required.

C. Hepatic Failure Patients.
1. Must increase the percentage of branched chain amino acids while reducing aromatic and straight chain amino acids.
2. Special formulas are indicated when encephalopathy is clinically evident or serum analysis reveals either hyperammonemia (>100 μg/dL) or an abnormal amino acid profile.

3. **Solutions available:**
   a. **Enteral:** Hepatic-Aid lacks electrolytes, vitamins, and minerals.
   b. **Parenteral:** Hepatamine and FreAmine HBC.

D. Glucose-Intolerant Patient.

1. Exclude sepsis as a cause of glucose intolerance.
2. Treat with regular insulin; use recombinant human insulin to minimize resistance on an immunologic basis.
3. Decrease carbohydrate load.
4. If enterally feeding, change to a formula with more complex carbohydrate.
5. Cautiously add fat as an energy source.
6. It may be necessary to withdraw support temporarily until sepsis is under control.

THE CENTRAL NERVOUS SYSTEM

13

I. GENERAL NEUROLOGIC EXAMINATION.

The examination is performed in a systematic manner, beginning with higher cortical functions and progressing to examination of the cranial nerves, and the testing of motor function, sensation, reflexes, and cerebellar function. As abnormalities are found, the examination is modified to attempt precise localization of the pathologic process responsible for the abnormality. The following is an outline of a complete neurologic examination, as would be performed on a normally awake patient. **Tests applicable to a comatose or uncooperative patient are italicized. Functions rarely tested are indicated with an asterisk.**

A. Mental Status.

1. *Response to external stimuli:* Is the patient awake, alert? Are the patient's eyes open spontaneously?
   a. Patient responds to verbal commands—opens eyes, shows fingers, answers questions.
   b. Patient does not respond to verbal commands but does respond to pain—localizes, withdraws, or postures.
   c. Patient does not respond to verbal commands or to pain.
2. **If the patient is alert, test general cognitive functions.**
   a. Orientation (person, place, and time).
   b. Speech (see Table 13–1).
      1) Verbalization—ability to speak (fluent), or inability to speak (nonfluent) aphasias.
      2) Comprehension—ability to follow simple commands.

517

TABLE 13-1.
Aphasias

Type	Spontaneous Speech	Comprehension	Repetition	Naming	Localization
Broca's	Nonfluent	Good	Poor	Poor	Broca's area (inferior dominant frontal lobe)
Wernicke's	Fluent	Poor	Poor	Poor	Wernicke's area (superior dominant temporal lobe)
Conductive	Fluent	Good	Poor	Poor	Arcuate fasciculus
Global	Nonfluent	Poor	Poor	Poor	Dominant perisylvian cortex
Anomic	Fluent	Good	Good	Poor	Not localized

    3) Repetition.

    4) Naming objects.

  3. **Memory and general intellectual function will vary according to patient's background and education.**

    a. Calculations.

    b. Perform serial sevens.

    c. Recollection of three objects at 5 minutes.

    d. Recitation of past Presidents.

B. Cranial Nerves (CN I–XII) and Brainstem Function.

  1. *Olfactory* **(CN I, smell):** Test ability to identify coffee or other available scent.

  2. *Optic* **(CN II, vision).**

    a. Visual acuity: Test with pocket card, newsprint, or finger counting.

    b. Visual fields: Test ability to detect objects at periphery of vision (Fig 13–1).

    c. Funduscopic examination—look for papilledema, hemorrhage.

  3. *Oculomotor* **(CN III, extraocular muscles except superior oblique and lateral rectus, pupillary constriction, levator palpebrae).**

    a. *Extraocular muscles except superior oblique and lateral rectus:* Test ability of patient to move eyes conjugately, up, down, and laterally (see pp 522–524).

    b. *Pupillary constriction:* Examine pupil size, symmetry, and reaction to light and accommodation.

    c. Levator palpebrae: Test ability to elevate eyelid.

  4. *Trochlear* **(CN IV, superior oblique muscle):** Test ability of patient to depress, intort, and adduct the globe. (*Note:* The patient with a CN IV palsy will tilt the head away from the affected side. See pp 522–524).

  5. *Trigeminal* **(CN V, facial sensation, corneal sensation, motor for muscles of mastication).**

    a. *Sensory for face:* Check all three divisions with light touch and pinprick.

    b. *Corneal sensation*—blink response to light touch of cornea with wisp of cotton (requires intact CN VII function and response to unilateral stimulation is bilateral).

    c. Motor—muscles of mastication. Palpate masseters and temporalis on biting, and note jaw deviation on

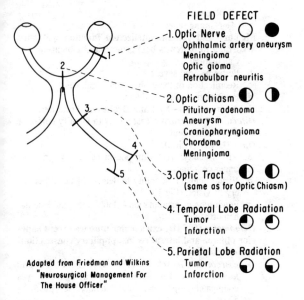

FIELD DEFECT

1. Optic Nerve
   Ophthalmic artery aneurysm
   Meningioma
   Optic gioma
   Retrobulbar neuritis

2. Optic Chiasm
   Pituitary adenoma
   Aneurysm
   Craniopharyngioma
   Chordoma
   Meningioma

3. Optic Tract
   (same as for Optic Chiasm)

4. Temporal Lobe Radiation
   Tumor
   Infarction

5. Parietal Lobe Radiation
   Tumor
   Infarction

Adapted from Friedman and Wilkins
"Neurosurgical Management For
The House Officer"

FIG 13–1.
Visual field defects. (Adapted from Friedman AH, Wilkins RH: *Neurosurgical Management for the House Officer*. Baltimore, Williams & Wilkins Co, 1984.)

opening mouth. (*Note:* Jaw deviates toward CN V motor deficit.)

6. *Abducens* (CN VI, motor for lateral rectus): Test abduction of eye (see section I.B.13).

7. *Facial* (CN VII, muscles of facial expression, taste, salivation and tearing, sensation of external auditory canal and tonsils, stapedius muscle motor innervation).

   a. Motor for muscles of facial expression: Test ability to wrinkle forehead, close eyes, smile, and check nasolabial fold symmetry. If only the lower face is weak, the lesion is "central or supranuclear," in the contralateral cerebral hemisphere. If the upper and lower face are weak, the lesion is in the ipsilateral facial nucleus or facial nerve ("peripheral or nuclear VIIth nerve palsy"). (*Note:* Facial weakness or asymmetry may be difficult to assess in cases of direct facial trauma.)

*b. Taste—anterior two thirds of the tongue.

*c. Tearing—may use Schirmer's test to distinguish between proximal and distal CN VII lesions. Taste sensation is absent in both lesions, but if the lesion is distal, tearing is preserved.

*d. Sensation of external ear, tympanic membrane, and tonsils.

*e. Stapedius innervation—tested by audiologists.

8. *Vestibulocochlear* **(CN VIII, hearing and vestibular function).**

   a. Auditory—history to include recent changes, speech discrimination, and tinnitus. Gross testing may be performed with a watch or by rubbing fingers near ear.

     1) **Weber test:** 512-Hz tuning fork placed at apex of skull will be heard as louder on the side of conductive hearing loss (external or middle ear), or less on side of sensorineural (inner ear) hearing loss. These may then be distinguished using:

     2) **Rinne test:** 512-Hz tuning fork is placed on the mastoid process until no longer audible, then placed near the external auditory meatus, to determine if air conduction (external and middle ear) is greater than bone conduction.

     3) Formal audiometry testing in case of deficit detected as above.

   b. Vestibular.

     1) In alert patient, look for nystagmus on extraocular movement testing or on ice water calorics (see pp 522–524).

     2) *In trauma patients or patients with decreased level of consciousness, may test with* **doll's eyes** *(after checking cervical spine films), or* **ice water calorics** *(after checking tympanic membranes)* (see pp 522–524).

*Indicates functions rarely tested.

9. *Glossopharyngeal* (CN IX, sensation for posterior tongue and pharynx, taste, salivation).
   a. Sensation of posterior one third of the tongue and pharynx: Test with gag reflex.
   *b. Taste—posterior one third of tongue.
   *c. Salivation—parotid gland.
   *d. Stylopharyngeus innervation.
10. *Vagus* (CN X, visceral and ear sensation, visceral parasympathetics, pharyngeal and laryngeal musculature).
    *a. Visceral and ear sensation.
    *b. Visceral parasympathetic innervation.
    c. *Pharyngeal and laryngeal musculature:* Test with gag reflex and palate elevation. Uvula deviates away from side of lesion.
11. *Accessory* (CN XI, motor for sternocleidomastoid, trapezius).
    a. Sternocleidomastoid: Test with contralateral head turning.
    b. Trapezius: Test with shoulder shrug.
12. *Hypoglossal* (CN XII, muscles of the tongue): Check for unilateral atrophy, or deviation of tongue on protrusion (toward side of lesion).
13. *Extraocular Movements (EOMs):* The action of the individual extraocular muscles is shown in Figure 13–2. The

*Indicates functions rarely tested.

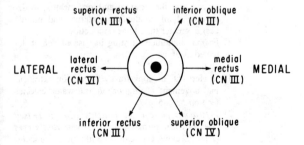

FIG 13–2.
The extraocular muscles (cranial nerve shown in parenthesis).

control of ocular movements is complex, involving the cerebral hemispheres, multiple cranial nerves, and brain-stem centers (Fig 13–3). Conjugate horizontal gaze is mediated through the paramedian pontine reticular formation (PPRF), which regulates the ipsilateral CN VI nucleus and the contralateral CN III nucleus. In addition, the frontal eye fields have input to the PPRF, driving the eyes to the contralateral side. In seizures with a frontal lobe focus, the eyes will deviate away from the side of the lesion during the seizure, but either following a seizure, or in the case of a destructive lesion of the frontal lobe, the eyes will deviate toward the side of the lesion.

a. **Evaluation of EOMs in the awake patient:** EOMs may be tested by having the patient look in all six cardinal directions, as shown in Figure 13–2, looking for asymmetry in movement or nystagmus.

b. **Evaluation of EOMs in the patient with decreased level of consciousness:** Examination of EOMs depends on the input of the vestibular system to the PPRF. The two common tests are the **doll's eye ma-**

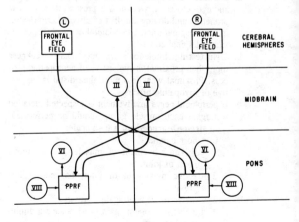

FIG 13–3.
Pathways for control of extraocular movements.

neuver (eyes move in direction opposite head movement), and **ice water calorics.** (*Note:* Prior to these
maneuvers, check for cervical fractures [doll's eyes]
or for perforation of the tympanic membranes [ice
water calorics].) The normal patient suppresses doll's
eye movements but develops nystagmus with the
slow component toward the side of irrigation with ice
water. (*Note:* This response requires intact semicircu-
lar canals, brainstem, and CN III, IV, VI, and VIII.)
In patients with absent cerebral function, the doll's
eye maneuver will be positive, and with ice water caloric testing, the eyes will remain deviated to the side
of irrigation (frontal eye field not functioning to drive
eyes back to midline). In patients with absent brainstem function, there is no eye movement with either
test.

C. **Motor Examination.**
Note muscle bulk and tone, look for asymmetry, atrophy,
fasciculations (lower motor neuron lesion) or increased tone,
spasticity (upper motor neuron lesion).

1. **Upper extremities.**
   a. **Pronator drift:** Extend arms with palms facing up
   and eyes closed. If weakness is present, there is slow
   pronation and downward drift of affected arm (lesion
   in corticospinal tract, contralateral hemisphere, or ipsilateral spinal cord).
   b. **Grip testing:** Look for asymmetry. Distal weakness
   more than proximal is suggestive of neuropathic process. Proximal weakness more than distal is suggestive of myopathic process.
   c. If peripheral nerve involvement is suspected, detailed
   testing of each muscle group should be performed,
   with **strength graded on a 0–5 scale:**
      0 = no movement.
      1 = flicker movement of muscle, but no move-
          ment of joint.
      2 = active movement of joint, but not against
          gravity.
      3 = active movement against gravity.
      4 = active movement against resistance but dimin-
          ished strength.
      5 = full strength.

2. **Lower extremities:** Easiest to test by observing gait, with normal and heel-and-toe walking.
   a. **Gait patterns.**
      1) Hemiparetic: Upper motor neuron weakness is manifested by external rotation of foot and circumduction of the affected lower extremity.
      2) Scissoring (hyperadduction of both lower extremities)—bilateral spasticity seen in spinal cord lesions.
      3) Trendelenburg: Hip weakness results in downward tilt of pelvis opposite weight-bearing leg.
   b. Examine lower extremities for atrophy, fasciculations, tone, spasticity, clonus. Examine and grade individual muscle groups as indicated.

D. **Sensory Examination.**
   The sensory examination is designed to test both of the primary afferent pathways (Fig 13–4).
   1. *Spinothalamic tract* (pain and temperature): Test with pinprick and hot or cold object. (*Note:* Pain and temperature fibers cross to the opposite side of the spinal cord within three spinal levels of their entry and form the lateral spinothalamic tract on the contralateral side of the cord. Therefore, spinal cord injuries cause contralateral deficits in pain and temperature sensation below the level of the lesion.)
   2. *Posterior columns* (fine touch, vibration, joint position sense): Test with wisp of cotton, tuning fork, and passive motion of joints, respectively. (*Note:* Fibers mediating touch, vibration, and joint position sense do not cross to the opposite side of the cord, but form the posterior columns on the ipsilateral side of the cord, to cross in the medulla. Therefore, spinal cord injuries cause ipsilateral deficits in posterior column functions below the level of the lesion. Lesions above the thalamus may not cause demonstrable deficits in the primary sensory modalities as discussed above, but may be manifest by decreased graphesthesia, stereognosis, or sensory extinction.)

E. **Reflexes.**
   Check deep tendon and superficial reflexes as appropriate, and look for pathologic reflexes (Table 13–2). Deep tendon reflexes are graded on a 0–4+ scale:

   0   = not elicitable.
   1+ = hypoactive.

ANTERIOR   POSTERIOR

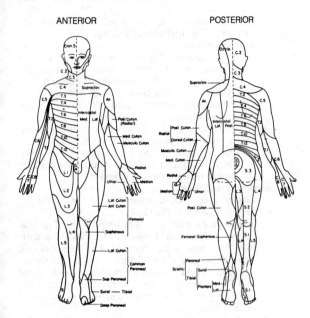

FIG 13–4.
Sensory dermatomes. (Duke Hospital Form H-0900.)

    2+ = normal.
    3+ = hyperactive.
    4+ = markedly hyperactive.
(*Note:* Grades 3+ and 4+ may be associated with either transient or sustained clonus.)

F. Cerebellar Testing.

A lesion in the cerebellar hemisphere (lateral) will cause a lateral deficit or intention tremor on the ipsilateral side. A lesion in the midline will cause a midline deficit (truncal ataxia and gait ataxia). Test upper extremities with finger-to-nose, finger-nose-finger (dysmetria), or rapid alternating movements (dysdiadochokinesis). Lower extremities may be assessed with gait (usually wide-based), heel-to-shin.

TABLE 13-2.
Reflexes

Reflex	Spinal Cord or Brain Innervation*	Peripheral or Cranial Nerve
1. Deep tendon reflexes		
Jaw jerk	V3	Mandibular division trigeminal nerve
Pectoralis	C5,6	Medial and lateral pectoral nerves
Biceps	C5,6	Musculocutaneous
Brachioradialis	C5,6	Radial
Triceps	C7,8	Radial
Patellar	L3,4	Femoral
Ankle jerk	L5,S1	Tibial
2. Superficial		
Abdominal	T6–L1	Intercostal
Cremasteric	L1,2	Ilioinguinal and genitofemoral
Superficial anal	S3–5	Inferior hemorrhoidal
Bulbocavernosus	S3,4	Pudendal
Plantar	L5–S2	Tibial
3. Pathologic		

Babinski: fanning of toes and dorsiflexion of great toe on stroking the sole of the foot (normal response is flexion of foot and toes); see Plantar reflex above

Frontal release signs: glabellar, snout, sucking, and grasp reflexes

*Key nerve root is italicized.

1. Anterior cerebellar lesion—ataxia of gait, impaired postural reflexes.
2. Vermian lesion—speech ataxia.

II. SPECIFIC CONDITIONS.

A. The Patient With Decreased Level of Consciousness

1. The *initial assessment* of the patient with altered level of consciousness should begin with the ABCs as described in Chapter 4. Should orotracheal intubation be required, the neck should not be extended prior to obtaining cervical spine films. After establishing an adequate airway and ensuring that the patient is adequately ventilated, attention is turned to the cardiovascular system. *Since shock only rarely occurs as the result of a head injury* (occasionally in infants with intracranial bleeding, patients with high cervical spinal cord or brainstem injuries, or hemorrhage from scalp lacerations or open skull fractures), *another etiology for shock should be sought and treated.* The patient with a **high cervical spinal cord lesion** who is hypotensive because of decreased sympathetic tone should be treated with volume expansion. **Persistent bleeding** from a scalp laceration or a compound skull fracture should be controlled and treated with volume replacement (preferably colloid, rather than crystalloid). Once the patient's vital signs are stabilized, a history of the alteration of consciousness should be obtained, including rate of onset, precipitating factors, duration, and associated amnesia. Although loss of consciousness associated with head injury is most likely due to concussion, other factors such as drug or ethanol intoxication, hypoglycemia, hypotension, hypoxemia, seizures, or even preceding intracranial hemorrhage should be considered and appropriate laboratory studies initiated. Past medical history and current medications should be elucidated, if possible. A brief physical examination should be performed next, looking for signs of trauma, e.g., raccoon eyes or Battle's sign (indicative of a basilar skull fracture). During the course of this examination, a brief mental status examination may be conducted, to determine if the patient is fully awake and alert, responding to verbal commands, somnolent but arousable, responsive only to pain, or unresponsive.

2. **The Glasgow Coma Scale (GCS)** was developed to assist in the evaluation of comatose patients (Table 13–3). The GCS has been standardized to limit interexaminer variability, but it has several important limitations. Eye opening may be hindered by periorbital edema or lacerations, and verbal responses may be limited owing to intubation or facial fractures. Also, the GCS does not completely assess the brainstem. The integrity of brainstem reflexes and motor response to pain can give vital information regarding the cause and site of neurologic dysfunction (Table 13–4). Because of the importance of pupillary light responses in assessing the patient with altered level of consciousness, do not give morphine or other narcotics (pupillary constrictors) and do not administer mydriatic agents to facilitate funduscopic examination.

3. **Appropriate neurologic examination:** Once the initial assessment is complete and any emergent therapeutic measures necessary are underway, a more detailed neu-

TABLE 13–3.

Glasgow Coma Scale*

	Response	
Eye opening (E)	Spontaneous	4
	To command	3
	To pain	2
	No response	1
Best motor (M)	Obeys verbal commands	6
	Localizes pain	5
	Withdraws to pain	4
	Abnormal flexion (decorticate)	3
	Extensor response (decerebrate)	2
	Flaccid	1
Verbal (V)	Oriented	5
	Confused conversation	4
	Inappropriate words	3
	Incomprehensible sounds	2
	No response	1

*Coma is defined as E + M + V ≤7 (E + M + V = 3–15).

TABLE 13–4.
Evaluation of Brainstem Function

Level of Lesion	Pupils	Ice Water Calorics	Respiration	Movement Response to Pain
None	Midposition reactive to light	Nystagmus	Rhythmic	Purposeful
Diencephalon	Small, reactive to light	Tonic, conjugate eye deviation	Cheyne-Stokes	Purposeful or decorticate
Midbrain	Midposition, unreactive to light	Dysconjugate eye deviation	Central neurogenic hyperventilation	Decerebrate
Pons	Pinpoint, reactive to light	None	Apneustic	Flaccid

rologic examination may be performed tailored to the neurologic status of the patient. To the extent possible, a **mental status examination** should be conducted and carefully documented—often a diminishing level of consciousness may be the first sign of progressive neurologic deterioration. If the patient is able to follow commands, a more detailed examination should be conducted. The examination of the unconscious patient is aimed at determining the level of brainstem dysfunction, and should include the items listed in section I as well as corneal, cough, and gag reflexes.

4. **Management.**

   a. As part of the initial assessment, **laboratory studies** should be obtained, including CBC, serum chemistries, ABG, type and crossmatch, clotting studies, ethanol level, and toxic screen of both blood and urine. If **hypoglycemia** is suspected, an **ampule of 50% dextrose** may be administered IV while awaiting the results of serum chemistries. If a **drug overdose** is suspected, an **ampule (0.4 mg) of naloxone HCl (Narcan)** may be administered IV.

   b. Clues to the etiology may be obtained through the history. If the history includes:

      1) **Trauma:** Intracranial hematoma must be ruled out. Common causes of decreased consciousness following trauma include concussion, brain shear injury, hypoxia, and intracranial hematoma. The patient who was awake and alert, and then rapidly deteriorates to unconsciousness with decerebrate posturing or hemiparesis may require a bur hole performed immediately, whereas the patient who has been unconscious for a period of time should undergo emergent CT scanning to be followed, if indicated, by craniotomy.

      2) **Sudden onset of severe headache:** Consider vascular etiology, such as subarachnoid hemorrhage (SAH) or intracerebral hemorrhage, and perform emergent CT scan.

B. **Increased Intracranial Pressure.**

The normal ICP in adults is 6–16 mm Hg. Because the cranial cavity is rigid, any increase in volume must be compensated by the displacement of one or more of the three intra cranial components: CSF, blood, and brain. Initially, a small change in intracranial volume results in only a minimal change in ICP. Volume changes seen with respiration or arterial pulsation may be compensated by displacement of CSF through the foramen magnum, compression of veins, or distention of the meninges. As the intracranial volume increases, however, these reserves are lost, and a small change in volume may result in a large change in ICP (Fig 13–5). As the ICP rises, the cerebral blood flow is diminished owing to decreased cerebral perfusion pressure (CPP):

$$CPP = MAP - ICP$$

The decreased cerebral blood flow results in cerebral vasodilation which may further increase ICP.

1. **Increased ICP** may be due to a discrete mass lesion (tumor, hematoma, abscess) or to a diffuse process such as cerebral edema.
   a. **Cytotoxic edema**—intracellular fluid collection, predominantly gray matter, commonly seen in stroke.
   b. **Vasogenic edema**—extracellular fluid collection, predominantly in white matter, commonly seen surrounding tumor or abscess, often responds to steroid therapy.

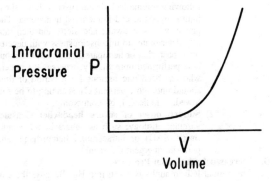

FIG 13–5.
Intracranial pressure-volume relationship.

    c. In addition to causing an increased ICP, a **mass lesion** may also cause a shift of the intracranial contents, resulting in further neurologic dysfunction.

2. **Diagnosis of increased ICP.**

    a. **Headache** is the cardinal presenting symptom of increased ICP. Usually, this type of headache is worse in the morning, or awakens the patient from sleep, and may be associated with nausea or vomiting.

    b. Patients with rapidly increasing ICP often demonstrate **systemic hypertension, bradycardia, and respiratory irregularities (Cushing's response).** In patients with longer-standing increased ICP, **papilledema** may be seen.

    c. In cases of herniation of the cerebellar tonsils into the foramen magnum, **nuchal rigidity** may be seen.

    d. In children with increased ICP, the head circumference may enlarge, one may see split sutures, or failure of fontanelle closure on films of the skull. Pressure on the tegmentum of the midbrain may result in paralysis of upward gaze ("setting sun sign").

3. **Monitoring:** If the evaluation demonstrates evidence of increased ICP, ICP monitoring may be beneficial. Becker et al., studying patients with either low or high density mass lesions on CT scan following severe head injury, found that **several factors were associated with the development of intracranial hypertension:**

    a. **Age** >40 years.

    b. **Systolic BP** <90 mm Hg.

    c. **Motor posturing,** either unilateral or bilateral.

    With two or more of these factors present, intracranial hypertension was present in 60% of patients, compared to only 4% when one or none of these factors was present. In the patient with motor posturing, ICP monitoring is crucial to the continued assessment of the patient, since the neurologic examination is extremely limited. ICP monitoring may be performed with either a ventricular catheter or a subarachnoid bolt. The ventricular catheter is the preferred method since it allows both recording of pressure, and drainage of CSF, to help lower increased ICP.

4. **Sustained ICP** ≥20 mm Hg should be treated as follows:

   a. **Elevate head of bed,** extending neck to facilitate venous drainage.

   b. **Hyperventilation**—to lower $PaCO_2$ to 25–30 mm Hg. Resultant vasoconstriction decreases intracranial volume and therefore pressure. If the patient fights the ventilator, pancuronium bromide (Pavulon) 0.04 mg/kg IV may be given. (*Note:* Because of its vasoconstricting effect, hyperventilation should be avoided in cases of ischemic cerebral disease.)

   c. **Steroids** stabilize blood-brain barrier, most effective in cases of vasogenic edema associated with brain tumors or postoperative swelling. Dexamethasone (Decadron) 10–100 mg IV, then 1–4 mg IV or po q.6.h. or methylprednisolone (Solu-Medrol) 1 g IV, then 40 mg IV q.6h. (*Note:* Cimetidine 300 mg IV or po q.6h., or ranitidine 50 mg IV q.8h. or 150 mg q.12h. po should be administered with steroids to prevent peptic ulcers.)

   d. **Diuretics.**

      1) **Mannitol** (osmotic agent): Monitor serum osmolarity, UO, to prevent overdehydration. Maximal dose 1 g/kg IV q.3h. Hold mannitol for serum osmolarity >305 mOsm/L.

      2) **Furosemide** (Lasix) 20 mg IV is not as potent as mannitol and is used less frequently.

   e. **CSF drainage:** If ventricular catheter is in place, may obtain large decrease in ICP with small volume of CSF drainage.

   f. **Lidocaine:** 100 mg IV bolus may reduce ICP through unknown mechanism.

   g. **Barbiturate coma**—thiopental 3–5 mg/kg IV, followed by 1–2 mg/kg/hr as needed to achieve desired reduction in ICP or burst suppression on EEG, taking care to avoid systemic hypotension. Because all brainstem reflexes except pupillary light responses are lost, ICP monitoring is essential.

   h. **Surgical techniques:**

      1) Resection of mass lesion.

      2) Resection of relatively silent region of brain, such as right anterior temporal lobe, or right

frontal lobe in extreme cases to achieve decompression when herniation (see below) has occurred.

C. **Herniation Syndromes.**

Brain herniation may occur through the foramen magnum or tentorial notch, or under the falx cerebri.

1. **Downward transtentorial herniation** may present in either of two distinct syndromes. In the early stages of herniation, neurologic deficits may be reversible, but once the deficit has spread to midbrain level with bilateral fixed pupils, dysconjugate caloric responses, and decerebrate posturing, secondary midbrain hemorrhage has usually occurred and the deficit is not reversible.

   a. **Central herniation**—diffusely increased ICP or centrally located mass lesion, with downward displacement of brainstem.

      1) Progressive **decrease in mental status** is earliest sign of central herniation. Impaired function of diencephalon results in Cheyne-Stokes respiration and small, reactive pupils. Decorticate posturing is seen along with Babinski plantar responses. To this point, neurologic deficits are usually reversible.

      2) Progressive midbrain dysfunction results in hyperventilation, decerebrate posturing, and midposition, fixed pupils.

      3) Continued herniation results in flaccidity, irregular respiration, and death. (*Note:* Herniation has occurred without a fixed and dilated pupil.)

   b. **Uncal herniation:** A lateral mass displaces the uncus of the temporal lobe medially, over the tentorial edge.

      1) **Ipsilateral pupillary dilation,** due to CN III compression, is most commonly the earliest presenting sign. (*Note:* Altered mental status may not necessarily be present in uncal herniation.)

      2) Continued herniation with pressure on midbrain results in decreasing level of consciousness and progressive midbrain dysfunction, with contralateral hemiparesis due to compression of ipsilateral cerebral peduncle. (*Note:* Ipsilateral hemiparesis may be seen with uncal herniation, secondary to

> compression of contralateral cerebral peduncle against the tentorial edge [Kernohan's notch], so the pupillary dilation is a more reliable indicator of laterality than is hemiparesis.)

    3) Bilateral decerebrate rigidity and hyperventilation occur, and with continued herniation, progressive brainstem dysfunction results in irregular respiration and flaccidity.

  2. **Posterior fossa mass lesions** may result in one of two syndromes:

    a. **Upward transtentorial herniation** may present with loss of upward gaze and rapid loss of consciousness.

    b. **Tonsillar herniation:** Cerebellar tonsils herniate downward through foramen magnum. May present with nuchal rigidity; compression of medulla may result in respiratory arrest.

  3. **Subfalcine herniation** may occur with displacement of the cingulate gyrus underneath the falx cerebri. This may result in enlargement of the contralateral lateral ventricle as the outflow via the foramen of Monro is occluded.

  4. **Herniation syndromes** are grave emergencies and are treated as described on p 534. In the presence of herniation, lumbar puncture is absolutely contraindicated. (*Note:* In the case of upward herniation, drainage of CSF with a catheter in the lateral ventricle may worsen the syndrome.)

D. Delirium.

Delirium is a transient disorder of global cognition, encountered frequently in hospitalized patients, especially in the intensive care setting. Delirium significantly increases patient morbidity and mortality, as an agitated, disoriented patient may inadvertently remove vital catheters, or damage wound dressings and sutures. The use of physical restraints and sedation may promote deep venous thrombosis, pulmonary embolism, and pneumonia.

  1. **Diagnosis:** A number of characteristic clinical features may present in a waxing and waning fashion, as assessed with serial mental status examinations.

    a. **Cognitive disorders:**

      1) Disorientation, especially for time.

      2) Confusion.

      3) Memory impairment.

4) Hallucinations—visual, auditory, tactile.
5) Delusions.
6) Inattention, distractability.
  b. **Behavioral disorders:**
1) Irritability.
2) Emotional lability.
3) Paranoia.
4) Increased or decreased motor behavior.
5) Agitation.
6) Combativeness.
7) Sleep-wake cycle disturbances—may see complete reversal.
  c. **Sympathetic nervous system hyperactivity** (tachycardia, hypertension, diaphoresis), especially in patients with drug or alcohol withdrawal.
2. **Etiology.**
  a. **Medications:** Lidocaine, digoxin, and cimetidine are commonly used in the SICU, and each may cause alterations in mental status. Drugs with anticholinergic side effects may have synergistic adverse effects on cognitive function. Drug interactions may result in impaired metabolism, with increased drug or metabolite levels contributing to cognitive dysfunction.
  b. **Electrolyte abnormalities,** especially Na^+, K^+, Ca^{2+}, Mg^{2+}.
  c. **Withdrawal** from alcohol or sedative-hypnotic drugs—onset of symptoms usually 24–72 hours after last ingestion.
  d. **Impaired gas exchange** and **acid-base disturbances**—hypoxia, hypercarbia, acidosis.
  e. **Cofactor deficiency**—Thiamine (alcoholics), cyanocobalamin (vitamin B_{12}), nicotinic acid.
  f. **Fever,** sepsis.
  g. **Endocrine abnormalities**—Disorders of glucose metabolism, as well as hypo- or hyperthyroidism, or hypo- or hyperadrenalism.
  h. **Hepatic or renal dysfunction.**
  i. SICU environment—intensive monitoring, altered sleep-wake cycles, sleep deprivation.
3. **Predisposing factors.**
  a. Advanced age is most important factor; increased risk > age 50.

    b. Prior cognitive impairment—previous cerebrovascular disease, underlying dementia.

    c. Sensory impairment—blindness, deafness.

    d. Major organ system failure—altered metabolism.

    e. Perioperative hypoxia, hypoperfusion, prolonged cardiopulmonary bypass.

    f. Trauma, especially to CNS.

4. **Evaluation:** Focus on detection of treatable physiologic abnormalities.

    a. **Physical examination.**

       1) VS.

       2) Assess major organ system function (CHF, hepatic dysfunction).

       3) Neurologic examination—mental status, focal neurologic signs, CT scan if indicated.

       4) Consider sepsis.

    b. **Laboratory studies**—CBCs, electrolytes (Na^+, K^+, Ca^{2+}, Mg^{2+}), glucose, creatinine, BUN, ABG, ECG, and arterial ammonia, bilirubin, endocrine testing as indicated.

    c. **Review medications:** Calculate cumulative doses, consider drug interactions.

    d. **Review pre- and intraoperative course,** history of alcohol or sedative-hypnotic drug use, predisposing factors.

5. **Treatment.**

    a. Correct or optimize physiologic abnormalities.

    b. Discontinue nonessential medications.

    c. Administer thiamine 100 mg IV or IM, followed by 100 mg IM or po daily for 3 days. Replace other vitamins or hormones as indicated.

    d. Environment.

       1) Minimize manipulations to allow as much uninterrupted sleep as possible.

       2) Orientation aids—calender, clock, family visits, familiar objects from home.

       3) Place patient in room with outside window, if possible, to aid in reestablishing normal day-night cycles.

    e. **Psychotropic medications:** When above measures are insufficient, consider pharmacologic approach.

       1) Mild symptoms—chloral hydrate or benzodiazepine at night to normalize sleep patterns.

2) **Antipsychotic medications.**
   a) **Low potency: Chlorpromazine** (Thorazine) acts through anticholinergic effects and α-receptor blockade. May cause orthostatic hypotension, urinary retention, and exacerbation of narrow-angle glaucoma.
   b) **High potency:** For most SICU patients **haloperidol** (Haldol) is the drug of choice owing to few hemodynamic side effects. Major side effects include extrapyramidal symptoms such as dystonic reactions, rigidity, late onset tardive dyskinesia. Dosage is 0.5–5.0 mg IM or 2–5 mg PO. Peak effect in 30 minutes (IM) or 3 hours (PO). Repeat dose until patient responds. Once patient is calm, maintenance dose of 2–5 mg IM or PO q.4–6h. with additional doses as needed. IM administration provides faster initial response but offers no advantage in maintenance, unless the patient is unable to take PO. After several days of normal cognitive function, taper over 2–3 days until discontinued.

f. **Alcohol or sedative-hypnotic withdrawal** is potentially fatal with 15% mortality in delirium tremens. Benzodiazepines are the drugs of choice, substituting for alcohol in the brain, allowing gradual withdrawal and raising the seizure threshold.

   1) **Thiamine:** Administer to all patients suspected of withdrawal.
   2) Volume repletion and correction of electrolyte and metabolic abnormalities.
   3) **Benzodiazepines** (for agitation, tremor, anxiety — chlordiazepoxide (Librium) 25–100 mg or diazepam (Valium) 5–10 mg PO (IM absorption erratic and should not be used) q.6h. for 24 hours. Begin tapering immediately, 25% of initial daily dose per day. Watch for oversedation. For extreme agitation, consider IV infusion of chlordiazepoxide 12.5 mg/min, or diazepam 2.5 mg/min until patient calm, then revert to oral dose.

E. **Seizures.**

Seizures should be considered a symptom of an underlying disease process, not a disease process in themselves. It is important to seek the underlying cause of the seizures.

1. **Etiology varies with age.**

   a. Infants—perinatal injury, inborn errors of metabolism, congenital malformation, infection.

   b. Children—infection, genetically inherited diseases, trauma.

   c. Adults—trauma, tumor, drugs (ethanol or barbiturate withdrawal).

   d. Elderly—tumor, vascular disease.

2. **Focal (partial) seizures** are always caused by focal cortical lesion.

   a. Elementary—no loss of consciousness.

   b. Complex—with altered consciousness.

   c. Focal seizures with secondary generalization.

   d. The location of the cortical focus will determine the initial seizure presentation. It is important to get a thorough seizure history from witnesses as well as the patient, as the patient may not recall the initial aspects of the seizure. Localizing signs include:

      1) Anterior frontal lobe—deviation of the head and eyes to contralateral side.

      2) Motor cortex—tonic-clonic movements of contralateral body and face.

      3) Sensory cortex—focal paresthesias in contralateral body and face.

      4) Occipital cortex—scintillations or transient visual field deficits in the contralateral visual field.

      5) Temporal cortex: Auditory, olfactory, visceral hallucinations.

      6) Temporary postictal neurologic deficits (e.g., Todd's paralysis) may help localize the origin of seizures.

3. **Complex partial seizures:** often initial temporal lobe aura, then altered consciousness with complex hallucinations or altered perception:

   a. Déjà vu.

   b. Automatisms.

   c. Mood changes, usually fear, depression.

   d. Hallucinations.

4. **Generalized seizures.**
   a. **Tonic-clonic:** May have prodrome, then patient loses consciousness, becomes rigid, with synchronous spasms of entire body. Postictally, patient is drowsy and confused for variable period of time.
   b. **Petit mal (absence):** Patient has brief lapse of consciousness during which he does not speak or understand speech. Commonly seen in childhood, EEG demonstrates 3/sec spike and wave pattern.
   c. **Akinetic seizures:** Patient loses postural muscle tone and falls to ground.
5. **Evaluation.**
   a. Serum electrolytes, glucose, Ca^{2+}, phosphate, ABG to rule out metabolic cause.
   b. Anticonvulsant levels, if indicated.
   c. Brain CT scanning to rule out mass lesions, especially in postoperative patient.
   d. Lumbar puncture (LP)—to be performed only after a CT scan, which shows no mass lesion, to rule out infection.
   e. EEG to help localize seizure focus.
6. **Treatment.**
   a. Of patients with penetrating head injury, 50% will develop seizures, and should be treated prophylactically. Of patients with nonpenetrating severe head injuries, 5% will have a single seizure, usually in the first week; 20% will develop late epilepsy.
   b. **Focal or generalized seizures:** Begin one drug at a time. Increase dose until seizures are eliminated or toxic levels reached, then add second medication, as necessary.
      1) **Phenytoin** 3–5 mg/kg/day IV or po (not to be given IM) to achieve serum levels of 10–20 μg/mL. Toxic effects include nystagmus, ataxia, gingival hyperplasia, blood dyscrasia.
      2) **Phenobarbital** 2–4 mg/kg/day to achieve serum level of 15–30 μg/mL. Toxic effects include ataxia, sedation, hyperactivity.
      3) **Carbamazepine** (Tegretol) 600–1,200 mg/day to achieve serum level of 4–8 μg/mL. Given po only. Toxic effects include diplopia, dizziness, drowsiness, blood dyscrasia.

7. **Status epilepticus.**
   a. ABCs as listed above.
   b. Blood workup as under section II.E.5 (p 541).
   c. **Diazepam** 10 mg IV bolus (short-acting).
   d. **Phenytoin** 50 mg/min IV bolus to total loading dose of 1 g for adult. Monitor BP and ECG (prolonged PR interval).
   e. If seizures continue, **phenobarbital** 120 mg IV bolus (25 mg/min) q. 15 min to 600 mg total. Monitor BP and ventilation.
   f. If seizures continue, **paraldehyde drip 4%** in NS. Titrate to control seizures. Monitor ventilation and IV site; infiltration may cause tissue necrosis.
   g. If all else fails, **general anesthesia** may be used to stop seizures.
8. Termination of treatment. If a patient has been seizure-free for 1–2 years, and EEG demonstrates no epileptiform activity, consider slowly withdrawing anticonvulsants over a period of several weeks.

F. Spinal Cord Injuries.

Spinal shock occurs following acute spinal cord injury, and may persist up to several weeks. Spinal shock is characterized by loss of reflexes in all segments below the lesion and atonic bladder.

1. **Syndromes of spinal cord injury** (Fig 13–6):
   a. **Central cord syndrome**—most commonly seen in trauma to patient with preexisting cervical spinal stenosis; loss of motor function greater in upper extremities than in lower extremities. Sensory loss is variable, may be in bandlike distribution. Recovery is first in lower extremities, then upper extremities.
   b. **Brown-Séquard syndrome** (hemisection of cord)—ipsilateral spastic paralysis below level of lesion, with ipsilateral loss of vibratory and position sense and contralateral loss of pain and temperature sensation, usually beginning one to two dermatomes below level of lesion.
   c. **Anterior cord syndrome**—most commonly vascular compression or occlusion of anterior spinal artery or major radicular artery secondary to atherosclerosis, aortic dissection; presents with complete paralysis, hypalgesia, and hypesthesia below level of lesion, but

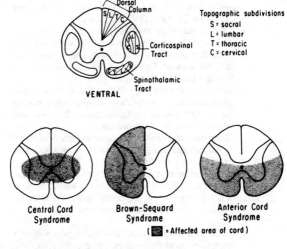

FIG 13–6.
Syndromes of spinal cord injury.

retained dorsal column function, i.e., intact vibratory and position sense.

2. **Treatment.**

a. Initial treatment is directed to **ABC**. If cervical fracture is suspected, the neck should not be moved and nasotracheal intubation or tracheostomy should be considered.

b. **Movement** of the patient with a suspected spine fracture and cord injury should be minimized, and spine should be moved as a unit, without rotation, flexion, or extension.

c. Recent studies with **high-dose methylprednisolone** demonstrate improved neurologic recovery if given within 8 hours of injury. Ideally, steroid therapy could begin in field or during transport to hospital. Therapy is begun with a bolus dose of 30 mg/kg IV given over 15 minutes followed by a 45-minute pause. A maintenance dose of 5.4 mg/kg/hr IV is then begun and continued for 23 hours, then discontinued.

d. Obtain **radiologic studies** (plain films, tomograms, CT) as needed to define fractures. Films of entire spine should be taken. In the patient with a higher-level fracture and associated neurologic deficit, a lower fracture may not be clinically evident.

e. If the observed neurologic deficit does not fit with documented fracture-dislocation, **myelography** may be necessary to rule out cord compression due to ruptured intervertebral disc or hematoma.

f. **Reduction** of a cervical fracture may be accomplished under radiographic guidance with cervical traction using a halo or cranial tongs.

g. **Stabilization** may be achieved with a cervical collar, halo vest, or cervical traction, for cervical fractures, or a corset or spica cast for thoracolumbar fractures. Internal fixation may be accomplished by a variety of techniques.

h. In the patient with a partial cord lesion, who is deteriorating, **surgical decompression,** may be required to remove bone fragments, disc material, or hematoma impinging on the cord.

i. The patient's **respiratory status** should be monitored closely. In high thoracic or cervical injuries, loss of intercostal muscle function may compromise ventilation. In addition, cervical cord injuries may involve the phrenic nerves (C3–5).

j. **BP** must be continuously monitored. Loss of sympathetic tone in spinal cord injuries should be treated with volume replacement (patient will diurese excess fluid as spinal shock clears). Elastic hose on the lower extremities and positioning the patient either horizontal or in Trendelenburg position may also assist in BP support.

k. **Bladder care:** Initially via Foley catheter, then as early as possible, switch to intermittent catheterization regimen. In conus or cauda equina injuries, bladder may remain hypotonic and bethanechol chloride (Urecholine) 10–50 mg po q.i.d. may help. To help prevent UTI, prophylactic antibiotics should be administered as long as catheterization is required (e.g., trimethoprim-sulfamethoxazole [Septra] two tablets b.i.d.).

l. **GI system:** Adynamic ileus may last several weeks. Use NG tube for gastric decompression, cimetidine 300 mg IV q.6h. or antacids to prevent ulcers. Bisacodyl (Dulcolax) suppositories given q.o.d. help regulate bowel movements.

m. **Deep venous thrombosis prophylaxis** with elastic stockings, external pneumatic compression stockings, and low-dose heparin (5,000 units SC q.12h.).

n. **Skin care** to prevent decubitus ulcers: "Log-roll" patient q.2h. Use egg crate mattress, sheepskin padding, rotating bed.

o. **Physical therapy** to prevent contractures.

p. Once patient's condition has stabilized, surgery may be performed to stabilize spine as needed. (Early surgery may cause increased neurologic deficit as the spinal cord is especially vulnerable in the immediate postinjury period.)

G. CNS Infections.

1. **Bacterial meningitis** may be seen in trauma, where the subarachnoid space has been exposed to contaminated areas (e.g., compound skull fractures), or with surgery or trauma extending into paranasal sinuses, mastoid air cells.

   a. **Etiology** varies according to source:

      1) Postcraniotomy or with open head trauma—*Staphylococcus aureus*.

      2) Postcraniotomy or posttrauma with CSF leak through paranasal sinuses—gram-negative rods (GNRs), *Escherichia coli, Pseudomonas; Streptococcus pneumoniae*.

      3) In spontaneous cases, most common etiology is related to age:

         a) 0–1 month—*E. Coli, Klebsiella, Str. pneumoniae*.

         b) 1 month–4 years—*Haemophilus influenzae, Neisseria meningitidis*.

         c) 4–30 years—*N. meningiditis, Str. pneumoniae*.

         d) 30–80 years—*Str. pneumoniae*.

b. **Diagnosis:**
   1) Symptoms and signs—fever, altered mental status, nuchal rigidity, other meningeal signs.
   2) LP. (*Note:* If focal neurologic examination, suspect focal lesion [e.g., localized infection] and obtain a CT scan. Do not perform LP if CT scan demonstrates a mass lesion.)

c. **Complications:** Cerebral edema, seizures, cortical venous thrombosis, subdural empyema, hydrocephalus.

d. **Treatment:** To be effective, antibiotics must cross the blood-brain barrier, and achieve therapeutic levels in CSF. Specific therapy should be targeted to the causative organism, and individually determined sensitivities. **Penicillin** is the drug of choice for meningitis of unknown etiology in adults and for pneumococcal or meningococcal meningitis. Because *H. influenzae* causes the majority of cases of meningitis in children over 2 months of age, **ampicillin-chloramphenicol** is the recommended initial treatment, until sensitivities are determined in culture isolates. In younger infants, **ampicillin plus gentamicin** will cover group B streptococci and GNRs—the common organisms in meningitis in this group. Several **third-generation cephalosporins** have an antibacterial spectrum and CSF penetration that make them useful for treatment of meningitis: moxalactam 8–12 g/day, or cefotaxime 12 g/day may be useful for gram-negative meningitis. **Aminoglycosides** have suboptimal CSF penetration, and intraventricular injection, via Ommaya or Rickham reservoir, may be required to achieve therapeutic levels in CSF.

2. **Shunt Infection.**
   a. **Ventriculoperitoneal shunts** have a 5%–10% infection rate. Most common organisms are skin flora including *Staphylococcus epidermidis, S. aureus,* or diphtheroids, although GNRs are also seen. Organisms may grow directly on the shunt and are shed into the CSF, causing ventriculitis and meningitis. Because the causative organisms are often low-grade pathogens, they may only cause a low-grade infection and the patient may present with low-grade fever with signs of shunt dysfunction or as acute sepsis. Because

the organisms grow directly on the shunt, CSF cultures may be negative in up to one third of cases, and obtaining fluid directly from the shunt reservoir will improve the yield on culture.

b. **Treatment:** Some patients may be successfully treated with a combination of systemic and intraventricular antibiotics; most often it is necessary to remove the shunt to cure the infection. After 1–2 weeks of antibiotic treatment with the shunt in place, the shunt may be removed and replaced at a different site, continuing antibiotics for 1–2 more weeks, depending on results of serial CSF sampling.

3. **Craniotomy wound infection** may involve scalp, bone, subdural, or subarachnoid spaces. Wound is tender, indurated, and erythematous. Treatment consists of antibiotics and wound debridement (including removal of devascularized bone flap). After removal of infected bone flap and successful treatment of the infection, a cranioplasty should be delayed for at least 1 year, to minimize changes of infecting the cranioplasty plate.

4. **Subdural empyema** may be seen with sinusitis, osteomyelitis, meningitis, infection of preexisting subdural fluid collection. Most common organisms are streptococci, staphylococci, GNRs.

   a. **Symptoms and signs**— headache, altered mental status, seizures, focal neurologic deficit, fever.

   b. **Diagnosis:**

      1) Plain films may demonstrate sinusitis or osteomyelitis.

      2) CT scan—low density extracerebral collection with an enhancing capsule.

   c. **Treatment:** This is a **neurosurgical emergency.**

      1) **Evacuate** purulent material through craniotomy or bur holes, taking care not to breach the arachnoid membrane. Remove primary source of infection, i.e., exenterate sinuses, remove infected bone. Subdural drain or wick is left in place.

      2) Broad-spectrum **antibiotics** until culture results available.

      3) In infants, serial subdural taps through the anterior fontanelle may replace craniotomy.

5. **Brain abscess.**
   a. **Source of infection:**
      1) **Parameningeal**—paranasal sinusitis spread to frontal lobes, mastoiditis to temporal lobe or cerebellum (streptococci, staphylococci).
      2) **Hematogenous spread,** especially in patients with right-to-left intracardiac shunts (various organisms).
      3) **Penetrating** cranial trauma or postcraniotomy, especially with retained foreign body or bone fragments (staphylococci).
   b. **Symptoms and signs**—headache, seizures, altered mental status with focal neurologic deficit, papilledema. Systemic signs of infection (fever, elevated WBCs) are typically absent unless there is a coexisting meningitis or other infection.
   c. **Diagnosis:**
      1) Plain films may demonstrate paranasal sinusitis.
      2) CT scan—mass lesion with enhancing rim around low density center with variable surrounding cerebral edema.
      3) LP will not make diagnosis of brain abscess and may lead to herniation if significant increased ICP or mass effect is present.
   d. **Treatment.**
      1) In early stages, with diffuse cerebritis, prior to formation of a discrete abscess, operation is not indicated and **antibiotic therapy** alone may eradicate the infection. Without cultures, begin penicillin (at least 20 million units/day) or nafcillin (12 g/day), chloramphenicol (3–4 g/day), and occasionally metronidazole (1,200–1,800 mg/day) for 4–6 weeks.
      2) **Surgical therapy**—if CT scan demonstrates well-formed abscess, may perform:
         a) Trephination with one or more taps, either freehand or with stereotactic guidance—may not drain loculated areas or satellite abscesses.
         b) Craniotomy for drainage of abscess without resecting capsule—may have recurrence.

 c) Craniotomy for excision of abscess in toto without opening abscess—may have more neurologic deficit with this method.

3) **Follow with serial CT scans.** Most abscesses require only one drainage with 4–6 weeks of antibiotics; 30%–70% will develop seizures within several years after onset.

6. **Spinal epidural empyema.** Hematogenous source, especially IV drug abusers, or postoperatively, *S. aureus* most common in either case.

a. **Symptoms and signs**—back pain with pain on percussion over spinous processes at level of infection. May have mild fever. As infection progresses, may see signs of cord or cauda equina compression.

b. **Diagnosis.**
1) LP: CSF reveals signs of parameningeal infection (see Chapter 22).
2) Plain films may show osteomyelitis.
3) Myelogram—partial or total epidural block.
4) CT scan with or without intrathecal contrast.
5) MRI scan.

c. **Treatment**—laminectomy for decompression and drainage of abscess with drains left in place; continue antibiotics for 4–6 weeks.

III. PERIOPERATIVE CARE.

A. Head Injuries.

Routine general principles of patient care including adequate fluid and caloric intake, oxygenation, except:

1. **Head of bed elevated 30 degrees** to reduce ICP, unless concomitant spine fractures.

2. **Restrict free water intake.** Follow serum electrolytes, osmolarity, urine specific gravity. Usually begin with D_5W ½ NS + 20 mEq/L KCl at 75 mL/hr (1,800 mL/day) for adults. **Hyponatremia** may be treated initially by restricting intake further to 500–1,000 mL/day. If Na falls to <120 mEq/L, may carefully diurese patient with furosemide or administer 3% NaCl 200 mL IV q.4h. by central line until Na is >130 mEq/l. Aim to correct Na by no more than 2 mEq/L/hr until Na of 125 is achieved in order to decrease risk of seizures and central pontine myelinolysis associated with too rapid correction of hyponatremia.

3. **Adequate caloric intake** is essential and nutrition should be addressed as soon as possible. A feeding tube should be placed and tube feeding begun as early as possible, with initial hypoosmolar feedings supplanted by hyperosmolar formulas as tolerated. Cimetidine to prevent peptic ulcers.

4. **Diabetes insipidus** may be treated as described under section III.B.6 (p 554).

5. **Pulmonary:** Avoid high PEEP (>12 cm H_2O) because of effect on ICP.

6. Skin care and positioning to prevent decubitus ulcer.

7. Control of ICP as described above.

8. **Check for signs of CSF leak**—CSF oto- or rhinorrhea, especially in basilar skull fractures. If present, head elevated 30 degrees will stop majority of cases. If not, check for hydrocephalus or increased ICP, watch for meningitis. Lumbar drain with slight negative pressure may stop leak. If leak persists, operative exploration and dural repair may be required.

9. **Deep venous thrombosis prophylaxis** with elastic stockings and external pneumatic compression stockings.

B. **Craniotomy.**

Similar to care of patients with head injuries, with details specific for given procedure.

1. **Preoperative orders (general).**

   a. NPO past midnight.

   b. Antibacterial shower (or sponge bath) and shampoo.

   c. Dexamethasone 10 mg po at midnight and at 6 A.M.

   d. On call to OR:

      1) Anti-thrombosis stockings/hose.

      2) Void.

      3) Diazepam 5–10 mg IM or IV.

   e. In induction room—for ventriculoperitoneal shunts and as desired for other cases, prophylactic antibiotics (e.g., vancomycin 1 g IV slowly over at least 1 hour to avoid side effects).

2. **General, routine postoperative orders.**

   a. VS with neurologic checks (level of consciousness, pupils, strength) per recovery room, then q.1h.

   b. Elevate head of bed 30 degrees.

   c. NPO until fully alert, then sips for first 12 hours after operation.

   d. D5 ½ NS IV + 20 mEq/L KCl at 75 mL/hr.

    e. Foley catheter to straight drain. Record intake and output q.1h.

    f. Medications:

       1) Dexamethasone 4 mg IV or q.6h. for 5 days.

       2) Methylprednisolone 40 mg IM on fourth postoperative day.

       3) Cimetidine 300 mg IV or PO q.6h. for 5 days.

       4) Acetaminophen 650 mg PO prn pain or temperature >38.5° C.

       5) Codeine 30 mg IM or PO q.4h. prn severe pain. Use with caution as neurologic examination is vital.

       6) Promethazine 25 mg IM or PO q.4h. prn nausea, vomiting.

       7) Anticonvulsants continued as preoperatively.

       8) Other preoperative medications continued, e.g., cardiac, antihypertensive, pulmonary drugs.

    g. Laboratory studies.

       1) CBC, serum chemistries, ABG in recovery room, on first evening and next morning.

       2) X-ray films to document hardware placement, e.g., for spinal fusions, shunts.

    h. Call house officer for temperature >38.5° C, UO <30 mL/hr for 2 hours, or declining neurologic status.

3. **Intracranial aneurysm.** Usually present with SAH, although may present as a mass lesion (third nerve palsy with posterior communicating artery aneurysm, chiasmal syndrome with anterior communicating artery aneurysm).

    a. **Preoperative care.**

       1) Attempt to avoid rebleeding (each episode of rebleeding associated with increased morbidity and mortality). Majority of episodes of rebleeding occur within 4 weeks of initial hemorrhage.

       2) Maintain cerebral perfusion in presence of spasm of cerebral vessels. Risk of vasospasm related to amount of blood in subarachnoid space surrounding vessels of circle of Willis. Vasospasm has onset around day 4, peaks at day 7, and usually resolves by day 21.

       3) These goals may be mutually limiting. Lowering pressure to decrease risk of rebleeding may lead to ischemia and increasing cerebral blood volume to

maintain perfusion may lead to aneurysm rerupture.

b. **Special orders** for patients with SAH secondary to aneurysm rupture:

1) **Elevate head of bed 10–15 degrees.** Promote venous drainage and CSF outflow since 10% develop communicating hydrocephalus. Avoid rapid decrease in ICP as this may lead to aneurysm rupture.

2) **SAH precautions**—quiet, darkened room; stool softeners; nothing per rectum, restricted visitation.

3) **Aminocaproic acid** 36 g/1,000 mL NS over 24 hours to prevent clot lysis in patients with documented aneurysm. If early operation is planned, may eliminate need for drug.

4) **BP control:** Use antihypertensives with caution owing to danger of ischemia with vasospasm. Acute hypertension often accompanies SAH and decreasing BP may exacerbate neurologic deficits.

5) **Vasospasm** is treated with plasma volume expansion. Plasma protein fraction, albumin, or blood may be used with caution to avoid rebleeding.

6) **Nimodipine** may be beneficial in the prevention of vasospasm secondary to SAH. Dosage is 60 mg PO q.4h. for 21 days.

7) Interventional neuroradiologic techniques utilizing **balloon angioplasty** may be used to directly dilate constricted cerebral arteries in patients with severe vasospasm with neurologic deficits unresponsive to volume expansion and nimodipine therapy.

8) In patients of good neurologic grade <4 days after SAH, with documented aneurysm and no vasospasm on arteriogram, **early surgery** for clip ligation of aneurysm and removal of some subarachnoid blood yields improved survival and eliminates risk of rebleeding, simplifying patient treatment. Operation during period of vasospasm, however, causes increased morbidity and mortality. In such cases, operation should

be deferred for 2 weeks, until vasospasm is resolving.

c. **Postoperative care:** Maximize cerebral perfusion,
therefore use routine craniotomy orders, except:
1) IV rate 100–150 mL/hr to maintain UO ≥50 mL/
hr.
2) Maintain BP at least at preoperative level.
3) Plasma protein fraction 250 mL IV q.6h. Gradually taper after 48 hours.
4) To monitor fluid status in case of vasospasm or
CHF, a PA catheter may be placed and PCWP
maintained at 15–29 mm Hg if the patient's heart
will allow, using plasma protein fraction, albumin, or blood.
5) Nimodipine: Continue 60 mg PO q.4h. for 21
days.
6) Aminocaproic acid should not be continued postoperatively.
7) Repeat arteriogram is obtained postoperatively to
document clip ligation of aneurysm.

4. **Arteriovenous malformation (AVM).**
a. As with aneurysm, may present with SAH or intra-
parenchymal hemorrhage; also with seizures, headache.
b. Preoperative care is similar to aneurysm but aminocaproic acid is not used. Vascular radiology may embolize AVM to reduce blood supply, making operation
easier.
c. Postoperative care—routine craniotomy orders.
Avoid hypotension, hypovolemia. Postoperative arteriogram will document extent of resection.

5. **Tumors**—preoperative studies to include CT scan, MRI,
or arteriography, as indicated. High-dose steroids to reduce cerebral edema preoperatively should be slowly tapered postoperatively.

6. **Transsphenoidal pituitary adenomectomy.**
a. **Preoperative evaluation** should include endocrine
evaluation to establish baseline, especially thyroid
function; visual fields; CT scan with coronal bone win-
dows of sphenoid sinus, or preferably MRI with axial,
coronal, and sagittal views to demonstrate positions of
carotid arteries in region of sella.

    b. **Preoperative orders:** Patients should be assumed to be panhypopituitary and should receive cortisone acetate 200 mg b.i.d. for 48 hours preoperatively.

    c. **Postoperative orders:**

      1) Elevate head of bed 30 degrees to minimize possibility of CSF rhinorrhea.

      2) Cortisone acetate tapered over 5–7 days to maintenance 25 mg in A.M. and 12.5 mg in P.M.

      3) Monitor intake and output, serum chemistries, and urine specific gravity for signs of **diabetes insipidus (DI)**. If urine output >200 mL/hr for 2 hours, with specific gravity <1.005, serum Na 150 mEq/L, give aqueous Vasopressin 5 units IM. Awake patients with intact thirst mechanisms may be able to keep up with their UO through PO intake, at least during the day. In patients unable to drink, it is best to base IV fluid administration on previous IV deficit using D5W. Often, DI is transient but if persistent, may require patient to continue on nasal desmopressin 2–4 μg prn.

      4) Cefazolin 1 g IV q.8h. until nasal packs removed.

      5) Monitor endocrine status—may require thyroid replacement.

C. Spinal Procedures.

  1. **Extradural** (e.g., anterior cervical discectomy and fusion [ACDF], cervical or thoracic laminectomies with or without fusion)—may consider preoperative steroids: dexamethasone 10 mg po at midnight and on morning of operation to protect spinal cord for ACDF, cervical laminectomies for spondylosis (do not need to continue postoperatively). In postoperative period, watch for signs of cord compression, e.g., epidural hematoma or CSF leak. After extensive cervical laminectomies for spondylosis in elderly patients, raise head of bed slowly over several days to avoid postural hypotension.

  2. **Intradural:**

    a. **Preoperative**—steroids used as for craniotomy cases.

    b. **Postoperative**—to minimize pressure on dural suture line and prevent CSF leaks:

      1) Head of bed elevated 30 degrees for cervical or upper thoracic cases.

2) Patient to remain flat in bed for 5 days for lower thoracic and lumbar cases.

3) Monitor patient for signs of cord compression, e.g., epidural hematoma.

SELECTED REFERENCES

NEUROLOGICAL EXAMINATION

DeJong RN: *The Neurological Examination. Incorporating the Fundamentals of Neuroanatomy and Neurophysiology,* ed 4. Hagerstown, Md, Harper & Row, 1979.

Fisher CM: The neurological examination of the comatose patient. *Acta Neurol Scand* 1969; 45:1.

Patten J: *Neurological Differential Diagnosis*. London, Harold Starke, 1977.

Plum F, Posner JB: *The Diagnosis of Stupor and Coma,* ed 3. Philadelphia, FA Davis Co, 1980.

INCREASED INTRACRANIAL PRESSURE

Bedford RF, Persing JA, Pobereskin L, et al: Lidocaine or thiopental for rapid control of intracranial hypertension? *Anesth Analg* 1980; 59:435.

Cottrell JE, Robustelli A, Post K, et al: Furosemide and mannitol-induced changes in ICP and serum osmolality and electrolytes. *Anesthesiology* 1977; 47:28.

Kosteljanetz M: Acute head injury: Pressure-volume relations and cerebrospinal fluid dynamics. *Neurosurgery* 1986; 18:17.

McGraw CP: Continuous intracranial pressure monitoring: A review of techniques and presentation of methods. *Surg Neurol* 1976; 6:149.

Narayan RK, Kishore PRS, et al: Intracranial pressure: To monitor or not to monitor? A review of our experience with severe head injury. *J Neurosurg* 1982; 56:650.

SEIZURES

Delgado-Escueta AV, Wasterlain C, Treiman DM, et al: Current concepts in neurology: Management of status epilepticus. *N Engl J Med* 1982; 306:1337.

Millichap JG: Drug therapy: Drug treatment of convulsive disorders. *N Engl J Med* 1972; 286:464.

Sutherland JM, Eadie MJ: The epilepsies: Modern diagnosis and treatment, Edinburgh, Churchill Livingstone, Ltd, 1980.

SPINAL CORD INJURY

Bracken MB, Shepard MJ, et al: A randomized, controlled trial of methylprednisolone or naloxone in the treatment of acute spinal cord injury. *N Engl J Med* 1990; 322:1405.

Feuer J: Management of acute spine and spinal cord injuries, old and new concepts. *Arch Surg* 1976; 111:638.

Gehweiler JA, Osborne RL, Becker RF: *The Radiology of Vertebral Trauma*. Philadelphia, WB Saunders Co, 1980.

Wagner FC: Management of acute spinal cord injury. *Surg Neurol* 1977; 7:346.

CNS INFECTIONS

Everett ED, Strausbaugh LJ: Antimicrobial agents and the central nervous system. *Neurosurgery* 1990; 6:691.

Samson DS, Clark K: A current review of brain abscess. *Am J Med* 1973; 54:201.

Wilson N: Infections of the nervous system. Philadelphia, FA Davis Co, 1979.

PERIOPERATIVE CARE

Allen GS, Ahn HS, Preziosi TJ, et al: Cerebral arterial spasm— a controlled trial of nimodipine in patients with subarachnoid hemorrhage. *N Engl J Med* 1983; 308:619.

Drake CG: Management of cerebral aneurysms. *Stroke* 1981; 12:273.

Horwitz NH, Rizzoli HV: Postoperative complications of intracranial neurological surgery. Baltimore, Williams & Wilkins Co, 1982.

Peerless SJ: Pre- and postoperative management of cerebral aneurysms. *Clin Neurosurg* 1979; 26:209.

Philippon J, Grob R, et al: Prevention of vasospasm in subarachnoid haemorrhage. A controlled study with nimodipine. *Acta Neurochir* 1986; 82:110.

THE ENDOCRINE   *14*
SYSTEM

I. DIABETES MELLITUS.
A. Preoperative Considerations.

Not only are diabetic patients at higher risk for coronary artery disease, renal failure, and peripheral vascular disease than nondiabetics, they require major surgical procedures more frequently and consequently have higher morbidity and mortality rates than nondiabetics. Other preoperative considerations include the propensity of diabetic patients to suffer acute tubular necrosis with dehydration and exposure to contrast agents for radiologic studies, and the abnormal responses of patients with diabetic autonomic neuropathy to anesthetic agents and other drugs. Poorly controlled diabetes results in an increased infection rate, poor wound healing, and susceptibility to osmotic diuresis and dehydration.

B. Glucose Monitoring.

Blood glucose should be monitored in all critically ill patients. Stress alters glucose metabolism which may aggravate preexisting glucose intolerance in overt or occult diabetics, but may also produce glucose intolerance in the previously normal patient. Methods to monitor blood glucose include:

1. **Blood glucose**—definitive, but one must wait for laboratory to report result. Usually values <140 mg/dL in the nonstressed patient and <175 mg/dL in the stressed patient are considered normal. May be spuriously elevated if blood sample is drawn proximal to an IV glucose infusion.

2. **Fingerstick**—immediate value obtainable. Must establish correlation with serum glucose and then can be used to follow trends. Values >400 mg/dL or <80 mg/dL require stat blood glucose determination.

3. **Urine sugar and acetone**—generally not reliable unless correlation with serum glucose is established and double-

voided specimen obtained. May not detect elevated blood glucose in the presence of renal insufficiency.

C. **Treatment of Hyperglycemia.**

Reasonable control of blood glucose is essential to prevent dehydration, avoid DKA, and promote anabolic actions of insulin. However, the dangers of iatrogenic hypoglycemia outweigh the risks of undertreatment and hyperglycemia. This is especially true in patients who are sedated, intubated, comatose, or unresponsive as the warning signs of hypoglycemia will be missed. Therefore, reasonable but not rigid control of blood glucose is sought with a target of maintaining levels **<250 mg/dL.** The initial steps to reduce blood glucose include eliminating glucose from IV solutions. This is rarely effective in the critically ill and insulin for blood glucose control is commonly required. Oral hypoglycemic agents are not indicated for control in the acute setting.

1. **Insulin types.**

Human insulin is used as the standard class of insulin. It is useful in the diabetic with antibodies to bovine or porcine-derived insulin. Short-acting or **regular insulin** is used in the acutely ill to allow for rapid responses. Other types of insulin are listed in Table 14–1.

2. **Insulin delivery.**

IV administration is desirable in the acutely ill patient because other methods of delivery rely on tissue perfusion which may be unpredictable in the unstable patient.

a. **IV bolus:** 5–10 units regular insulin IV bolus provides rapid response, accurate dosing. Requires supplemental insulin because of short $T\frac{1}{2}$.

b. **IV infusion:** 1–2 units/hr regular insulin IV administered by infusion pump is typical starting dose (25

TABLE 14–1.

Pharmacokinetics of Subcutaneously Administered Insulin

Insulin	Action	Onset (hr)	Peak (hr)	Duration (hr)
Regular (Semilente)	Short	0.5–1.0	2–4	6
			4–8	12–16
NPH (Lente)	Intermediate	1–2	8–12	18–24
Protamine (Ultralente)	Long	4–8	12–24	36

units/250 mL NS at 10–20 mL/hr). Blood glucose is monitored q.h. with titration of insulin infusion to maintain blood glucose <250 mg/dL.

c. **Intramuscular:** 5–10 units regular insulin IM has intermediate absorption and a longer $T\frac{1}{2}$ than an IV bolus.

d. **Subcutaneous:** SC is least reliable in hypoperfused patient, but advantageous in well-perfused patient because of longer $T\frac{1}{2}$ (see Table 14–1).

3. **Insulin dosage.**

In the SICU, insulin is usually administered in response to measured blood glucose levels. Various guidelines to initiate therapy are listed; however, administration of insulin requires repeated determinations of blood glucose to monitor its effect. In general, the amount of insulin required in the nonstressed or preoperative setting serves as a guide to the baseline amount of insulin required. For example, if a patient required 40 units/24 hr preoperatively, he will probably need **at least** that amount postoperatively. Exceptions are patients with exacerbated glucose intolerance due to infection who have surgical drainage of that infection, whose total postoperative insulin requirements may be less than preoperative requirements. **Guidelines to administer IV or SC insulin** based on measured blood glucose are given in Tables 14–2 and 14–3. Individual responses vary and blood glucose monitoring at 1–2-hour intervals until glucose levels approach 250 mg/dL is suggested in the critically ill. If blood glucose levels are persistently elevated, the total amount of insulin required the previous day is administered in four divided doses in ad-

TABLE 14–2.

Intravenous Administration of Regular Insulin (25 units in 250 mL NS)

Blood Glucose (mg/dL)	Infusion Rate (mL/hr)	Insulin Rate (units/hr)
0–100	0	0
100–200	5–20	0.5–2.0
200–300	20–30	2.0–3.0
300–400	30–40	3.0–4.0
400+	10 + supplement	4.0 + supplement

TABLE 14-3.

Subcutaneous Administration of
Regular Insulin Every 6 Hours
(Sliding Scale)

Blood Glucose (mg/dL)	Regular Insulin
0-100	0
100-200	0
200-300	5 units
300-400	10 units
400+	10 units + supplement

dition to the sliding scale. For example, if a patient received 4 × 10 units of insulin q.6h. by sliding scale and blood glucose levels remained 300-400 mg/dL, in the next 24 hours, 10 units (40/4) of regular insulin is administered SC q.6h. *in addition* to the sliding scale.

D. Preoperative Management

1. Preoperative glucose control required prior to elective surgery.

2. Preoperative electrolyte abnormalities, especially hypokalemia, must be corrected.

3. Adequate hydration must be maintained.

4. Patients with non-insulin-dependent diabetes (NIDDM) undergoing relatively nonstressful surgical procedures rarely require exogenous insulin replacement. Patients requiring preoperative insulin and patients who are controlled with oral hypoglycemics undergoing major surgical procedures require postoperative blood glucose management with exogenous insulin.

E. Management of Non-IDDM Patients Undergoing Major Surgery.

1. Patients with diabetes mellitus controlled with diet or oral hypoglycemic agents undergoing the stress of major surgical procedures usually require exogenous insulin to control blood sugar intraoperatively and postoperatively. Few patients require long-term insulin after the acute stress of the surgical procedure.

2. Preoperative orders:
   a. NPO after midnight.
   b. Start IV of D5 ½ NS + 20 mEq/L KCl at 75–100 mL/hr the night prior to surgery.
   c. 5 units regular insulin SC at 6 A.M.
3. Postoperative orders: Postoperatively, the goals are to maintain blood glucose at ≤ 250 mg/dL and to avoid ketosis.
   a. Stat blood glucose (Chem CS) in recovery room.
   b. Intravenous fluid: D$_5$ ½ NS + 20 mEq/L KCl at 75–100 mL/hr.
   c. Fingerstick or blood glucose q.6h.
   d. Regular insulin SC q.6h. by sliding scale.
4. As the patient resumes oral feedings, convert to preoperative regimen.

F. **Management of Insulin-Dependent Diabetic Patients (IDDM) Undergoing Minor Surgical Procedures.**
   1. The diabetic patient undergoing operation not expected to cause major stress should receive **one-half** the usual dose of insulin SC on the morning of operation.
   2. Preoperative orders:
      a. NPO after midnight.
      b. Start IV of D5 ½ NS + 20 mEq/L KCl at 75–100 mL/hr the night prior to surgery or at 6 A.M.
   3. Postoperative orders: Postoperatively, the goals are to maintain blood glucose at ≤ 250 mg/dL and to avoid ketosis.
      a. Stat blood glucose (Chem CS) in recovery room.
      b. IVF: D$_5$ ½ NS + 20 mEq/L KCl at 75–100 mL/hr.
      c. Fingerstick or blood glucose q.6h.
      d. Regular insulin SC q.6h. Total daily insulin required preoperatively is administered as regular insulin q.6h. with supplemental insulin administered by sliding scale. For example, if total daily insulin requirement was 40 units, administer 10 units SC q.6h. with supplemental sliding scale insulin.
   4. The patient is maintained with a daily insulin regimen until an oral diet is tolerated at which point the usual insulin regimen is instituted.

G. **Management of IDDM Patients Undergoing Major Surgical Procedures.**
   1. The IDDM patient is managed either with regular insulin q.6h. plus a sliding scale or with a continuous IV insulin

infusion. IV infusion has the advantage of more precise blood glucose control and less risk of hypoglycemia. The infusion is started either in the OR or immediately postoperatively. The patient must receive IV dextrose via a separate IV access when receiving IV insulin.

2. Preoperative orders:
   a. NPO after midnight.
   b. Start IV of D_5 ½ NS + 20 mEq/L KCl at 75–100 mL/hr the night prior to surgery or at 6 A.M.
   c. ½ total regular insulin dose SC at 6 A.M.

3. Postoperative orders:
   a. Stat blood glucose.
   b. 25 units regular insulin in 250 mL NS at 10 mL/hr.
   c. Via separate IV D_5 ½ NS + 20 mEq/L KCl at 100 mL/hr.
   d. Blood glucose after 1 hour and q.2h. (until blood glucose stabilizes, then at least q.4h.).

4. The insulin infusion may be increased to 40 mL/hr (4 units/hr) to control persistent hyperglycemia. The infusion is stopped after 24–48 hours with conversion to either a q.6h. insulin regimen with supplemental sliding scale insulin, or if the patient is taking oral feedings, to the usual insulin dose.

H. Management of Diabetic Ketoacidosis.

1. DKA is the most severe form of insulin deficiency characterized by hyperglycemia, dehydration, ketosis, and anion gap acidosis.

2. Decreased insulin levels lead to decreased peripheral glucose uptake, and accelerated hepatic glycogenolysis and gluconeogenesis, leading to **hyperglycemia, osmotic diuresis, dehydration, and electrolyte abnormalities.** With decreasing insulin, adipose tissue lipolysis occurs to release FFAs and glycerol. FFAs are converted into ketone bodies in the liver. **Metabolic acidosis** results from the release of H^+ from the liver along with 3-hydroxybutyrate and acetoacetate. This depletes plasma bicarbonate levels causing the characteristic anion gap acidosis.

3. **Therapy consists of low-dose insulin and volume replacement.** Low-dose insulin is used to avoid hypoglycemia and vigorous fluid and electrolyte replacement is emphasized. DKA is often precipitated by an infection or other acute illness. Underlying pathologic conditions

should be sought and managed during resuscitation and treatment.

  a. **Insulin therapy:** IV loading dose of 10–20 units regular insulin followed by continuous infusion of 5–10 units/hr. The insulin infusion is decreased to 1–5 units/hr when the blood glucose reaches 250 mg/dL. At this point dextrose is added to the infusate. Serum glucose levels should decrease at a rate $\leq$ 100 mg/dL/ hr to avoid cerebral edema.

  b. **Fluid therapy:** Fluid replacement to replace a volume deficit of 5–10 L is started with NS. The IV fluid is changed to D_5NS when the serum glucose is < 250 mg/dL. The presence of other medical problems may be an indication for CVP monitoring but should not prevent aggressive fluid resuscitation.

  c. **Potassium replacement:** Total body K^+ is depleted despite artificially elevated serum K^+ levels secondary to acidosis. Insulin treatment and correction of acidosis compound hypokalemia as K^+ is taken up by cells. Average K^+ requirements over the first 24 hours range from 200–350 mEq/L.

  d. **Bicarbonate therapy:** Replace HCO_3^- if arterial pH < 7.2

  e. **Phosphate therapy:** Replace phosphate if marked hypophosphatemia is present.

4. **Summary of management of DKA.**

  a. **Diagnosis and monitoring:**

    1) Hemodynamic monitoring as indicated.

    2) ABG, blood glucose, serum electrolytes, PO_4^{2-}, Mg^{2+} stat.

    3) ABG, blood glucose, K^+ q.1h. × 4, then q.2h.

  b. **Volume replacement:**

    1) Anticipate 5–10 L volume deficit

    2) NS + 10 mEq/L KCl at 500 mL/hr (if infusion via central venous line, increase KCl to 20 mEq/L).

    3) When serum glucose <250 mg/dL, convert IV to dextrose-containing fluid (D_5NS).

    4) When serum Na >150–155 mEq/L, convert IV to hypotonic fluid (½ NS).

  c. **Insulin:**

    1) 10 units regular insulin IV stat.

    2) Infusion of 50 units regular insulin in 500 mL NS at 50 mL/hr.

        3) Decrease infusion to 1–5 units/hr when blood glucose <250 mg/dL.

   d. **Potassium:**

      1) Replace by supplementing IV fluid with 10–20 mEq/L KCl until serum K^+ >5.0.

      2) Replace with K_2HPO_4 if hypophosphatemia present.

   e. **Acid-base:**

      1) If arterial pH <7.1 or $NaHCO_3$ <5 mEq/L, give two ampules $NaHCO_3$ (44–88 mEq/L).

      2) If arterial pH <7.0, give three ampules $NaHCO_3$.

   f. $PO_4{}^{2-}$: Replace if <2.0 mg/dL.

   g. Mg^{2+}: Replace if <1.5 mg/dL.

I.   **Management of Hyperosmolar Nonketotic Diabetic Coma.**

   1. **Hyperosmolar nonketotic diabetic coma (HNDC)** is characterized by severe hyperglycemia with attendant dehydration, electrolyte depletion, dehydration, serum hyperosmolarity (often > 350 mOsm/L), minimal ketosis or acidosis. Abnormal neurologic function is common.

   2. The **neurologic dysfunction** is apparently due to the hyperosmolarity. The reasons why patients with HNDC fail to develop significant ketosis despite apparent relative insulin deficiency remain unclear.

   3. **Treatment involves fluids, insulin, and potassium.** Patients are usually more volume-depleted than those with DKA. Hemoconcentration is common with Hcts as high as 90%. As with DKA, HNDC is often precipitated by infection or other acute illness. Underlying pathologic conditions should be sought and managed during resuscitation.

   a. **Fluid therapy:** Fluid replacement to replace a volume deficit of 5–15 L is started with ½ NS. The IV fluid is changed to D5 ½ NS when the serum glucose < 250 mg/dL. Isotonic saline may be used in hypotensive patients. CVP monitoring is often required in the elderly.

   b. **Insulin therapy:** Patients with HNDC may be extremely sensitive to insulin and IV continuous infusion of regular insulin 5–10 units/hr is used. The insulin infusion is discontinued when blood glucose reaches 250 mg/dL. At this point dextrose is added. Serum glucose levels should decrease at a rate $\leq$ 100 mg/dL/hr to avoid cerebral edema.

c. **Potassium replacement:** Total body K^+ is depleted despite artificially elevated serum K^+ levels secondary to acidosis. Insulin treatment and correction of acidosis compound the problem as K^+ is taken up by cells. Average K^+ requirements over the first 24 hours range from 200–350 mEq/L.

4. **Summary of management of HNDC.**
   a. **Diagnosis and monitoring:**
      1) Hemodynamic monitoring as indicated.
      2) ABG, blood glucose, serum electrolytes, PO_4^{2-}, Mg^{2+} stat.
      3) ABG, blood glucose, K^+ q.1h. × 4, then q.2h.
   b. **Volume replacement:**
      1) Anticipate 5–15 L volume deficit
      2) ½ NS + 10 mEq/L KCl at 500 mL/hr (if infusion via central venous line, increase KCl to 20 mEq/L).
      3) When serum glucose < 250 mg/dL, convert IV to dextrose-containing fluid (D_5 ½ NS).
      4) If hypotensive, switch to isotonic fluid (NS).
   c. **Insulin:**
      1) Infusion of 50 units regular insulin in 500 mL NS at 50 mL/hr.
      2) Decrease infusion to 1–5 units/hr when blood glucose <250 mg/dL.
   d. **Potassium:** Replace by supplementing IV fluid with 10–20 mEq/L KCl until serum K^+ >5.0.

II. ACUTE ADRENAL INSUFFICIENCY.

A. **Acute adrenal insufficiency (AAI)** is a life-threatening metabolic emergency due to inadequate amounts of adrenocorticosteroids to support the patient. This deficiency may be caused by destruction of the adrenal cortex or inadequate secretion of ACTH which may be occult until the stress of major illness or surgical procedure increases the demand for corticosteroids. This relative lack of corticosteroids may result in AAI (addisonian crisis) which is catastrophic if unrecognized. Many cases of adrenal crisis may occur in patients with chronic primary adrenal insufficiency (Addison's disease), but **the most common cause is increased stress in a patient with adrenal suppression from taking exogenous corticosteroids for various conditions.** Less commonly, acute adrenal hemorrhage due to anticoagulation or meningococcal sepsis may cause AAI. The normal adrenal gland secretes 20–30 mg/day of cortisol, but this may be increased to 300–400 mg/day during stress. Cortisol deficiency can result in multisystem failure. **Hypotension** results from decreased vascular tone, **hyponatremia** from inadequate free water clearance by the kidney, **hyperkalemia** and **metabolic acidosis** from inadequate mineralocorticoid action on the kidney. **Hypoglycemia** is due to absent glycogenolytic and gluconeogenic effects of cortisol. Nonspecific symptoms and signs are listed in Table 14–4.

B. **Diagnosis of AAI.**

 1. **The diagnosis of AAI** should be suspected in any patient with unexplained hypotension, particularly if accompanied by nausea, vomiting, and fever. A history of steroid use, adrenal insufficiency, hypopituitarism, or pituitary or adrenal surgery should be sought. Other clues include signs and symptoms related to underlying diseases including meningococcemia.

 2. **Tests for AAI include:**

  a. Serum cortisol.

   1) A.M. normal 8–25 μg/dL.

   2) P.M. normal 5–15 μg/dL.

   3) <5 μg/dL in A.M. suggests insufficiency.

  b. **ACTH stimulation.**

   1) 0.25 μg IV cosyntropin and plasma cortisol measured at 30 minutes and, 1 and 2 hours

   2) Peak level at 30–60 minutes should be > 18 μg/dL.

TABLE 14–4.

Symptoms and Signs of Acute Adrenal Insufficiency

Symptoms	Signs	Laboratory Diagnosis
Weakness	Fever	Hyponatremia
Apathy	Hypotension	Hyperkalemia
Anorexia		Acidosis
Weight loss		Hypoglycemia
Nausea		Eosinophilia
Vomiting		Lymphocytosis
Abdominal pain		Low cortisol
Diarrhea		

        3) If cortisol doubles or exceeds 30 µg/dL, primary adrenal insufficiency is excluded.

C. Treatment.

1. **Treatment** includes adrenocorticosteroid replacement, IV fluids, and electrolyte repletion. Corticosteroid replacement begins with a preparation incorporating both glucocorticoid and mineralocorticoid activity such as hydrocortisone (Solu-Cortef) (Table 14–5).

2. **Methylprednisolone and dexamethasone** should be avoided.

3. **Treatment** must begin prior to definitive evidence of adrenal insufficiency (low serum cortisol). Empiric therapy in patients clinically suspected of having AAI should begin immediately.

4. From the knowledge that the normal adrenal gland is thought to secrete 300–400 mg/day of cortisol under stress, appropriate replacement doses can be calculated (see Table 14–5). Cortisone and prednisone require hepatic conversion to the biologically active relatives cortisol (hydrocortisone) and prednisolone. A solution of 5% glucose in NS is used to restore plasma volume, correct hypotension, replace Na^+ and correct hypoglycemia. **The initial treatment includes:**
   a. 200 mg hydrocortisone IV stat.
   b. 100 mg hydrocortisone IV q.6h. (for a daily dose of 400 mg).
   c. D_5NS 1 L IV/1 hr.
   d. D_5NS + 20 mEq/L KCl at 250 mL/hr until rehydration is complete.
   e. Frequent serum Na^+ and K^+ levels.

5. **Maintenance therapy:** When stability is achieved, substitute one of the longer-acting glucocorticoids. Hydrocortisone contains sufficient mineralocorticoid activity to reverse hyperkalemia and promote Na retention, but other preparations may need supplements. A mineralocorticoid such as desoxycortisone acetate (Doca) 5 mg IM b.i.d. or fludrocortisone acetate (Florinef) 0.1–0.2 mg/day po is administered if hypokalemia or hypotension persist. Maintenance therapy:
   a. Prednisone 5 mg PO in A.M., 2.5 mg po in P.M.
   b. Fludrocortisone acetate 0.1–0.2 mg po in A.M.
   c. Adjust dosage based on BP and electrolytes

TABLE 14-5.
Steroid Preparations

Name	T1/2 (hr)	Glucocorticoid Potency Relative to Cortisol*	Mineralocorticoid Activity Relative to Cortisol*	Equivalent Glucocorticoid Dose (mg)
Glucocorticoids				
Cortisol	8–12	1	1	20
Cortisone	8–12	0.8	0.8	25
Prednisone	12–36	4	0.8	5
Prednisolone	12–36	4	0.8	5
6α-Methylprednisolone	12–36	5	0.5	4
Triaminolone	12–36	5	0	4
Betamethasone	36–72	10	0	2
Dexamethasone	36–72	25	0	0.6
Paramethasone	36–72	30	0	0.75
Mineralocorticoids				
Desoxycorticosterone		+	++	
Fludrocortisone		+	++	

*+ = some activity; ++ = considerable activity.

D. Treatment of Patients on Preoperative Steroid Therapy.

1. Unless patients taking steroids for various medical diseases are treated with appropriate pre- and postoperative steroid replacement, the stress of a major surgical procedure will likely result in acute adrenal insufficiency.

2. Any patient on chronic oral steroid therapy in the 3 months prior to admission should have the dose increased or converted to IV therapy prior to major surgical procedures. The IV infusion may be either continuous or intermittent and should continue postoperatively until the patient can once again be converted to oral prednisone.

3. **Intermittent:**

   a. Hydrocortisone 100 mg IV at 6 A.M. on day of procedure and 100 mg IV q.6h. until recovery from initial stress.

   b. Wean from stress dose hydrocortisone to preoperative dose over a 6-day period. For example, in a patient taking prednisone 5 mg PO q.d. preoperatively, a steroid taper (Table 14–6) would consist of:

TABLE 14–6.
Steroid Taper

Postoperative Day	Drug/Dosage
1	Hydrocortisone 100 mg IV q.8h.
2	Hydrocortisone 80 mg IV q.8h.
3	Hydrocortisone 60 mg IV q.8h. (or prednisone 18 mg po q.12h.)
4	Hydrocortisone 40 mg IV q.8h. (or prednisone 12 mg po q.12h.)
5	Hydrocortisone 20 mg IV q.8h. (or prednisone 6 mg po q.12h.)
6	Hydrocortisone 10 mg IV q.8h. (or prednisone 5 mg PO q.d.)
7	Prednisone 5 mg po q.d.*

*Prednisone is given when patient is tolerating po diet.

4. **Continuous:** Hydrocortisone 100 mg in 250 mL D_5W at 10 mL/hr until patient able to tolerate po fluids, then convert to an equivalent prednisone dose given q.12h. and rapidly taper to preoperative dose.

III. PHEOCHROMOCYTOMA.

A. The control of hypertension is the goal of preoperative and intraoperative management in patients with pheochromocytoma. Therapy is directed toward the blockade of catechol-amine receptors on end organs.

B. α-Adrenergic Receptor Blockade.

1. The drug of choice for preoperative preparation is the α-adrenergic antagonist **phenoxybenzamine.** Phenoxybenzamine produces a cumulative noncompetitive α-receptor blockade. The dosage is:
   a. Phenoxybenzamine 10 mg po q.12h.
   b. Increase in 10-mg increments until BP control is obtained.
2. Patients should have a normal BP on a fixed dose of phenoxybenzamine prior to invasive diagnostic or surgical procedures. High doses of phenoxybenzamine cause postural hypotension.

C. β-Adrenergic Receptor Blockade. The β-antagonist **propranolol** is a useful adjunct in patients with tachyarrhythmias following adequate α-blockade with phenoxybenzamine. Patients with pheochromocytoma are sensitive to propranolol. The dosage is propranolol 10 mg po t.i.d.

D. Steroids. Preoperative steroids are recommended by some, especially if the tumor is familial and bilateral adrenalectomy is anticipated. If unilateral adrenalectomy is performed, steroid replacement is not necessary and steroids are halted.

E. Intraoperative Management.

1. Avoid $MgSO_4$, meperidine as they cause catechol release. Atropine is avoided as it causes tachycardia. Enflurane, droperidol, N_2O, and thiopental appear to work well.
2. Arterial line and CVP line with or without PA monitoring are indicated.

F. Postoperative Management.

1. Patient may require massive fluid resuscitation postoperatively due to loss of peripheral catecholamine stimulation and α-stimulated vascular tone.
2. This effect is less frequent in patients with good pre-operative α-adrenergic blockade.
3. After successful resection of a pheochromocytoma, some patients may remain transiently hypertensive because of excessive catecholamine stores in sympathetic nerve endings. This postoperative hypertension is best controlled with **IV sodium nitroprusside.**

IV. THYROID DYSFUNCTION.

A. It is difficult to assess thyroid function in the acutely ill patient, owing to drug effects on hormones, effects of acute and chronic disease, effects of profound malnutrition, and other factors. Common thyroid function tests are listed in Table 14–7.

B. The effects of common drugs on thyroid hormone metabolism are shown in Table 14–8.

C. Effect of illness on thyroid hormone metabolism.

1. It is a challenge to exclude thyroid disease in an acutely ill patient with markedly abnormal test results.

2. In **starvation,** there is a decrease in total and free T_3 levels in the blood, associated with an increase in reverse T_3 levels within 1–3 days. Total and free T_4 and TSH concentrations and the TSH response to TRH are minimally affected by starvation.

3. **Postoperatively,** T_3 falls but returns to normal after 1 week. T_4 levels remain constant. TSH levels fall transiently on the first postoperative day.

4. Many **chronic illnesses,** such as chronic hepatic disease, are associated with decreased conversion of T_4 to T_3 and decreased serum T_3 levels. For this reason serum T_3 determinations are less useful in assessing thyroid function in the acutely ill.

5. **Nonthyroidal diseases,** such as hepatic cirrhosis, are associated with decreased levels of TBG, so total T_4 levels are reduced. Free T_4 index values should remain normal, but nonthyroidal diseases can also affect free T_4 determinations. Fortunately, hypothyroidism in patients with low free T_4 indices can usually be excluded by measurement of TSH, which should be elevated in hypothyroidism.

TABLE 14–7.

Thyroid Function Tests in Primary Thyroid Disease

Test	Hypothyroid	Hyperthyroid
Total T_4	Decreased	Increased
Resin T_3 uptake	Increased	Decreased
Free T_4 index	Decreased	Increased
TSH	Increased	Decreased

TABLE 14–8.

Effects of Drugs on Thyroid Hormone Metabolism

Drug	Level	Effect
Dopamine	Pituitary	Decrease TSH/inhibit TSH response to TRH
L-Dopa		
Bromocriptine		
Cyproheptadine		
Opiates		
Corticosteroids		
Metaclopramide		Increase TSH; increase TSH response to TRH
Chlorpromazine		
Haloperidol		
Cimetidine		
Iodide	Thyroid	Decrease thyroid hormone release
Lithium		
Nitroprusside		
Clomiphene		
Methimazole		Decrease thyroid hormone formation
Propylthiouracil		
Co-trimoxazole		
Estrogens		Increase levels of TBG
Clofibrate		
5-Fluorouracil		
Opiates		
Androgens	Transport proteins	Decrease levels of TBG
Danazol		
Salicylates	Binding to transport proteins	Displace T_4 and T_3 from binding proteins in vivo
Heparin		
Diazepam		
Sulfonylureas		
Fenclofenac		
Carbamazepine	Induction of enzymes	Increase metabolism of T_4 and T_3, lower blood levels
Phenobarbital		
Phenotoin		
Propranolol	Inhibition of peripheral T_4–T_3 conversion	Decrease T_3 levels, may increase T_4 levels
Glucocorticoids		
Amiodarone		
Propylthiouracil		
Iodine-containing contrast medium		

6. Acutely ill patients often have decreased T_3 levels for a variety of reasons. T_4 indices are more useful in the acutely ill patient. In a study of patients admitted to a medical ICU, 25% percent had decreased total T_4 levels, 18% had decreased free T_4 index, and 10% had decreased free T_4. In virtually all cases hypothyroidism can be excluded by TSH measurements which are elevated in hypothyroidism, but TSH will be lowered in patients with pituitary hypothyroidism or in those receiving dopamine or high-dose corticosteroids. In most cases the correct thyroid status can be ascertained by the use of T_4, T_3 resin uptake, and TSH measurements.

D. Management of Myxedema Crisis.

1. **Myxedema crisis** is an acute, life-threatening complication of what may otherwise be mild, stable hypothyroidism. Although rare, it remains highly lethal, with mortality rates approaching 50%. The majority of cases appear to be precipitated by a factor such as tranquilizer or narcotic administration, CO_2 narcosis, and febrile infectious illness.

2. Myxedema crisis is an acute exacerbation of underlying hypothyroidism. **CNS depression** is due to the lack of thyroid hormone's direct effect on the brain and from complicating and precipitating factors. **Infection** is a common precipitating factor and should be sought in all patients with this condition. Pulmonary dysfunction, including CO_2 retention and CO_2 narcosis, may lead to coma. Delayed metabolism of drugs may cause myxedma crisis, as slowed metabolism is characteristic of hypothyroidism and therapeutic doses may need to be reduced, especially sedatives, sleeping pills, and narcotics. Iodide in small amounts inhibits the release of thyroid hormone and may precipitate crisis. Hyponatremia may also contribute to the obtundation seen.

3. **Diagnosis.**

   a. The diagnosis is usually made on **clinical** grounds, given the usual delay in the return of thyroid function tests. A history of known hypothyroidism is helpful, as is evidence of symptoms of hypothyroidism: cold intolerance, weight gain, hair loss, hoarseness, constipation, apathy, lethargy.

b. **Physical findings** of hypothyroidism include coarse, dry skin, alopecia, enlarged tongue, goiter, bradycardia, decreased deep tendon reflexes, and decreased heart sounds.

c. **Laboratory** and other findings include hyponatremia, hypercarbia, hypercholesterolemia, low voltage on ECG, pericardial or pleural effusion on CXR, high protein concentration in CSF.

4. **Treatment.**

   a. Rapid thyroid hormone replacement.

   b. T_4 300–500 µg IV in a single dose, followed by a 100 µg/day IV for days to weeks, until the patient is taking oral medications.

   c. Metabolic effects of rapid T_4 administration become evident after 24 hours. Normal T_4 levels in the blood appear rapidly, prior to metabolic effects.

   d. Many recommend treating with stress doses of corticosteroids for the first several days of treatment, because pituitary function is abnormal for 10 days after therapy is started.

   e. **Systemic support:**

      1) Hypothermia should not be treated with warming blankets, since peripheral vascular collapse can occur during replacement therapy.

      2) Hyponatremia will occasionally respond to fluid restriction, but in hypotensive patients isotonic and rarely hypertonic solutions are administered.

      3) Infectious precipitating cause should be specifically treated.

      4) Pericardial and pleural effusions usually resolve spontaneously.

      5) Respiratory failure requires mechanical ventilation.

      6) Ileus, urinary retention, and hypoglycemia are treated appropriately.

E. **Management of Thyrotoxic Crisis.**

1. **Thyrotoxic crisis** is a life-threatening augmentation of the symptoms of hyperthyroidism, differing qualitatively from hyperthyroidism in that **fever** is almost invariably present. The incidence has declined significantly owing to improved management of thyroid disease but, a mortality of 10%–20% persists. Thyrotoxic crisis most frequently occurs in patients with underlying Graves' disease (thyrotox-

icosis, diffuse goiter, infiltrative exophthalmos) who are stressed by an acute illness or a major surgical procedure.

2. Thyrotoxic crisis is often provoked by an **infectious disease or other stress** such as an operation. The syndrome resembles that of severe, prolonged β-adrenergic agonist overload, although catecholamine levels and metabolism are relatively normal.

3. **Diagnosis.**

   a. Thyrotoxic crisis is differentiated from uncomplicated thyrotoxicosis by clinical assessment. Fever is crucial, and rectal temperature <101° F suggests another diagnosis. The clinical manifestations of thyrotoxicosis in a patient with known Graves' disease or with goiter establish the diagnosis, and treatment should begin immediately. **Signs and symptoms are:**

1) **Systemic**	Fever (may be 39° C), profuse sweating
2) **Cardiovascular**	Tachycardia
	Worsening angina
	Atrial flutter or fibrillation
	High output CHF, hypotension (preterminal)
3) **GI**	Nausea, vomiting, abdominal pain, hepatic congestion
4) **CNS**	Delirium, apathy, stupor, coma, tremulousness

   b. The **treatment** of thyrotoxic crisis should not await the confirmation of thyroid function tests. The blood levels of thyroid hormones are no different from those in compensated hyperthyroidism.

4. **Treatment** of thyrotoxic crisis includes inhibition of thyroid hormone synthesis, inhibition of thyroid hormone release, inhibition of peripheral β-adrenergic activity, and systemic support.

   a. **Inhibition of hormone synthesis:** Propylthiouracil (PTU): 200 mg po or via NG tube q.4h. (inhibits hormone synthesis and peripheral conversion of T_4 to T_3). Decreases T_3 levels to about 50% within 24 hours. Does not inhibit thyroid hormone release from the gland, which would continue for several days if only PTU is used.

b. **Inhibition of thyroid hormone release:** Supersaturated potassium iodide (SSKI): Five drops PO or via NG tube q.6h. or KI 1 g IV/30 min q.8h. SSKI inhibits release of hormone from thyroid, but should be given 1 hour after starting PTU since iodide can contribute to hormone synthesis unless synthesis is blocked. Although hormone release will be blocked immediately, the $T^{1}/_2$ of circulating T_4 is about 1 week and metabolic effects will persist for several days. A rapid-acting thyroid hormone antagonist is needed. Since no specific antagonist exists β-adrenergic antagonist for immediate effect is used.

c. **Inhibition of peripheral β-adrenergic activity:**
   1) **Propranolol:** 40–80 mg PO or via NG tube q.6h. titrated to clinical response, or IV propranolol 1 mg IV q. 10 min until clinical response is up to 10 mg (IV dosing with adequate ECG monitoring). Propranolol inhibits peripheral effects of thyroid hormones and can be used with caution in patients with tachycardia and high output CHF. If propranolol is contraindicated or ineffective, reserpine and guanethidine may be useful.
   2) **Reserpine** 2.0–2.5 mg IM q.4–6h.
   3) **Guanethidine** 50–150 mg PO q.d. may be used if reserpine is unsuccessful. May take several days for maximal effect.

d. **Systemic support:**
   1) Control of hyperpyrexia with external cooling and acetaminophen (aspirin may cause release of thyroid hormones from carrier proteins and should be avoided).
   2) Fluid resuscitation with glucose-containing electrolyte solutions (the great majority of patients are severely dehydrated from sweating, vomiting, and diarrhea)
   3) Treatment of secondary complications such as CHF with O_2, diuretics and possibly digitalis.
   4) Thorough search for infection. Some advocate use of broad-spectrum antibiotics, but this is controversial.
   5) Corticosteroids are recommended by many. Hydro-

cortisone 200 mg IV initially and then 100 mg q.6h. Steroids provide both support for possible adrenal insufficiency and inhibit release of hormones from thyroid.

V. DIABETES INSIPIDUS (DI).

A. DI is the failure of water homeostasis. Pituitary DI is due to a deficiency in vasopressin (ADH) release in response to increased serum osmolality. Seventy percent of patients with diabetes insipidus have either an intracranial neoplasm or trauma secondary to an accident or cranial surgery. DI can either be transient with resolution after the acute injury phase or permanent.

B. Diagnosis

1. **Clinical:**
   a. Polyuria.
   b. Thirst.
   c. Polydipsia.
2. **Laboratory:**
   a. Hypernatremia.
   b. Urine specific gravity <1.005.
   c. Urine osmolality <200 mOsm/kg H_2O.
   d. Serum osmolality >290 mOsm/kg H_2O.
   e. Normal GFR.
   f. Increase in urine osmolality of $\geq$ 10% with vasopressin 5 units SC after overnight H_2O deprivation.

C. Treatment.

1. A patient with free access to H_2O can prevent the clinical manifestations of volume depletion and this may be all that is necessary in patients with vasopressin deficiency.
2. In patients with complete hormone deficiency, the requirement of up to 10 L/day of H_2O and invariable nocturia require hormone replacement. The goal of treatment is to decrease urine volume and prevent nocturia.
3. In the early postoperative period, vasopressin 5 units SC q.4h. is the treatment of choice.
4. Desmopressin is the drug of choice for long-term management of DI. Desmopressin 2–4 μg intranasally b.i.d. is the usual dose. The drug is titrated to the prevention of nocturia and may be combined as one dose per day (see p 554).

SELECTED REFERENCES

Cobb WE, Spare J, Reichboin S: Neurogenic diabetes insipidus: Management with DDAVP. *Ann Intern Med* 1978; 88:183.

Croxson MS, Hall TD, Nicoloff JT: Combination drug therapy for treatment of hyperthyroid Graves disease. *J Clin Endocrinol Metab* 1977; 45:623.

Engelman K: Pleochromocytoma. *Clin Endocrinol Metab* 1977; 6:769.

Podolsky S: Management of diabetes in the surgical patient. *Med Clin North Am* 1982; 66:1361.

Rush DR, Hamburger SC: Endocrine metabolic emergencies. *South Med J* 1984; 77:220.

THE HEMATOLOGIC SYSTEM

15

I. PATIENT EVALUATION.

A. Routine Preoperative Evaluation.

1. **History:**

   a. Has patient ever bled for a long time after a minor injury (e.g., laceration, tongue bite) or minor procedure (e.g., tooth extraction, skin biopsy)?

   b. Does patient bruise easily or develop large bruises without being able to remember how?

   c. Has patient ever had renal failure, liver disease, cancer, blood clots?

   d. What medications has patient taken in the past 7–10 days? Include warfarin, aspirin, dipyridamole, NSAIDs.

   e. Has any blood relative had a problem with unusual bruising, bleeding, clotting? Were blood transfusions required to control bleeding?

2. **Physical examination:** Look for signs of abnormal hemostasis including petechiae, purpura, ecchymoses, hematuria, and heme-positive stool.

3. **Laboratory tests:** Based on screening history, physical examination, and planned operative procedure, four levels of increasing concern and need for preoperative testing can be reached:

   a. **Level I:** Negative screening history and minor operation (e.g., tooth extraction, excisional biopsy). No screening tests required.

   b. **Level II:** Negative screening history and major operation (e.g., cholecystectomy, bowel resection). Platelet count and PTT are recommended.

    c. **Level III:** Either the screening history raises the possibility of defective hemostasis, or patients with a negative screening history are undergoing an operation which may impair hemostasis (e.g., open heart surgery). These patients should have platelet count, bleeding time (BT), PT, and PTT (Table 15–1).

    d. **Level IV:** Screening history is suspicious for hemostatic abnormality. Operation may be minor or major. The initial screening evaluation is the same as for level III. If tests are negative, consider performing additional tests:

        1) Give 650 mg aspirin and repeat BT. Consider platelet aggregation tests.

        2) Measure factor VIII and IX coagulant activity. These help rule out hemophilia A and B.

        3) Perform a thrombin clotting time (TCT), utilizing a thrombin concentration that gives a time of 15–20 seconds in normal plasma.

  4. Screen for hypercoagulable status in patients prior to infrainguinal arterial reconstruction, especially if history is suggestive.

B. Evaluation of Bleeding Patient.

  1. The evaluation of any bleeding patient must include consideration of the three components of normal hemostasis:

    a. **Vascular integrity.**

      1) Inspect for surface bleeding.

      2) Inspect for internal bleeding (endoscopy, angiography, possibly surgery).

      3) Control hypertension.

    b. **Platelets.**

      1) **Abnormal platelet count:**

        a) If $<20,000/mm^3$, transfuse to prevent spontaneous bleeding

        b) If $<50,000/mm^3$, transfuse only if patient is bleeding

      2) **Abnormal platelet function:** If no mechanical source of bleeding is apparent and platelet count, PT, and PTT are normal, consider abnormality in platelet function. Check BT; if abnormal, consider platelet transfusion. Consider

TABLE 15-1.
Diagnosis of Bleeding Disorders Based on Screening Tests

	PT, PTT Normal	PT Abnormal, PTT Normal	PT Normal, PTT Abnormal	PT, PTT Abnormal
BT normal	Factor XIII deficiency	Factor VII deficiency Malnutrition Liver disease Warfarin	Factor VIII, IX or XI deficiency Heparin	Factor I, II, V, or X deficiency Malnutrition Warfarin Heparin Liver disease
BT abnormal Normal platelet count			VWD	Afibrinogenemia Dysfibrinogenemia Primary fibrinolysis DIC
Low platelet count				

BT = bleeding time; VWD = Von Willebrand disease.

        cryoprecipitate or desmopressin (DDAVP) in uremic patients.

c. **Coagulation system.**

  1) If PT and PTT normal, no therapy.

  2) If PT abnormal, PTT normal, consider vitamin K deficiency, malnutrition, liver disease, warfarin excess. Treat with FFP, vitamin K.

  3) If PTT abnormal, PT normal, consider factor VIII, IX, XI deficiency, heparin excess. Treat with FFP or factor concentrates.

  4) If PT and PTT abnormal:

    a) Measure thrombin time.

      i) If normal, consider problems outlined in c.2 and c.3 above. Treat with FFP.

      ii) If abnormal, measure fibrinogen level.

    b) Fibrinogen level.

      i) If low, consider DIC, primary fibrinolysis, or massive blood transfusion. Treat with FFP, cryoprecipitate, or aminocaproic acid as appropriate (see section II. B, 589).

      ii) If normal, measure FDP.

    c) FDP.

      i) If elevated, consider DIC. Treat with FFP.

      ii) If normal, consider circulating heparin. If present, treat with protamine sulfate.

2. Several common causes of postoperative bleeding are summarized in Table 15–2.

C. **Laboratory Tests.**

1. **Prothrombin time (PT):**

  a. Tissue thromboplastin (a factor VII activator) and calcium are added to test plasma and clotting time is determined. Factors II, V, VII, X, and fibrinogen are measured.

  b. PT is a useful screening test of the extrinsic coagulation pathway (see Fig 15–1) and is used to monitor warfarin therapy. It may be abnormal in liver disease, malnutrition, and vitamin K deficiency.

2. **Activated partial thromboplastin time (PTT):**

  a. Platelet-poor test plasma is incubated with a platelet membrane substitute (phospholipid) and a factor XII

TABLE 15–2.
Common Etiologies of Postoperative Bleeding

Etiology	Platelet Count	PT	PTT	TCT	Fibrinogen	Fibrinolysis
Dilution	Low	Normal/prolonged	Normal	Normal/low	Absent	
DIC	Low	Prolonged	Prolonged	Prolonged	Low	Absent/present
Primary fibrinolysis	Normal	Normal/prolonged	Normal/prolonged	Normal/prolonged	Normal/low	Present
Circulating heparin	Normal	Normal/prolonged	Prolonged	Prolonged	Normal	Absent

activator and then recalcified. The clotting time is measured. All factors except VII and XIII are measured.

b. PTT is a useful screening test of the intrinsic coagulation pathway and is used to monitor heparin therapy.

3. **Thrombin clotting time (TCT):**
   a. A standard concentration of thrombin is added to test plasma and clotting time is measured. TCT assesses fibrinogen concentration.
   b. TCT is prolonged by hypofibrinogenemia, dysfibrinogenemia, presence of FDP, and heparin. TCT is used to monitor fibrinolytic therapy.

4. **Fibrinogen assay:** Fibrinogen levels may be measured using a modified TCT.

5. **Fibrin D-dimer assay:** Test plasma is mixed with latex beads coated with an antibody to the D-dimer domain of fibrin. This assay measures FDP and is useful in the evaluation of DIC, primary fibrinolysis, and thrombolytic therapy.

6. **Specific factor assays:**
   a. Test plasma is diluted with specific factor-deficient plasma and the clotting time is measured. The degree of correction in the clotting time is proportional to the amount of the specific factor present in the test plasma.
   b. Specific factor assays are available for factors II (thrombin), V, VII–XIII.

7. **Factor VIII–ristocetin cofactor assay** (von Willebrand's factor):
   a. Fixed platelets are mixed with test plasma and ristocetin is added. Platelet agglutination is monitored. The time required for agglutination is related to the amount of ristocetin cofactor.
   b. This is a sensitive and specific test for von Willebrand's disease (VWD).

8. **Bleeding time (BT):**
   a. BT is performed with a commercial device to ensure standardization and reproducibility. Vessel integrity and platelet *function* are measured.
   b. BT is prolonged when platelet counts are <50,000/mm^3. BT >10 minutes with a normal platelet count

indicates either a qualitative disorder of platelets (e.g., aspirin effect, uremia) or VWD.

9. **Activated clotting time (ACT):**
    a. ACT is used to monitor heparinization and heparin reversal during cardiac surgery. A normal ACT is 90–120 seconds. From a dose-response curve, the amount of heparin needed to produce a desired prolongation of the clotting time can be determined. Also, if the ACT is known, the amount of heparin in the circulation can be calculated and the dose of protamine needed to reverse the heparin can be determined.
    b. To construct a dose-response curve (Fig 15–1):
        1) Measure a baseline ACT (Fig 15–1, point A).
        2) Administer heparin 2 mg/kg and measure the ACT again (Fig 15–2, point B).
        3) Draw a straight line between points A and B.

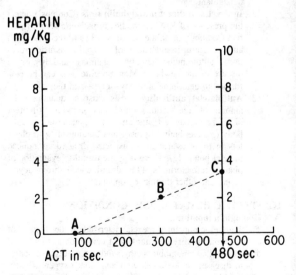

FIG 15–1.
Activated clotting time *(ACT)* dose-response curve.

        4) Determine by extrapolation (point *C*) the amount of heparin (mg/kg) needed to achieve desired ACT (e.g., 480 seconds, or ~5 × control).

        5) Heparin reversal—measure ACT, determine from the curve the level of circulating heparin, and calculate the neutralizing dose of protamine (heparin level × 1.3).

10. **Euglobulin lysis time** measures the fibrinolytic activity of test plasma. A normal whole blood clot does not lyse for over 24 hours.

11. **Assays for acquired anticoagulants (50:50 mix):** In a patient with an abnormal PT or PTT in whom antibodies to a coagulation factor are suspected as the cause rather than a factor deficiency, repeat the PT and PTT with a 50:50 mixture of normal plasma and patient plasma. If clotting time corrects, consider a factor deficiency. If clotting time does not correct, consider a circulating anticoagulant.

12. **Indirect and direct antiglobulin tests** (Coombs') detect the presence of RBC antibodies in patient's serum (indirect Coombs') or on the patient's RBCs (direct Coombs') and are useful in evaluation of delayed transfusion reactions, autoimmune hemolytic anemias, and hemolytic disease of the newborn. More specific tests can be performed to determine antibody isotype and titer.

13. **Antiplatelet antibodies:** Tests exist to quantitate the amount of free (serum) antiplatelet antibodies (indirect platelet antibody test), the amount of platelet-bound antibody (platelet-bound Ig test), and binding of Ig to platelets in the presence of a suspected drug (drug-induced platelet-bound Ig). These tests are useful in evaluation of platelet refractoriness, ITP, drug-induced thrombocytopenia, and other thrombocytopenias.

II. SPECIFIC HEMATOLOGIC CONDITIONS.

A. Hemoglobinopathies.

The hemoglobinopathies are characterized by production of an **abnormal quality or quantity** of hemoglobin. Sickle cell disease, sickle hemoglobinopathy syndromes, unstable hemoglobin disease, hemoglobins with abnormal oxygen affinity, and the M hemoglobins are structural abnormalities of hemoglobin (qualitative disorders). The thalassemia syndromes result from decreased production of normal globin chains (quantitative disorders).

1. **Sickle cell disease** is an inherited, chronic hemolytic anemia which affects 1 in 500 black infants born in the United States. Patients with sickle cell anemia (homozygous, Hb SS) typically have a hemoglobin of 8–10 g/DL in the first year and 6–9 g/DL in later childhood. Sickle cell trait (heterozygous, Hb SA) is found in 8%–11% of the black population, and sickle crises occur only during extreme conditions of deoxygenation. **Hemoglobin electrophoresis** is utilized to detect the specific hemoglobin abnormality. The **sickle preparation** detects Hb S by inducing sickling with sodium metabisulfate. The following are complications of sickle cell disease (Hb SS).

   a. **Acute infections:** Young children are at risk for overwhelming infection by encapsulated organisms such as *Streptococcus pneumoniae* and *Haemophilus influenzae*. Pneumonia or sepsis is treated with ampicillin (200 mg/kg/day). Sickle cell patients should receive Pneumovax and *H. influenzae* vaccine during infancy.

   b. **Aplastic crisis** occurs when decreased RBC production, usually following a viral or bacterial infection, is superimposed on the preexisting shortened RBC survival. This results in a rapid drop in Hct and symptoms of anemia (pallor, fatigue tachycardia). Treatment includes transfusion of PRBCs and supportive care.

   c. **Sequestration** is the rapid accumulation of large volumes of blood in the sinusoids of the spleen, producing hypovolemia, shock, and death. It is usually seen in patients under the age of 5 years (spleens are still intact) and produces pallor, listlessness, abdominal fullness, and abdominal pain. Physical examination reveals a large tender spleen. Treatment includes hemodynamic support with IV fluids and PRBC transfusions. Since recurrence is common, splenectomy is recommended after the second episode.

   d. In young children, **painful crises**, due to occlusion or infarction of small blood vessels, often occur in the hands and feet, accompanied by fever. Older children experience abdominal crises characterized by abdom

inal distention and tenderness and vomiting, which
may be difficult to differentiate from an acute surgical
abdomen. Treatment consists of IV hydration, O_2,
analgesics (narcotics, NSAIDs, sedatives), correction
of acid-base disturbances, and workup to exclude
other acute abdominal problems.

e. **Chronic complications** result from repeated episodes
of vaso-occlusion and subsequent tissue infarction
and include cerebral infarction and intracerebral hemorrhage, retinopathy, aseptic necrosis of bones, osteomyelitis, leg ulcers, priapism, pulmonary embolism
and infarction, sickle nephropathy, and cholelithiasis
(pigment stones secondary to hemolysis).

f. **Perioperative care** of patients with sickle cell disease:

　　1) Careful preoperative preparation is particularly
important in these patients. **Transfuse blood** to
achieve Hct >35% and a Hb A level
>65%–70%.

　　2) **Adequate hydration** (1.5 × maintenance)
should be given throughout the perioperative period since dehydration predisposes to RBC
sludging and sickling.

　　3) **Supplemental O_2** in the postoperative period
and early ambulation are essential.

2. *Thalassemias* are genetic disorders characterized by un-
derproduction of at least one of the normal globin pep-
tide chains (α or β) resulting in deficient hemoglobin accumulation. *Thalassemia trait* (heterozygous state) produces a mild to moderate hypochromic, microcytic anemia that may be confused with iron deficiency anemia.
Generally, no treatment is required. Patients with *thalassemia major* (homozygous state) usually die of cardiac
disease in childhood, though some survive into adult-
hood. RBC transfusions are necessary but should be
minimized in order to delay iron overload (hemochroma-
tosis) with resultant hepatosplenomegaly, cirrhosis, diabetes mellitus, and cardiomyopathy. **Deferoxamine** may
help. Splenectomy may be useful when splenomegaly
causes mechanical pressure symptoms or when hypersplenism with sequestration is documented by increasing
RBC requirements, leukopenia, or thrombocytopenia.

Splenectomized patients are susceptible to sepsis with encapsulated organisms, so delay splenectomy until after age 4 if possible, remember Pneumovax, and treat fevers early with ampicillin.

B. Coagulopathies.

The coagulation cascade is depicted in Figure 15–2.

1. **Congenital disorders of coagulation.**

   a. **Hemophilia A (classic hemophilia).**

      1) **Cause:** Hemophilia A is a failure to synthesize normal *factor VIII*. It is inherited as an X-linked recessive trait with spontaneous mutations accounting for 20% of patients. The incidence is 1:10,000 births (about five times more frequent than hemophilia B).

      2) **Clinical manifestations:**

         a) The clinical course parallels the factor VIII:C level:

            i) Severe (0%–5%): many spontaneous bleeds.

            ii) Moderate (5%–10%): occasional spontaneous bleeds.

            iii) Mild (10%–40%): rare spontaneous bleeds.

         b) The most common sites of bleeding are intraarticular, IM, urinary tract, intracranial.

      3) **Diagnosis:** Severe cases are usually noted in childhood. Typically, there is either a personal or family history of bleeding in a male child. The PTT may be prolonged with severe deficiency of factor VIII while the PT remains normal. The definitive test is a factor VIII assay.

      4) **Treatment:**

         a) The basis of treatment is replacement with factor VIII concentrate. The biologic $T_{1/2}$ is 8–12 hours and the minimal hemostatic level for joint, muscle, or other hemorrhagic lesions is 50%.

         b) For operation, levels of 80%–100% should be achieved preoperatively as prophylaxis by giving 40–50 units/kg of factor VIII prior to surgery (each unit of factor VIII infused per kg body weight yields a 2% rise in

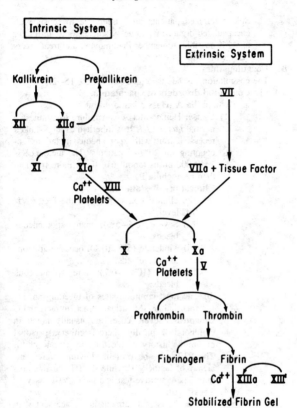

FIG 15-2.
Coagulation cascade.

plasma factor VIII level). Postoperatively, levels >30% should be maintained for 10-14 days.

    b. **Hemophilia B** (Christmas disease).

        1) **Cause:** Hemophilia B is a deficiency in *factor*

IX and is inherited as an X-linked recessive trait.

2) **Clinical manifestations** are identical to hemophilia A. The findings correlate with the degree of factor IX deficiency.

3) **Diagnosis:** A family history of bleeding is often obtained. In severe factor IX deficiency, PTT is prolonged and PT is normal. Assay of factor VIII:C is normal while the level of factor IX is low.

4) **Treatment:**

   a) Both the treatment of severe bleeding and prophylaxis for surgery are managed with factor IX–containing prothrombin complex concentrates. These have a $T\frac{1}{2}$ of 24 hours (dose q. 16–24 h.).

   b) For surgery, a factor IX level of 60% preoperatively and >20% for 10–14 days postoperatively is needed. The preoperative loading dose is 60 units/kg IV. Levels can be monitored by factor IX assay.

c. **Von Willebrand's Disease.**

   1) **Cause:** VWD is characterized by *defective platelet adhesion* to vascular surfaces caused by abnormal synthesis of von Willebrand factor (VWF)–VIII protein. VWD is inherited as an autosomal dominant trait and has an incidence equal to hemophilia.

   2) The **clinical features** include petechiae and purpura, identical to a platelet-vascular disorder. Mucosal and cutaneous hemorrhages are common. Menorrhagia is frequently excessive in the postpartum period. Excessive bleeding may also follow dental or surgical procedures.

   3) **Diagnosis:** BT is prolonged and platelet count is normal. Measurement of VWF is a sensitive and specific test.

   4) **Therapy** of choice is cryoprecipitate (CP). FFP may be used if CP is unavailable. The goal of transfusion is a factor VIII level of 30%–50%. A rough guideline is 1–3 units/day/kg of CP. Preoperatively, the patient should receive 3 units of CP/10 kg.

2. **Acquired coagulation disorders** are usually associated with *multiple* deficiencies in clotting factors. The diagnosis is often suggested by associated clinical features and by the results of screening tests, such as the platelet count, PT, PTT, and TT. Avoid aspirin-containing medicines in patients with these disorders.

   a. **Vitamin K deficiency.**

      1) **Cause:** Vitamin K is required for the *hepatic synthesis of factors II, VII, IX, and X.* Causes of vitamin K deficiency include:

         a) Dietary inadequacy.

         b) TPN.

         c) Biliary obstruction or fistula (causing fat malabsorption).

         d) Malabsorption syndromes (e.g., cystic fibrosis, sprue, ulcerative colitis or regional ileitis, and short-bowel syndrome).

         e) Parenchymal liver disease.

         f) Broad-spectrum antibiotic use (e.g., moxalactam).

         g) Warfarin therapy.

      2) **Treatment:**

         a) Correct underlying cause of the disorder.

         b) Give 10–20 mg/day of vitamin K (phytonadione) IM for 3 days to treat the deficiency. For emergency operations, give 10–20 mg vitamin K IV and 10–15 mL/kg of FFP.

   b. **Liver disease:** One or more derangements of the coagulation mechanism are commonly seen in liver disease. Troublesome or severe bleeding may occur following trauma or surgery or with local lesions such as esophageal varices or peptic ulcers. Severe bleeding may also be seen following portasystemic shunts.

      1) The **causes** of the hemostatic defect in liver disease include:

         a) *Defective synthesis of vitamin K–dependent clotting factors (II, VII, IX and X)* is probably the most important cause and demonstrated by prolonged PT.

         b) Impaired fibrinogen synthesis.

         c) Increased fibrinolytic activity.

         d) Thrombocytopenia.

2) **Treatment of bleeding:** The basis of therapy is infusion of FFP. Administer vitamin K as above. If significant fibrinolysis is present, the use of aminocaproic acid may be indicated (see section IV.I, p 614).

c. **Renal failure:** Uremia produces reversible platelet dysfunction. Cryoprecipitate or desmopressin (DDAVP) may improve platelet function in severe patients with normal BT but not in patients with normal BT (see p 614).

d. **Massive transfusion syndrome:** See p 607.

e. **Disseminated intravascular coagulation.**

   1) **Cause:** The intravascular release of thromboplastic substances causes diffuse intravascular thrombosis and thrombolysis, resulting in a hemostatic defect due to consumption of clotting factors and platelets ("consumption coagulopathy"). DIC is most commonly associated with the following:

      a) Obstetric events (amniotic fluid embolism, placental abruption, eclampsia, intrauterine fetal death).

      b) Intravascular hemolysis (hemolytic transfusion reactions, minor hemolysis, massive transfusions).

      c) Bacteremia or sepsis (usually gram-negative, occasionally gram-positive) or viremia.

      d) Malignancy (carcinoma of prostate, pancreas, or lung; acute myelogenous leukemia).

      e) Burns, crush injuries, aortic aneurysms, tissue necrosis.

      f) Collagen-vascular diseases.

      g) Surgery (prostatic operations, extracorporeal circulation).

   2) Nonspecific **clinical manifestations** include fever, hypotension, acidosis, proteinuria. More specific signs include petechiae and purpura, wound bleeding (especially from a traumatic or surgical wound), oozing from venipunctures and intraarterial lines, hemoptysis, and GI bleeding.

   3) **Diagnosis:** Laboratory findings include throm-

bocytopenia ($<50,000/mm^3$ in half of patients), hypofibrinogenemia, elevated FDP, prolonged PT, and microangiopathic blood smear.

    4) ***Treat the underlying condition.*** Replacement therapy with FFP and platelets is usually necessary. If bleeding continues despite replacement therapy (e.g., ongoing, nonpreventable release of tissue thromboplastin), consider IV heparinization (controversial). A hematologist should be consulted prior to initiating heparin therapy for DIC.

  f. **Primary fibrinolysis.**

    1) **Cause:** An inherited or acquired increase in fibrinolytic activity in the apparent absence of intravascular coagulation.

    2) **Clinical manifestations** are similiar to DIC.

    3) **Diagnosis** must differentiate primary fibrinolysis from DIC using the platelet count (normal in hyperfibrinolysis and decreased in DIC), precipitation of citrated blood with protamine (negative in former and positive in latter), and euglobulin lysis time (decreased in former and normal in latter).

    4) Treatment: Aminocaproic acid (see p 614).

C. Thrombocytopathies.

  1. **Thrombocytopenia** is the most common disorder of platelets in surgical patients and the most common underlying cause of bleeding in general.

    a. **Cause:** Thrombocytopenia may be the result of decreased platelet production (marrow failure or replacement), platelet sequestration (hypersplenism), or increased platelet destruction (autoantibody, prosthetic valves, DIC). If the platelet count decreases >25% in 24 hours in the absence of blood loss, platelet destruction rather than decreased marrow production is the most likely cause. A bone marrow aspirate and biopsy may be required to assess platelet production. Decreased numbers of megakaryocytes suggest decreased platelet production; normal or increased numbers imply platelet destruction.

    b. **Spontaneous bleeding** occurs when platelet counts

are $<20,000/mm^3$. Although the platelet concentration that allows the safe performance of an operation has not been firmly established, a count $>60,000-100,000/mm^3$ is generally preferred.

c. **Specific causes** of thrombocytopenia include:

1) **Immune thrombocytopenic purpura:** Initial treatment is prednisone (1–3 mg/kg/day) until platelet count is $>100,000/mm^3$ and then slowly taper. If steroids cannot be tapered without a concomitant drop in platelet count, add azathioprine (Imvran) (200 mg/day). With failure of medical therapy or with life-threatening hemorrhage at presentation, splenectomy may be necessary. In preparation for surgery, attempt to induce remission with prednisone and transfuse platelets intraoperatively to obtain a platelet count $>50,000/mm^3$. Postsplenectomy thrombocytosis may occur but rarely requires treatment.

2) **Other immune thrombocytopenias:** In general, immune thrombocytopenias associated with diseases such as SLE, chronic lymphocytic leukemia, or lymphoma are treated with corticosteroids and immunosuppressive agents in a manner similar to ITP. Therapy must also be directed at the underlying disease. Splenectomy is indicated for some patients with splenic sequestration and unmanageable bleeding.

3) **Thrombotic thrombocytopenic purpura** is a rare syndrome characterized by thrombocytopenia, microangiopathic hemolytic anemia, and fluctuating neurologic abnormalities, often with fever and renal dysfunction. TTP may progress and be lethal. Treatment may include FFP, aspirin, dipyridamole, steroids, vincristine, plasmapheresis, and plasma exchange. Avoid platelet transfusions.

4) **Hypersplenism** (enhanced filtration and phagocytosis of the cellular elements of the blood, resulting in variable degrees of anemia, leukopenia, and thrombocytopenia.) can be primary (hypertrophy due to hereditary spherocytosis or elliptocytosis or autoimmune anemia or

thrombocytopenia) or secondary (cirrhosis with congestive splenomegaly, inflammatory disorders, leukemia, lymphoma). In patients with cirrhosis, portal hypertension, and splenic sequestration, splenectomy is indicated only in the setting of unmanageable bleeding.

5) **Transfusion-associated purpuras:** Thrombocytopenia may follow massive transfusion (due to dilutional platelet loss) or extracorporeal circulation (due to mechanical platelet destruction). It typically persists 3–5 days and may be treated with platelet transfusions.

6) **Posttransfusion purpura (PTP)** is a rare condition seen primarily in women approximately 5–10 days following a blood transfusion. It is due to antibodies to platelet antigen $P1^{A1}$ and is clinically indistinguishable from ITP or drug-induced thrombocytopenia. It is usually self-limiting (lasts 2–6 weeks), but if treatment becomes necessary owing to low platelet counts ($<10,000/mm^3$), either a partial exchange transfusion with whole blood or plasmapheresis is the treatment of choice. Steroids and platelet transfusions are ineffective.

7) **Thrombocytopenia in surgical patients** is commonly due to a medication-induced decrease in platelet production or increase in platelet destruction. The latter mechanism is usually immune-mediated. Commonly implicated drugs include quinidine, quinine, sulfonamides, indomethacin, thiazide diuretics, cimetidine, ranitidine, estrogens, ethanol, gold, and heparin. In most cases, discontinuing the drug is adequate treatment.

8) **Heparin-associated thrombocytopenia and thrombosis (HATT)** is a rare but serious drug-induced thrombocytopenia. The development of an antibody against a heparin-platelet membrane complex induces intravascular platelet aggregation in the presence of heparin. Widespread platelet aggregation leads to thrombocytopenia and major vessel thrombosis. **Patients receiving**

heparin should have platelet counts monitored every 1–2 days. In vitro platelet aggregation studies confirm the diagnosis. When thrombocytopenia develops, heparin should be discontinued and anticoagulation of another type (e.g., warfarin) should be instituted if necessary. The defibrinating agent anerod has been used with success in Canada but is not yet available in the United States. When signs of vascular thrombosis appear, treatment with antiplatelet drugs (aspirin and dipyridamole) should be instituted.

2. **Platelet function disorders.**
   a. **Cause:** a failure of platelet adhesion or aggregation. *A very common cause of abnormal platelet aggregation in surgical patients is ingestion of aspirin.* Platelet aggregation is abnormal for as long as 1 week after 650 mg of aspirin. Other disorders of platelet adhesion include VWD, Bernard-Soulier syndrome, hypergammaglobulinemia, and medications (thiazides, NSAID).
   b. **Clinical manifestations:** abnormal skin or mucous membrane bleeding.
   c. **Diagnosis:** prolonged BT despite normal platelet count.
   d. **Treatment:** Transfusion of platelets may be necessary.

3. *Thrombocytosis.*
   a. **Cause:** Thrombocytosis (platelet count >740,000/mm^3) can be primary (myeloproliferative disorders) or secondary (iron deficiency, inflammatory disorders, malignancies, postsplenectomy).
   b. **Clinical manifestations:** rarely symptomatic (1%–5%).
   c. **Treatment:** Except in the setting of myeloproliferative disease or paroxysmal noctural hemoglobinuria, therapy with anticoagulants or antiplatelet agents is rarely required. When diffuse hemorrhage, thrombocytosis, and no other underlying cause of bleeding are present, consider platelet pheresis or hydroxyurea (0.5–2.0 g PO q.d.).

D. **Hypercoagulable States.**
   The coagulation cascade (see Fig 15–2) is downregulated by at least three mechanisms: AT-III, proteins C and S, and t-

PA. Inherited deficiencies of these proteins produce hypercoagulable states associated with recurrent venous thromboses (superficial venous thrombosis, deep venous thrombosis [DVT] pulmonary embolism [PE]).

1. *Antithrombin III deficiency.*
    a. **Cause:** AT-III inactivates thrombin and other coagulation factors. AT-III deficiency may be congenital or acquired (secondary to massive thrombosis, DIC, heparin therapy, liver disease, or protein-losing disorders of the kidney and GI tract).
    b. **Clinical manifestations:** Patients with congenital AT-III deficiencies have a markedly increased risk of venous thrombosis and PE. The prevalence of hereditary AT-III deficiency in a general patient population with thrombotic events is 3%–4%.
    c. **Laboratory tests** demonstrate low AT-III levels with normal global tests of coagulation and normal BT.
    d. **Treatment:** oral anticoagulation (warfarin) or antiplatelet therapy (aspirin plus dipyridamole).

2. **Protein C Deficiency.**
    a. **Cause:** Protein C is a major inhibitor of the procoagulant system (it degrades factors V and VIII). Its synthesis in the liver requires vitamin K. An inherited deficiency of protein C has been described with homozygous individuals dying in infancy of massive venous thrombosis and purpura fulminans (ischemic necrosis of skin and digits) and heterozygous individuals displaying variable penetrance.
    b. When present, **clinical manifestations** include recurrent DVT and PE beginning in the late teenage years. Congenital protein C deficiency may account for up to 10% of all patients presenting with venous thrombosis or PE.
    c. **Diagnosis** is made by demonstrating low levels of protein C.
    d. **Treatment:** Symptomatic individuals are heparinized briefly and then placed on warfarin.

3. **Protein S deficiency:** Protein S is a vitamin K–dependent hepatic protein that is a cofactor in protein C activation. Congenital deficiency of protein S (autosomal dominant) causes a thrombotic disorder that is manifested and treated like protein C deficiency.

III. BLOOD COMPONENT THERAPY.

A. Indications.

The indications for blood component transfusion are to (1) provide adequate *blood volume,* (2) increase *oxygen-carrying capacity* of blood, and (3) replace *platelets or clotting factors* to maintain hemostasis. The different components of blood available for transfusion are described below (B–M). Those used to replace platelet and coagulation factors are summarized in Table 15–3. Transfusion reactions and other complications of transfusion therapy are described under N.

B. Whole Blood.

1. Blood is collected in the anticoagulant CPDA-1 (citrate phosphate dextrose adenine) and stored at 4° C. The shelf life is 35 days. In this interval, at least 70% of the RBCs will survive and function normally after transfusion.

2. The *only established indication* for transfusion of whole blood is *massive, acute blood loss* (50%–60% decrease in blood volume) necessitating a large-volume resuscitation and an increase in oxygen-carrying capacity. In an emergency, when ABO group and Rh type are not known, transfuse O-negative blood. When ABO group and type are known (typing requires 5–10 minutes), transfuse type-specific blood. Screening for RBC anti-

TABLE 15–3.

Platelet and Coagulation Factor Replacement Therapy

Factor	Surgical Requirement	Plasma T$\frac{1}{2}$	Replacement*
Fibrinogen (I)	>200 mg/dL	120 days	WB, FFP, CP, fibrinogen
Prothrombin (II)	>50%	80–120 hr	WB, FFP, PC
V	>50%	15–24 hr	FFP
VII	>50%	4–8 hr	WB, PC
Antihemophilia factor (VIII)	80%–100%	8–12 hr	FFP, CP, F-VIII
Christmas factor (IX)	>60%	24 hr	WB, FFP, CP, PC
Stuart factor (X)	>50%	45–60 hr	WB, FFP, PC
XI	>50%	60 hr	WB, FFP
Platelets	>100,000/mm^3	6 days	Platelet concentrate

*WB = whole blood; FFP = fresh frozen plasma; CP = cryoprecipitate; PC = prothrombin complex; F-VIII = factor VIII concentrate.

bodies (present in 2%–3% of the population) and cross-matching of blood requires ~1 hour (longer if problems with antibodies arise).

3. Banked blood is a poor source of platelets and factors I, V, and VIII. FFP and platelets may be required with massive transfusions (see p 607).

C. **Packed Red Blood Cells**

1. PRBCs are prepared by removing supernatant plasma from whole blood. The Hct is ~65%–70% and the volume is ~300–350 mL/unit. The shelf life is 42 days.

2. PRBCs are the product of choice for the improvement of oxygen-carrying capacity without extensive blood volume expansion. The Duke Transfusion Service recommends transfusion for either a Hct <21% or a Hct <30% with symptoms of anemia.

3. In a normal adult, 1 unit of PRBC should raise the hemoglobin level ~1 g/dL or the Hct ~3%–4%.

4. The use of washed PRBCs may be indicated in patients experiencing "allergic reactions" to plasma components.

D. **Frozen (Deglycerolized) RBCs.**

1. Frozen RBCs are prepared by suspension in glycerol and freezing. Frozen RBCs are thawed and washed of glycerol prior to transfusion.

2. Advantages include the preservation of rare RBC types, improved RBC viability, maintenance of ATP and 2,3-DPG concentrations, and a reduction in WBCs and donor plasma in the RBC unit.

3. Disadvantages include high cost and the need for transfusion within 24 hours of thawing.

E. **Leukocytes.**

Leukocyte transfusions are rarely used in surgical practice. They are occasionally given in septic neonates or septic, neutropenic adults (absolute neutrophil count <500/mm^3) not responding to antibiotic therapy. Their use may require hematology consultation or special approval.

F. **Platelet Concentrates.**

1. Platelet concentrates are derived by the differential centrifugation of whole blood within 6 hours of collection. They may be stored under continuous gentle agitation at 22°–24° C for 3–5 days or at 4°C for 48 hours. There are approximately 7×10^{10} platelets in a unit of random single-donor platelets (~50 cc). This is enough to raise

the platelet count ~10,000/mm³. Six to 10 units are frequently pooled and transfused together (one "adult pack" of platelets)

2. Platelet transfusion is indicated for platelet counts <20,000/mm³ (to prevent spontaneous bleeding), counts <60,000/mm³ in patients undergoing surgery, massive blood transfusions (>10 units of blood or >1 blood volume), open heart surgery with pump times >2 hours, pediatric open heart cases requiring extracorporeal circulation. Transfusion is probably contraindicated in TTP, PTP, and ITP (see pp 595–596).

3. Platelets can be transfused without regard to ABO group and survive in the circulation with a T½ of ~6 days (varies with age of platelets). Survival is shorter in the presence of continued platelet consumption. Previously sensitized patients may require *single-donor, HLA-matched* platelets.

G. Fresh Frozen Plasma.

1. FFP is prepared by centrifugation (to remove platelets) of plasma remaining after the preparation of PRBC. It is stored at 20° C (to preserve the activity of factors V and VIII) and takes 20–30 minutes to thaw. FFP transfusion requires ABO typing but not crossmatching. The volume of a unit of FFP is ~200–250 cc.

2. FFP is indicated for rapid treatment of the bleeding patient with a coagulation defect caused by liver disease, vitamin K deficiency, warfarin therapy, DIC, or dilutional coagulopathy (massive RBC transfusions), or any bleeding patient with a PT ratio >1.2. It may also be used for patients who have a congenital deficiency of factors II, V, IX, or XI. FFP can serve as a colloid volume expander but should not be used primarily for this purpose.

H. Cryoprecipitate.

1. Cryoprecipitate is prepared by freezing plasma to −90° C and then allowing it to slowly warm to 4° C. The precipitate which forms is separated with a small amount of plasma. Each unit of cryoprecipitate contains about 200 mg fibrinogen, 150 units of factor VIII:VWF, and 100 units of factor VIII.

2. Despite its small volume (15–25 mL), a unit will significantly expand the circulating blood volume

3. Cryoprecipitate is *indicated in* patients with (1) *fibrinogen deficiency* with fibrinogen level <100 mg/dL (dysfibrinogenemia, hypofibrinogenemia, consumption coagulopathies); (2) hemophilia A (factor VIII level <50%), (3) *VWD,* and (4) acquired platelet defects (uremic patients with prolonged BTs or active bleeding, and platelet function abnormalities after cardiopulmonary bypass [CPB]).

I. **Factor VIII Concentrate.**
   1. Human factor VIII concentrates are prepared from large pools of donor plasma which are enriched for factor VIII. Because of donor pooling, the risk of disease transmission (primarily hepatitis) is high.
   2. Factor VIII concentrate is the *product of choice for* patients with moderate to severe *hemophilia A,* particularly when bleeding occurs. Acquired factor VIII deficiencies and the presence of factor VIII inhibitors can also be treated with human factor VIII concentrates.

J. **Prothrombin Complex.**
   1. Prothrombin complex is a lyophilized powder that is rich in factors II, VII, IX, and X.
   2. It is primarily intended for the *treatment of* congenital factor IX deficiency *(Christmas disease)* but may also be used for either congenital or acquired deficiencies of factors II, VII, or X.
   3. The major side effects are thrombosis and hepatitis (high risk).

K. **Rh Immune Globulin (RhIG).**
   RhIG is a concentrated solution of IgG anti-D derived from human plasma. It is indicated pre- and postpartum for Rh-negative women with Rh-positive fetuses or infants. It may also be indicated in Rh-negative women in the trauma setting.

L. **Autotransfusion (Autologous Blood).**
   1. The use of autologous blood virtually eliminates transfusion reactions and the risk of disease transmission. There are four approaches to autotransfusion:
      a. *Preoperative removal and storage* (predeposit autologous transfusion):
         1) Blood is removed before elective operation, stored, and then made available to the same person at the time of surgery.

2) If stored in the liquid state, blood must be used within 35 days; freezing allows safe storage for 2 years.

3) This technique is particularly valuable in patients with multiple antibodies or rare blood types.

4) Guidelines for safe preoperative phlebotomy include a Hct >34%, removal of no more than 10% of the estimated blood volume at a single donation, and donations at least 4 days apart (usually ≥1 week apart).

5) Alert the blood bank early that autologous blood is available.

b. **Immediate preoperative phlebotomy and hemodilution:**

1) This technique is most commonly used in open heart surgery. It involves the simultaneous infusion of a hemodiluent (crystalloid or colloid) into one vein and phlebotomy from another vein to produce a state of normovolemic anemia. The withdrawn blood is later reinfused as needed. Platelets and coagulation factors remain relatively intact.

2) The rationale for this procedure in cardiac surgery is to make available for reinfusion autologous blood that has not been exposed to the injury associated with CPB. Also, the blood lost intraoperatively has a lower Hct, thus decreasing the loss of RBCs.

c. *Intraoperative autotransfusion:*

1) Two options are available for intraoperative autotransfusion. Blood may be collected, filtered, and reinfused as whole blood, or it may be collected, processed, and reinfused as washed PRBCs.

2) Advantages of whole blood autotransfusion are that it is fast, simple, and inexpensive. Platelets and plasma proteins are infused along with the RBCs.

3) Disadvantages are the potential inclusion of debris, irrigation solutions, activated factors, anticoagulants, and free hemoglobin. This approach

is therefore contraindicated when blood is contaminated with stool, bacteria, or malignant cells.

4) Some methods require systemic heparinization while others use CPD (citrate phosphate dextrose) mixed with blood at the suction tip; in techniques using cell washing, heparin is added as the blood is aspirated.

d. **Postoperative autotransfusion:** Mediastinal blood which is shed after open heart procedures is often collected from the chest tubes, filtered, and reinfused. No heparinization is required since this blood contains no fibrinogen and does not clot.

M. **Directed Donations.**

1. A *directed donation* is blood deposited for a specific patient from family members or friends of that patient.

2. Directed donations do not appreciably improve the safety of blood transfusions and are therefore not generally recommended.

N. **Complications of Transfusion Therapy.**

1. **Acute hemolytic transfusion reaction.**

a. **Cause:** intravascular antibody and complement-mediated hemolysis due to *ABO* incompatibility is *usually due to clerical error.* Incidence is ~0.06:1,000 transfusions.

b. **Presentation:** Manifestations occur early in the transfusion (first 50–100 cc) and include severe headache, chest pain, dyspnea, flank and back pain, fever, chills, tachycardia, restlessness. The reaction may progress to hemoglobinemia and hemoglobinuria, ARF, DIC, bleeding, shock. The only early signs in an anesthetized patient may be fever, tachycardia, and excessive bleeding.

c. **Therapeutic and investigative procedures** are initiated immediately if a hemolytic transfusion reaction is suspected.

1) *Discontinue the transfusion immediately.*

2) *Hydrate the patient* with crystalloid solutions to maintain a urine output of >100 mL/hr. Insert a Foley catheter.

3) Give 25–50 g of mannitol IV or furosemide to *initiate diuresis.*

    4) Begin vasopressors if hypotension develops despite support with fluids

    5) Follow electrolytes, BUN and creatinine, DIC panel.

    6) Recheck both patient and blood identification.

    7) Save remaining donor blood for analysis.

    8) Draw a sample of venous blood for repeat cross-matching. A hemolytic antibody is sought by direct and indirect Coombs' tests.

    9) Obtain a urine sample and check for free hemoglobin.

   10) Draw blood from arm opposite transfusion site and examine for hemolysis.

2. *Delayed hemolytic transfusion reaction.*

    a. **Cause:** incompatibility of *minor blood group antigens* (Rh, Kell, Duffy, Kidd, etc.).

    b. **Presentation:** Occurs several days to weeks post-transfusion, and includes fever, chills, abdominal pain, anemia, indirect hyperbilirubinemia, jaundice, hemoglobinuria, and elevated LDH.

    c. **Treatment:** Give fluids, diurese, monitor renal function, avoid nephrotoxic agents, give antipyretics. Report reaction to transfusion service.

3. *Leukoagglutinin reaction* ("febrile transfusion reaction").

    a. **Cause:** recipient antibodies to donor *leukocyte antigens* (leukoagglutinins) due to previous allogeneic blood exposure (transfusion or pregnancy). Incidence is <2%.

    b. **Presentation:** Usually occurs late in the transfusion (30 minutes–2 hours). Symptoms include fever, chills, headache, flushing. Signs include tachycardia, hypo- or hypertension.

    c. **Treatment:** Stop transfusion, give IV fluids, antipyretics (acetaminophen), and rule out an acute hemolytic reaction. Transfusion may continue if there is no change in BP, if symptoms are mild and occur at the end of the transfusion, if plasma and urine show no evidence of hemolysis, and if patient is known to have a history of febrile nonhemolytic reactions to blood. Report to the transfusion service. Consider WBC poor products or the use of WBC filters (cheaper and effective) for future transfusions.

4. *Allergic transfusion reactions.*
   a. **Cause:** recipient antibodies to donor *plasma antigens*. The incidence is ~0.2–1.0:1,000.
   b. **Presentation:** urticaria (most common), fevers, chills, flushing, pruritus, and rarely anaphylaxis with bronchospasm and vascular collapse.
   c. **Treatment:** Stop the transfusion, give IV fluids, diphenhydramine 50 mg IM or PO. If effective, restart transfusion slowly and continue unless symptoms recur. Severe reactions may require epinephrine, steroids, bronchodilators, pressors, or intubation. Report to the transfusion service. Consider washed PRBCs for future transfusions.
5. *Noncardiogenic pulmonary edema.*
   a. **Cause:** probably due to antibodies to donor WBCs.
   b. **Presentation:** dyspnea, hypotension, normal cardiac pressures, interstitial edema on CXR, ARDS.
   c. **Treatment:** Stop transfusion, give O_2, intubate if necessary. Use WBC-poor products for future transfusions.
6. *Cardiogenic pulmonary edema (fluid overload).*
   a. **Cause:** patients with borderline cardiac status who cannot tolerate the volume of a transfusion.
   b. **Presentation:** symptoms and signs of CHF.
   c. **Treatment:** Give diuretics (e.g., furosemide IV). Transfuse cautiously.
7. *Infectious complications.*
   a. **Hepatitis:** The incidence of posttransfusion hepatitis is ~10%. Non-A, non-B hepatitis is the most common cause (78%–100% of all cases) with hepatitis B responsible for most of the remaining cases. Of those infected, between a quarter and a third develop chronic liver disease. Whole blood, PRBCs, platelets, and FFP carry a similar hepatitis risk. Cryoprecipitate, factor VIII concentrates, and prothrombin complex have a higher risk of hepatitis transmission because of donor pooling. Albumin and plasma protein fractions have essentially no risk of hepatitis.
   b. **Human immunodeficiency virus infection:** The risk of HIV infection from a single transfusion is estimated to be extremely low (~1:150,000 units). Whole blood, PRBCs, and FFP are equally capable

of transmitting HIV infection. Pooled products carry an increased risk. Factor VIII and IX concentrates can also transmit infection, though heat treatment of these products may inactivate the virus.

c. Other transmissible infectious agents include CMV, EBV, HTLV-I and -II, papovavirus, malaria, toxoplasmosis, and babesiosis.

d. Donated blood is screened for antibodies to HBsAg, HBcAg, HCV, HTLV-I, and HIV.

8. **Complications of massive transfusion:**

a. The term *massive transfusion* implies either a single transfusion >2,500 mL or the replacement of one or more blood volumes (~75 mL/kg, or ~5000 mL in a 70-kg adult) over a 24-hour period. Metabolic and hemostatic derangements may accompany massive transfusion.

b. The *coagulopathy* that results from massive transfusion is due to dilutional thrombocytopenia, impaired platelet function, and deficiencies of factors V, VIII, and XI. Ideally, the transfusion of platelets and coagulation factors should be guided by appropriate laboratory values. If this is not possible, the transfusion of ~1–2 units of FFP for every 5 units of blood and one "adult pack" of platelets for every 10 units of blood may be helpful.

c. *Citrate toxicity* is rare but can be caused by the binding of serum calcium by the citrate in banked blood, resulting in hypocalcemia. Administer calcium IV as needed (often ~one ampule per 4–5 units of blood).

d. *Hyperkalemia* is due to the relatively high potassium content of banked blood (12 mEq/l K^+ after 7-day storage). Massively transfused patients with adequate renal function should excrete excess potassium in the urine. In patients with renal failure, fresh blood products should be transfused to minimize the potassium load.

e. *Decreased 2,3-DPG-* Stored blood, depleted in 2,3-DPG, is less efficient in releasing O_2 to body tissues. Patients requiring normal levels of 2,3-DPG for O_2 transport may be transfused either with blood that is <1 week old or with frozen RBCs.

f. *Metabolic acidosis* is due to a combination of hypoperfusion and the low pH of stored blood (pH 6.9 after 2-day storage). An initial metabolic acidosis may occur during massive transfusion, but the rapid metabolism of citrate produces HCO_3^- which causes metabolic alkalosis. If necessary, treat the acidosis with IV bicarbonate.

g. *Hypothermia,* due to transfusion of cold blood products, is relatively common and has adverse effects on platelet function, coagulation, acid-base balance, and cardiovascular function. Hypothermia may be prevented by warming all blood products and fluids during massive transfusions. Treat with warmed fluids and increased ambient temperature (heat lamps, overhead heaters, blankets).

IV. PHARMACOLOGIC THERAPY.

Pertinent agents include anticoagulants (heparin, warfarin), thrombolytics (streptokinase, urokinase, t-PA), antiplatelet agents (aspirin, dipyridamole), heparin antidotes (protamine), antithrombolytics (aminocaproic acid), and vasopressin analogues (desmopressin).

A. Heparin.

Before beginning anticoagulant therapy with heparin or warfarin, weigh the risks of hemorrhage against the risk of thrombosis or embolism.

1. **Effect:** *Augments the activity of antithrombin III,* thereby inhibiting *new* thrombus formation. Prolongs PTT, TT, and to a lesser extent PT. T$\frac{1}{2}$ is ~1–3 hours. Degraded in the liver with degradation products excreted in the urine.

2. **Indications:** *acute* treatment of venous thrombosis, PE, atrial fibrillation, thromboembolic stroke, acute MI, peripheral arterial occlusion, DIC (controversial), and prophylaxis of postoperative DVT or PE (controversial).

3. **Relative contraindications:** active bleeding, bleeding tendencies or disorders, severe hypertension or retinopathy, cerebrovascular hemorrhage, pregnancy.

4. **Usage.**

   a. Initiation of therapy:

      1) Obtain a baseline Hct, platelet count, PT, PTT.

      2) Administer 5,000–10,000 units as an IV bolus injection.

      3) Begin continuous infusion at a rate of 1,000 units/hr.

  b. Monitoring therapy:

    1) Obtain a PTT 6–8 hours after start of heparin infusion. The therapeutic anticoagulant effect of heparin usually corresponds to PTT values 1.5–2 × baseline (approximately 50–80 seconds). The heparin infusion rate is adjusted if the observed PTT is outside this range.

    2) If the PTT is <50 seconds, increase the heparin infusion rate to ~1,200 units/hr. A second IV bolus of 2,000–5,000 units may be necessary if the PTT is <40 seconds.

    3) If the PTT is >80 seconds, decrease the heparin infusion rate to ~800 units/hr. It may be necessary to hold the heparin infusion for 1 hour before resuming at the lower rate.

    4) Obtain a PTT ~6 hours after each change in the infusion rate.

    5) Change infusion rates by increments of ~100–200 units/hr depending on PTT.

    6) Monitor PTT at least once per day, the Hct and platelet count every 1–2 days, and the plasma heparin level in patients who are unusually sensitive or resistant to heparin (some patients require >2,000 units/hr).

  5. **Adverse effects:** Observe for hemorrhage (the most common adverse effect), thrombocytopenia and arterial thromboembolism (HATT), fever, urticaria, osteoporosis, skin necrosis.

B. Warfarin Sodium (Coumadin).

  1. **Effect:** It *inhibits the hepatic synthesis of factors II, VII, IX, X* (and proteins C and S). It is well absorbed orally, is ~97% albumin-bound, and has a T$\frac{1}{2}$ of 36–72 hours. It is degraded in the liver to inactive metabolites that are excreted into the bile, reabsorbed, and excreted into the urine.

  2. **Indications and contraindications:** similiar to heparin, though used for *chronic* therapy, crosses placenta.

  3. **Usage:**

    a. Before beginning therapy, obtain a baseline PT, PTT, Hct, and platelet count. Weigh the risks of therapy vs. nontherapy.

b. Initiation of therapy: Give 10–15 mg PO q.d. for 1–3 days.

c. Monitoring therapy:

1) Obtain PT values daily after the first one to two 10-mg/day doses.

2) Adjust daily doses on the basis of the observed PT values. Changes in dosage require approximately 2 days before they are reflected in the PT.

3) Desired PT ratios are 1.4–1.8 times control in DVT and PE, and 1.6–2.1 times control in arterial thrombosis. The values required in patients with prosthetic heart valves may be lower.

4) Maintenance doses are usually in the range of 2–10 mg PO q.d.

5) Once the PT has stabilized, it may be followed every 2–3 days (inpatients) or every 1–4 weeks (outpatients). Patient compliance is important.

6) The Hct should also be monitored.

4. **Adverse effects:**

a. Hemorrhage (the most common adverse effect), skin necrosis, nausea, vomiting, diarrhea, urticaria, alopecia, and teratogenic effects may occur.

b. Warfarin overdosage is treated with vitamin K (10–20 mg IV or PO) and blood products (primarily FFP).

c. Enhanced anticoagulant responses may be seen in patients with liver disease, vitamin K deficiency, hyperthyroidism, and drug interactions (see below).

5. **Drug interactions**

a. **Drugs that cause a decreased PT:** adrenocorticosteroids, antacids, alcohol, aminogluthethamide, antihistamines, barbiturates, carbamazepine, chloral hydrate, chlordiazepoxide, cholestyramine, ethchlorvynol, glutethimide, griseofulvin, haloperidol, meprobamate, oral contraceptives, paraldehyde, primidone, ranitidine, rifampin, trazodone, vitamin C.

b. **Drugs that cause an increased PT:** alcohol, allopurinol, aminosalicylic acid, amiodarone, anabolic steroids, anesthetics (inhalation), antibiotics, bromelains, chlorpropramide, chymotrypsin, cimetidine, clofibrate, dextran, D-thyroxine, diazoxide, diflunisal, disulfiram, ethacrynic acid, glucagon, ibuprofen, indomethacin, influenza virus vaccine, MAOIs, methyldopa, methylphenidate, metronidazole, nalidixic acid, naproxen, narcotics, pentoxifylline, phenylbutazone, phenytoin, pyrazolones, quinidine, quinine, ranitidine, salicylates, sulfinpyrazone, sulfonamides, sulindac, tamoxifen, thyroid drugs, tolbutamide.

  c. Warfarin increases the anticonvulsant blood levels of phenobarbital and phenytoin and increases the hypoglycemic effect of chlorpropamide and tolbutamide.

C. Streptokinase (SK)

1. **Effect:** converts plasminogen to plasmin, which degrades fibrin and fibrinogen.
2. **Indications:** DVT, PE, arterial thrombosis or embolism.
3. **Contraindications:** recent (past 2 months) stroke, intracranial or intraspinal surgery or neoplasm, active bleeding. Relative contraindications include recent (past 10 days) surgery, GI bleed, or trauma; severe hypertension; left heart thrombus; SBE; coagulopathies; pregnancy; cerebrovascular disease; diabetic retinopathy; septic thrombophlebitis.
4. **Systemic streptokinase therapy.**
   a. Initiating therapy:
    1) Obtain baseline Hct, platelet count, DIC panel, and TCT.
    2) Administer 250,000 units IV bolus over 30 minutes, then 100,000 units/hr continuous IV infusion for 24–72 hours.
    3) To minimize the risk of hypersensitivity, administer 50 mg diphenhydramine IV or 100 mg hydrocortisone IV before the start of therapy and then q. 12–24 h.
   b. Monitoring therapy:
    1) Obtain the first treatment TCT 2–4 hours after starting therapy. A good fibrinolytic response is associated with a TCT two to five control.
    2) Other tests which can be used to monitor fibrinolytic therapy are fibrinogen, fibrin split products, PTT, and PT.
    3) Monitor TCT values at least once per day. If observed TCT and fibrinogen levels remain un

changed, discontinue SK and consider urokinase (UK).

5. Adverse effects include hemorrhage, fever, allergic reactions, urticaria, anaphylactic shock, nausea, vomiting, headache, muscle pain.

6. Should massive bleeding occur during therapy, stop SK, transfuse PRBCs, infuse 5 units of cryoprecipitate (fibrinogen) until bleeding stops, and infuse aminocaproic acid 4 g IV followed by 1 g/hr IV until bleeding stops.

D. Urokinase

1. Effect, indications, and contraindications are similiar to SK.

2. **Dosage.**

   a. Systemic therapy: Load with 4,400 units/kg IV bolus over 10 minutes, then infuse at 4,400 units/kg/hr for 12–24 hours.

   b. Local therapy (treatment of peripheral arterial occlusion): Load with 50,000 units IV bolus into the occluded vessel, then infuse at 50,000 units/hr.

3. Adverse effects include hemorrhage, fever, allergic reactions.

E. Tissue Plasminogen Activator

1. **Effect:** t-PA is a recombinant glycoprotein (serine protease) which forms a complex with plasminogen and fibrin and then activates the plasminogen that is complexed with fibrin, thereby allowing specific fibrin lysis.

2. **Indications:** acute MI.

3. **Contraindications:** history of a stroke; recent (past 2 months) intracranial or intraspinal surgery, or trauma; intracranial neoplasm, arteriovenous malformation (AVM), or aneurysm; active bleeding; known bleeding diathesis; severe uncontrolled hypertension

4. **Dosage:** 100 mg IV over 3 hours (60 mg/hr × 1 hour, then 20 mg/hr × 2 hours). For smaller individuals, give 1.25 mg/kg over 3 hours as above.

5. **Adverse effects:** Bleeding (internal and surface) is the most common (~10%); mild hypersensitivity reactions, nausea and vomiting, hypotension, and fever are less common.

F. Aspirin.

1. **Effect:** irreversibly inactivates cyclooxygenase, thus inhibiting synthesis of prostaglandins and thromboxanes.

Inhibition of platelet thromboxane production eliminates one important stimulus for platelet aggregation and release. Effects persist for the 7–10-day life span of the platelets exposed to aspirin. Therefore, aspirin must be discontinued 10 days prior to surgical procedures.

2. **Indications:** antiplatelet therapy (cerebrovascular, coronary, peripheral atherosclerosis), anti-inflammatory (arthritis, rheumatic diseases), antipyretic, analgesic (minor aches and pains).

3. **Contraindications and relative contraindications:** salicylate hypersensitivity, gastric ulcers, asthma, warfarin therapy, thrombolytic therapy, bleeding disorders.

4. **Dosage:** 325–1,000 mg po q.4h. up to ~4000 mg/24 hr. Measure salicylate levels as needed.

5. **Adverse effects:** salicylate hypersensitivity (rhinitis, urticaria, angioedema, bronchospasm, vasomotor collapse), gastric ulcers, GI disturbances, tinnitis and deafness, hepatotoxicity, renal dysfunction, irritability, elevated serum transaminases and alkaline phosphatase.

G. Dipyridamole.

1. **Effect:** platelet adhesion inhibitor (mechanism of action not fully elucidated). Well absorbed orally, two half-lives (75 minutes and 10 hours), highly protein-bound, and metabolized in liver and excreted in bile.

2. **Indications:** sometimes given with aspirin for antiplatelet therapy.

3. **Contraindications:** none known.

4. **Dosage:** 75–100 mg po q.i.d. for cardiac valve replacement, 25–75 mg po t.i.d. for treatment of ASPVD

5. **Adverse effects:** usually minimal and transient, may include dizziness, abdominal distress, headache, rash.

H. Protamine Sulfate.

1. **Effect:** Small basic proteins react with heparin (which is acidic) to form an inactive salt complex. A weak anticoagulant in the absence of heparin. Onset of action within 5 minutes of IV dose.

2. **Indications:** heparin antagonist, for heparin overdosage or reversal.

3. **Usage:** Give 1% protamine 1.0–1.5 mg 1%/100 units IV heparin given in the previous 4 hours, or calculate the needed dose using the ACT (see p 585). Use conserva-

tive estimates of dose needed and monitor response carefully, since protamine has anticoagulant effects itself. Administer at rate of 5 mg/min IV with maximum rate of 50 mg/10 min or 200 mg/2 hr (rarely give >100 mg). Monitor continuously for hypotension during infusion.

4. **Adverse effects:** hypotension, bradycardia, pulmonary hypertension, allergic reactions and anaphylaxis, incompatibility with penicillins and cephalosporins, dyspnea, flushing, rebound anticoagulation (30 minutes–18 hours after heparin reversal).

I. Aminocaproic Acid.

1. **Effect:** inhibits plasminogen activator substances and, to lesser degree, plasmin, thereby inhibiting fibrinolysis. Rapid oral absorption and rapid renal excretion (75% unmetabolized).

2. **Indications:** bleeding due to *primary fibrinolysis but not DIC*. Must differentiate primary fibrinolysis from DIC (see pp 593–594).

3. **Dosage:** Load with 4–5 g po or IV (in 250 mL crystalloid diluent over 1 hour), then 1.0–1.25 g po or IV (in 50 mL) q.h. × 8 hours or until bleeding stops (maximum 30 g/24 hr). Monitor for hypotension, bradycardia, dysrhythmias.

4. **Adverse effects:** intrarenal thrombosis and obstruction in patients with upper urinary tract bleeding; cardiac and skeletal muscle injury; hypotension, bradycardia, and dysrhythmias with rapid infusion; prolonged BT (apparently clinically insignificant).

J. Desmopressin Acetate (DDAVP).

1. **Effect.**
   a. Increases plasma levels of factor VIII.
   b. Increases renal water conservation.

2. **Indications.**
   a. Hemophilia A and VWD chronic renal failure: effective in patients with mild or moderate factor VIII deficiency (levels >5%; occasionally justified with levels 2%–5%) with spontaneous or traumatic bleeding or surgery (give 30 minutes preoperatively).
   b. Follow factors VIII, VIII:C, VIII:VWF, BT.
   c. Central DI, including posttraumatic and postoperative.

3. **Dosage.**
   a. IV (for either indication): 0.3–0.4 µg/kg over 10 minutes. Has biphasic half-lives of 8 and 75 minutes. Dose q. 2–3 d. (more frequent dosing results in decreased effect of factor VIII activity).
   b. Intranasal (for outpatient management of central DI): 0.1–0.4 mL/day, divided into one to three doses (usual dose is 0.1 mL b.i.d.).
4. **Adverse effects:** slight elevation in BP (infrequent), water intoxication and hyponatremia; occasionally headache, abdominal cramps, local erythema, facial flushing.

V. RADIATION THERAPY AND CHEMOTHERAPY.
A. Principles of Radiation Therapy.
1. **Megavoltage**—used to treat deeply situated lesions. X-rays have a sharply defined beam, and result in decreased radiation to surrounding tissues. There is also a relative skin-sparing, decreased absorption in bone relative to soft tissues, and a greater penetration of tissues.
2. **Brachytherapy**—interstitial or intracavitary radiation, with a rapid decrease in dose with distance from the radiation source.
3. **Units for describing radiation doses:**
   a. Roentgen (R)—unit of exposure.
   b. Gray (Gy)—unit of absorbed dose. Developed since different tissues will absorb different amounts of radiation when exposed to the same beam of radiation. 1 Gy represents the absorption of 1 J/kg of matter, and is equivalent to 100 rad.
4. **Method of cellular injury:**
   a. Radiation causes the loss of reproductive integrity, or the ability to divide indefinitely.
   b. Chromosomal DNA is the primary target for radiation-induced lethality.
   c. A specified dose of radiation will kill a constant fraction of irradiated cells.
   d. *Therapeutic ratio* is defined as the damage to tumor–damage to normal cells.
   e. Tumor response depends on the balance between new cell growth and radiation-induced cell death. In general, a given dose of radiation is more effective when given as a single dose, vs. the same dose given in

multiple exposures. The total dose for multiple doses may have to be two to five times greater than a single dose to produce the same effect.

    f. Well-oxygenated cells are 2.5–3.0 times more radio-sensitive than anoxic cells.

B. Complications of Radiation Therapy.

Early complications occur in rapidly dividing cells which are also exposed to the radiation dose, such as GI epithelium and skin. Late complications result primarily from injury to the supporting structures, such as vascular endothelium and connective tissue. Vascular injury leads to endarteritis and obliteration of capillary lumen, leading to atrophy, fibrosis, and ulceration.

  1. **Acute radiation syndrome** is typically seen after exposure of most of the body to an external source of ionizing radiation.

    a. **Hematologic form** is manifested at 1–3 weeks after exposure, with falling granulocytes, lymphocytes, and platelets. Clinical signs include:

      1) Fever due to inability to adequately fight infection.

      2) Abscesses.

      3) Petechiae, purpura, bleeding.

    b. **GI form:**

      1) Anorexia, nausea, vomiting, diarrhea, occurring within hours after exposure.

      2) May progress to fulminant enterocolitis.

    c. **CNS and cardiovascular forms:**

      1) Manifested by disorientation, ataxia, prostration, shock.

      2) Alternates between CNS excitability and CNS depression, leading to coma and fatal outcome in 24–48 hours.

  2. **Radiation injury to the skin:**

    a. Erythema, comparable to a first-degree burn, occurring at 2–3 weeks.

    b. Epilation, begins after exposures of approximately 300 rad.

    c. Transepidermal injury (dermatitis), comparable to a second-degree burn, occurring at 1.5–3.0 weeks after exposures of 1,000 rad.

3. **Radiation injury to GI tract:**
   a. Damage to the small intestine and colon may occur during radiation therapy for pelvic or abdominal malignancies.
   b. Damage occurs most commonly after total doses exceed 5,000 rad, with small bowel affected more commonly than colon.
   c. Hyperemia and ulceration of mucosa are common. More severe injury is characterized by diffuse edema, followed by ischemia and fibrosis.
   d. Abscesses and fistulas may develop between loops of intestine or between intestine and neighboring organs; late changes result in stricture formation.
   e. Symptoms include:
      1) Diarrhea, malabsorption, rectal bleeding.
      2) Small intestine symptoms result from fibrosis with obstruction or fistulization and abscess formation.
   f. Treatment consists of:
      1) An elemental diet free of milk protein and lactose.
      2) Steroid retention enemas for severe rectal bleeding with transfusions as indicated.
      3) Dilation of rectal strictures.
      4) Resection of fistulas with draining of any abscesses. Bowel resections with primary reanastomosis are hazardous because of impaired blood supply.

4. **Radiation injury to the lung:**
   a. Commonly results after radiation therapy for thoracic malignancies.
   b. Most predominant injury occurs in alveolar type II cells (surfactant producers), capillary endothelial cells, and bronchial epithelial cells as these are the most rapidly dividing.
   c. Rare with total doses <2000 rad; common when radiation dose >4,000 rad.
   d. Acute changes occur 1–2 months after radiation, and are characterized by dyspnea and cough.
   e. Permanent changes of fibrosis take 6–24 months to develop, and usually remain stable after 2 years if no

further injury occurs. Injury results in restrictive lung disease.

5. **Radiation injury to nervous system:**
   a. Usually seen when radiation has been directed at neoplasms of the brain or at other head and neck tumors.
   b. The spinal cord can also be injured by radiation directed at a primary cord tumor or at tumors overlying the spine and paraspinal regions.
   c. Damage to the brain occurs with approximately 6,000 rad; the radiation tolerance of the spinal cord is lower. Peripheral nerves are relatively radioresistant.
   d. Symptoms occur approximately 1 year after radiation, and are associated with nerve cell damage, demyelination, and vascular changes.
   e. Onset is insidious, and rate of progression unpredictable.
   f. Clinical differentiation between radiation injury and tumor recurrence may be difficult.

6. **Radiation injury to the heart:**
   a. Clinically apparent in approximately 5% of patients receiving >4,000 rad.
   b. Manifested as pericardial disease, including acute pericarditis, chronic effusion, or chronic constrictive pericarditis.
   c. Less commonly, myocardial fibrosis may occur and can result in conduction disturbances.

7. Most common problem arising during radiation therapy is maintenance of adequate food and fluid intake. Patients, especially those irradiated around the head or neck, often lose their appetite because of changes in saliva and impaired taste sensation. Patients with bowel complications may require special diets.

8. Cancer patients are subject to numerous concomitant medical problems, including MI, acute appendicitis, perforation of peptic ulcer, and other major medical or surgical problems. The tendency to ascribe all complaints to irradiation must be resisted, so all patients are thoroughly evaluated and definitive therapy is not delayed.

C. **Principles of Chemotherapy.**
   1. The basic goal is the development of agents with selective toxicity against replicating tumor cells, sparing replicating host tissues. Chemotherapy is based on the quan-

titative differences in the proliferative kinetics of normal and neoplastic cell growth. Stimulated normal tissue which is proliferating as rapidly as neoplastic tissue will be effected to the same extent as neoplastic tissue.

2. Two types of agents:
   a. Cell cycle–specific—only effective against actively proliferating cells engaged in DNA synthesis and mitosis.
   b. Cell cycle–nonspecific—kill both normal and tumor cells regardless of their proliferative state.

3. Any tissue, normal or neoplastic, manifests an early logarithmic phase of exponential growth during which most cells are in active mitosis. When a certain bulk is obtained, there is a transition to a later steady-state plateau growth phase during which a lesser fraction of cells is in the proliferative cycle. To maximize the effects of cell cycle–specific agents, resting cells must be induced to proliferate without increasing vulnerability of normal tissues. This implies a reduction in tumor growth with a reentry into the exponential growth phase. Methods for reducing tumor bulk include treatment with cell cycle–nonspecific agents, radiation, or removal of gross tumor masses at surgery.

4. The goal of chemotherapy can be either curative or palliative. The degree of toxicity that is acceptable depends on the goal.

D. Chemotherapeutic Agents and Their Complications.

    1. Hormones.

        a. **Glucocorticoids:**

            1) Exert a "lympholytic" effect useful in the treatment of leukemias and lymphomas and also useful in the treatment of hormonally sensitive tumors (breast, prostate).

            2) They improve cerebral edema associated with brain tumors, correct hypercalcemias associated with malignancies, and can palliate hemolytic anemias associated with lymphomas and leukemias.

            3) Complications of therapy:
                a) Metabolic—hyperglycemia, sodium retention, potassium wasting.
                b) GI—peptic ulceration.

       c) Immunosuppressive—increased susceptibility to infection.
  b. **Estrogens:**
       1) Useful in prostatic cancer.
       2) Side effects include:
            a) Fluid retention.
            b) Feminization of males.
            c) Uterine bleeding.
            d) GI disturbances, including nausea and vomiting.
  c. **Androgens:**
       1) Useful for breast cancer.
       2) Side effects include:
            a) Virilization of women.
            b) Fluid retention.
            c) Cholestatic jaundice (oral preparations).
  d. **Antiestrogens:**
       1) Antagonize estrogen stimulation of hormone-dependent tumors (breast).
       2) Toxicity minimal (nausea, vomiting, hot flashes).
2. **Alkylators:**
  a. Form cross-links at the guanine residues of double-stranded DNA. Alkylators are cell cycle–nonspecific and affect both resting and dividing cells, normal and malignant cells.
  b. Examples include nitrogen mustard, cyclophosphamide (Cytoxan), chlorambucil (Leukeran), L-phenylalanine mustard (Alkeran), busulfan (Myleran) and thiotepa.
  c. Toxicity is related to effects on rapidly dividing tissue (GI, gonadal, skin, hematopoietic); bone marrow suppression is predominant. Alkylators also cause nausea and vomiting, hypospermia, menstrual irregularities, fetal anomalies.
  d. Side effects associated with specific alkylators include:
       1) Alopecia and hemorrhagic cystitis (cyclophosphamide).
       2) Melanosis and pulmonary fibrosis (busulfan).
3. **Nitrosoureas:**
  a. Cell cycle–nonspecific agents similar to alkylators, with greater lipid solubility.

    b. Examples include carmustine (BCNU), lomustine (CCNU), and semustine (methyl-CCNU).

    c. Toxicity includes nausea and vomiting, prolonged marrow suppression, local phlebitis.

4. **Antimetabolites:**

    a. Compounds resemble substrates normally utilized by cells for metabolism and growth. Structural analogues interfere with nucleic acid synthesis and impair proliferation of normal and neoplastic cells, making the compounds cell cycle–specific.

    b. Methotrexate:

        1) Inhibits dihydrofolate reductase.

        2) Toxicity includes mucositis, gastroenteritis, dermatitis, marrow suppression, hepatitis.

        3) Side effects may be alleviated by the administration of folinic acid (citrovorum factor).

    c. Fluorouracil (5-FU):

        1) Thymidine analogue interferes with thymidylate synthetase, an enzyme involved in the generation of thymidylic acid, a DNA precursor.

        2) Side effects include dermatitis, gastroenteritis, mucositis, marrow depression.

        3) Erythema of buccal mucosa is an early sign of mucosal toxicity and is usually associated with ulcerations in GI tract; hold therapy until erythema or ulceration heals.

5. **Cytotoxic antibiotics:**

    a. Cell cycle–nonspecific.

    b. Dactinomycin:

        1) Inhibits DNA-dependent synthesis of RNA by ribosomes.

        2) Toxicity includes marrow suppression, ulcerative stomatitis, gastroenteritis, and local tissue necrosis if extravasated.

    c. Doxorubicin (Adriamycin):

        1) Tumoricidal antibiotic that intercalates between adjacent base pairs of double-stranded DNA.

        2) Toxicity includes marrow suppression, alopecia, mucitis, delayed cardiac toxicity.

        3) Changes in cardiac function can be detected at doses of 300 mg/m^2 and no patient should receive >550 mg/m^2.

    d. Bleomycin:
        1) Impairs cell division by scission of DNA strands or inhibition of ligase.
        2) The most serious side effects are interstitial pneumonitis and fibrosis, which are usually dose-related and occur at doses exceeding 150 mg/m^2. Generally older patients and those with preexisting lung disease are most susceptible.
        3) Hypersensitivity pneumonitis with eosinophilia may occur at any dosage and responds to steroid administration.
        4) Additional toxicity includes dermatitis with hyperpigmentation and desquamation, acute febrile reactions, and stomatitis.
        5) The drug is marrow-sparing.
        6) Management includes minimizing O_2 administration which exacerbates pulmonary fibrosis. Use minimal concentration of O_2.
    e. Any preoperative patient with a history of receiving doxorubicin or bleomycin should have a careful evaluation of cardiac and pulmonary function.
6. **Plant alkaloids:**
    a. Cell cycle–specific agents which bind to cytoplasmic precursors of the mitotic spindle, causing polymerization and compromise of the mitotic spindle.
    b. Vinblastine:
        1) Primarily causes marrow suppression, but also gastroenteritis, neurotoxicity, alopecia.
        2) Severe local ulcer forms if the drug extravasates.
    c. Vincristine:
        1) Primarily neurotoxic, and may induce peripheral, autonomic, or cranial neuropathies.
        2) Mild form consists of paresthesias in fingers and toes. Progression to involve the PIP joints; hyporeflexia or muscle weakness necessitates discontinuation of therapy.
        3) Constipation is the most common symptom of autonomic neuropathy, and all patients should receive stool softeners and cathartics to prevent impaction.
        4) Alopecia is also common.
7. **Miscellaneous compounds:**
    a. Procarbazine:

1) MAOI causes both oxidation and alkylation of cellular components.
2) Toxicity includes marrow suppression, gastroenteritis, dermatitis, CNS abnormalities.

  b. Etoposide:
  1) Causes breakage in single-stranded DNA.
  2) Toxicity is mainly marrow suppression.

  c. Interferon-α: Toxicity includes flulike symptoms (fever, chills, malaise), CNS symptoms (somnulence, confusion), hypotension, granulocytopenia.

8. **Late complication** of chemotherapy is the increased risk of developing a second malignancy, most commonly acute leukemia. Incidence is 2% in patients treated with MOPP for Hodgkin's disease. Certain drugs (e.g., melphalan, procarbazine) are more carcinogenic than others.

SELECTED REFERENCES

Donaldson MC, Weinberg DS, Belkin M, et al: Screening for hypercoagulable states in vascular surgical practice: A preliminary study *[see comments]*. *J Vasc Surg* 1990;6:825–831.

Mannucci PM: Desmopressin: A monotransfusional form of treatment for congenital and acquired bleeding disorders. *Blood* 1988;72:1449–1455.

Rappaport SI: Preoperative hemostatic evaluation: Which tests, if any? *Blood* 1983;61:229.

Reisner EG, Telen MJ, Issitt L, et al: *Transfusion Service Manual*. Durham, NC, Duke University Medical Center, 1990.

Rohrer MJ, Michelotti MC, Nahrwold DL: A prospective evaluation of the efficacy of preoperative coagulation testing. *Ann Surg* 1988;208:554–557.

Rudolph R, Boyd CR: Massive transfusion: Complications and their management. *South Med J* 1990;83:1065–1070.

Vander-Woude JC, Milam JD, Walker WE, et al: Cardiovascular surgery in patients with congenital plasma coagulopathies. *Ann Thorac Surg* 1988;46:283–288.

Ware R, Filston HC, Schultz WH, et al: Elective cholecystectomy in children with sickle hemoglobinopathies. Successful outcome using a preoperatie transfusion regimen. *Ann Surg* 1988;208:17–22.

Webster MW, Chesebro JH, Fuster V: Platelet inhibitor therapy. Agents and clinical implications. *Hematol Oncol Clin North Am* 1990;4:265–289.

TRANSPLANTATION *16*

I. BRAIN DEATH DIAGNOSIS.

A. The first phase of transplantation of any organ commonly begins in the SICU with the diagnosis of brain death. Organ procurement remains the major limitation for transplantation. Physicians are now required by law to inquire regarding anatomical gifts in all in-hospital patient deaths, with few exceptions such as patients with AIDS, rabies, active hepatitis, or Creutzfeldt-Jakob disease. Moreover, it is important to remember that functional cornea, bone, skin, and cardiac valve grafts can be obtained in the absence of any cardiovascular function.

B. Throughout the United States and Canada, there are minor interhospital and legal variations of the **Uniform Determination of Death Act.** This act states: "An individual who has sustained either (1) irreversible cessation of circulatory and respiratory functions or (2) irreversible cessation of all functions of the entire brain, including the brain stem, is dead. A declaration of death must be made in accordance with accepted medical standards."

C. Realistically, the most important aspect of brain death is the **irreversible absence of all brain and brainstem functions.** The coma must be deep and its cause sufficient to account for the observed loss of brain function.

   1. **Irreversible loss of function requires:**

      a. An adequate core temperature $> 32.2°$ C ($90°$ F).

      b. The absence of all sedation.

      c. The absence of metabolic causes of coma (hepatic encephalopathy, hyperosmolar coma, preterminal uremia).

      d. The absence of neuromuscular blockade.

      e. The absence of shock.

   2. **A toxin screen** may be necessary to assure the absence of depressant drugs.

3. **Absent cephalic reflexes that need documentation** include:
   a. Pupillary light response.
   b. Oculocephalic (doll's eyes testing).
   c. Oculovestibular (caloric testing).
   d. Oropharyngeal (gag reflex testing).
   e. Respiratory reflexes (apnea testing).

4. **Respiratory reflexes are tested by apnea observation.**
   a. The patient is ventilated with 100% O_2 for 10 minutes and the ventilator replaced by high flow O_2 continuous positive airway pressure (CPAP).
   b. Care should be taken not to hyperventilate the patient in the initial phase (keep $PaCO_2$ $\geq$40 mm Hg).
   c. Hypercarbia stimulates the respiratory effort within 30 seconds when $PaCO_2$ >60 mm Hg.
   d. The $PaCO_2$ usually rises 3 mm Hg for every minute of apnea. Usually 10 minutes of apnea is sufficient to achieve this level of hypercarbia, and should be confirmed by ABG.
   e. Spontaneous respiratory efforts during an adequate examination indicate residual function of part of the brainstem.

5. **Spinal reflexes** may persist (including the nonpurposeful withdrawal to pain). *True decerebate or decorticate posturing or seizures are inconsistent with the diagnosis of death.*

6. **In infants and children <5 years old,** particular caution should attend the application of criteria for brain death because of increased resistance to injury and the ability to recover function.

7. Each hospital should have a **brain death committee** available at all times to help with consultation regarding the determination of brain death.

8. It is most important that the diagnosis of death and its time be clearly **recorded in the medical record.** (An "examination consistent with brain death" is not a pronouncement of death.)

9. Individual institutions and states may have specific criteria for determination of brain death. The Duke University Medical Center algorithm for determination of brain death is given in Table 16–1.

TABLE 16–1.

Duke University Criteria for Determination of Brain Death

The patient is normothermic (core temperature >32.2° C), normotensive (systemic BP >80 mm Hg), and must be comatose, apneic, and without cephalic reflexes, *and* the case meets the conditions specified in A *or* B *or* C below:

A. This state is present for at least 3 days.

B. 1. The primary condition is known to be an irreparable lesion of the brain.
   2. The patient, by appropriate examinations, must be shown to have for at least 30 mins:
      a) Electrocerebral silence on EEG *or*
      b) Absence of cerebral blood flow (quantitative CSF, four-vessel angiogram, isotopic angiogram, bolus passage of IV isotopes, or absent midline echo) *or*
      c) No cerebral metabolism (CMR O_2 < 1 mL/g/min, AV DO_2 < 2 vol %, or lactic acid > 6 mEq/L).

C. 1. The primary condition, not a known irreparable lesion of the brain, has not responded to appropriate treatment.
   2. a) The patient's EEG must be isoelectric for 2 days *or*
      b) At least 6 hr after the ictus, the conditions of B.2 are met.

D. *Communication with the family* of an organ donor regarding brain death is a very sensitive process and can affect indelibly how they will respond to organ donation. The clinician with the greatest rapport and the most senior available member of the primary service should be present with the patient's nurse and chaplain or social worker as indicated. All the diagnostic findings should be reviewed. The irreversibility of the process should be emphasized. The fact that brain death has been diagnosed, by whom, and at what time should be firmly established. The finality of this diagnosis should be emphasized in terms appropriate to the family's understanding (e.g., "He is dead now just as surely as if his heart had stopped instead of his brain.").

E. Most important, take care to avoid any implication of guilt or misconduct to the family of an organ donor. Explain that the ventilator and drips will be stopped and hypotension and asystole will follow, the medical examiner will be contacted, and why, etc. The family should be offered the opportunity to view the body before or after the discontinuation of support but it should be clear that this cannot affect the termination of support.

F. The family has a choice in cases in which the patient is not known to be an organ donor. By this stage, organ donation should not be entirely new to the family. If they have been kept accurately informed of the patient's course and the reason for proceedings surrounding the determination of brain death, the possibility of organ donation should have been mentioned. If it has not, or if the family is suspected to be negatively inclined, then the assistance of an organ procurement coordinator may be helpful during this conversation.

G. The **required request** for organ donation provides a ready reason to begin discussion of this topic. The options should be articulately and dispassionately discussed and written consent obtained. Again, it should be clear that death has already occurred. Usually the family has formed the decision before organ donation is discussed. In situations of indecision, a favorable outcome can be expected when the time is taken to explain the importance of organ donation to the lives of others. It is useless to try to dissuade a family set against organ donation.

II. PHYSIOLOGIC MAINTENANCE OF THE BRAIN-DEAD CADAVER.

A. As soon as the possibility of brain death is reasonably entertained, the transplant coordinator or organ procurement officer should be contacted. Early contact of the procurement coordinators will allow them to initiate tissue typing and viral antibody studies and to begin coordinating transplant activities. In addition, they provide valuable advice in the physiologic management of the brain-dead cadaver to support graft function to the time of organ harvest.

B. To the moment that brain death occurs, all resuscitative efforts must be directed to O_2 delivery to the brain and reduction of brain edema, as addressed in Chapter 13. Optimal neurologic management usually includes treatments detrimental to blood flow to other (transplantable) organs. At the time of brain death in the organ donor, intensive care changes from neurologic concerns to optimization of blood flow and O_2 delivery to potential donor organs.

C. The goals of donor maintenance therapy are outlined in Table 16–2.

D. The acceptance of criteria for brain death has come in large part from the demonstration that cardiovascular collapse oc

TABLE 16–2.

Goals of Maintenance of Organ Donor

Plan to deliver the donor to the OR
with:
  PaO_2 >100 mm Hg
  Systolic BP > 100 mm Hg on < 10
    μg/kg/min dopamine
  UO > 100 mL/hr
  Normal LFTs
  Normal serum creatine
By treating:
  Hypothermia
    Warm inspired gas to 37° C.
    Warm all infusions
    Overhead heater/heating mattress
    Blankets
  Hypoxemia
    Adequate preload
    Increase FIO_2
    PEEP
    Maximize Hct
    Bronchodilators, pulmonary toilet
  Hypotension
    Optimize preload
    Dopamine 10 μg/kg/min
    Treat bradycardia only if
      hypotensive
    ? Glucagon, ? neosynephrine
  Metabolism
    Correct electrolyte imbalance
    Check urine Na^+, K^+
    Replace urinary losses
    Normalize blood glucose
    ? Consider vasopressin if
      significant DI

---

curs without exception following irreversible cessation of all brain function. The only variable is the rapidity with which subsequent loss of thermoregulatory, cardiovascular, metabolic, and pulmonary reflexes occurs as swelling proceeds to brainstem herniation. The following considerations may help maintain donor graft function provided the defects are recognized and treated early.

E. ***Donor hypothermia*** is due to loss of hypothalamic thermo-regulatory and brainstem vasomotor centers. The goal of therapy is maintenance of normothermia to avoid the cardio-vascular instability associated with hypothermia and to aid brain death certification.

1. Reduce heat loss by increasing room temperature and providing insulating warm blankets.

2. Especially if still hyperventilating the patient, warm inspired airway gases with a heater attached to the ventilator.

3. Exogenous heat may be delivered by overhead warmers and heating mattresses

4. *All* IV fluids, especially blood products, should be warmed prior to administration.

5. In general, hypothermia is easier to prevent than to reverse once it occurs.

F. ***Donor hypoxemia*** may be due to thoracic injury, aspiration, VQ mismatch with shunt physiology, and neurogenic PE.

1. **FIO_2 and PEEP** should be increased to achieve a PaO_2 >100 mm Hg

2. **V_T and rate** should be adjusted to achieve $PaCO_2$ of 24–40 mm Hg. Cerebral swelling that may accompany reversal of hyperventilation may so adversely affect cardiovascular responses that it may be preferable to maintain hypocarbia.

3. A patient requiring FIO_2 >0.40, PEEP >10 cm H_2O, or peak airway pressures >30 cm H_2O may not be a suitable lung or heart-lung donor. However, if adequate oxygenation can be maintained, other organs may be suitable for transplantation.

4. Often a pulmonary contusion or aspiration is present and vigorous **pulmonary toilet** with frequent suctioning is advisable.

5. **Bronchodilators** are indicated for the treatment of reactive airway disease.

6. **Pulmonary edema** may cause hypoxemia and can be the result of either overly vigorous volume resuscitation or CNS injury. If PE is present, a PA catheter will simplify diagnosis and allow monitoring of efficacy of treatment.

a. **Normal to low filling pressures,** with impaired oxygenation and nonsegmental pulmonary infiltrates on CXR, suggests neurogenic PE which should be managed by additional PEEP and inspired O_2.

   b. **Elevated filling pressures** imply a cardiac cause and
      should be managed with diuretics to relieve preload
      and dopamine to support contractility as indicated by
      systemic BPs.
7. With modest hypoxemia, O_2 delivery can be maintained
   by **PRBC transfusions** to increase O_2 carrying capacity.
   a. The Hct should be maintained at or above 30%, and
      if associated with hypoxemia, to 40%–45%.
   b. The usual large-volume crystalloid resuscitation
      which occurs to support the brain-dead cadaver will
      mandate some transfusion to maintain the Hct.
G. *Donor hemodynamic instability* is managed by a reorienta-
   tion from aggressive neurologic support to vigorous volume
   resuscitation.
   1. At the declaration of brain death, and not before then,
      diuretic therapy should be terminated, the donor reposi-
      tioned into Trendelenburg's position, if necessary, to im-
      prove venous return to the heart. Intravascular volume
      should be increased with crystalloid and PRBCs to
      achieve a normal CVP (and PCWP if available).
   2. As CVP and PCWP return to normal, CO should return
      to normal, and can be verified with a mixed venous
      blood gas or thermodilution CO. Persistent hypotension
      with a normal CVP indicates the need for additional
      PCWP and SVR data which can be obtained by insertion
      of a PA catheter.
   3. Usually **vigorous restoration of preload** will maintain
      normal hemodynamics. Precipitous drops in BP may oc-
      cur as further brainstem herniation results in loss of re-
      sidual vasomotor tone. A quick check of CVP (and
      PCWP and SVR, if available) will confirm the problem,
      which should respond to volume resuscitation. Such epi-
      sodes of hypotension are often premorbid.
   4. **Bradycardia** is generally of no significance unless ac-
      companied by hypotension.
      a. After correcting preload, if hypotension remains, the
         bradycardia may be treated with **atropine 1.0 mg
         IV.** In theory, the brain-dead cadaver has no vagal
         tone and should not respond to atropine. In practice,
         in many cases there is residual vagal tone, presum-
         ably of single synapse origin or originating in the ax-
         ons distal to the nucleus.

  b. **Isoproterenol 1 mg/250 mL IV infusion,** titrated to
     achieve the desired rate, is useful especially because
     of its splanchnic and renal vasodilator effect. How-
     ever, β-adrenergic vasodilation may result in an even
     lower BP despite improved rate, as may be con-
     firmed by SVR determinations.
  c. **Transvenous pacing** is rarely required.
  5. **Inotropic support** is frequently indicated. Many patients
     will be on inotropic agents at the time of declaration of
     brain death. The goal of inotropic therapy is to support
     perfusion until adequate preload can be established, and
     then weaned.
     a. **No more than 10 µg/kg/min of dopamine** should
        be used unless absolutely necessary to support CO
        after adequate volume resuscitation. Dopamine di-
        lates the renal vasculature directly and has a vaso-
        constrictor effect on the splanchnic circulation only
        in its α-adrenergic range.
     b. **Dobutamine,** though not known to adversely effect
        renal or splanchnic flow, lacks the vasodilating char-
        acteristics of dopamine, which is preferred.
     c. **Epinephrine and phenylephrine** constrict both
        splanchnic and renal vascular trees and are contrain-
        dicated.
     d. Some institutions are cautiously using **phenyleph-
        rine 40 mg/250 mL IV infusion at low dose (1–2
        µcg/kg/min)** to achieve sufficient increase in SVR as
        needed to easily support the circulation. This agent
        can reduce CO and maintain renal and splanchnic
        flow with diuresis by increasing diastolic (and mean)
        BP.
     e. **Glucagon 1 mg IV bolus** has an uncertain role al-
        though it improves splanchnic perfusion.
     f. The procurement officer should be notified at first
        contact of present inotropic support and advised at
        once of any increased requirements.
H. *Donor metabolism* may be significantly altered by aggressive
   neurologic management.
   1. **Serum electrolytes** including Ca^{2+}, Mg^{2+}, and $PO_4{}^{2-}$
      should be determined and corrected as indicated to
      achieve normal values.

2. Hypokalemia, hypocalcemia, hypomagnesemia, and hypophosphatemia are frequent findings in heavily diuresed patients and should be corrected with IV infusions.

3. **Na$^+$ and K$^+$ replacement** are simplified by knowing urine Na$^+$ and K$^+$ concentrations. Knowing the hourly UO, one can then calculate the minimum replacement required.

4. **Loss of ADH secretion results in DI,** occasionally with massive diuresis.

   a. Mild degrees of DI are well tolerated and easily managed by replacing UO with ½ NS with appropriate K$^+$ repletion. Knowledge of urine electrolytes will simplify this task.

   b. When it becomes difficult to maintain intravascular volume or serum K$^+$ with this approach (UO usually >500 mL/hr), the procurement officer should be informed and vasopressin given.

      1) **Vasopressin 1–5 units IV bolus** is given and an infusion begun (25 units/250 mL) at 1 unit/hr and titrated to maintain UO at 200–500 mL/hr.

      2) Vasopressin is a powerful renal and splanchnic vasoconstrictor and should be used cautiously.

      3) Concomitant use of low-dose dopamine (5 μg/kg/min) should be considered.

      4) At the first indication of UO <100 mL/hr, vasopressin should be immediately discontinued.

5. **Hyperglycemia** should be managed with the usual measures and an infusion of insulin started, if necessary. Normoglycemia will significantly decrease urinary osmolar load and reduce diuresis to more easily manageable levels.

III. IMMUNOSUPPRESSIVE THERAPY IN TRANSPLANT RECIPIENTS.

A. Improvements in transplant survival have paralleled development of new immunosuppressive agents and regimens. Nearly all current immunosuppressive protocols are based on **multiple agents** with the aim of minimizing toxicity while maximizing control of rejection. Many protocols now are divided into an initial **induction phase** utilizing potent agents to maximize immunosuppression while avoiding nephrotoxic agents such as cyclosporine, followed by a **maintenance**

phase where biologic agents are discontinued and cyclosporine therapy is begun. A gradual taper of corticosteroids still is a part of most immunosuppressive protocols.

B. The ability to **monitor blood levels** of agents such as cyclosporine has allowed more accurate dosing despite individual differences in metabolism. At some centers measurements of active components of the immune response, such as specific lymphocyte subsets and lymphokines, are being evaluated in hopes of providing more exact suppression of the response to an allograft.

C. The need to transplant the increasing numbers of **sensitized recipients** will likely require specific peritransplant therapy directed at removing or neutralizing circulating antibodies that would otherwise lead to hyperacute rejection.

D. Advances in recognition of rejection episodes has allowed earlier administration of **antirejection therapy,** reversing most instances of acute cellular rejection. Table 16–3 lists the types and mechanism of the major types of rejection.

    1. Clinically, **rejection usually presents as one of three situations:**

        a. The recipient will have stable good graft function which suddenly deteriorates.

        b. The recipient will have poor postoperative function and the renal scans or graft biopsies will show rejection

TABLE 16–3.
Types of Allograft Rejection

Type	Time to Appear	Mechanism
Hyperacute	Minutes	Preformed antibodies to donor tissue cause graft destruction almost immediately after reperfusion
Accelerated	Days	Rejection due to second set (anamnestic) response in previously sensitized recipient.
Acute (cellular)	Any time	Cellular immune response to graft that is usually reversible with therapy
Chronic (humoral)	mo–yr	Often slow destruction caused by immunoglobulin deposition in the small vessels of the graft.

        c. The recipient, while resolving postoperative poor function, will have slower improvement in function than anticipated.

    2. **The graft should be biopsied** to establish the diagnosis of rejection. A Tru-Cut needle biopsy is done at the bedside or wedge biopsy or endomyocardial biopsy in the OR. Fine needle aspiration cytology is also being used for kidney grafts. Short of histologic confirmation of acute rejection, however, all other indications of rejection are relative.

E. Protocols for immunosuppression vary from institution to institution and change with time. The transplant nurse clinician is a good resource for determining the correct protocol.

F. Specific Immunosuppressive agents.

    1. **Corticosteroids inhibit T cell proliferation.**

        a. Used at least initially in nearly all protocols. The introduction of agents such as cyclosporine has allowed a more rapid taper and the use of lower doses of corticosteroids.

        b. **Methylprednisolone** administered in high dose (250 mg–2 g) perioperatively is rapidly tapered to about 0.5 mg/kg during the first week with a more gradual taper after switching to oral prednisone over the following weeks and months (4 mg IV methylprednisolone = 5 mg PO prednisone).

        c. **Side effects** include glucose intolerance, psychosis, acne, sodium and fluid retention, and increased susceptibility to bacterial and fungal infections.

        d. Chronic use can lead to adrenal suppression, growth retardation, cataract formation, and osteoporosis with aseptic necrosis.

    2. **Purine analogues** (6-mercaptopurine, azathioprine) inhibit lymphocyte proliferation by altering purine nucleotide synthesis and metabolism.

        a. **Loading dose** of azathioprine is 500 mg for adults (8.5 mg/kg for children and small adults) over 3 days, usually 200, 150, and 150 mg/day.

        b. **Usual maintenance dose** is 1–3 mg/kg/day adjusted for WBC count:

            1) Reduce dose for WBC <7,000/mm^3.

            2) Hold daily dose for WBC <3,500/mm^3.

        c. **Excretion** is via the kidney. Decrease dose by one half if patient is dialysis-dependent.

d. **Toxicity** includes bone marrow suppression and hepatotoxicity. Increased hepatocellular enzymes is an indication to switch to cyclophosphamide

3. **Cyclosporine** has become the mainstay of most immunosuppressive protocols.

   a. **Oral bioavailability** is 33% so oral dosage is three times IV dosage.

   b. **Loading dose** varies from 1–4 mg/kg IV depending on type of transplant and protocol. To minimize nephrotoxicity, cyclosporine is often withheld in renal transplantation until good graft function is observed.

   c. **Dose is adjusted** by measuring trough cyclosporine levels by high-performance liquid chromatography (only parent drug measured) or by RIA (parent drug plus active metabolites measured). **Usual dose is 1.5 mg/kg PO.**

   d. Optimal level varies with protocol and type of transplant. Usual levels for renal transplant are 100–200 μg/mL

   e. **Many drug interactions** can lead to elevated or lowered cyclosporine levels:

      1) **Drugs which may lower cyclosporine levels:**
         a) Trimethoprin IV.
         b) Rifampin.
         c) Isoniazid.
         d) Carbamazepine.
         e) Phenobarbital.
         f) Phenytoin.

      2) **Drugs which may elevate cyclosporine levels:**
         a) Anabolic steroids.
         b) Erythromycin.
         c) Ketoconazole.
         d) High-dose methylprednisolone.
         e) Calcium channel blockers (diltiazem, nifedipine, etc.).

   f. **Primary toxicity is impaired renal function** from vasoconstriction that alters renal hemodynamics and can lead to progressive renal fibrosis. Renal toxicity may require discontinuation of the drug.

   g. **Other side effects** include hypertension, hyperkalemia, hirsutism, gingival hypertrophy, alterations in serum cholesterol levels, and increased incidence of B cell lymphomas.

4. **FK-506 is a macrolide antibiotic** recovered from soil fungus culture that is being used in a limited number of centers for solid organ transplantation.

   a. It inhibits lymphocyte activation by inhibition of the synthesis and expression of IL-2 and other cytokines, but with a lower incidence of toxicity.

   b. Early reports have shown superior graft survival and a reduced need for corticosteroids when compared to regimens based on cyclosporine.

5. **Heterologous serum preparations** such as ATG and ALG are used to deplete circulating lymphocytes.

   a. These agents may be used prophylactically at the time of transplant or for rejection episodes at a dose of 15 mg/kg/day.

   b. **Skin tests** are often used initially to test for hypersensitivity to these preparations that are prepared in horses, goats, or other animals. The possibility of reaction to the heterologous serum increases with subsequent treatments.

   c. Other agents, particularly cyclosporine, must be reduced or withheld during treatment with ALG or ATG to avoid serious infections.

   d. **Side effects** include thrombocytopenia, leukopenia, fever, rash, serum sickness.

6. **Monoclonal antibodies** hold the promise of more specific therapy. The only commercially available preparation to date, **OKT3** (Orthoclone), is a mouse monoclonal antibody that reacts with a surface marker (CD3) present on all T lymphocytes.

   a. **Administration of 5 mg IV** leads to prompt disappearance of circulating T lymphocytes, followed in most cases by reversal of rejection.

   b. The usual **course of therapy** is 10–14 days for acute rejection.

   c. Some protocols use OKT3 initially as prophylaxis against rejection episodes. Many patients will develop antibodies to the mouse immunoglobulin which may limit effectiveness of subsequent treatments.

d. Doses of other immunosuppressive agents, particularly cyclosporine, must be decreased while patients are being treated with OKT3 to avoid serious infections from too vigorous immunosuppression.

e. **Side effects** include fever, chills, pulmonary edema.

IV. GENERAL CARE OF THE IMMUNOSUPRESSED.

A. Antacids.

Used aggressively, especially with high-dose steroid administration as prophylaxis against gastric ulceration. Aluminum tends to constipate; magnesium tends to loosen stools.

1. **Amphojel:** 320 mg $Al(OH_3)_3/5$ mL = 7 mEq OH^-; 440 mg $Al(OH)_3$/tablet = 9 mEq OH^-; 15 mL or two tablets q.6h.

2. **Basaljel:** 546 mg $Al_2 (CO_3)_3/5$ mL or tablet = 14 mEq OH; 15 mL or two tablets q.6h.

3. **Maalox:** 225 mg $Al(OH_3)$ +200 mg $Mg(OH)_2/5$ ml = 13 mEq OH^-; 200 mg Al $(OH)_3$ + 200 mg $Mg(OH)_2$/ tablet = 9 mEq OH^-; 15 mL or two tablets q.6h.

4. **Mylanta:** 200 mg $Al(OH)_3$ + 200 mg $Mg(OH)_2/5$ mL or tablet = 12 mEq OH; 15 mL or two tablets q.6h.

5. **Phosphaljel:** 233 mg $Al(PO)_4/5$ mL = 6 mEq OH; 15 mL po q.6h.

B. Antibiotics.

1. **For renal transplants,** cefazolin (Ancef) while npo, and doxycycline (Vibramycin) 50 mg po q.i.d. when taking po for 4 weeks postoperatively.

2. **For liver recipients,** cefamandole q.6.h. for 3 days. Some patients with choledochoenterostomies may receive doxycycline as above.

3. **Cardiac recipients** receive cefazolin until the chest tubes are removed.

C. *Candida.*

Mycostatin 50,000 units, swish and swallow q.i.d., is among routine orders to minimize oral colonization.

D. Herpes.

Blistex and viscous lidocaine or Cepastat. Acyclovir ointment 5% to lesions q.6.h. while awake.

V. INTENSIVE CARE OF TRANSPLANT PATIENTS.

A. The Transplant Team

Organ transplantation utilizes a team approach. The nephrologist, hepatologist, cardiologist, hematologist, infectious disease consultant, endocrinologist, transplant physician, and transplant surgeon work in concert to provide care for the patient and ensure the best results. In addition, the perioperative care of transplant patients is facilitated by the involvement of anesthesiologists with a particular interest in transplantation. Transplant nurse clinicians provide valuable assistance in keeping up with protocols, scheduling tests, and communicating with families.

B. Transplant Recipient Evaluation.

1. **Living-related donor (LRD) renal recipients** are admitted at least 24 hours prior to elective transplantation in order to prepare them for a major operation. Communicate with the team and transplant surgeon and order appropriate additional studies and consults if the history, physical, or laboratory studies demonstrate unexpected abnormalities

2. **Cadaveric (CAD) transplantation** is an urgent, but elective procedure requiring an expeditious, but thorough, evaluation. In any potential transplant recipient particular attention should be paid to any **immediate medical problems such as uncontrolled hypertension or diabetes with hyperglycemia.** A careful inquiry and examination looking for any **active infectious process** is vitally important as its presence may preclude transplantation at that time. Immediately notify the transplant surgeon of any significant abnormalities as soon as they are discovered.

C. Renal Transplantation:

1. **Preoperative Assessment:**
   a. Pathogenesis of CRF.
   b. Site and status of dialysis access, method and schedule of dialysis, and most recent dialysis.
   c. Usual creatinine, "dry weight," and average daily UO.
   d. Location and fate of any previous transplants.
   e. Results of previous GU workup, if any.
   f. Stool guaiac and rectal examination.
   g. HBsAg status.

2. **Laboratory studies:**
   a. **The crossmatch is usually the rate-limiting step** (about 4 hours) prior to CAD renal transplantation. Send two large red top (serum) and one lavender top

(EDTA) stat to the tissue typing laboratory. The crossmatch tests for the presence of preformed cytotoxic antibodies in the recipient's blood against the donor organ. A *negative* crossmatch is necessary prior to transplant.

b. **Other necessary preoperative studies** include, CXR, ECG, CBC with differential, PT, PTT (draw 2 hours or more after last dialysis), HBsAg, electrolytes, BUN, creatinine, type and crossmatch 2–4 units PRBCs.

3. **Preoperative immunosuppression** should be administered according to appropriate protocol. Often this is delayed in CAD recipients until after a negative crossmatch is reported.

LRD _____   CAD _____

_____   _____

_____   _____

_____   _____

4. **Preoperative antibiotic** is administered (1 g cefazolin) and usually a CVP line is inserted.

5. **Procedure:**

The donor kidney is usually transplanted to the iliac vessels through an extraperitoneal approach.

a. Shortly before perfusion of the organ, furosemide and mannitol are given to induce diuresis.

b. Postoperative function is directly related to the duration of warm ischemia as well as preservation time and donor factors. In general, <10 minutes of warm ischemia is associated with immediate function upon restoration of blood flow, 30–60 minutes often leads to ATN, while >60 minutes often results in acute cortical necrosis.

c. The ureter is implanted into the bladder after placement of a stent. A Foley catheter drains the bladder.

6. **Postoperative intensive care:**

a. **Maintenance of adequate intravascular volume** is the primary goal of early SICU management.

b. Clinical evaluation (JVD, oxygenation, etc.) and often measurement of the CVP are performed frequently.

c. The **UO and IV fluid intake** are measured and adjusted hourly.

    d. An example of IV fluid orders based on UO is shown in Table 16–4. The goal is to avoid CVP values <5–6 cm H_2O.

    e. It should be remembered that the patient received diuretics in the OR which may lead to a tapering diuresis.

    f. A brisk diuresis (100–1,000 mL/hr) can ensue, despite relative hypovolemia, from:

        1) Proximal tubular damage from graft ischemia.

        2) Osmotic load secondary to uremia or high glucose concentrations in IV fluids (use D2.5 or less).

        3) Total body fluid and electrolyte overload in CRF.

    g. **If immediate UO does not occur, ATN is presumed to have occurred.** Keep IV fluids to a minimum (30–50 mL/hr) to avoid fluid overload. Dialysis may be required.

    h. **Monitor electrolytes and glucose closely (q.4.h.).** Urine electrolytes help in diuresing large volumes. Adjust fluids as needed (NS to treat hyponatremia or elevated glucose). Insulin may be required.

TABLE 16–4.

Postoperative Fluid Orders After Renal Transplantation*

Urine Output/hr (mL)	IV Intake/hr
<75	Output + 50 mL and reassess patient
75–100	Output + 50 mL
100–200	Output + 25 mL
200–300	Output
300–400	Output − 50 mL
400–600	Output − 100 mL
600–800	Output − 200 mL
>800	Output − 50 mL and reassess patient

*Use D2.5 ½NS.

    i. **Perioperative immunosuppression** is given per individual protocol.

    ————————————————————

    ————————————————————

    ————————————————————

    j. To avoid kinking vessels or displacing the graft, the **patient lies supine or on the transplant side only** and allowed to sit with the head of bed elevated no higher than 45 degrees for 72 hours.

    k. **Prophylactic antibiotic** is continued for 24 hours or until drain is removed, then patient is placed on po urinary antibiotic (doxycycline 50 mg b.i.d.).

    l. Clear liquids when bowel sounds present, usually postoperative day 1. Advance to appropriate diet as tolerated.

7. **Creatinine:** The limits of laboratory interassay variability of serum creatinine are ± 0.2 of normal (1–3 mg/dL). At higher levels, proportionately greater errors are applicable. Thus, an increase of ≥ 0.2 mg/dL requires at least a stat repeat determination on a new sample.

8. **Oliguria** in the transplant patient has a wide differential including hypovolemia, rejection, and technical problems. An algorithm for diagnosis and treatment is shown in Figure 16–1.

9. **Fine-needle aspiration:** A fine needle is placed into the graft and the inflammatory cells and parenchymal cells in the aspirated mixture of blood and urine are counted. From this differential count is subtracted the background peripheral blood (drawn simultaneously) differential count, and an inflammatory score is calculated. This is useful in differentiating ATN, cyclosporine nephrotoxicity, and rejection.

10. **Nuclear medicine renal battery:** ^{99m}Tc DTPA is bolus-injected IV and the lower abdomen is scanned. Phases of study include arterial imaging, graft perfusion, graft function (filtration and tubular activity), and ureteral patency and course. These studies are affected by the state of hydration and it is advisable to schedule *before dialysis* if both are to occur on the same day. This is presently our only noninvasive test for rejection during ATN.

11. **Stentogram:** A ureteral fistula is associated with very high morbidity and mortality. Usually on postoperative

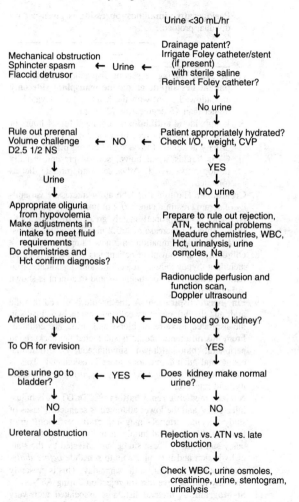

Urine <30 mL/hr
↓
Drainage patent?
Irrigate Foley catheter/stent
  (if present)
  with sterile saline
Reinsert Foley catheter?
↓
No urine
↓
Mechanical obstruction
Sphincter spasm   ← Urine ←
Flaccid detrusor

Rule out prerenal
Volume challenge   ← NO ←   Patient appropriately hydrated?
D2.5 1/2 NS   Check I/O, weight, CVP
↓   ↓
Urine   YES
↓   ↓
Appropriate oliguria   NO urine
from hypovolemia   ↓
Make adjustments in   Prepare to rule out rejection,
  intake to meet fluid   ATN, technical problems
  requirements   Meadure chemistries, WBC,
Do chemistries and   Hct, urinalysis, urine
  Hct confirm diagnosis?   osmoles, Na
                             ↓
                             Radionuclide perfusion and
                               function scan,
                               Doppler ultrasound
                             ↓
Arterial occlusion   ← NO ←   Does blood go to kidney?
↓   ↓
To OR for revision   YES
                             ↓
Does urine go to   ← YES ←   Does kidney make normal
  bladder?   urine?
↓   ↓
NO   NO
↓   ↓
Ureteral obstruction   Rejection vs. ATN vs. late
                               obstuction
                             ↓
                             Check WBC, urine osmoles,
                               creatinine, urine, stentogram,
                               urinalysis

FIG 16–1.
Diagnosis and treatment of low urine output in renal transplant patients.

day 5 the ureter and ureteroneocystostomy are checked with contrast injection, and if without leak or obstruction, the stent can be removed.

12. **Rejection in renal transplant recipients** occurs most often in the weeks immediately following transplantation, but may occur at any time. Features include:
    a. Increased serum creatinine.
    b. Decreased UO.
    c. Fever.
    d. Tender, enlarged kidney.
    e. Increased diastolic BP.
    f. Renal biopsy showing acute cellular infiltrate.

13. **Antirejection therapy can** consist of pulse steroids (1 g methylprednisolone IV q. d. × 5), OKT3, ALG, or ATG, depending on severity of rejection and current protocol. Check with transplant surgeon before starting therapy.

14. **Cyclosporine toxicity** may be difficult to distinguish from rejection. Treatment consists of decreasing the dose. Differentiating diagnostic features include:
    a. Rising creatinine.
    b. Absence of oliguria and fever.
    c. Renal tubular epithelial cells on urinalysis.
    d. Elevated cyclosporine levels.
    e. Hyperkalemia.
    f. Tremor.
    g. Hypertension.

D. Pancreas Transplantation.

1. Most pancreas transplant recipients also receive a **concomitant kidney transplant,** but, an increasing number of diabetics are undergoing isolated pancreas transplantation.

2. **Additional preoperative evaluation should include:**
   a. Duration of diabetes and end-organ manifestations.
   b. Diet and insulin regimen.
   c. Baseline glycosylated hemoglobin and amylase determinations.

3. **Preoperative medications:**
   a. Immunosuppression per current protocol.

_____
_____
_____

    b. Insulin drip begun for good glucose control.

    c. Dipyridamole and aspirin for anticoagulant effect.

    d. Preoperative antibiotics per current protocol.

4. **Procedure:** The pancreas is placed in the iliac fossa via either a retroperitoneal or transabdominal approach. Exocrine drainage is usually through the pancreatic duct into a small portion of donor duodenum that is anastomosed to the bladder. A Foley catheter drains the bladder.

5. **Postoperative intensive care:**

    a. **Fluid management** is similar to that of kidney recipients. The IV fluid of choice is D2.5 ½ NS with two ampules (88 mEq) of $NaHCO_3$ to make up for loss of $HCO_3{}_-$ from the transplanted pancreas into the bladder.

    b. **An insulin drip** is administered to all patients with the goal of maintaining the blood sugar as close to 100 mg/dL as possible to avoid stimulating the pancreas.

        1) A low blood sugar is a sign of a functioning graft and should be treated by increasing the quantity of glucose being given to the patient rather than decreasing the insulin drip <2 units/hr.

        2) The infusion is stopped 24–96 hours after transplantation.

    c. **Venous thrombosis** is an early complication of pancreas transplantation. This is prevented by prophylaxis with aspirin, dipyridamole, and a dextran infusion.

    d. Patients are kept at **bed rest for 72 hours** to prevent shifting of the transplanted organ.

    e. **Monitoring graft function** is done by measurements of urinary amylase. A decline is indicative of loss of graft function.

    f. **Postoperative immunosuppression**

    _____

    _____

    _____

    g. **Antirejection therapy** is similar to that used for kidney transplant rejection and depends on the current protocol.

   h. **Unique complications** include activation for proenzymes by microorganisms in the bladder leading to cystitis as well as low serum CO_2 from chronic alkali loss in urine.
E. **Liver Transplantation.**
   1. **Preoperative evaluation should include:**
      a. Pathogenesis of liver failure, bilirubin, albumin, PT,PTT.
      b. Document dry weight and mental status.
   2. **Preoperative studies should include:**
      a. CXR, ECG, CBC with differential, chemistries (including liver studies), albumin, PT, PTT, calcium, and urinalysis. A BT may be requested.
      b. Blood for the blood bank is of primary importance (three large red tops and two blue tops)
   3. **Preoperative immunosuppression** per current protocol.

   _____
   _____
   _____

   4. **Procedure** is complex. Note should be made of:
      a. Total ischemic time.
      b. Total blood component replacement.
      c. Degree of coagulopathy.
      d. Stablity of the venous bypass phase.
      e. Special attention should be paid to the details of arterial and biliary anatomy and reconstruction. A T tube is used to stent the biliary anastomosis.
   5. **Postoperative intensive care.**
      a. **Fluid resuscitation:**
         1) **Hepatic blood flow** is maximized and hepatic lymph flow minimized at lower CVP (3–6 cm H_2O). Nearly all patients receive a significant positive operative fluid balance but will have 24–48 hours of oliguria. Overly vigorous crystalloid and colloid resuscitation can produce PE and diminished graft function.
         2) **Most patients receive FFP** to complete correction of the coagulation parameters, initially 100 mL/hr, until the coagulation profile is acceptable, to maintain the CVP and promote diuresis.
         3) **Albumin 10 mL/hr** is administered while synthetic function is poor and hypoalbuminemia exists.

   4) **Concentrated factors** in the form of cryoprecipitate are given if significant hypofibrinogenemia
is present.

   5) **Platelets and PRBCs** are given as required.

   6) **Diuretics** are used to stimulate UO and maintain
fluid balance.

   7) Production of bile from the T tube, LFTs, coagulation profiles, glucose, calcium, and albumin
provide the best overview of graft performance.

b. **Postoperative immunosuppression.**
   _____
   _____
   _____
   _____

c. **Acute rejection therapy.**
   _____
   _____
   _____
   _____

d. **The patient is kept supine for 48 hours** and then
gradually allowed to have the head of the bed progressively elevated. By day 4, most patients are sitting in a chair without difficulty.

e. **Prophylactic antibiotics** for biliary tract penetration
are maintained for 5 days or as indicated.

f. **A T tube study** will be performed as indicated by
early graft function. This may be obtained as early as
several days posttransplant if suspicious of an early
leak, or may be postponed to a routine check at
7–10 days postgraft.

g. **Metabolism:**

   1) Close attention (q. 4–6 h.) is paid to **serum glucose** and supplemental glucose is given to maintain it well >100 mg/dL. Rarely is insulin
needed.

   2) **Hypocalcemia** from massive transfusion needs
correction to maintain cardiovascular function
and coagulation system performance.

   3) **Hypo- and hyperkalemia** are frequent problems. Hypokalemia is best managed by bolus IV
potassium, adjusted to need.

4) A citrate-induced (from transfused blood products) **metabolic acidosis** is occasionally seen and accompanies poor graft function.

h. **Hypertension:**

1) This common problem is treated with hydralazine, labetolol or propranolol, minoxidil, clonidine, and captopril.

2) **Nifedipine** (10 mg sublingually) can be useful for rapid control.

3) Methyldopa is hepatotoxic and should be avoided, as should sodium nitroprusside. Sodium nitroprusside is metabolized to cyanide which may be detrimental to the recently ischemic liver.

i. **Primary graft nonfunction** occurs in ~5% of patients. Urgent retransplantation provides the only good outcome. The patient with a failed liver graft is supported with glucose, FFP to correct coagulapathy, and minimal sedation to reduce metabolic encephalopathy. Early dialysis is used to support renal function.

j. **Vascular thrombosis of arterial or portal vein supply:**

1) This early severe complication is especially frequent in children.

2) In the SICU, thrombosis will present as sudden deterioration of graft function or a leak from an ischemic bile duct anastomosis.

3) Ascites indicates portal vein thrombosis with portal hypertension. The diagnosis is confirmed with Doppler ultrasound of the hepatic artery and portal vein flow as well as an arteriogram.

4) The acutely failed liver graft is treated in the same fashion as failure from primary nonfunction.

k. **ARF** is not uncommon and should be treated with early dialysis to allow nutrition and best healing.

l. **Hepatitis** can be caused by CMV, hepatitis B, adenovirus, and herpes virus following transplantation. The diagnosis is confirmed by increases in viral antibody titers or by positive viral culture. The treatment involves judicious reduction of immunosuppression

(CMV is immunosuppressive in and of itself). Acyclovir can be applied to symptomatic lesions. **Ganciclovir** 5 mg/kg IV g. 8 h. can be used to treat CMV diagnosed by biopsy.

m. **Graft vs. host disease:** In ABO-mismatched grafts, the mild and self-limiting hemolysis occurs 5–8 days following transplantation and lasts 1–3 weeks. One to 2 weeks after transplantation, antirecipient ABO antibodies can be detected on circulating RBCs.

n. **Biliary complications** of stricture or leak usually occur later, outside the SICU. SICU management of biliary leak, confirmed by cholangiogram, is generally by percutaneous catheter drainage. Definitive management of biliary stricture requires operative revision of the anastomosis.

o. **An algorithm** is for diagnosis and management of early complications in liver transplantation is given in Table 16–5.

F. Cardiac Transplantation.

1. **Preoperative assessment:**
   a. Etiology of heart failure.
   b. Present medications.
   c. Pressures from most recent PA catheterization.
   d. Usual dry weight

TABLE 16–5.

Diagnosis and Management of Early Complications After Liver Transplantation

Worsening LFTs, increased bilirubin, transaminases, PT, APTT, decreased glucose, albumin
If not improved postoperatively: consider primary nonfunction or thrombosis
If complications occur after improved function: consider rejection, thrombosis, hepatitis, biliary complication
Arterial and portal flow by Doppler ultrasound: not thrombosis
No flow: proceed to arteriogram
Cholangiogram normal: not biliary complication
Abnormal: drain or dilate obstruction as indicated
Tru-cut needle biopsy: hepatitis or rejection
Viral studies: Hepatitis A, B (C?), herpes serology, CMV, adenovirus, herpes culture

    e. Laboratory workup.

    f. LVAD use.

2. **Preoperative immunosuppression.**

   _____

   _____

   _____

3. **Intraoperative procedure:** Special attention should be given to:

    a. Intraoperative PA pressures and catheter position.

    b. Cardiac output.

    c. Location of pacing wires and their thresholds.

    d. Degree of hemostasis and status of heparin reversal.

4. **Postoperative intensive care:**

    a. **Hemodynamic management** of the heart transplant recipient is similar to that for other postoperative cardiac patients with a few notable differences.

      1) The transplanted heart, with its rate controlled by the donor SA node, is free of direct autonomic nervous system input. Thus, **CO is very rate- and preload-dependent.**

      2) **Isoproterenol** (1–2 mg/250 mL) infusion or pacing is used to maintain the rate at approximately 100 bpm.

      3) In most recipients, **the pulmonary vascular resistance (PVR) is elevated** as a consequence of terminal LV failure. Great care should be taken to avoid elevation of PVR. PEEP should be adjusted as necessary. Dobutamine or isoproterenol (which decreases PVR) or dopamine (no effect on PVR) is used for inotropic support.

      4) The transplanted organ is **usually dependent on inotropic support** initially to maintain LV and RV output. This support is very slowly weaned as the denervated heart is quite sensitive to IV catecholamines and preload.

      5) Oral isoproterenol may be given if necessary to wean the patient off IV drips.

    b. **Postoperative immunosuppression.**

   _____

   _____

   _____

    c. **Strict reverse isolation** is maintained in the SICU. ET tubes, central and arterial lines, and the Foley catheter are removed as soon as possible. Standard **prophylactic antibiotics** are given.

    d. **Gradual changes in patient position** will avoid sudden changes in preload. Sitting in a chair is encouraged by postoperative day 2 and progressive ambulation instituted as tolerated.

    e. **Endomyocardial biopsies** are obtained at regular intervals beginning the first week following transplantation. This protocol is continued on a regular schedule for a year or as indicated by unexplained fever, malaise, or signs of right heart failure. Biopsy remains the most accurate method of diagnosing asymptomatic rejection.

    f. **Mechanical assist of ventricular function** may be required for poor ventricular function.

G. Heart-Lung Transplantation.

  1. The presence of either secondary or primary pulmonary hypertension precludes cardiac transplantation owing to the inability of the normal RV of the donor organ to pump against the high pressures of the recipient pulmonary circuit. Such patients are considered for combined heart-lung transplantation.

  2. **Operative technique** is similar to cardiac transplantation. The donor trachea is attached to the recipient trachea just above the bifurcation.

  3. **Immunosuppression** usually includes axathioprine, cyclosporine, and ALG. Steroids are withheld during the first week following transplantation in order to aid in healing of the airway anastomosis.

  4. Close attention is paid to volume status, with care taken to avoid volume overload and subsequent edema in the lungs.

  5. **Rejection is common,** particularly in the early phases of transplantation, and may involve heart or lungs alone. Transbronchial biopsy and bronchoalveolar lavage may be useful for diagnosis.

  6. **Pulmonary infections** are treated aggressively with broad-spectrum antibiotics. Prophylactic drugs (trimethoprim-sulfamethoxazole) have been used to prevent opportunistic infections.

Subjective:	Pain, malaise, fever, chills, stool quality, bladder cramps?
Objective:	Intake good (125–150 mL/hr for good renal function, less for poorer function)
	Output good (100–125 mL/hr for good renal function, less for poorer function)
	Wound check, graft nontender?
	Weight/temperature, BP, Creatinine, LFTs, glucose, cyclosporin A level, WBC, Ca, PO_4, electrolytes
Impression:	Graft function: good or poor, improving or decreasing? Evidence of rejection: present or absent? Evidence of infection: present or absent? Evidence of metabolic imbalance: present or absent? Evidence of therapeutic toxicity: present or absent?
Medication:	Immunosuppression: appropriate doses? Follow protocols Antacids: Appropriate anions, cations? Antibiotic: Renew, if indicated
Plans:	Based on above information.

IS YOUR TRANSPLANT PATIENT TUCKED IN?

1. Did the patient receive appropriate immunosuppression?

2. Did the patient receive antirejection therapy?

3. Is it time to adjust immunosuppression for A.M.?

4. Did the ward clerks enter the protocol laboratory work? Special studies for A.M.?

5. Are you confident that rejection and infection are absent?

   IF NOT: Is the appropriate workup complete or pending? Are the orders for additional studies or treatments written and nurses informed?

FIG 16–2.
Transplant rounds checklist.

H. Pulmonary Transplantation.

1. Single lung transplantation can be utilized to treat pulmonary fibrosis or primary pulmonary hypertension as well as some older patients with emphysema. Double lung transplantation has been used to treat cystic fibrosis and younger patients with emphysema.

2. The bronchial anastomosis is wrapped in omentum to aid in healing. Immunosuppression is similar to heart-lung transplantation.

3. Bacterial, viral, and fungal infections are common. Prophylactic therapy is routine and usually includes trimethoprim-sulfamethoxazole, acyclovir, and oral nystatin. Aggressive treatment of any pulmonary infiltrate is standard.

4. Bronchoscopy with biopsy as well as lung perfusion scans are used to diagnose rejection, which usually occurs early.

5. **Chronic rejection** usually presents as progressive airway obstruction (bronchiolitis obliterans).

I. Transplant Rounds (Fig 16–2).

REFERENCES

Bach FH, Sachs DH: Transplantation immunology. *N Engl J Med* 1987; 317:8.

Cooper JD: The evolution of techniques and indications for lung transplantation. *Ann Surg* 1990; 212:249.

Kahan BD: Cyclosporine. *N Engl J Med* 1989; 321:1725.

McCarthy PM, Starnes VA, Theodore J, et al: Improved survival after heart-lung transplantation. *J Thorac Cardiovasc Surg* 1990; 99:54.

Rubin RH, Wolf JS, Cosimi AB, et al: Infection in the renal transplant patient. *Am J Med* 1981; 70:405.

Starzl TE, Demetris AJ (eds): *Liver Transplantation*. Chicago, Mosby-Year Book, Inc, 1990.

Sutherland DER, Dunn DL, Goetz FC, et al: A 10-year experience with 290 pancreas transplants at a single institution. *Ann Surg* 1989; 210:274.

INFECTIONS 17

I. **FEVER AND DISORDERS OF TEMPERATURE HO-MEOSTASIS.**
A. **Normal Temperature Homeostasis.**
   1. **Normal range:**
      a. Core temperature: 36.7–37.6° C.
      b. Superimposed on this range is a **normal diurnal variation,** ±0.7–1.5° C, usually peaking in the evening, and a menstrual variation in females, ±0.5° C, usually peaking at ovulation.
   2. **Normal homeostatic mechanisms:**
      a. Thermal control originates from the preoptic nucleus of the anterior hypothalamus which directs the autonomic nervous system to regulate cutaneous vasomotor tone, perspiration, cutaneous muscular tone, and endocrinologic effectors of metabolic activity.
      b. Nonshivering thermogenesis, exaggerated metabolic activity of brown fat (significant in neonates only) and skeletal muscle (adults and neonates) can increase heat production 40%–100%.
   3. **Measurement:**
      a. Ideal measurement of core temperature in the SICU is via a thermal sensor-equipped PA catheter.
      b. Esophageal probes are suited only for unconscious patients.
      c. Rectal temperature is the best noninvasive method.
      d. Oral measurement is suitable for patients able to maintain an oral seal.
      e. Automated devices for tympanic membrane (external canal) monitoring.
B. **Fever.**
   1. **Pathophysiology:** In response to noxious stimuli (endotoxin, complement activation, immune complexes, tissue injury, etc.) activated macrophages or lymphocytes release cytokines (primarily IL-1,-2 and -6, TNF, and

653

INF-α, -β, and -γ) which ultimately raise the hypothalamic thermal set point.

2. **All fevers warrant clinical evaluation** (see pp 659–662).

3. **Fever need only be treated** per se to reduce the discomfort of associated myalgias, etc., or when the increased metabolic activity stresses a compromised cardiovascular system.

   a. **Drugs affecting prostaglandin synthesis** (acetaminophen, NSAIDs) should be used.

   b. **Topical cooling** does not reduce fever, and actually increases metabolic demand unless the hypothalamic driven effectors of temperature regulation are blocked. This can be accomplished in extreme instances by sedation and pharmacologic paralysis (pancuronium, vecuronium).

   c. **Specific treatment** should be directed to the underlying infection or damaged tissue.

4. **Complications:**

   a. In general, major complications related to fever are the result of the causative agent or illness, not the elevated temperature.

   b. **Febrile seizures** rarely, if ever, occur after the age of 6 years, and, even in childhood, are usually benign.

   c. **Patients with marginal cardiovascular reserve can suffer serious consequences** (stroke, MI, dysrhythmia, CHF, acute PE) if unable to meet the increased O_2 consumption (7% increase in O_2 consumption for each 1° C fever) or decreased SVR of pyrexia. **Aggressive treatment is indicated in these instances.**

C. **Hyperthermia.**

1. **Examples** include malignant hyperthermia (MH; see section I.D), thyroid storm, dehydration, heat stroke, and hypothalamic injury (e.g., trauma, tumor, infarction).

2. **Clinical evaluation:**

   a. Hyperthermia cannot be distinguished from fever based on the magnitude of pyrexia. Certain clinical situations produce a readily apparent diagnosis (e.g., heat stroke), but endocrinologic and hypothalamic disorders can require extensive testing.

   b. Clinical evaluation is the same as with fever. In the absence of an obvious or infectious cause, consider drug-induced hyperthermia.

3. **Treatment:**
    a. Therapy is directed to the underlying disorder.
    b. Offending drugs are withdrawn.
    c. Hydration is maintained.
    d. Specific pharmacotherapy (e.g., dantrolene, propyl-thiouracil) is employed when indicated.
    e. Topical cooling (paralysis is not needed) for temperatures $>40°$ C.
4. **Complications** depend on the underlying disorder. In primary heat stroke, mortality approaches 70% unless promptly treated.

D. **Malignant Hyperthermia.**
  1. **Definition:**
     a. **The clinical syndrome** of acute and uncontrolled increase in exothermic metabolic activity usually in response to volatile anesthetics (halothane, enflurane, isoflurane) or depolarizing muscle relaxants (succinylcholine).
     b. **The incidence** of fulminant MH is 1 in 250,000 anesthetics (1 in 62,000 when only volatile or depolarizing agents are considered) and the incidence of suspected MH is 1 in 16,000 anesthetics (1 in 4,200 with the above agents). It occurs most commonly in pediatric patients, where its incidence is 1 in 12,000 anesthetics.
     c. **Mortality,** even in treated patients, is 10%.
  2. **Pathophysiology:** MH is a genetic myopathy of skeletal muscle producing an acute loss of intracellular control of calcium in response to provoking stimuli. Increases in intracellular calcium initiate intense metabolic activity to regain homeostasis while at the same time provoking muscular contracture. Aerobic metabolism and glycolysis produce heat as well as increases in lactic acid, apparently in the absence of hypoxia.
  3. **Clinical presentation and diagnosis:**
     a. MH may occur during induction or be delayed up to 25 hours. It may present in the recovery room or SICU in nonanesthetized, awake patients.
     b. **Early signs** include a hypermetabolic state with tachycardia, metabolic acidosis, hypoxemia, increased end-expiratory CO_2 general anxiety.
     c. Skin mottling, cyanosis, and unstable BP are common.

    d. Masseter stiffness progressing to whole body rigidity, tachycardia, and hypertension soon follow.

    e. **Pyrexia** (which may exceed 43° C) occurs relatively late.

    f. Metabolic exhaustion, generalized edema (including cerebral edema), DIC, and multisystem failure result in death.

    g. Prior uneventful anesthesia does not rule out MH.

4. **Treatment:** By the time the diagnosis is obvious, irreversible damage is likely. Prompt, aggressive treatment is warranted as soon as MH is suspected.

    a. **Discontinue** anesthetic agents.

    b. **Hyperventilate** with 100% O_2. Use an anesthetic machine not exposed to anesthetic agent.

    c. **Give dantrolene 2.5 mg/kg IV immediately** and q. 5 min up to 10 mg/kg until the syndrome abates.

        1) The drug comes in 20-mg vials which must be diluted in sterile water (without dextrose or electrolytes). As this task is time-consuming and absolutely vital, one person should be assigned this duty separate from all other responsibilities.

        2) Repeat the 2.5-mg/kg dose q. 12 h. for 48 hours.

    d. **Monitor UO and urine myoglobin** via bladder catheterization. Maintain urine flow with hydration and mannitol 12.5 g IV as prophylaxis against ATN.

    e. Start arterial line.

    f. **Treat metabolic acidosis** with IV $NaHCO_3$.

    g. Follow blood gas, serum potassium, serum glucose, and DIC panel determinations frequently. Treat with IV insulin as needed.

    h. **Control pyrexia** with surface cooling if temperature >39° C and remains elevated despite dantrolene administration.

    i. In patients who have had an episode of MH or those thought to be susceptible, triggering agents should be avoided. Caffeine and halothane contractive tests involve biopsy of a 1-in. sample of muscle and are the gold standard for susceptibility. Although no anesthetic regimen is completely safe, **certain drugs are considered relatively free from triggering action:**

       1) Barbituates, ketamine, vercuronium, atracurium, pancuronium, opioids, benzodiazepines, local anesthetics.

       2) Some recommend pretreatment with dantrolene 2.5 mg/kg 15–30 minutes prior to anesthetic induction or 3 mg/kg/day for 2 days preoperation.

    j. **Procaine or procainamide** should be used to control ventricular arrythmias.

    k. **Follow serial CPK enzymes** until remission of the episodes.

E. Hypothermia.

  1. **Differential diagnosis:**

    a. The most **common causes** of hypothermia (core body temperature <35° C) in the SICU are prolonged intraabdominal surgery, cooling during CPB, sepsis, and environmental exposure following burns or trauma.

    b. **Metabolic causes** include hypoglycemia, hypopituitarism, hypothyroidism, hypothalamic dysfunction.

    c. Ethanol, barbiturates, phenothiazines, and anesthetics all can lower core temperature.

  2. **Complications:**

    a. The most important problems stem from dysfunction of excitable tissues:

       1) **Ventricular fibrillation,** which occurs at 30–32° C, is the most common cause of death.

       2) **Depressed mentation** progressing to a flat EEG around 20° C.

    b. **Coagulation factors** work poorly <35° C, substantially complicating trauma resuscitation and recovery from cardiopulmonary bypass (CPB).

    c. A leftward shift in the O_2 dissociation curve prevents adequate unloading of O_2 at the tissues.

    d. **Brain death cannot be declared** in any potential organ donor with hypothermia.

  3. **Treatment:**

    a. **Passive rewarming is used if temperature is >30° C** and the patient's homeostatic regulatory mechanisms (e.g., shivering) are intact.

       1) Monitor ECG and core temperature.

       2) Administer 100% O_2.

       3) Warm the room and close the door (if practical).

      4) Utilize heat lamps or overbody warmers.

      5) Warm all IV fluids and inspired gases to 39° C.

      6) Raise the core temperature 1.0–1.5° C/hr, stopping at 35° C.

  b. **Active rewarming is used for temperatures <30° C** or when normal regulatory mechanisms are impaired.

      1) Continue passive rewarming.

      2) Consider gastric, colonic or peritoneal lavage with 39° C lactated Ringer's solution.

      3) Consider warming via CPB or hemodialysis.

  c. **Complications of rewarming:** Sudden vasodilation can cause severe hypotension and a washout of previously nonperfused vascular beds precipitating lactic acidosis. Also, as cold blood returns from the extremities, a paradoxical decrease in core temperature can initially occur.

II. SURGICAL INFECTIONS.

Two general categories of surgical infections are (1) those which require surgical intervention (e.g., necrotizing fasciitis) and (2) those which occur postoperatively or posttraumatically. Postoperative infections include those treated medically (e.g., postoperative pneumonia) as well as surgically. Clinical management and specific therapy depend upon the nature of the infection and the clinical situation.

A. Signs and Symptoms.

  1. **A surgical infection** may manifest itself clinically as fever, leukocytosis, and local signs such as inflammation, wound drainage, or foul sputum.

  2. **Signs of a localized soft tissue infection** are heat, redness, swelling, and tenderness. The classic signs of infection, however, are not always present, especially in immunocompromised patients.

  3. **Infection** should be considered in patients with:

    a. Tachycardia.

    b. Tachypnea, hypoxemia.

    c. Ileus.

    d. Hyperglycemia (insulin resistance).

    e. Altered mental status.

    f. Hypotension.

    g. Hypovolemia.

h. DIC.

i. Hypothermia.

4. **Risk factors** which increase the likelihood and severity of infections include advanced age, diabetes, malnutrition, immunocompromise (steroids, burns, AIDS), and multisystem organ failure (MSOF).

5. **Risk factors for MSOF** include multiple trauma, burns, pancreatitis, hemodynamic instability, complex elective operations, major postoperative complications, and overwhelming infections, especially intraabdominal.

B. **Clinical Management.**

1. **Fevers** in the SICU are conveniently grouped into those occurring within 48 hours of trauma or surgery, and those occurring after 48 hours. Physical examination is based on time of occurrence.

a. **Within 48 hours,** atelectasis, clostridial, or streptococcal wound infections; infections related to anastomotic leak; and generalized immune activation following major trauma can all produce significant fever.

1) **Fever in the first 48 hours postoperatively is usually caused by atelectasis.** Measures to prevent this include providing adequate analgesia, encouraging deep breathing, early ambulation, ET suctioning, and IPPB. CXR may demonstrate platelike densities. The fever should resolve with pulmonary toilet.

2) **Early cellulitis** is due to either streptococcal or clostridial infection. The wound should be examined to exclude this cause of early fever.

3) **An anastomotic leak or perforation** may cause fever in the early postoperative period. Usually these patients are hypovolemic and may appear systemically ill.

4) **The presence of a preoperative infection** may be the cause of early postoperative fever.

5) **Consider malignant hyperthermia** if associated signs are present.

b. **Beyond 48 hours, more extensive evaluation is required.**

1) **All wounds** should be examined, including all sites of transcutaneous catheters.

2) **A thorough HEENT examination** for signs of otitis, sinusitis, or meningitis is especially important in patients with an instrumented naso- or oropharynx.

3) **Thoracic examination** should aim to detect areas of pulmonary consolidation, effusions, or bronchospasm. Presence of a new cardiac murmur or rub may be indicative of endo- or pericarditis, respectively.

4) **Abdominal examination** should aim to rule out cholecystitis, pancreatitis, intraabdominal abscess, and intestinal obstruction.

5) Prostatitis and perirectal abscess should be ruled out by **rectal examination.**

6) **Signs of thrombophlebitis** should be sought.

7) **Laboratory studies** should include CBC, differential, urinalysis, and two sets of blood cultures drawn during the febrile episode from separate sites.

8) **CXR** (PA and lateral, if possible) should be obtained.

9) **More extensive testing** (e.g., abdominal CT scan, ventilation-perfusion scan, lumbar puncture, sinus films, echocardiogram) are performed as indicated.

10) Tumor (especially lymphoma and lung carcinoma) and autoimmune (e.g., SLE, vasculitis)-related fever should be considered when appropriate.

2. **In the hemodynamically stable patient:**

 a. A diagnostic evaluation can proceed prior to initiating therapy.

 1) History and physical examination are the key to diagnosis.

 2) Evaluation includes laboratory and radiographic studies.

 3) Blood cultures, Gram's stain, and appropriate fluid cultures are obtained prior to beginning antibiotics.

    b. If infectious source identified:
        1) Initiate treatment appropriate for diagnosis.
        2) The clinical response is the standard by which therapy is assessed. The patient is reassessed to exclude errors in diagnosis or omissions.
        3) Antibiotics are altered as culture and sensitivity results become available.
    c. If infectious source is not obvious:
        1) The surgeon needs to decide if empiric therapy is warranted. Both the clinical situation and the risk factors of the patient need to be considered. Empiric therapy is based on the most likely diagnosis.
        2) Alternatively, therapy may be withheld pending culture results or repeat examination. The patient must be reassessed as necessary.
3. **Fever in the hemodynamically unstable patient:**
    a. **Patients with surgical infections may present in septic shock.**
        1) Sepsis usually presents in adults as fever (temperature >38.5° C), tachycardia (pulse >100 bpm), tachypnea (respiration rate >20), and at least one manifestation of organ dysfunction.
        2) A patient with multiple risk factors for infection is more likely to present with respiratory or cardiovascular instability.
    b. **Resuscitation is the first line of therapy of the patient in shock.**
        1) **Intubation** may be required in patients with respiratory insufficiency.
        2) Hypotension should be treated with **volume resuscitation and cardiovascular agents** as appropriate.
        3) **A PA catheter** may be helpful in guiding resuscitation in patients with poor cardiac function or who are at risk of developing MSOF.
        4) Patients in septic shock normally have a low SVR and elevated CO. Phenylephrine or norepinephrine can be used to increase SVR.
    c. **After resuscitation and stabilization,** begin diagnostic evaluation for infection.

    d. When the source of infection is known a specific treatment based on the most likely pathogens can begin. However, the source of infection is often not obvious and **empiric therapy should be instituted in the unstable patient.**

        1) **Broad-spectrum antibiotics should be started when all cultures have been obtained.**

            a) Ampicillin, gentamicin, and clindamycin are often started as empiric therapy.

            b) Vancomycin is indicated when line sepsis is felt to be the source.

            c) Third-generation cephalosporins and imipenem can also be used as broad-spectrum therapy, especially if renal insufficiency is present.

        2) **Specific surgical therapy is instituted as indicated** (e.g., debridement in gas gangrene). Rarely is it necessary to perform an exploratory laparotomy in a patient without a specific diagnosis.

        3) Use of **high-dose steroids** have not been shown to be of benefit. Use of **naloxone** is uncommon.

C. Pathogens.

Pathogens are usually identified by Gram's stain and culture. A likely pathogen may be suspected based on the nature of the infection. Not all organisms are necessarily pathogens; e.g., a granulating wound may be colonized with microbes which in the absence of a wound infection should not be treated.

    1. **Gram-positive cocci:**

        a. *Staphylococcus aureus* is often a cause of wound- and catheter-related infections. Treat with nafcillin or oxacillin.

        b. **Methicillin-resistant *S. aureus* (MRSA)** has same virulence as *S. aureus* but requires treatment with vancomycin. Hospitalized patients colonized with MRSA require reverse isolation to avoid spreading the bacteria to other patients.

        c. *Staphylococcus epidermidis* is often associated with infections of prosthetic materials. Since the organism is part of normal skin flora it may appear as a contaminant in blood cultures. Treat with vancomycin.

d. **Streptococci** are often a cause of cellulitis and endo-carditis. Group A are causative in scarlet fever, ery-sipelas, and impetigo, and may lead to rheumatic fever. Treat with penicillin G.

e. **Enterococci** are often associated with infections involving IV devices and biliary sepsis. Treat with ampicillin and gentamicin.

2. **Gram-positive rods.**

   a. *Clostridium:*

      1) *C. tetani* **and** *C. perfringens* are anaerobic bacteria which cause tetanus and gas gangrene, respectively. Treatment requires debridement and penicillin G.

      2) *C. difficile* is the major cause of pseudomembranous colitis and is usually treated with po vancomycin or po or IV metronidazole.

   b. *Bacillus anthracis* is the causative organism in anthrax. Treat with penicillin G.

   c. *Corynebacterium diphtheriae* is the causative organism in diphtheria. Prevention is by immunization with diphtheria toxoid which is usually given with tetanus toxoid. Treat with diphtheria antitoxin and penicillin G.

3. **Gram-negative cocci:**

   a. *Neisseria gonorrhoeae* causes gonorrhea. Treat with penicillin.

   b. *Neisseria meningitidis* causes meningitis and septic shock. Treat with penicillin.

4. **Gram-negative rods:**

   a. *Bacteroides* are anaerobic bacteria often involved in mixed anaerobic-aerobic infections of the GI tract with *B. fragilis* most eminent. Treat with metronidazole or clindamycin. Ampicillin and gentamicin are usually added in mixed infections to treat aerobes.

   b. **Enterobacteriaceae family** includes *Escherichia coli, Klebsiella, Enterobacter, Serratia,* and *Proteus.* These organisms are involved in biliary, urinary, and GI-related infections. Treat with gentamicin or amikacin. Alternatively, a second- or third-generation cephalosporin may be used.

   c. *Haemophilus* organism is usually *H. influenzae* type b which may cause meningitis, epiglottitis, or pneu

monia. Treatment is with third-generation cephalosporin (e.g., ceftriaxone) since ampicillin-resistant
strains are now common.

d. **Pseudomonas aeruginosa** is common in nosocomial
infections. Wound infections typically have greenish
exudate with fruity odor. Treat with two synergistic
drugs to avoid resistance (usually mezlocillin and
gentamicin).

5. **Acid-fast organisms** are mostly *Mycobacterium* which
are responsible for tuberculosis. *M. avium-intracellulare*
(MAI) is often found in AIDS patients. Treat with combination of isoniazid, rifampin, and ethambutol.

6. **Fungal infections:**

a. **Pathogens** are usually *Candida* sps. *Cryptococcus,
Histoplasma, Mucor,* and *Aspergillus* are also seen.

b. *Candida* **infections** are associated with:

1) Immunosuppression, including patients on steroids or those with T cell dysfunction.

2) Long-term illnesses.

3) Long-term antibiotic use, especially broad-spectrum antibiotics.

4) Recurrent or persistent fistulas.

5) Continued respiratory failure.

c. **Evaluation of fungal infections** involves physical
examination, culture, and Gram's stain.

1) Obtain sputum, stool, urine, drain sites, and
blood cultures for fungus. Usually six blood cultures are obtained over a 48-hour period.

2) Funduscopic examination to identify *Candida*
chorioretinitis.

d. **The decision to treat a presumed fungal infection**
is based upon the clinical setting in conjunction with
laboratory results. Several common clinical settings
exist:

1) When **positive blood culture is drawn through
an indwelling catheter,** catheter should be
changed and catheter tip sent for culture.

2) **Persistent positive blood cultures after catheters have been changed or removed.** This usually necessitates parenteral amphotericin B or
fluconazole.

3) *Candida* **endophthalmitis** is an indication for systemic therapy.

4) *Candida* **isolated from more than three separate sites** with negative blood cultures, usually necessitates empiric amphotericin B therapy for presumed disseminated candidiasis.

5) **Symptomatic urinary tract infection** with cultures of *Candida:*

  a) If a Foley catheter is present, an attempt should be made to remove foreign bodies from the urinary tract. If Foley catheter drainage is mandatory, treatment of positive fungal cultures is usually based upon symptomatic urinary tract infection including fever and symptoms localized to the urinary tract. Treatment can include amphotericin bladder irrigation or oral fluconazole for more severe infections.

  b) If no catheter is present, symptomatic urinary tract infections are usually treated by bladder irrigation.

6) **Oral or esophageal candidiasis:**

  a) Prophylaxis against oral candidiasis is best performed using nystatin PO.

  b) Candidiasis may be treated with either oral nystatin or fluconazole.

7. *Entamoeba histolytica* infection (amebiasis) may cause dysentery, colitis, or hepatic abscess. Treat with metronidazole in combination with chloroquine and diloxanide. Hepatic abscess requires drainage.

8. **Viruses:**

   a. **Hepatitis B** is transmitted by blood, blood products, or sexual contact and can result in chronic active hepatitis and cirrhosis. Needle sticks from carriers can be treated by **hepatitis B immune globulin (HBIG) 0.06 mL/kg** and vaccination. Prevention is best managed by immunization with hepatitis vaccine.

   b. **HIV (the agent of AIDS):**

   1) Needle sticks from seropositive patients carry risk of infection of 1 in 250 to 1 in 300.

   2) Exposure to blood of seropositive patients should be managed by serotesting the health

  care worker and repeated testing at 6 weeks, 3,
  6, and 12 months after exposure.

  3) Contact hospital infectious disease consultant.
  Protocols exist for use of AZT in exposed health
  care workers (AZT 250 mg PO q. 4 h. × 6–7
  weeks). The initial dose of AZT should be administered immediately after exposure.

 c. The risk of developing **rabies** after animal bite depends upon status of animal. If animal is proved negative by observation or pathologic examination, then
  no treatment is necessary. Bites from rabid animals or
  wild animals are treated with rabies immune globulin
  (RIG) 20 IU/kg IM and human diploid cell rabies
  vaccine (HDCV) as 1-mL doses on days 0, 3, 7, 14,
  and 28.

 d. **Herpesviruses:**

  1) **CMV infection** is usually seen in immunocompromised patients, especially in bone marrow
  and organ transplant patients. Inoculation is usually through blood transfusion or organ transplantation. Attempts to limit transmission have
  included organ depletion of WBCs which harbor
  the virus and screening donors for CMV sero-
  logic markers.

   a) Diagnosis is by viral titer, inclusion bodies
   seen on biopsy, viral culture, or detection of
   CMV DNA by polymerase chain reaction.

   b) Severe infections are treated with ganciclovir (5 mg/kg).

  2) **Herpes simplex** causes oral and genital skin
  eruptions, pneumonitis, and encephalitis. Treat
  with acyclovir.

  3) **Varicella-zoster (VZV)** is the causative agent in
  both chickenpox (primary) and zoster (reactiva-
  tion). VZV pneumonia can also occur, especially in adults. Treat with acyclovir.

D. Prevention of Surgical Wound Infections.

 1. **Bacterial contamination:**

  a. The presence of infection prior to surgery increases
  the risk of wound infection. Elective surgery should
  be postponed until the infection has been treated.

  b. Antiseptic showers prior to surgery decrease wound
  infection rate. Skin is prepared with chlorhexidine or

povidone-iodine. Hair should not be shaved until immediately before surgery.

c. **Prophylactic antibiotics are** chosen to combat bacteria likely to be present in the operative field. No antibiotics should be given for clean cases in which there is minimal contamination (e.g., thyroidectomy). Most abdominal procedures necessitate the use of antibiotics to cover anaerobes and gram-negative aerobes (cefoxitin). Operations which require prosthetics should be effective against skin contaminants (cefazolin, vancomycin). Antibiotics are given 30 minutes preoperatively and stopped several hours after operation.

d. **A mechanical preparation** (magnesia of citrate or PEG with clear liquids for 2 days) combined with an antibiotic (neomycin-erythromycin base for several doses) will significantly reduce bacterial counts in the colon.

e. **Wound infection rates** depend upon type of operation.

1) **Clean:** no gross contamination (e.g., hernia, thyroidectomy, mastectomy). Wound infection rate is ~1%.

2) **Clean-contaminated:** minor contamination (e.g., gastric and biliary surgery). Wound infection rate is ~2%–5%.

3) **Contaminated:** Major contamination (e.g., gross spillage from unprepared bowel). Wound infection rate is 5%–30%.

4) **Infected:** contamination from infected source (e.g., drainage of appendiceal abscess). Wound infection rate is >30%.

2. **Patient risk factors:**

a. **Hyperglycemia** interferes with WBC function. Control with insulin.

b. **Steroids** are immunosuppressive and their use is associated with increased wound infection rates and poor healing. Rapidly taper.

c. **Advanced age** is associated with poor wound healing due to systemic abnormalities such as vascular disease.

d. **Wound healing is impaired in malnutrition.** Nutritional support (enteral or TPN for 7–10 days) may be necessary.

    e. **Renal failure** causes poor wound healing.

    f. **Obese** patients have higher wound infection rates which may be related to poorly vascularized fat.

    g. **Radiation and chemotherapy** interfere with normal wound healing processes. Neutropenia results in increased risk of wound infection.

3. **Operative technique:**

    a. Sterile technique and sterilization of instruments with either autoclaving or treatment with gaseous ethylene oxide.

    b. Retained foreign body is associated with increased wound infections. Foreign bodies include permanent suture material and care should be taken to leave as little suture as possible.

    c. Fluid collections (hematoma, seroma) can serve as a growth media for bacteria. Drains may be necessary. Closed drainage systems (Jackson-Pratt) are better able to maintain sterility than open drains (Penrose).

    d. Necrotic tissue may also lead to infections and care should be taken to debride dead tissue. Excessive use of cautery injures tissue and increases infection rates.

    e. **In contaminated cases** it may be preferable to leave the skin open to allow healing by secondary intention rather than risk wound infections. Three general methods are used to treat wounds at risk for infections.

        1) **Open:** The wound may be left open and dressing changes performed.

        2) **Delayed primary closure:** The wound is left open with a gauze pack and is examined on postoperative day 5. If there is no sign of infection the wound is closed with nylon sutures placed at the time of surgery, or with skin tapes.

        3) **Wicks:** The wound is compartmentalized with gauze wicks between skin sutures. The wicks are usually removed in 3–5 days.

E. **Postoperative Infections.**

The presence of a postoperative infection usually manifests itself by fever (see pp 659–662). Leukocytosis with a left shift, tachycardia, and signs of toxemia may be present.

1. **Respiratory infections** are common in postoperative patients. Prolonged intubation and underlying lung disease are associated with an increased risk of pneumonia.

a. **Sputum production,** pleuritic chest pain, and auscultatory findings of consolidation are usually present.

b. **Gram's stain of sputum** should reveal large amounts of WBCs. The predominant organism found in the area of WBCs should be the suspected organism. Culture results will aid in diagnosis and should allow alteration of antibiotic therapy.

c. **CXR** may reveal a pulmonary infiltrate.

d. **Treatment** involves aggressive pulmonary toilet and appropriate antibiotics. The choice of antibiotics is guided by the clinical situation and the Gram's stain results. *Pseudomonas,* a leading cause of nosocomial pneumonia, is treated with two synergistic drugs.

2. **Urinary tract infections** may occur any time during hospitalization. Urinary retention and instrumentation predispose to urinary infections.

a. Dysuria, frequency, hesitancy, and inability to void are frequent symptoms of cystitis. Flank pain, high fevers, and ileus may be due to pyelonephritis.

b. **Urinalysis and urine culture** should be performed. The presence of pyuria, WBC esterase, nitrates, and bacteriuria should be noted. A positive culture is reported as >100,000 colonies per milliliter of urine of a specific organism.

c. **Treatment** includes adequate urinary drainage and appropriate antibiotics. Usual organisms are gram-negative rods.

3. **Wound infections** are usually evident by physical examination. Erythema, drainage and the presence of crepitus should be noted.

a. **Cellulitis** is manifest by a tender, warm erythematous wound without drainage or fluctuance. Treat with antibiotics, usually cefazolin.

b. **Wound infections associated with drainage or fluctuance** should be opened bluntly and loculations broken up. Superficial wound infections of abdominal incisions can lead to fascial dehiscence if left undrained. Open drainage and dressing changes are usually all the treatment that is needed. Antibiotics are used only if there is a component of cellulitis.

c. **Dehiscence of abdominal wounds classically presents as drainage of clear fluid on postoperative day 5–7.** Inspection after opening the skin incision reveals fascial dehiscence, often with evisceration of abdominal contents. Keep abdominal contents moist with sterile saline-soaked gauze. **Reoperation** is required to close defect.

d. **Infection over vascular grafts require expert care.** Graft removal may be required and the operating surgeon should be notified immediately.

   1) **Wound infection** over prosthetic graft may be treated with dressing changes and antibiotics.

   2) **If anastomosis is visible** in field, graft removal may be indicated.

   3) **Massive bleeding** may occur and is treated by application of pressure. Injury to adjacent structure may occur by application of clamps. Urgent transport to the OR is required for definitive care.

4. **Indwelling IV catheters** should be changed q. 3–4 d. to avoid line sepsis.

   a. Fever workups should first include routine examinations and tests.

   b. If no other source can be found, the catheter should be checked for infection by **drawing a blood culture through it.** This must be done with extreme care as a false-positive culture will result in unwarranted removal of the catheter.

   c. **A peripheral blood culture** *must* be obtained at the same time as the central catheter is cultured. If both are positive the catheter should be left in place and antibiotics given. If only the central catheter is positive, it should be removed.

   d. Attempts at sterilizing the central catheter are discouraged.

5. **Peritonitis:**

   a. In the appropriate clinical setting an **anastomotic leak** may be the cause of peritonitis.

   1) These patients usually have the picture of an ileus, hypovolemia, and free air.

   2) **Free air** can normally be seen in patients after abdominal exploration for up to a week postoperatively.

   3) **A bile leak** after biliary surgery will also present as peritonitis and is usually associated with nau-

sea and vomiting. Ultrasound may reveal a fluid collection.

4) Patients with a suspected anastomotic leak are best evaluated with a water-soluble contrast study. If a leak is demonstrated reoperation may be necessary.

5) **A fistula** may become evident by enteric contents draining from the wound. Small bowel fistulas may resolve without operation.

b. **Intraabdominal abscess** usually presents with localized tenderness and spiking fevers.

1) **A CT scan** is the study of choice to evaluate the possibility of an abscess. The abscess can then be drained either percutaneously by CT guidance or operatively.

2) In the clinical setting where an abscess is likely but cannot be localized by CT, laparotomy may be necessary for diagnosis.

3) **Broad-spectrum antibiotics** are indicated. Triple coverage with ampicillin, gentamicin, and metronidazole is standard.

c. A postoperative patient can develop an **abdominal process not directly related to the surgery.** Perforated ulcer can present as diffuse peritonitis. Acalculous cholecystitis can occur in debilitated patients. Treatment depends upon the diagnosis being considered.

d. **Peritoneal signs of infection associated with peritoneal dialysis** are cloudy peritoneal fluid containing inflammatory cells and the presence of bacteria on Gram's stain or culture.

1) **First occurrence** in a stable patient can be treated with IP antibiotics, vancomycin 1 g/L load and tobramycin 1.7 mg/kg, and heparin 2,000 units/L with a dwell time of 3 hours, followed by 1-L exchanges q. 6 h. containing vancomycin 30 mg and tobramycin 8 mg for 48 hours. Culture results should guide antibiotic therapy when available.

2) **Catheter removal is indicated** for persistent tunnel tract infection, multiple episodes of peritonitis caused by the same organism, or fecal

peritoneal drainage which also necessitates laparotomy. Catheters should not be replaced for 2–3 weeks.

   e. Peritoneal signs of infection may be due to nonoperative causes and these should be excluded. Common causes are pancreatitis, sickle cell crisis, cystitis, zoster, and pneumonia.

6. **Meningitis** should be excluded as a cause of postoperative fever. This is usually evident on physical examination. A spinal tap is performed when meningitis is suspected.

7. **Endocarditis** may be a cause of persistent fever. It most often occurs in patients with a history of valvular disease. Echocardiography should be performed to search for vegetations. **Antibiotic prophylaxis should be given to all patients at risk** (e.g., valvular heart disease, prosthetic valves) who are undergoing instrumentation of the oral, respiratory, GI, and urinary tracts.

   a. **Oral and respiratory:** Penicillin V 2.0 g PO 1 hour before operation and 1.0 g 6 hours later or erythromycin 1.0 g PO 2 hours before and 0.5 g PO 6 hours later.

   b. **GI or urinary:** Amoxicillin 3.0 g PO 1 hour before operation and 1.5 g PO 6 hours later or vancomycin 1.0 g IV and gentamicin 1.5 mg/kg IV given 30 minutes before.

   c. **Prosthetic valves:** Ampicillin 2.0 g IV and gentamicin 1.5 mg/kg IV given 30 minutes before operation.

8. **Sinusitis** is commonly seen in patients with prolonged nasal intubations (ET or NG tubes). Diagnosis is made by sinus films. Treatment is with antibiotics and nasal vasoconstrictors.

9. **Noninfectious causes of fever** in the postoperative period are due to drug reactions, tumor, thyrotoxicosis, diencephalic storm, and factitious.

F. **Surgical Infections Associated With Soft Tissue Inflammation.**

Infection associated with soft tissue inflammation usually requires surgical intervention. The patient often presents with fever, leukocytosis, and a specific area of inflammation which may be either a de novo localizing process or a site of surgical wound. The site should be examined for inflammatory reaction, fluctuance, crepitus, and tissue necrosis.

1. **Superficial inflammation:**
   a. The presence of erythema without fluctuance or drainage and no devitalized tissue is most likely cellulitis.
   b. An area of erythema occurring over a vein associated with a palpable cord may be **thrombophlebitis.**
   c. Linear red streaks proximal to an inflammatory reaction of a distal limb represent lymphangitic spread.
   d. **Treatment** includes warm soaks, elevation, and antibiotics. Usual antibiotics are either penicillin G or penicillinase-resistant penicillin (nafcillin, methicillin, dicloxacillin).
   e. Failure to improve rapidly should lead one to suspect a resistant organism, abscess, or phlebothrombosis.

2. **Deep inflammation** is characterized by the presence of local inflammation associated with fluctuance, drainage, or sinus tracts. **Needle aspiration** with a large-bore needle (16 gauge) and a small syringe (1 mL) may be helpful to determine if an undrained collection is present.
   a. **No collection:** An abscess may not as yet have formed, or an unconsidered diagnosis may exist.
   b. **Collection present:** An abscess is resistant to the action of antibiotics and requires surgical drainage and possibly debridement.
   c. **Phlebothrombosis** is treated with operative debridement and excision of the vein.

3. **The presence of devascularized skin, deep necrosis, and crepitus** should alert one to the possibility of a more serious soft tissue infection.
   a. **A history** of crush injury with devitalized tissue, foreign body, systemic signs of toxemia, muscle necrosis, and gram-positive rods are signs of clostridial myositis (gas gangrene).
      1) **Extensive debridement** is necessary and often requires limb amputation.
      2) **Aggressive circulatory support** is needed to maintain tissue perfusion.
      3) **Penicillin G** 12–24 million units/day IV is given.
      4) **Hyperbaric O$_2$** has been shown to be helpful. However, treatment by debridement has priority over transfer to hyperbaric O$_2$ chamber.

b. The presence of a rapidly spreading infection, mixed organisms on Gram's stain, necrotic fascia, and thrombosis and obliteration of subcutaneous vessels are signs of **necrotizing fasciitis.** As part of a spectrum of necrotizing infections is gram-negative synergistic necrotizing cellulitis. This can present as a necrotizing infection of the abdominal wall. **Fournier's gangrene** is a necrotizing infection of the scrotum.

   1) **Extensive debridement** of necrotic fascia is necessary but limbs can usually be salvaged.
   2) **High-dose penicillin G and gentamicin** are given.
   3) **Circulatory support** is necessary to maintain perfusion.

G. Tetanus.

Tetanus should always be considered when treating puncture wounds or wounds with devitalized tissue. The causative organism is *Clostridium tetani.* Nervous irritability and muscular rigidity are mediated by a neurotoxin produced by the bacterium.

1. **Asymptomatic acute injury:** All patients who are not allergic to toxoid should be prophylactically immunized. Active immunization is usually given in childhood.

   a. **Clean lacerations** (e.g., a knife or glass) are not prone to tetanus.
      1) **Previously immunized:** No tetanus treatment is necessary. If last booster was given >10 years ago, give tetanus toxoid and diphtheria booster (dTet) 0.5 mL IM.
      2) **Not previously immunized** (or inadequate previous immunization): Give dTet 0.5 mL IM. Plans to complete the series should be made if the patient has not previously been immunized.

   b. **Puncture wounds, wounds with devitalized tissue, wounds caused by missiles, burns, frostbite, crush injury, and wounds with foreign body are at increased risk for tetanus.**
      1) **Previously immunized:** No tetanus treatment is necessary. If last booster was given >5 years ago, give dTet 0.5 mL IM.
      2) **Not previously immunized** (or inadequate immunization): Give dTet 0.5 mL IM, with plan to

complete the series and tetanus immune globulin (TIG) 250 units IM.

2. **Symptomatic tetanus:** Tetanus can occur as early as 1 day after injury or as late as several months (average, 1 week). **Symptoms** include pain in the area of injury associated with spasm and rigidity of the facial muscles (risus sardonicus) and of the jaw (lockjaw). Laryngospasm and spasm of the back muscles can occur. Chest and diaphragmatic spasm require intubation and mechanical ventilation. Diaphoresis and tachycardia may be present.

   a. **Neutralize the tetanus toxin** with TIG 3,000–6,000 units injected IM. TIG is best administered in the extremity proximal to the injury.

   b. **Perform extensive debridement** of the wound. The wound is left open.

   c. **Sedation** with diazepam may be helpful in controlling spasm.

   d. **Respiratory compromise** is treated with intubation and induced paralysis (curarization). Usually such patients require tracheostomy for long-term mechanical ventilation.

   e. **Penicillin** G 12–24 million units/day IV.

H. Infection in the Immunocompromised Host.

The immunocompromised host is any patient with impaired host defenses who is at increased risk of developing infection. Such infections are likely to be of greater severity than in the normal host. The increasing prevalence of immunocompromised patients is due to (1) advances in cancer chemotherapy, organ transplantation, and immunosuppressive therapy of nonmalignant disease, and (2) AIDS. Infection is the most common immediate cause of death. Infection is likely to be due to opportunistic pathogens. Since the host's ability to mount an inflammatory response is impaired, **signs of serious systemic infection may be nonspecific or absent.**

1. **Management.**

   a. **Evaluation** of potential infection in the immunocompromised host is similar to that in the normal patient except:

     1) The subtle and atypical nature of symptoms and signs demands a **high index of clinical suspicion,** willingness to intervene early, and persis-

tence in search for potential causative organisms by rigorous and repeated septic workups.

2) **Minimal symptoms** demand complete evaluation.

3) **All nonspecific signs** (clinical deterioration, hypothermia, hypotension, glucose intolerance, low-grade pyrexia) demand full septic workup.

4) Identification of infectious agent must be prompt and precise.

5) **Consider early** use of invasive diagnostic procedures (transbronchial or open lung biopsy).

b. **Therapeutic intervention requires knowledge of:**

1) Presence of immunologic deficiencies in the compromised host.

2) Infections the patient is susceptible to on basis of impaired host defenses (see below).

c. **Therapy:**

1) Drainage or debridement of localized collections of infected material.

2) Specific antibiotics.

3) Reconstruction of deficient antimicrobial defenses (FFP for complement deficiencies, immune serum globulin for IgG deficiency, reduction or cessation of immunosupressive therapy, CSFs, WBC transfusion).

d. **Empiric antibiotic therapy:**

1) Broad-spectrum regimen against potential major gram-positive and gram-negative pathogens.

2) Use of synergistic antibiotic combinations rather than single-agent–Nonsynergistic combinations reduces morbidity and mortality (neutropenic patients) (e.g., vancomycin + ticarcillin + amikacin, ceftazidime + amikacin).

3) If a febrile, neutropenic patient is unresponsive to antibacterial treatment, consider amphotericin B.

e. **Prevention of infection:**

1) Avoid damage to physical barriers (repeated venipuncture, indwelling venous or urinary catheters)

2) Bolster host defenses (immune serum globulin, hyperimmune varicella-zoster immune globulin,

vaccination against *Pneumococcus, Haemophilus, Meningococcus*)
3) Maintain optimal nutritional status.
4) Avoid acquisition of new potential pathogens (sterility, isolation).
5) Suppression of colonizing flora:
    a) Gut sterilization and prophylactic systemic antibiotics for endogenous bacteria and fungi (80% of infections in neutropenic patients).
    b) Prophylaxis of specific infections with high incidence in certain populations (trimethoprim-sulfamethoxazole and aerosolized pentamidine protect against *Pneumocystis carinii* pneumonia in patients with AIDS).

2. **Defects in host defenses.**
  a. **Two types:**
    1) **Nonspecific** (nonimmunologic) host defenses: body's barrier systems, complement, phagocytosis.
    2) **Specific** (immunologic) host defenses:
      a) Humoral immune responses.
      b) Cellular immune responses.
  b. **Granulocytopenia.**
    1) Absolute granulocyte count $<500/\mu\text{L}$.
    2) Quantitative or qualitative defect in phagocytosis.
    3) Incidence or severity of infection related to:
      a) Absolute granulocyte count.
      b) Rapidity of onset of granulocytopenia.
      c) Duration of granulocytopenia.
    4) Etiology:
      a) Leukemia, lymphoma, collagen-vascular disease.
      b) Cytotoxic chemotherapy or radiation therapy for malignant disease.
      c) Immunosuppressive therapy for autoimmune disease and posttransplantation (corticosteroids, azathioprine, cyclophosphamide).
    5) Organisms:
      a) Gram-positive: *S. aureus, S. epidermidis.*
      b) Gram-negative: *E. coli, Klebsiella pneumoniae, P. aeruginosa*

c) Fungal: *Candida albicans, Aspergillus, Mucors.*

d) Viral: herpesviruses.

6) Myelosuppression and radiation therapy will cause concurrent damage to other host defenses (e.g., mucosal barriers) allowing portal of entry for organisms.

c. **Cellular immune dysfunction.**

1) Etiology:

a) Hodgkin's disease, non-Hodgkin's lymphoma.

b) AIDS.

c) Autoimmune disease (SLE, vasculitis).

d) Organ transplant recipients (corticosteroids, immunosupressive therapy).

2) Organisms:

a) Bacterial: *Listeria monocytogenes, Salmonella* sp., *Nocardia asteroides, Legionella* sp., mycobacteria.

b) Fungal: *Cryptococcus neoformans, Candida* sp., *Histoplasma capsulatum, Coccidioides immitis.*

c) Viral: VZV, CMV, HSV.

d) Parasitic: *P. carinii, Toxoplasma gondii, Giardia lamblia, E. histolytica, Cryptosporidium enteritis, Strongyloides stercoralis.*

d. **Humoral immune dysfunction:**

1) Etiology:

a) Multiple myeloma, chronic lymphocytic leukemia, sickle cell disease.

b) Chemotherapy.

2) Organisms: *Streptococcus pneumoniae, H. influenzae.*

3. **Infections in the solid organ transplant recipient.**

a. **Factors predisposing to infection:**

1) Immunosuppression: Net state of immunosuppression defined by immunosuppressive drug therapy; presence of leukopenia; metabolic factors, including uremia and hyperglycemia; co-infection with viruses with immunomodulating effects (CMV, EBV).

    2) **Technical complications:** increased risk of infection in presence of seroma, uroma, necrotic tissue, and anastomotic dehiscence.

    3) **Epidemiologic exposure** to pathogens: endogenous, allograft, environment, food and water.

b. **General considerations in transplant patients:**

    1) Reduction of risk of rejection by optimal tissue typing and matching of donor organ to potential recipient.

    2) Careful procurement and preservation of donor organ, optimal preparation of recipient.

    3) Meticulous attention to surgical technique.

    4) Precise management of immunosuppressive regimen to prevent allograft rejection while minimizing depression of host defenses against infection.

    5) Prompt empiric therapy, early diagnosis, and specific therapy of recognized infections.

    6) Immunosuppressive therapy may need to be discontinued in severe infection, thus increasing the risk of graft rejection.

c. **Evaluation of infection following transplantation is dependent on time following organ transplant.**

    1) **First posttransplant month** (phase of maximal leukopenia) infections usually involve common bacterial pathogens:

        a) **Pretransplant infections** present in patients with CRF, hepatic, or cardiac failure. Pneumonias and bacteremias must be effectively treated pretransplant.

        b) If an infection is present in the donor prior to harvest of the organ, pathogens may infect the recipient (allograft infection). **Cultures from the graft and graft perfusates are routinely obtained** and antibiotics given if cultures are positive.

        c) **Perioperative infections** are often due to common bateriologic pathogens and are associated with a high incidence of technical complications including dehiscence, hematomas, seromas, etc.

    d) **Opportunistics infections** usually do not occur during the first posttransplant month. A careful evaluation of the SICU environment is warranted to exclude an unusual source of infection.

    e) **Endogenous infections** may be due to unrecognized latent infections in the recipient. *Mycobacterium tuberculosis* may remain latent until the cellular immune response is depleted.

2) **Posttransplant months 1–6** is the time of greatest risk of life-threatening infections to:

    a) The long duration of immunosuppression leads to significant compromise in host defenses.

    b) Episodes of graft rejection may have occurred prior to this period requiring acute antirejection therapy (commonly high-dose steroids or administration of monoclonal antibodies against lymphocytes) leading to a profound decrease in host defenses.

    c) Immunosuppressive viral infections, including CMV and EBV, commonly occur in this period.

    d) **Opportunistic infections** include *Pneumocystis carinii* pneumonia, herpes zoster infections.

3) **Posttransplant >6 months** (chronic immunosuppression):

    a) **Low-risk patient:** good graft function, low levels of immunosuppression, no acute antirejection therapy. Infectious disease problems similar to those in general community.

    b) **Middle-risk group:** good graft function but chronic viral infection (CMV, EBV). Progressive disease due to interaction of chronic infection and chronic immunosuppressed state.

    c) **High-risk patient:** chronic rejection, poor graft function, high levels of antirejection therapy.

4. **Fever** can be the first clue to rejection or impending sepsis. Transplant patients' immunosuppression necessitates the urgent and thorough evaluation of any fever. A brief check list is provided in Table 17–1.

5. **Specific Infections** in transplant patients–immunocompromised host.

   a. **UTI:**

      1) Most UTIs are prevented by perioperative antibiotic prophylaxis. Mycostatin is administered simultaneously to minimize *Candida* colonization.

      2) Factors contributing to UTI include indwelling bladder catheter, intraoperative renal trauma, and immunosuppressive therapy.

      3) The majority of bacteremias in patients following renal transplant are related to the urinary tract.

      4) Infections are often associated with pyelonephritis, bacteremia, and a high rate of relapse when treated with conventional 10–14-day courses of antibiotics. Majority are eliminated by the use of antibiotic prophylaxis during the high-risk period.

   b. **Pneumonia:**

      1) Most common form of life-threatening infection observed in transplant patients. Pneumonia occurs in 20% of transplant patients at some time in their course. Rapid diagnosis and prompt, effective intervention are key.

         a) Bacterial pneumonias usually develop <24 hours; viral, fungal, or protozoan infections usually require days to weeks before clinical presentation.

         b) The pattern of pulmonary abnormalities seen on CXR may provide an etiologic clue.

            i) Consolidation suggests bacteria, fungus, *Nocardia,* or tuberculosis.

            ii) Interstitial infiltrate suggests *Pneumocystis.*

            iii) Nodular infiltrate suggests fungus, *Nocardia,* tuberculosis.

         c) The patient's possible exposure to mycobacterium or fungi may provide clues to etiology.

TABLE 17-1.
Evaluation of Fever in the Transplant Recipient

Subjective	Physical Examination*	Laboratory Studies*	Plan
Infection ?Pain, sore throat, cough, dysuria, diarrhea, malaise	Skin, HEENT, chest, abdomen, wound, extremities, neurologic, IV sites	WBC with differential; CXR; urinalysis with micro; sputum, blood, and urine C & S, fungal C & S, viral C & S	Appropriate antibiotic and adequate drainage
Rejection Malaise, tender graft	Body weight, intake and urine output, graft site	Creatinine, K^+, BUN, urinalysis, urine Na^+, biopsy,	Treat rejection
Allergy Temporal relation to ATG or antibiotic	Rash	Eosinophilia	D/C causative agent, if possible
Thrombophlebitis Risk factors, history	Chest, extremities, IV sites	VQ scan	Anticoagulant

*Micro = microscopic examination; C & S = culture and sensitivity; D/C = discontinue; VQ = ventilation-perfusion.

2) **Evaluation of fever and pulmonary infiltrate:**
   a) Exclude noninfectious source of infiltrate (PE, pulmonary infarct, hemorrhage).
   b) Routine bacteriologic studies include sputum Gram's stain and culture, and blood cultures. Serum is obtained for viral antibodies.
   c) If bacterial infection is suspected, treatment with broad-spectrum antibiotics should be initiated. If the response is poor after 24 hours' IV antibiotics, invasive diagnostic procedures should be considered.
   d) If diagnosis is not apparent and the patient is stable, consider bronchoscopy, bronchoalveolar lavage, or percutaneous biopsy. One may perform an open lung biopsy if these are nondiagnostic.
   e) If the diagnosis is not apparent and the patient is in distress, one may also consider open lung biopsy for diagnosis.

c. **Bacteremia and candidemia** are major causes of morbidity and mortality in the transplant patient and can be divided into the following categories: IV line sepsis, urosepsis, GI sepsis, CNS sepsis.

   1) **IV line sepsis** is similar to that in other patients in that staphylococci, aerobic gram-negative rods, and *Candida* are often pathogens. However, the consequences of bloodstream invasion are much greater in transplant patients. Candidemia in nonimmunocompromised hosts as a result of a contaminated central venous line may be effectively treated by removal of the contaminated line. In contrast, immunocompromised patients with candidemia may have metastatic seeding and systemic antifungal therapy is required in >50% of patients. IV and arterial lines should be reduced to a minimum using strict antiseptic technique.

   2) *Candida* **pyelonephritis,** which is associated with fungus obstruction at the UPJ or ureterovesical junction, may lead to disseminated candidiasis. This usually occurs in patients with diabetes, poorly functioning bladders, and those who have stents or catheters replaced because of

technical complications. Candiduria in a transplant patient requires both antifungal therapy and abdominal ultrasound to exclude obstructive uropathy.

3) **Diverticulitis and perforation of a gastric or duodenal ulcer** are common causes of sepsis. Clinical manifestations may be minimized and an aggressive evaluation of a transplant patient presenting with distention, ileus, pain, or fever is essential. Cholecystitis and appendicitis are unusual in this population. Bacteremias following liver transplantation may be due to technical complications of the biliary anastomosis leading to spontaneous bacterial peritonitis. *Candida* colonization of the UGI tract in such patients presumably has a significant role in the high rate of invasive candidiasis.

4) **Meningitis and brain abscess** may occur and *Toxoplasma* and *Cryptococcus* are known to cause CNS infections in immunocompromised patients. In renal transplant patients, *Listeria* has emerged as a major cause of bacteremia and CNS infection. *Listeria* is acquired by the ingestion of organisms followed by colonization of the GI tract and bloodstream invasion with a particular tropism for the CNS.

III. ANTIBIOTICS.

A. Principles of Antimicrobial Therapy.

1. Mechanisms of action (Table 17–2):
   a. **Bacteriostatic:** prevention of growth and multiplication of bacteria (bacteria not killed). Host defenses clear infection.
   b. **Bactericidal:** bacterial killing; mandatory in immunocompromised host.
2. Use of multiple antibiotics:
   a. Possible or proven multiple organisms (e.g., gram-negative septicemia).
   b. Prevention of emergence of resistant strains (e.g., pseudomonads, mycobacteria).

TABLE 17–2.
Mechanisms of Action of Antibiotics

Penicillins, cephalosporins, bacitracin, vancomycin, novobiocin	Inhibition of cell wall synthesis (bactericidal)
Aminoglycosides, tetracyclines, chloramphenicol, erythromycin, lincomycin, clindamycin	Inhibition of protein synthesis (bactericidal, bacteriostatic)
Sulfonamides, trimethoprim, nalidixic acid rifampicin, para-aminosalicylic acid	Inhibition of nucleic acid synthesis (bacteriostatic)
Polymyxins, imidazoles, amphotericin B	Inhibition of cell membrane function (bactericidal)

3. Antimicrobial synergy (see pp 687–704):
   a. Potentiation at a biochemical level.
   b. Assistance to cellular penetration (e.g., action of penicillins at cell wall level interferes with the ability of *Streptococcus faecalis* to resist penetration by aminoglycosides).
   c. Protection (e.g., clavulanic acid [broad-spectrum enzyme inhibitor] protects amoxicillin against degradation by β-lactamases).
4. **Antibiotic incompatibilities** (see pp 687–704): Bacteriostatic agents (tetracyclines) interfere with mechanism of action of β-lactam antibiotics on cell wall synthesis.
5. **Monitoring of serum levels** (see pp 687–704):
   a. Guide to drug dosage (ensure therapeutic levels, minimize complications).
   b. Mandatory if renal function impaired.
   c. Steady-state levels achieved after fifth dose.
   d. Peak levels measured 1 hour after IV or IM administration.
   e. Trough levels measured immediately prior to next dose.
   f. Important for agents with known toxicity, dose-related complications, narrow therapeutic range:
      1) Aminoglycosides.
      2) Vancomycin.
      3) Ketoconazole.
      4) Chloramphenicol.

6. **Side effects, complications** (see pp 687–704).
   a. Incidence is 5%, most of minor significance.
   b. **General:**
      1) Local irritation, phlebitis (with IV infusion).
      2) GI disturbances (oral administration).
      3) High sodium content of many antibiotics may precipitate CHF, especially if renal function is impaired.
      4) Hepatic or renal dysfunction may lead to accumulation of antibiotics or their metabolites with toxic side effects.
      5) Antibiotics may induce hepatic enzyme activity, increasing metabolism of concurrently administered drugs.
   c. **Hypersensitivity reactions:**
      1) Most frequently seen with β-lactam agents.
      2) Cross-sensitivity with cephalosporins of 6%–9%.
      3) Immediate: nausea, vomiting, urticaria, anaphylaxis.
      4) Delayed: skin rashes (generalized maculopapular).
   d. **Supression of normal gut flora** (superinfection):
      1) Candidiasis (nystatin PO, miconazole IV).
      2) *S. aureus* enterocolitis (cloxacillin PO).
      3) *C. difficile* (pseudomembranous) enterocolitis (vancomycin PO).
   e. Neurotoxicity: aminoglycosides.
   f. Encephalitic reactions: high-dose penicillins, cephalosporins, nalidixic acid.
   g. Peripheral neuropathy: isoniazid, chloramphenicol, metronidazole, nitrofurantoin.
   h. Neuromuscular blockade: aminoglycosides.
   i. Marrow toxicity:
      1) Sulfonamides, co-trimoxazole.
      2) Chloramphenicol: aplastic anemia (mortality 50%).
      3) Penicillins: hemolytic anemia.
      4) Ampicillin, methicillin, carbenicillin: granulocytopenia.

B. **Specific Agents.**
  1. **Aminoglycosides.**
    a. **Activity:**
      1) Bactericidal against most aerobic and facultative anaerobic gram-negative bacilli.
      2) Moderate activity against gram-positive cocci.
      3) No anaerobic activity.
    b. **Adverse reactions:**
      1) Narrow therapeutic margin, monitoring of serum levels required.
      2) Nephrotoxicity is rare on initial administration, usually dose-dependent reversible ATN. Prolonged dosage intervals permit use in established renal failure.
      3) Ototoxicty: vestibular or auditory dysfunction due to seventh cranial nerve injury.
      4) Neuromuscular blockade: anticholinesterase effect.
    c. **Drug interactions:**
      1) Cephalosporins: synergistic nephrotoxicity.
      2) Diuretics may potentiate oto- and nephrotoxicity due to volume contraction.
      3) Penicillin: inactivation of aminoglycosides (clinical significance unknown).
    d. **Specific agents:**
      1) **Gentamicin, tobramycin:** Similar spectrum, gentamicin slightly more nephrotoxic.
      2) **Amikacin:** active against many strains resistant to gentamicin or tobramycin.
      3) **Netilmicin:** less nephrotoxic and ototoxic but may cause hepatic toxicity.
      4) **Kanamycin:** oral preparation used for bowel sterilization.
    e. **Pharmacokinetics** (Table 17–3).
      1) Risk factors in aminoglycoside toxicity (Table 17–4).
        a) Age.
        b) Sustained high trough, elevated peak concentration.
        c) Cumulative dose, duration of treatment.
        d) Concurrent toxic drugs.

TABLE 17–3.
Pharmacologic Features of Aminoglycosides

	Routes	Dose (mg/kg)		Therapeutic Serum Levels (µg/mL)	Half-Life (hr)	
					Normal	Anephric
Gentamicin	IM, IV	1.0–1.7	q. 8 h.	4–10	1.2–5.0	21–70
Amikacin	IM, IV	5	q. 8 h.	8–16	0.8–2.8	28–87
		7.5	q. 12 h.			
Tobramycin	IM, IV	1.0–1.7	q. 8 h.	4–8	1.0–2.0	27–70
Netilmicin	IM, IV	1.3–2.2	q. 8 h.	0.5–10	2.0–2.5	32–52
		1.5–3.25	q. 12 h.			
Kanamycin	Oral, IM, IV	7.5	q. 12 h.	8–16	2.0–2.5	40–96

TABLE 17-4.

Risk Factors in Aminoglycoside Toxicity

Age
Sustained high trough, elevated peak concentration
Cumulative dose, duration of treatment
Prior aminoglycoside exposure
Concurrent toxic drugs
Dehydration
Dialysis

       e) Dehydration.

       f) Dialysis.

2. **Penicillins.**

  a. **Bactericidal against majority of:**

    1) Gram-positive cocci.

    2) Gram-negative cocci.

    3) Gram-positive bacilli.

  b. **Adverse reactions:**

    1) Hypersensitivity: fever, rash, serum sickness, anaphylaxis.

    2) Neurotoxicity: convulsions, encephalitis, encephalopathy.

    3) Nephrotoxicity: interstitial nephritis.

    4) Hemotologic: Coombs'-positive hemolytic anemia.

    5) Hypercalcemia: following high dosage with renal insufficiency.

  c. **Drug interactions:**

    1) Aminoglycosides inactivated by penicillins.

    2) Probenicid, aspirin, indomethacin may block renal tubular secretion of penicillins leading to high serum levels.

  d. **Specific agents:**

    1) **Penicillin G:** most active against streptococci.

    2) **Ampicillin:** enterococcus, *H. influenzae.*

    3) **Methicillin:** penicillinase-resistant staphylococci develop; may be associated with interstitial nephritis.

    4) **Nafcillin:** penicillinase-resistant; less nephrotoxic than methicillin; may be associated with neutropenia, phlebitis.

    5) **Oxacillin:** penicillinase-resistant; may be associated with hepatotoxicity.

    6) **Expanded penicillins:**

        a) **Azlocillin, mezlocillin, piperacillin** (uriedopenicillins): broad spectrum against gram-negative organisms with activity against *E. coli, Proteus, Enterobacter,* and many strains of *Pseudomonas.* Mezlocillin and piperacillin are also active against some strains of *Klebsiella* and *Serratia.* Adverse reactions similar to carbenicillin.

        b) **Carbenicillin, ticarcillin** (carboxypenicillins): highly active against gram-negative organisms, including pseudomonads; may be associated with hepatitis, hypokalemia, and decreased platelet aggregation.

  e. **Pharmacokinetics are given in Table 17–5.**

3. Cephalosporins.

  a. **Activity** (see specific agent below and Table 17–6).

  b. **Adverse reactions:**

    1) Large safety margin and high therapeutic margin.

    2) Hypersensitivity: Cross-sensitivity to penicillin-allergic patients is 6%–9%. Avoid use in patients with history of anaphylaxis or penicillin hypersensitivity.

    3) Nephrotoxicity: interstitial nephritis.

    4) Neurotoxicity: convulsions, confusion.

    5) Hematologic: Coombs'-positive anemia, thrombophlebitis, inhibition of platelet aggregation, suppression of vitamin K–dependent clotting factors.

  c. **Specific agents** (generations based on gram-negative sensitivity; Table 17–7):

    1) **First generation:** effective against gram-positive and some gram-negative bacteria.

    2) **Second generation:** increased gram-negative but less gram-positive activity.

TABLE 17–5.
Pharmacologic Features of Penicillins

	Routes	Peak Level (µg/mL)	Na (mEq/g)	Dose (Normal creatinine)
Penicillin V	Oral	—	2.6	125–500 mg q. 6 h.
Penicillin G Na	Oral, IM, IV	60	2/million units	100,000–200,000 units/kg/day
Penicillin G K	Oral, IM, IV	60	0.3/million units	100,000–200,000 units/kg/day
Ampicillin	Oral, IM, IV	20	3	0.25–1.0 g q. 6 h. (15–200)
Penicillinase-resistant				
Methicillin	IM, IV	30–45	3	1–3 g q. 4–6 h.
Nafcillin	Oral, IM, IV	90	2.9	0.5–1.0 g q. 4 h. (50–150)
Oxacillin	Oral, IM, IV	95	2.8	0.5–1.0 g q. 4–6 h.
Extended spectrum				
Carbenicillin	Oral, IM, IV	50	4.7–5.0	30–40 g q.d. (400–500)
Ticarcillin	IM, IV	45	5.2	3 g q. 3–6 h (200–300)
Mezlocillin	IM, IV	16–42	1.85	3–4 g q. 4–6 h (100–300)
Piperacillin	IM, IV	16	1.85	3–4 g q. 4–6 h (100–300)
Azlocillin	IV	25–45	2.17	3–4 g q. 4–6 h (100–300)
Amdinopenicillin				
Amdinocillin	IM, IV	5–10	2.17	0.5–1.0 g q. 4–6 h. (40–60)

TABLE 17–6.
Pharmacologic Features of Cephalsporins

	Routes	Dosage (g)		Half-Life (hr)	Sodium (mEq/g)	Protein Binding (%)
First generation						
Cefazolin (Ancef, Kefzol)	IM, IV	0.25–2.0	q. 4–8 h.	1.4	2.0–2.1	75
Cephalexin (Keflex)	Oral	0.25–0.5	q. 6–8 h.	0.8	—	—
Cephalothin (Keflin)	IM, IV	0.5–2.0	q. 4–6 h.	0.6	2.8	65
Cephapirin (Cefadyl)	IM, IV	0.5–2.0	q. 4–6 h.	1.3	2.4	8–17
Second generation						
Cefaclor (Ceclor)	Oral	0.25–0.5	q. 8 h.	—	—	—
Cefamandole (Mandol)	IM, IV	0.5–2.0	q. 4–6 h.	0.5	3.3	75
Ceforanide (Precef)	IM, IV	0.5–1.0	q. 12 h.	2.9	0	80
Cefoxitin (Mefoxin)	IM, IV	1–2	q. 4–8 h.	0.8	2.3	70
Cefuroxime (Zinacef)	IM, IV	0.75–1.5	q. 8 h.	1.3	2.4	50
Third generation						
Cefoperazone (Cefobid)	IM, IV	2–4	q. 4–12 h.	2.0	1.5	85
Cefotaxime (Claforan)	IM, IV	1–2	q. 4–6 h.	1.0	2.2	30
Cefotetan	IM, IV	1–3	q. 12 h.	3.0	3.5	88
Ceftazidime (Fortraz)	IM, IV	0.5–2.0	q. 8–12 h.	1.7	2.3	17
Ceftizoxime (Cefizox)	IM, IV	1–2	q. 8 h.	1.7	2.6	30
Ceftriaxone (Rocephin)	IM, IV	1–2	q. 12–24 h.	8.0	3.6	90
Moxalactam (Moxam)	IM, IV	1–2	q. 4–8 h.	1.7	3.8	45

3) **Third generation:** main effect is on gram-negative bacteria.

4) Pharmacokinetics (see Table 17–7).

4. **Antianaerobic agents:**

a. **Metronidazole:**

1) **Activity:** bactericidal against *Trichomonas, Giardia* sp., *E. histolytica,* and anaerobic bacteria including *Bacteroides* sp.

2) **Adverse reactions:**

a) Nausea, vomiting, metallic taste.

b) Headache, ataxia, vertigo, neuropathy, seizures.

3) **Dose:** 30 mg/kg / 24hr t.i.d.–q.i.d. (500 mg IV q. 6 h.).

b. **Clindamycin:**

1) **Activity:** gram-positive and gram-negative anaerobes, including *Bacteroides*.

2) **Adverse reactions:**

a) Diarrhea occurs in 20%–30%.

b) Hepatotoxic.

3) **Dose:** 30–40 mg/kg /24hr t.i.d.–q.i.d. (600–900 mg IV q. 6–8 h.).

c. **Chloramphenicol:**

1) **Activity:** gram-negative bacteria, especially when resistant to conventional agents (rickettsial disease, psitticosis, lymphogranuloma venereum).

2) **Adverse reactions:** Bone marrow supression (aplastic anemia).

3) **Dose:** 0.25–1.0 g PO q.6.h. (500 mg); 0.5–1.0 g IV q. 6 h.

4) **Monitored serum levels:**

a) Peak: 20 μg/mL.

b) Trough: 2 μg/mL.

5. **Other agents.**

a. **Vancomycin:**

1) **Activity:** bactericidal against gram-positive bacteria, methicillin-resistant *staphylococci;* treatment of pseudomembranous colitis.

2) **Adverse reactions:**

a) Ototoxicity: associated with high serum levels.

TABLE 17-7.

Organisms Susceptible to Cephalosporins (%)*

Organism	1st-Generation Cephalosporin			
	Cz	Cx	Cl	Cr
Acinetobacter anitratus	<20	20–50	<20	<20
Acinetobacter calicoaceticus	<20	20–50	20–50	<20
Citrobacter diversus	50–80	80–95	80–95	0
Citrobacter freundii	20–50	<20	20–50	0
Enterobacter aerogenes	<20	<20	<20	<20
Enterobacter agglomerans	50–80	50–80	50–80	<20
Enterobacter cloacae	<20	<20	<20	<20
Escherichia coli	80–95	80–95	80–95	80–95
Klebsiella oxytoca	80–95	95+	80–95	50–80
Klebsiella pneumoniae	80–95	95+	80–95	50–80
Bacteroides fragilis	0	0	<20	0
Bacteroides, other	0	0	0	0
Clostridium difficile	<20	<20	<20	<20
Clostridium perfringens	0	0	0	0
Clostridium, other	0	0	0	0
Fusobacterium	0	0	0	0
Peptococcus	0	0	0	0
Peptostreptococcus	0	0	0	0
Propionibacterium	0	0	0	0

Veillonella	0	0	0
Morganella morganii	<20	<20	<20
Proteus mirabilis	95+	80–95	80–95
Proteus vulgaris	<20	20–50	<20
Providencia	50–80	20–50	0
Pseudomonas aeruginosa	<20	<20	<20
Pseudomonas fluorescens	<20	<20	<20
Pseudomonas maltophilia	<20	<20	<20
Salmonella	50–80	50–80	50–80
Serratia marcescens	<20	<20	<20
Shigella	20–50	80–95	80–95
Haemophilus influenzae	80–95	50–80	20–50
Neisseria gonorrhoeae	95+	95+	80–95
Neisseria meningitidis	95+	95+	95+
Listeria monocytogenes	<20	<20	<20
Streptococcus agalactiae	95+	95+	95+
Streptococcus faecalis	<20	<20	<20
Streptococcus pneumoniae	95+	95+	95+
Streptococcus pyogenes	95+	95+	95+
Streptococcus viridans	80–95	80–95	80–95
Staphylococcus aureus	95+	95+	95+
Staphylococcus epidermidis	95+	<20	95+

(Continued.)

TABLE 17-7 (cont.).

Organism	2nd-Generation Cephalosporin				
	Cc	Cm	Cef	Co	Cu
Acinetobacter anitratus	<20	<20	<20	<20	<20
Acinetobacter calcoaceticus	50–80	20–50	<20	20–50	<20
Citrobacter diversus	95+	80–95	95+	80–95	80–95
Citrobacter freundii	50–80	50–80	50–80	<20	80–95
Enterobacter aerogenes	50–80	50–80	80–95	<20	50–80
Enterobacter agglomerans	80–95	50–80	20–50	50–80	50–80
Enterobacter cloacae	20–50	50–80	20–50	<20	50–80
Escherichia coli	95+	95+	80–95	95+	95+
Klebsiella oxytoca	95+	50–80	0	95+	95+
Klebsiella pneumoniae	95+	95+	95+	95+	95+
Bacteroides fragilis	<20	20–50	0	80–95	20–50
Bacteroides, other	95+	95+	0	80–95	50–80
Clostridium difficile	<20	<20	0	<20	<20
Clostridium perfringens	0	95+	0	95+	95+
Clostridium, other	0	95+	0	95+	80–95
Fusobacterium	0	95+	0	95+	50–80
Peptococcus	95+	95+	0	95+	80–95
Peptostreptococcus	95+	95+	0	95+	80–95
Propionibacterium	95+	95+	0	95+	80–95

Veillonella	0	95+	0	80-95
Morganella morganii	20-50	80-95	<20	80-95
Proteus mirabilis	95+	95+	95+	95+
Proteus vulgaris	<20	50-80	20-50	80-95
Providencia	20-50	95+	50-80	95+
Pseudomonas aeruginosa	<20	<20	<20	<20
Pseudomonas fluorescens	<20	<20	<20	<20
Pseudomonas maltophilia	<20	<20	<20	<20
Salmonella	50-80	80-95	0	95+
Serratia marcescens	<20	20-50	<20	<20
Shigella	80-95	95+	0	80-95
Haemophilus influenzae	95+	95+	80-95	95+
Neisseria gonorrhoeae	95+	95+	95+	95+
Neisseria meningitidis	95+	95+	95+	95+
Listeria monocytogenes	<20	20-50	<20	<20
Streptococcus agalactiae	95+	95+	0	95+
Streptococcus faecalis	<20	<20	<20	<20
Streptococcus pneumoniae	95+	95+	80-95	95+
Streptococcus pyogenes	95+	95+	95+	95+
Streptococcus viridans	95+	95+	0	95+
Staphylococcus aureus	95+	95+	80-95	95+
Staphylococcus epidermidis	95+	80-95	0	95+

(Continued.)

TABLE 17-7 (cont.).

Organism	Ct	Ca	Ce	Cq	Ci	Ct	Mo
Acinetobacter anitratus	<20	50-80	<20	80-95	50-80	<20	20-50
Acinetobacter calicoaceticus	<20	80-95	20-50	80-95	50-80	20-50	20-50
Citrobacter diversus	95+	95+	95+	95+	95+	95+	95+
Citrobacter freundii	80-95	80-95	50-80	50-80	80-95	50-80	95+
Enterobacter aerogenes	95+	95+	20-50	50-80	80-95	50-80	95+
Enterobacter agglomerans	95+	95+	80-95	80-95	95+	80-95	95+
Enterobacter cloacae	80-95	95+	20-50	50-80	80-95	50-80	95+
Escherichia coli	95+	95+	95+	95+	95+	95+	95+
Klebsiella oxytoca	80-95	95+	95+	95+	95+	95+	95+
Klebsiella pneumoniae	95+	95+	95+	95+	95+	95+	95+
Bacteroides fragilis	50-80	20-50	50-80	<20	20-50	<20	80-95
Bacteroides, other	95+	50-80	50-80	50-80	50-80	20-50	80-95
Clostridium difficile	<20	<20	<20	<20	<20	<20	<20
Clostridium perfringens	95+	95+	95+	20-50	95+	95+	80-95
Clostridium, other	95+	95+	95+	<20	<20	95+	50-80
Fusobacterium	95+	95+	95+	80-95	95+	95+	95+
Peptococcus	95+	95+	95+	95+	80-95	95+	95+
Peptostreptococcus	95+	95+	95+	95+	95+	95+	20-50
Propionibacterium	95+	95+	95+	95+	95+	95+	95+

Organism							
Veillcnella	95+	95+	95+	95+	95+	95+	95+	95+
Morganella morganii	95+	95+	95+	95+	80–95	80–95	95+	95+
Proteus mirabilis	95+	95+	95+	95+	95+	95+	95+	95+
Proteus vulgaris	95+	95+	95+	95+	95+	95+	95+	95+
Providencia	80–95	95+	95+	95+	95+	95+	95+	95+
Pseudomonas aeruginosa	80–95	50–80	<20	80–95	<20	<20	<20	50–80
Pseudomonas fluorescens	20–50	<20	<20	80–95	<20	<20	<20	<20
Pseudomonas maltophilia	<20	<20	<20	20–50	95+	95+	95+	80–95
Salmonella	95+	95+	95+	95+	95+	95+	95+	95+
Serratia marcescens	80–95	80–95	80–95	95+	95+	95+	80–95	95+
Shigella	95+	95+	95+	95+	95+	95+	95+	95+
Haemophilus influenzae	95+	95+	95+	95+	95+	95+	95+	95+
Neisseria gonorrhoeae	95+	95+	95+	95+	95+	95+	95+	95+
Neisseria meningitidis	95+	95+	95+	95+	95+	95+	95+	95+
Listeria monocytogenes	20–50	<20	<20	<20	<20	<20	20	50–80
Streptococcus agalactiae	95+	95+	95+	95+	95+	95+	95+	95+
Streptococcus faecalis	<20	<20	<20	<20	<20	<20	<20	<20
Streptococcus pneumoniae	95+	95+	95+	95+	95+	95+	95+	95+
Streptococcus pyogenes	95+	95+	95+	95+	95+	95+	95+	95+
Streptococcus viridans	95+	50–80	50–80	95+	95+	95+	95+	95+
Staphylococcus aureus	80–95	80–95	80–95	80–95	80–95	80–95	80–95	80–95
Staphylococcus epidermidis	80–95	80–95	20–50	<20	50–80	50–80	50–80	50–80

*Cz = cefazolin; Cx = cephalexin; Cl = cephalothin; Cr = cephradine; Cc = cefaclor; Cm = cefamandole; Cef = ceforanide; Co = cefonicid; Cu = cefuroxime; Cf = cefoperazone; Ca = cefotaxime; Ce = cefotetan; Cq = ceftizoxime; Ci = ceftazidime; Cf = ceftriaxone; Mo = moxalactam; 0 = not done.

  b) Nephrotoxicity: infrequent.
  c) Hypotension: associated with rapid infusion.
  d) Hypersensitivity.
  3) **Dose:** 20–30 mg/kg/24 hr b.i.d.–t.i.d. (1 g IV q. 12 h.).
  4) **Monitored serum levels:**
    a) Peak: 35 µg/mL.
    b) Trough: 5 µg/mL.

b. **Erythromycin:**
  1) **Activity:** bacteriostatic (bactericidal in high doses) against gram-positive bacteria; good substitute for penicillin in allergic patient.
  2) **Adverse reactions:**
    a) Nausea, vomiting, epigastric discomfort, diarrhea.
    b) Cholestatic jaundice (>10-day course, repeated courses).
    c) Thrombophlebitis.
  3) **Dose:** 0.25–1.0 g PO q. 6 h. or IV q. 6 h. in 30–60-minute saline infusion.

c. **Clavulanic acid:**
  1) β-Lactamase inhibitor.
  2) Extends spectrum of amoxicillin or ticarcillin by protecting against β-lactamase degradation.
  3) **Dose:**
    a) Amoxicillin 1 g IV q. 6–8 h.
    b) Ticarcillin 3 g IV q. 4–6 h.

d. **Imipenem-cilastatin:**
  1) Broad spectrum of activity against pseudomonads, *Serratia, Enterobacter,* enterococcus, anaerobes.
  2) May cause seizures, nausea, vomiting.
  3) **Dose:** 0.5–1.0 g IV q. 6–8 h.

e. **Quinolones:**
  1) Active against most aerobic gram-positive and gram-negative bacteria, mycobacteria, mycoplasmas, chlamydia.
  2) Useful for UTI, enteric infection.
  3) May cause nausea, vomiting, dizziness, seizures.
  4) **Dose:**
    a) Norfloxacin 400 mg PO q. 12 h.
    b) Ciprofloxacin 200–300 mg IV q. 12 h.; 750 mg PO q. 8–12 h.

f. **Trimethoprim-sulfamethoxazole:**
1) Active against *Pneumocystis, Shigella,* gram-negative bacilli, except pseudomonads.
2) May cause nausea, vomiting, blood dyscrasias (agranulocytosis, thrombocytopenia, hemolytic anemia).
3) **Dose:** IV trimethoprin 80 mg–sulfamethoxazole 400 mg/5 mL; PO trimethoprin 40 mg–sulfamethoxazole 200 mg/5 mL; 10–50 mg/kg/24 hr b.i.d.–t.i.d.

g. **Aztreonam:**
1) Bactericidal against gram-negative aerobes, including pseudomonads.
2) May cause nausea, vomiting, phlebitis.
3) **Dose:** 1–2 g IV q. 6–8 h.

h. **Tetracyclines:**
1) Bacteriostatic against a variety of gram-positive and gram-negative bacteria, rickettsia, mycoplasmas, chlamydia.
2) High incidence of bacterial resistance limits use.
3) May cause hepatotoxicity, GI upset, thrombophlebitis.
4) **Dose:** 250–500 mg PO q. 6 h.; 500 mg IV q. 12 h. (5-mg/mL infusion: 2 mL/hr).

6. **Antifungal agents.**
a. **Amphotericin B:**
1) Active against most fungi, including *Histoplasma, Coccidioides, Candida, Aspergillus, Blastomyces, Cryptococcus, Sporotrichum,* Phycomycetes.
2) **IV administration only.** Most potential toxicity of all anti-infective agents; infusion-related reaction occurs in 20% of patients.
3) **Dose:**
   a) Dilution in D5 to concentration of 10 mg/dL stable for 24 hours.
   b) Severe febrile reactions require **1-mg** test dose given over 30 minutes with observation for 1 hour. Monitor for fever, hypotension, tachycardia.

       c) Slow IV infusion over 6 hours with monitoring.

          i) First day: 0.25 mg/kg IV over 6 hours.

          ii) Increase dose by 0.1 mg/kg/day to dose of 0.5–0.7 mg/kg/day.

          iii) Never >1.5 mg/kg/day.

  b. **Total dose of amphotericin B** is usually 6 mg/kg and should not usually exceed 8 mg/kg (total dose of 3–5 g prescribed for more severe or persistent infections).

  c. **Monitor** BP, pulse, respiratory rate, and temperature q. 30 min during treatment.

  d. **Discontinue** treatment or reduce dose if temperature >38.9° C; systolic BP <100 mm Hg, or fall in systolic BP of >30 mm Hg pretreatment; pulse >130.

  e. **Febrile or hypotensive reaction** may be ameliorated by premedicating with 125 mg hydrocortisone IV 30 minutes before treatment. Diphenhydramine and acetaminophen or meperidine may help.

    1) **Adverse reactions:**

      a) **Nephrotoxicity** is dose-related. Most patients experience 30% decrease in GFR with standard treatment. Volume loading reduces renal toxicity.

      b) **Chills,** fever, headache, anorexia, weight loss, nausea, vomiting (50%–80%).

      c) **Thrombophlebitis,** anemia, hypersensitivity.

      d) **Arachnoiditis,** auditory neurotoxicity.

    2) **Amphotericin B bladder irrigation:**

      a) Amphotericin B 50 mg in 1 L NS infused through Foley catheter over 8 hours as continuous bladder irrigation.

      b) Irrigation is usually continued for 7–10 days.

      c) Following cessation of bladder irrigation, urine is recultured for fungal culture.

 f. **Flucytosine:**

    1) Active against *Candida, Cryptococcus,* chromomycoses.

    2) May cause diarrhea, colitis, allergic rash, neutropenia, thrombocytopenia, hepatotoxicity.

    3) High incidence of resistance when used as single agent; used in combination with amphotericin B to reduce dose of latter.

       4) **Dose:**
         a) Amphotericin B 0.3 mg/kg/day PO.
         b) Flucytosine 37.5 mg/kg q. 6 h. PO.

g. **Fluconazole:**
   1) Indications: oral, pharyngeal, and esophageal candidiasis, cryptococcosis, and coccidioid meningitis.
   2) Adverse reactions: hepatic toxicity; monitoring of liver function tests recommended.
   3) **Dose:**
     a) **Oral:** excellent absorption following oral administration. Recommended dose for oral pharyngeal candidiasis is 200 mg on day 1 followed by 100 mg PO q. 6 h. Doses of up to 400 mg/day may be used for severe esophageal candidiasis or cryptococcal meningitis.
     b) **Parenteral administration** (doses per PO administration) is by IV infusion. Maximum rate: 200 mg/hr.

h. **Nystatin:**
   1) For use in oral candidiasis.
   2) **Dose:** nystatin liquid 5 mL PO q. 6 h. (swish and swallow); nystatin tablets one or two PO q. 6 h. (dissolve in mouth).

i. **Griseofulvin:**
   1) Active against dermatophytic fungi (tinea).
   2) May cause GI upset, hypersensitivity, headache, confusion, syncope, leukopenia, proteinuria.
   3) **Dose:** 0.5 – 1.0 g/day PO, single or divided doses.

j. **Miconazole:**
   1) Second-line antifungal agent, used when there is intolerance or resistance to amphotericin B. Active against coccidioidomycoses, candidiasis, paracoccidioidomycoses, cryptococcal meningitis.
   2) May cause pruritus, anemia, nausea, hyponatremia, phlebitis.
   3) **Dose:** 0.4 – 1.2 mg q. 8 h. PO or IV.

k. **Ketoconazole:**
   1) Active against *Candida, Coccidioides, Histoplasma, Blastomyces, Paracoccidioides,* dermatophytes.

        2) May cause GI upset, hepatotoxicity, hepatic necrosis, pruritus, dizziness, somnolence.

        3) **Dose:** 400 mg/day PO.

  7. **Antiviral agents.**

    a. **Acyclovir:**

      1) Active against herpesviruses HSV-1, HSV-2, VZV, EBV. Inactive against human CMV.

      2) **Dose:**

        a) IV: 5–10 mg/kg q. 8 h.

        b) PO: 50–200 mg PO q. 4–8 h. (suppression, therapy).

        c) Topical: 5% ointment, four to six applications per day.

    b. **Ganciclovir:**

      1) Markedly increased activity against CMV.

      2) **Dose:** 5 mg/kg q. 12 h. IV × 14–21 days, then 5 mg/kg/day maintenance.

    c. **Vidarabine:**

      1) Active against HSV-I, HSV-2, VZV, EBV.

      2) **Dose:** 10–30 mg/kg/day IV, 12-hour infusion.

    d. **Azidothymidine** (AZT, zidovudine).

      1) Inhibition of HIV-1 replication.

      2) Dose: 200 mg PO q. 4 h.; reduce to 200 mg PO q. 8 h. if toxic.

    e. **Amantadine, rimantadine:**

      a) Influenza A prophylaxis and treatment.

      b) **Dose:** 200 mg/day, one or two divided doses.

    f. **Topical antivirals:**

      a) Idoxuridine (IUDR): herpesviruses, poxviruses.

      b) Trifluorothymidine (TFT): herpesviruses.

      c) Vidaribine.

      d) Acyclovir.

SELECTED REFERENCES

FEVER

Balkwill FR, Burke F: The cytokine network. *Immunol Today* 1989; 10:299.

Brengelmann GL: Body temperature regulation, in Patton (ed): *Textbook of Physiology.* Vol 2: *Circulation, Respiration, Body Fluids, Metabolism and Endocrinology,* ed 21, Philadelphia, WB Saunders Co, 1989.

Gronert GA, Schulman SR, Mott J: Malignant hyperthermia, in Miller RD (ed): *Anesthesia,* ed 3. New York, Churchill Livingston Inc, 1990.

LeGall JR, Fagniez PL, Meakins J, et al: Post-laparotomy fever: A prospective study of 100 patients. *Br J Surg* 1982; 69:452.

Swartz MN, Simon HB: Pathophysiology of fever and fever of undetermined origin, in *Medicine,* vol 2. New York, Scientific American Inc, 1989.

INFECTIONS

Feld R: The compromised host. *Eur J Cancer Clin Oncol.* 1989; 25 (suppl 2):S1.

Rubin RH, Young LS (eds): *Clinical Approach to Infection in the Compromised Host,* ed 2. New York, Plenum Medical Book Co, 1988.

Sanford JP: *Guide to Antimicrobial Therapy 1990,* ed 19. West Bethesda, Md, Antimicrobial Therapy Inc., 1990.

Schwartz SI: *Principles of Surgery.* New York, McGraw-Hill Book Co, 1984.

Way LW: *Current Surgical Diagnosis and Treatment.* East Norwalk, Conn, Appleton & Lange, 1988.

Wilmore DW, et al: Care of the surgical patient, in *Medicine.* New York, Scientific American, Inc, 1989.

ANTIBIOTICS

Bergamini TM, Polk HC Jr: Pharmacodynamics of antibiotic penetration of tissue and surgical prophylaxis. *Surg Gynecol Obstet* 1989; 168:283.

Gorbach SL, et al: *Manual of Surgical Infections.* Boston, Little, Brown & Co, 1984.

Keighley MRB, Giles GR: The investigation and treatment of surgical infections, in Cuschieri A, Giles GR, Moossa AR (eds): *Essential Surgical Practice,* ed 2. Bristol, England, John Wright, 1988.

Wilson JD, et al (eds): *Harrison's Principles of Internal Medicine,* ed 12. New York, McGraw-Hill Inc., 1991.

PEDIATRIC SURGERY   *18*

I. MANAGEMENT OF THE PEDIATRIC SURGICAL PATIENT.

A. Pediatric Vital Signs and Monitoring.

As in the adult patient, the pediatric SICU patient should have various physiologic parameters such as vital signs, urinary output, cardiac rhythm, and O_2 saturation continuously monitored and recorded on the flow sheet.

1. **Vital signs** (Table 18–1):
   a. The Doppler ultrasound technique of monitoring cuff BP is the most accurate noninvasive method.
   b. In very sick infants and children, arterial BP should be monitored directly. This is most commonly performed with a radial artery catheter placed either percutaneously or via cutdown. Other options include the temporal artery or dorsalis pedis artery.
   c. In neonates, an umbilical artery catheter may be placed for BP monitoring.

2. **Oxygenation and ventilation:**
   a. Patients being artifically ventilated should have frequent ABG determinations.
   b. Noninvasive methods of measuring respiratory function include pulse-oximetry to monitor O_2 saturation, or transcutaneous electrode monitoring of peripheral O_2 and CO_2 concentrations.
   c. In the stable ventilator patient, it may be difficult to obtain ABG determinations, and noninvasive monitoring methods may be adequate. In addition, such methods may be adequate in weaning a patient whose ventilatory status is improving.
   d. The transcutaneous CO_2 monitor must be moved at least q. 4 h. in order to prevent skin burns.

TABLE 18–1.

Normal Vital Signs of Children

Age (yr)	Pulse (bpm)	Blood Pressure (mm Hg)	Respirations (min)
0–1	120	80/40	40
1–5	100	100/60	30
5–10	80	120/80	20

3. **Urinary output:**
   a. Urinary output is a useful parameter in monitoring fluid management and can be monitored continuously either with an indwelling Foley catheter or with a bag placed over the urethral opening in smaller infants.
   b. An appropriate urinary output is 1–2 mL/kg/hr.
4. **Body weight:**
   a. Frequent measurement of body weight is especially useful in managing neonates and young infants.
   b. Acute changes reflect changes in total body water, and serial measurements are therefore useful guides in fluid replacement.
   c. It should be noted that newborns undergo significant diuresis on the first day of life which results in a normal loss of total body water and weight.
5. **Temperature:**
   a. Skin probes should be used to continuously monitor the body temperature of neonates and infants. These patients are vulnerable to hypothermia because of their relatively large body surface area and lack of subcutaneous tissue.
   b. Neonates are unable to shiver and therefore respond to cold stress by mobilizing brown fat deposits. Continued exposure to cold results in peripheral vasoconstriction and subsequent decreased tissue perfusion.
   c. Body temperature should be maintained by the use of overhead radiant heaters or warming lamps.
B. **Fluid and Electrolytes.**
   1. **Normal fluid requirements:**
      a. The normal daily requirements for children are relatively larger than those of adults, because of increased insensible losses, and a relative inability of the infant kidney to maximally concentrate urine.

   b. The daily fluid requirements for infants and children are
      listed in Table 18–2. In addition, the daily fluid re-
      quirements (mL/kg) may be estimated by:

   Daily fluid required mL/kg = [3 × (age in years)]

2. **Electrolyte requirements:**
   a. In general, the pediatric patient's daily electrolyte re-
      quirements will be met if the proper amount of IV fluid
      is given as 5% or 10% dextrose and 0.25% saline with
      20 mEq/dL KCL/deciliter as a maintenance solution.
   b. Potassium and sodium requirements are in the range of
      2–3 mEq/kg/day.
   c. The electrolyte concentration of measured drained fluids
      such as NG drainage is the same as that in the adult.

3. **Postoperative fluid management:**
   a. For patients who are NPO following an operation, in-
      sensible fluid losses and urinary requirements are
      matched by administration of IV fluids in accordance
      with the requirements listed in Table 18–2.
   b. Additional fluid as a balanced salt solution (i.e. lactated
      Ringer's) should be given to replace estimated third-
      space losses. As an initial approximation, the total fluid
      administered should be increased by 25% of the calcu-
      lated maintenance fluid requirements for each quadrant
      of the peritoneal cavity which is entered.
   c. Twenty-four hours postoperatively, albumin at a final
      concentration 5% solution may be added as an aid in
      maintaining plasma osmotic pressure.

TABLE 18–2.

Daily Fluid Requirements in
Infants and Children

Weight (kg)	Volume
0–10	100 mL/kg
11–20	1000 mL + 50 mL/kg over 10 kg
>20	1500 mL + 20 mL/kg over 20 kg

d. Total fluid administration rates should be adjusted to maintain urinary output between 1–2 mL/kg/hr.
e. If the child has a central line, CVP may be monitored to accurately assess volume status.

C. Nutritional Support.

1. Requirements:

a. Nutritional requirements are increased in younger children and infants relative to adults. Nutritional requirements of children may be calculated from the data in Table 18–2 (in children, kcal/kg/hr = mL/kg/hr).

b. Alternatively, the following equation may be used to estimate the caloric requirements of children:

$$kcal/day = 100 - 3 \times (age\ in\ years) \times (weight\ in\ kg)$$

c. Daily nutritional requirements may be increased in stress states such as sepsis, trauma, or fever.

d. As a general rule, 50% of calories should be provided as carbohydrates, 35% fat, and 15% protein.

2. Enteral feeding:

a. As in the adult population, if the GI tract is functioning properly, fluid and nutritional requirements should be given enterally. Breast milk is a preferred substrate for the newborn. Table 18–3 lists the composition of a number of the more commonly used infant formulas.

b. Postoperatively, enteral feedings may be started when the postoperative ileus is resolved, as evidenced by:
   1) Passage of meconium or stool.
   2) Reduction of NG tube drainage to <2 mL/hr.
   3) Disappearance of bilious green color of NG tube drainage.

c. Because of poor swallowing coordination and the increased work of feeding, infants are generally fed via gavage or gastrostomy tube in the early postoperative period.

d. Feedings in neonates are initiated and advanced as follows:
   1) Begin with 10–15 mL Pedialyte q. 2–3 h.
   2) Increase by 2–5 mL increments over the next 12–24 hours until infant is receiving 30–45 mL of Pedialyte q. 3 h.

TABLE 18–3.

Composition of Infant Formulas

Formula	Kilocalories (kcal/mL)	Na (mEq/L)	K (mEq/L)	Ca (mg/L)	P (mg/L)	Fe (mg/L)	Osmolarity (mOsm/L)
Breast milk	0.67	7	14	340	162	1.5	100
Cow's milk	0.67	25	35	1,240	950	1	270
Enfamil	0.67	11	19	546	462	Trace	285
Nutramigen	0.67	14	17	630	473	13	460
Portagen	0.67	14	21	630	473	13	210
Pregestimil	0.67	14	17	630	473	13	311
ProSobee	0.67	18	19	788	525	13	250
Similac 20	0.67	11	19	580	430	Trace	285

     3) The patient is then begun with half-strength formula for 24 hours followed by full-strength formula q. 3–4 h. at volumes calculated to meet the child's fluid and caloric requirements.

  e. Hyperosmolar feeding often produces diarrhea.

  f. In the early postoperative period, non–lactose-containing formulas such as Isomil or ProSobee may be better tolerated.

3. **Parenteral nutrition.**

  a. Indications for TPN:

    1) TPN may be performed with the central infusion of hypertonic solution, or the infusion of less hypertonic solutions through a peripheral vein.

    2) Newborns and infants should be started on TPN if they are expected to be without nutrition for 4–5 days

    3) Older children may tolerate a slightly longer period of inadequate nutrition.

    4) The most common indications for TPN therapy in the pediatric patients are listed in Table 18–4.

  b. Because of the inflammation resulting from hyperosmolarity, solutions with a glucose concentration >12.5% should not be infused in peripheral veins. For this reason, peripheral parenteral nutrition is generally appropriate only for very short-term total nutrition or partial parenteral nutrition.

  c. Central venous access for TPN is generally achieved by percutaneous placement of a catheter into the subclavian vein or venous cutdown and placement of a catheter into the external jugular vein. Fluoroscopy is used to

TABLE 18–4.

Common Indications for Total Parenteral Nutrition

Short-bowel syndrome
Necrotizing enterocolitis
Crohn's disease with fistula
Gastroschisis
Omphalocele
Intestinal atresia

---

ensure that the end of the catheter resides in the superior vena cava at its junction with the RA. Such catheters should only be placed by persons experienced in pediatric vascular access.

   d. Initiation of TPN:

      1) Initially, protein is usually given at the rate of 1 g/kg/day, and slowly increased to 1.5–3 g/kg/day.

      2) Glucose administration should start at approximately 7 g/kg/day and increase over several days to 17–20 g/kg/day.

      3) Lipid (10%–20% fat emulsion) is given from 1–4 g/kg/day to attain total caloric support.

   e. For patients requiring long-term parenteral nutrition, TPN infusions may be cycled to run for 12 hours at night, and the line may be capped during the day.

   f. Complications of TPN:

      1) Electrolyte abnormalities.
      2) Cholestatic jaundice.
      3) Hyperlipidemia.
      4) Trace element deficiencies.
      5) Catheter sepsis.
      6) Fluid overload.
      7) Hyperammonemia.
      8) Hepatic dysfunction.

   g. Patients on TPN should be monitored closely to prevent serious metabolic complications. Early after the initiation of TPN, and during periods of irregularity, serum electrolytes, protein, liver enzymes, and triglycerides should be measured daily. Once the patient has stabilized, the following parameters should be monitored:

      1) Weight (daily).
      2) Serum electrolytes (twice weekly).
      3) Serum triglycerides, albumin, liver enzymes, calcium, phosphorus, magnesium (weekly).
      4) Vitamins A, D, B_{12}, folate, calcium, phosphorus, zinc (monthly).

D. Shock and Circulatory Failure.

   1. In children, shock results most commonly from either hypovolemia or sepsis. The specific diagnosis can usually be made on the basis of the history, e.g., a history of vomiting and diarrhea leads one to suspect that the patient is hypovolemic.

2. Children are better able to compensate for circulatory failure than adults. Peripheral resistance increases to maintain normal BP. This may result in ischemia of the peripheral tissues, with resulting lactic acidosis. Consequently, in the pediatric patient, hypotension may be a very late finding and may signify a decompensation just prior to cardiac arrest.
   a. Early signs of circulatory failure:
      1) Anxiety and irritability.
      2) Tachycardia.
      3) Pallor.
      4) Cool extremities.
   b. Late signs:
      1) Tachypnea.
      2) Oliguria.
      3) Metabolic acidosis.
      4) Hypotension.
      5) Somnolence.
3. **The aim of treatment in circulatory failure is to increase tissue perfusion.** Initial resuscitation measures are designed to ensure an adequate airway, adequate ventilation, and improve DO_2.
   a. Administer O_2 by face mask or intubation as appropriate.
   b. Establish IV access. Options include:
      1) Peripheral venous cannula.
      2) Saphenous vein cutdown.
      3) Tibial interosseous infusion.
      4) Central venous catheter. These lines should only be placed by persons experienced in establishment of such access in pediatric patients.
   c. Bolus infusion of 20 mL/kg of lactated Ringer's solution, which may be repeated once before further measures are taken. If there is no improvement after the initial fluid administration of 40 mL/kg, the following measures should be taken:
      1) Placement of an indwelling urinary catheter.
      2) ABG measurement.
      3) Consider whole blood transfusion if there is a possibility of blood loss.
      4) Treatment of acidosis with $NaHCO_3$. For a pH <7.20, an initial dose of 2 mEq/kg is indicated.

       5) Consider placing central venous catheter to monitor filling pressures.
- d. Continue fluid administration until CVP is >5 mm Hg. Consider use of a 5% albumin solution.
- e. Consider blood transfusion if there is a history of hemorrhage.
- f. Begin dopamine infusion at $5-10$ µg/kg/min if hypotension and poor tissue perfusion persist.
- g. Consider echocardiogram to evaluate for a possible cardiac etiology of shock.

  4. Further evaluation:
- a. If sepsis is a likely etiology for the patient's hemodynamic collapse, then blood, urine, sputum, and CSF samples should be obtained and the child started on broad-spectrum antibiotics.
- b. A search should also be made for other etiologies of the shock state including underlying cardiac disease, occult trauma (child abuse), drug overdose, etc.

E. Respiratory Failure.

1. Children who are septic or following major surgical procedures often have hypoxemia because of a capillary leak syndrome (noncardiogenic pulmonary edema) and often need ventilatory support. The goal of assisted ventilation is to maintain the pH between 7.25 and 7.45, PaO_2 between 50 and 85 mm Hg, and PCO_2 between 35 and 50 mm Hg. Management of pediatric patients with respiratory failure differs little from the management of adult patients. An exception is that in neonates and preterm infants, assisted ventilation is usually performed with pressure ventilators rather than volume ventilators.

2. **Indications for assisted ventilation:**
- a. Respiratory acidosis with a pH <7.2–7.25.
- b. Severe hypoxemia (PaO_2 < 64 with FIO_2 of 70%–100%).
- c. Neonatal apnea.

3. **Assisted ventilation:** Infants and larger children are generally supported with volume-cycled ventilators. The use of these machines is described on pp 263–264. There are no significant differences between the management of children and adults. For children, the initial TV should be set from 7–10 mL/kg. In this section, the management of neonates and preterm infants using pressure cycled ventilators is em-

phasized. Suggested initial ventilator settings for neonates with both normal lungs and those having respiratory distress syndrome (RDS) are presented in Table 18–5.

4. **Ventilator parameters:**
   a. Peak inspiratory pressure (PIP) determines the pressure differential which occurs between the onset and end of inspiration, therefore determining the delivered TV. Increasing PIP results in increased TV, increased CO_2 elimination, and may improve oxygenation.
   b. Positive end-expiratory pressure (PEEP) prevents alveolar collapse, maintains lung volume, and ameliorates ventilation-perfusion mismatch. Increasing PEEP decreases the pressure gradient between inspiration and expiration, thus *decreasing* ventilation and increasing PCO_2. Increasing PEEP results in increased oxygenation because of alveolar recruitment. PEEP decreases venous return to the heart and may decrease CO.
   c. Increasing *frequency* results in increased alveolar ventilation and reduced PCO_2. Frequency changes do not substantially affect PO_2.
   d. The inspiratory to expiratory (I:E) ratio may be altered to improve oxygenation without increasing peak airway pressures, thereby resulting in less barotrauma. Reversal of the I/E ratio will increase the mean airway pressure and may cause barotrauma.
   e. Increasing the FIO_2 will result in an increased hemoglobin oxygen saturation. However, the use of high FIO_2 may lead to worsening atelectasis and in the long term an increased incidence of bronchopulmonary dysplasia (BPD).

TABLE 18–5.

Suggested Initial Ventilator Settings

	Normal Lungs	Respiratory Distress Syndrome
PIP	12–18 cm H_2O	20–25 cm H_2O
PEEP	2–3 cm H_2O	4–5 cm H_2O
Frequency	10–20/min	20–40/min
I/E ratio	1:2–1:10	1:1–1:3

5. Complications resulting from ventilatory support in pre-term infants and neonates relate to toxicity from elevated FIO_2 and barotrauma from positive pressure ventilation. Chronic lung disease, or BPD, results from the combination of high FIO_2 and positive ventilation in preterm infants. Thus, complications associated with assisted ventilation in preterm infants and neonates can be reduced by reductions in FIO_2 and peak airway pressures to the lowest values consistent with adequate oxygenation and ventilation. Radiographic manifestations of barotrauma include pneumothorax, pulmonary interstitial emphysema, pneumopericardium, and subcutaneous emphysema.

6. In some centers, high frequency ventilation (HFV) is used in the treatment of patients with the RDS who have failed conventional ventilatory methods. This technique is experimental, and further studies are awaited. A theoretical advantage is improved oxygenation at lower peak pulmonary pressures, resulting in decreased incidence of barotrauma and BPD.

7. Some centers are beginning to utilize extracorporeal membrane oxygenation (ECMO) in patients failing conventional ventilatory methods (see pp 721–730).

F. **Specific Pediatric Surgical Conditions.**

1. **Necrotizing enterocolitis (NEC)** is the single most common surgical emergency in newborns. The clinical spectrum ranges from mild abdominal distention, ileus with occult blood in the stools, and pneumatosis intestinalis to fulminant sepsis and shock resulting from intestinal necrosis with peritonitis.

   a. Pathogenesis: NEC is thought to result from bacterial colonization and intestinal ischemia. Oral feeding formula may be a substrate for bacterial growth and breast milk may be protective against development of NEC. In most cases, NEC occurs in preterm infants below the age of 35–36 weeks' gestational age.

   b. Diagnosis:

      1) The mean gestational age of NEC patients is 31 weeks and the mean growth weight is 1,400 gm.

      2) Initial findings include:

         a) Abdominal distention with increased gastric aspirate.

         b) Gross or occult GI bleeding.

        c) Abdominal wall erythema, warmth, and induration with abdominal tenderness.

        d) Pneumatosis intestinalis or free intraperitoneal air on abdominal radiographs.

    3) In advanced disease, there is marked abdominal distention, and often bowel perforation or necrosis with clinical deterioration and shock.

c. Medical treatment: As soon as the diagnosis of NEC is suspected, the following measures should be taken:

    1) Discontinue oral feedings.

    2) Orogastric tube decompression of the GI tract.

    3) Fluid resuscitation to maintain adequate urinary output of 1.5–2 mL/kg/hr.

    4) Systemic antibiotic therapy should be instituted. Anaerobic coverage is unnecessary in children <10 days old.

    5) Institution of parenteral nutrition.

    6) Strict infection control measures.

    7) Antibiotics and bowel rest should be continued for 10–14 days after resolution of pneumatosis intestinalis.

d. Surgical treatment: Nearly 50% of patients with NEC will ultimately require surgery. Surgery is indicated for signs of peritonitis and in patients with frank bowel perforation or with abscess formation. Other indications include:

    1) Progressive edema, hyperemia, and tenderness of the abdominal wall on maximal medical therapy.

    2) Failure to clinically stabilize after 12–24 hours of medical treatment with the development of worsening sepsis.

    3) The presence of a palpable abdominal mass.

    4) In some centers an abdominal tap is performed to confirm the presence of intestinal gangrene.

    5) Surgical management usually includes resection of the gangrenous bowel and the formation of an ostomy and mucous fistula.

2. **Diaphragmatic hernia (Bochdalek's hernia).**

a. This congenital anomaly is a failure in the development of the posterior aspect of the diaphragm (most commonly on the left side). Severe hypoplasia of one or both lungs may result from the evisceration of the abdominal contents into the chest during development, which may result in respiratory distress at birth.

  b. Diagnosis: Depending on the severity of the respiratory distress, the child may present with severe collapse within minutes to hours of birth. In less severe cases, the diagnosis may be incidentally made later in life. Physical findings include:

    1) Respiratory distress including dyspnea and cyanosis.
    2) Decreased breath sounds usually in the left chest
    3) Scaphoid abdomen.
    4) Abdominal and chest films are usually diagnostic with the finding of abdominal viscera in the left chest.

  c. Treatment:

    1) An orogastric tube should be passed to decompress the GI tract.
    2) ET intubation and assisted ventilation.
    3) Consideration should be given to bilateral tube thoracostomies to prevent tension pneumothorax.
    4) The patient should be hyperventilated to maintain a $PaCO_2$ of <25 mm Hg and a pH of 7.45–7.50 to offset the tendency of the hypoplastic lung vasculature to vasoconstriction. When the patient becomes hemodynamically stable, definitive surgical therapy may be considered.
    5) Consider ECMO therapy if standard assisted ventilation does not improve the patient's condition (see p 721–731).

3. **Omphalocele and gastroschisis.**

  a. These conditions present with the evisceration of some or all of the abdominal contents through an abdominal wall defect. The embryology differs significantly. The goal of definitive treatment is to ultimately restore the viscera to the peritoneal cavity with closure of the abdomen.

  b. Diagnosis: Omphalocele consists of a translucent sac of peritoneum and amniotic membrane at the base of the umbilical cord, ranging in size from a few centimeters to a huge sac containing the entire midgut including the liver. In gastroschisis, the intestines protrude through a defect in the abdominal wall adjacent to umbilicus. The

bowel in this case has been exposed to amniotic fluid
and is therefore covered by a membrane of inflamed
peritoneum. The liver is always in the abdomen in gastroschisis. With an omphalocele, there is a high incidence of associated cardiac or other congenital anomalies.

  c. Resuscitation and definitive therapy:
     1) Place an orogastric tube.
     2) Cover eviscerated abdominal contents with warm
        gauze moistened with saline. **Extreme care must
        be taken to ensure that the eviscerated intestine
        is not strangulated secondary to volvulus or by
        the fascial defect.**
     3) Place the child within a sterile plastic bag from the
        neck down to maintain body temperature and re-
        duce fluid losses from exposed viscera.
     4) Institute O_2 therapy with intubation and mechanical
        ventilation if necessary.
     5) Consider broad-spectrum antibiotic coverage.
     6) Placement of an IV cannula and fluid resuscitation.
        In gastroschisis, because of the inflamed bowel and
        consequent large fluid losses, the patient should be
        given an initial IV bolus of 20 mL/kg of D5LR fol-
        lowed by a continuous infusion at a rate equal to
        three to four times the normal maintenance rate un-
        til the urinary output is adequate.

  d. Whenever possible, definitive closure of the abdominal
     wall defect is the preferred initial procedure.
     1) Washing out the meconium from the distal bowel
        with saline enemas and retrograde flushing of the
        bowel through the stomach tube decreases the vol-
        ume of the abdominal contents, increasing the like-
        lihood of closure at the initial operation.
     2) The main factor in determining whether complete
        closure is possible is the compromise of respiratory
        function resulting from the increased intraabdomi-
        nal pressure.
     3) Patients often will need ventilatory support for sev-
        eral days until the intraabdominal pressure de-
        creases. If the defect is too large to allow initial
        permanent closure, a Silastic silo is sewn to the ab-
        dominal wall, and the viscera are gradually reduced
        into the abdomen over a period of 3–4 days.

4. **Esophageal atresia.**

  a. In most cases, a distal tracheoesophageal fistula (TEF) is associated with esophageal atresia. Thus, the stomach is usually connected to the distal airway, resulting in reflux and aspiration of gastric contents.

  b. Diagnosis:

    1) Neonates usually present with markedly increased oral secretions.

    2) Coarse lung sounds and rhonchi.

    3) Abdominal distention is usually evident when a TEF is present.

    4) The diagnosis is confirmed by the gentle passage of an orogastric tube until it stops, and after insufflation with 10 mL air, a plain film will demonstrate the proximal esophageal pouch. Radiopaque contrast is contraindicated.

  c. Initial management:

    1) The tube in the proximal esophageal pouch should be placed on continuous suction.

    2) Position the patient in the prone position with the head elevated (anti-reflux position).

    3) Provide O_2 and ventilatory assistance as needed.

    4) Administer broad-spectrum antibiotics.

  d. Surgical therapy should be undertaken or a staging gastrostomy performed. In general, with multiple anomalies, pneumonia, or prematurity, survival is improved if definitive esophageal repair is delayed and initial gastrostomy is performed under local anesthesia to decompress the GI tract. This prevents regurgitation of gastric contents into the airway until the definitive procedure is performed.

5. **Intestinal malrotation.**

  a. **Because of the danger of volvulus with subsequent strangulation of the small intestine, a symptomatic malrotation constitutes a surgical emergency. Further, any obstruction of the alimentary tract must be considered a malrotation until absolutely ruled out.**

  b. Diagnosis:

    1) Neonates with proximal obstruction usually present with bile-stained emesis.

    2) A history of maternal hydramnios suggests the presence of a complete obstruction proximal to the mid-jejunum.

3) The abdominal plain film may show high-grade proximal obstruction. In normal infants air should fill the colon by 8–12 hours after birth.

4) A UGI contrast study usually will demonstrate duodenal obstruction or right-sided ligament of Treitz in cases of malrotation.

5) A barium enema may be useful if complete intestinal obstruction is seen on plain film showing abnormal positioning of the cecum.

6) In the face of obstructive symptoms, if either the UGI study or barium enema is abnormal, surgery should be performed immediately.

c. **In cases of proximal intestinal obstruction, if malrotation has not been ruled out, the patient should undergo an urgent exploratory laparotomy.** The goal is to prevent catastrophic infarction of the small bowel resulting from volvulus.

II. EXTRACORPOREAL MEMBRANE OXYGENATION.
A. Indications and Patient Selection.
1. **Initial evaluation:**
   a. ECMO is indicated for newborns and children with acute respiratory failure that is refractory to conventional management. An objective evaluation of the mortality risk of respiratory failure is the *oxygenation index* (OI) which is calculated as follows:

$$OI = \frac{[\text{mean airway pressure} \times FIO_2]}{PaO_2} \times 100$$

   b. When treated by conventional management alone, patients with an OI of 25 have a predicted mortality >50%, and an OI of 40 predicts a mortality of 80%. Currently, patients are considered candidates for ECMO after demonstrating three of five OIs >40 on maximal conventional therapy within a 4-hour period.

   c. Cerebral and cardiac anomalies must be ruled out by echocardiography and cranial ultrasonography.

   d. Newborns under 34 weeks' gestation or <2 kg are usually excluded from ECMO. Mechanical ventilation with high FIO_2 for >5 days is a relative contraindication and >10 days is an absolute contraindication to ECMO owing to the likelihood of irreversible lung damage.

2. **Common indications.**
   a. **Meconium aspiration syndrome** (MAS).
      1) During delivery, meconium-stained amniotic fluid indicates fetal distress and results from sustained hypoxemia that causes hyperperistalsis and sphincter relaxation. At birth, the neonate may aspirate meconium into the distal airways, causing airway obstruction, inflammation, and chemical pneumonitis.
      2) Infants who aspirate meconium may have mild, moderate, or severe respiratory distress at birth. Patients with MAS and severe respiratory distress refractory to conventional therapy are the most common candidates for ECMO.
   b. **Persistent pulmonary hypertension of the newborn** (PPHN).
      1) In the newborn lung, severe pulmonary vasoconstriction often occurs in response to factors such as hypoxia, hypercarbia, and acidosis. The resultant elevation in pulmonary vascular resistance can cause right-to-left shunting of blood flow away from the lungs and through the ductus arteriosus and foramen ovale. As this negative cycle perpetuates, the neonate becomes severely hypoxemic and acidotic. Standard therapy for PPHN consists of mechanical ventilation, induced respiratory alkalosis, and various pharmacologic agents. However, approximately 2%–5% of neonates fail to respond to this therapy and are considered for ECMO.
   c. **Congenital diaphragmatic hernia.**
      1) During the embryonic formation of the diaphragm, a defect may result from incomplete closure of the posterolateral communication between the abdominal and thoracic cavities. This most commonly occurs on the left. With incomplete development of the posterior diaphragm, abdominal contents herniate into the chest cavity and interfere with lung development and prevent inflation after delivery. Severe respiratory distress presents as PPHN and surgical repair is required.
      2) Postoperatively, neonates experience a "honeymoon period" of improved pulmonary function, often fol-

lowed by intractable respiratory failure. ECMO is indicated in patients failing conventional treatment after a honeymoon period.

3) The absence of this honeymoon period is considered evidence of pulmonary hypoplasia and is therefore a contraindication to ECMO.

d. **Postcardiac surgery:** Venoarterial ECMO can also serve as a form of mechanical assist or "assistance" in patients with severe cardiac failure. This may be applied preoperatively or postoperatively in patients with correctable cardiac anomalies who experience reversible mechanical failure due to severe pulmonary hypertension or depressed myocardial function.

B. ECMO Protocol.

1. After obtaining informed consent, the ECMO team is mobilized. This team usually consists of a select group of respiratory therapists, perfusionists, nurses, and physicians who have combined to establish a safe and reliable protocol for initiating, maintaining, and concluding extracorporeal life support.

2. ECMO is performed by draining venous (deoxygenated) blood, pumping it through an artificial lung where CO_2 is removed and O_2 is added, and returning the blood to the circulation via an artery (venoarterial ECMO) or a vein (venovenous ECMO).

   a. **Venoarterial (VA) ECMO:**

      1) In VA ECMO, the functions of both the heart and lungs are partially or totally replaced.

      2) Deoxygenated blood is drained from the RA via a cannula inserted into the right internal jugular (RIJ) or femoral vein while oxygenated blood is pumped through a cannula placed into the right common carotid (RCC) artery.

      3) VA ECMO is the standard configuration for neonatal ECMO and is the backup method when other techniques (VV ECMO) are insufficient.

   b. **Venovenous (VV) ECMO:**

      1) VV ECMO provides gas exchange but no cardiac support. Venous drainage and infusion cannulas are placed into the RA or venae cavae via the RIJ or femoral veins. Alternatively, a single specially designed double-lumen catheter may be positioned in

the RA through the RIJ vein for both drainage and infusion.

2) In either case, blood is drained from and returned to the venous circulation at the same rate. Therefore, ECMO candidates who are hemodynamically unstable and require cardiovascular support should be placed on VA ECMO.

3) In addition, a portion of newly oxygenated blood is removed by the drainage catheter in VV ECMO and this recirculation fraction increases with the circuit blood flow.

3. **Initiation and management of ECMO.**
   a. **The ECMO circuit:**
      1) The components of a standard ECMO circuit are illustrated in Figure 18–1. Deoxygenated blood drains passively into a distensible silicone bladder which operates as the control point of a servo-regulated roller pump that draws blood from the bladder.
      2) If the pump flow exceeds the passive venous return, the bladder will collapse and the roller pump will automatically slow down or shut off until it reexpands.
      3) Blood is then pumped through a silicone rubber membrane lung which is specifically designed for the extended periods of ECMO. After passing through a countercurrent heat exchanger, the warmed, oxygenated blood is returned to the patient via the arterial or venous infusion cannula.
      4) A tubing bridge is created between the drainage and perfusion catheters to allow recirculation of the ECMO circuit during priming and weaning.
      5) Heparin and fluids are infused into the circuit immediately before the bladder.

   b. **Cannulation.**
      1) Cannulation is performed by cutdown and ligation of vessels under strict sterile technique at the SICU bedside with an OR team and a complete set of instruments.
      2) In the neonate, a 12F or 14F venous and 10F or 12F arterial (for VA ECMO) are inserted into the

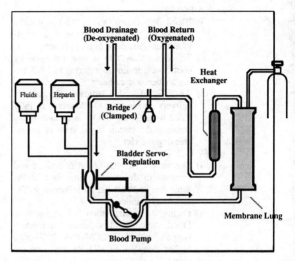

FIG 18–1.
ECMO circuit schematic drawing. Deoxygenated blood drains passively to a sealed bladder. If negative pressure occurs within the bladder, the roller pump is automatically shut off. After passing through the membrane lung, oxygenated blood is circulated through a countercurrent heat exchanger and back to the patient. Heparin and other infusions are delivered into the circuit immediately before the bladder.

RIJ vein and RCC artery, respectively, after a heparin loading dose of 100 units/kg.

3) Since circuit blood flow is limited by the available venous drainage, the venous drainage cannula should be as large as possible.

c. **Circuit management.**

1) The blood flow setting of the ECMO circuit is determined by the O_2 delivery requirements of the patient. Typical blood flow rates are 100–150 mL/kg/min in neonates and 80–120 mL/kg/min in children.

    a) VA ECMO:

        i) Blood flow during VA ECMO is usually 80% of the total CO, resulting in a diminished but observable pulse pressure.

        ii) The exact flow rate is best managed by continuous, in-line monitoring of $S\bar{v}O_2$ using a fiberoptic catheter.

        iii) An $S\bar{v}O_2$ of $\geq 75\%$ indicates adequate O_2 delivery. Inadequate O_2 delivery, as indicated by a falling $S\bar{v}O_2$, is treated by increasing the circuit blood flow or by increasing the Hct.

    b) VV ECMO:

        i) During VV ECMO, blood is drained and returned to the venous circulation at the same rate and thus has no influence on CO or hemodynamics.

        ii) Owing to recirculation of oxygenated blood, the circuit flow for total respiratory support with VV ECMO is 20%–50% higher than VA ECMO for the same patient.

        iii) Also, with recirculation, the $S\bar{v}O_2$ will be falsely elevated and less reliable to assess adequacy of O_2 delivery. Continuous pulse oximetry provides better information for determining adequate blood flow during VV ECMO.

2) Oxygenation is controlled by the FIO_2 of the gas connected to the membrane lung. In both VA ECMO and VV ECMO, a postoxygenator PO_2 of 200–300 mm Hg is maintained.

    a) VA ECMO: The systemic PO_2 during VA ECMO results from the combined bypass and nonbypass O_2 delivery. In most conditions (80% bypass and poor native lung function) the patient's hemoglobin will be fully saturated with a PaO_2 of 150–250 mm Hg.

    b) VV ECMO: Owing to the recirculation of VV ECMO, the patient's systemic SaO_2 will range from 85%–90%, with a PaO_2 of 60–80 mm Hg. Patients undergoing VV ECMO may appear slightly cyanotic, although O_2 delivery is usually adequate if CO and hemoglobin are maintained in their normal ranges. If O_2 delivery is inadequate during maximal settings on VV ECMO, extracorporeal support should be converted to the VA mode.

3) The patient's $PaCO_2$ is maintained at a value of 35–50 mm Hg by adjusting the "sweep" flow of gas. Frequently, however, 5% CO_2 is added to the lung gas flow owing to the high efficiency of CO_2 removal characteristic of membrane lungs.

4) Heparinization:
   a) A continuous heparin infusion of 15–60 units/kg/hr is required throughout the ECMO course. To monitor heparinization, the ACT is measured hourly.
   b) ACT is normally 100 seconds, and during ECMO the heparin infusion is titrated to maintain an ACT of 180–220 seconds.
   c) Owing to the constant heparin infusion, no IM injections should be given, and chest tubes, central lines, etc, should not be removed while on ECMO.

d. **Patient care during ECMO:**
   1) During ECMO support, ventilator management should be adjusted to minimal settings to provide lung rest and optimum conditions for pulmonary recovery. Ventilator settings should be reduced to an FIO_2 of 0.21, peak airway pressure of 20 cm H_2O, and a respiratory rate of 5–10. A PEEP of at least 3–5 cm H_2O should be maintained to prevent profound atelectasis. Aggressive pulmonary toilet should be performed several times per day and a CXR should be ordered daily.

   2) Medications and fluids:
      a) An accurate record of fluid balance and daily weights is essential.
      b) Blood is transfused to maintain a Hct of 40%–45%.
      c) Platelets are routinely administered at the initiation of ECMO and daily thereafter to maintain a count >100,000/mm^3.

      d) Prophylactic antibiotics are usually given daily while on bypass.

      e) Full nutrition should be administered throughout ECMO support.

      f) Patients requiring ECMO are usually hypervolemic upon initiation of support. In these cases, pharmacologic diuresis is instituted to remove excess fluid and return the patient dry weight. If diuretics are insufficient, a small, hollow-fiber hemofilter may be placed into the ECMO circuit to supplement urinary output and provide hemoconcentration.

      g) A mild to moderate level of sedation is usually maintained during ECMO. Any seizure activity must be treated promptly.

   3) Laboratory studies:

      a) Prior to initiation of ECMO, baseline CBC, electrolytes, liver function tests, and coagulation parameters must be obtained.

      b) During ECMO, CBC, electrolytes, and coagulation parameters are measured q. 8 h.

      c) Blood gasses are obtained q. 4–8 h. and a pulse oximeter is monitored continuously.

      d) In addition, a daily head ultrasound is performed on neonates to rule out intracranial hemorrhage.

4. Weaning and decannulation from ECMO.

   a. ECMO support is usually maintained for 4–5 days. Indications of lung recovery include an increasing $S\overline{v}O_2$ and systemic PaO_2, or decreasing $PaCO_2$ while ECMO flow and ventilator settings are constant. Other signs of improvement are noted by increased pulmonary compliance and normalization of the CXR. Cardiac recovery is noted by increased pulse pressure, CO, and $S\overline{v}O_2$, in addition to improved contractility as monitored by serial echocardiography.

   b. Weaning from VA ECMO: Upon documenting significant improvement in native lung or cardiac function, VA ECMO blood flow is gradually reduced over a period of hours. When the native lung and heart can provide adequate O_2 delivery and gas exchange at 20% of baseline VA ECMO flow, a brief trial off bypass (cannulas clamped, bridge open) is attempted on moderate ventilator settings. If successful, VA ECMO is restarted and the patient is prepared for the sterile decannulation procedure.

c. Weaning from VV ECMO: A trial wean from VV ECMO consists of decreasing and capping the gas flow to the membrane lung while continuing extracorporeal flow. If the native lungs provide adequate gas exchange, ECMO can be discontinued and the cannulas removed.

5. **Emergencies and complications during ECMO.**
   a. **Infrequently, an emergent situation, such as circuit disruption or air embolism, may occur that requires immediate exclusion from the ECMO circuit. If this situation develops, the following steps must be followed sequentially:**
      1) **Clamp venous drainage line.**
      2) **Open tubing bridge.**
      3) **Clamp infusion line.**
      4) **Increase patient ventilator settings to full support.**
      5) **Disconnect gas line to membrane lung.**
      6) **Repair or replace source of emergency.**
      7) **Evaluate need for restarting ECMO.**
   b. **Complications:**
      1) Mechanical complications occur in approximately one third of applications. These range from frequent minor events such as cracks in connectors and kinking of tubing to rare major problems such as oxygenator failure and raceway rupture. While the direct effect of these technical problems on survival has been about 5%, physiologic instability may be significant until the difficulty has been corrected.
      2) Medical:
         a) Bleeding: Owing to continuous systemic anticoagulation, bleeding is the most common complication. Intracranial hemorrhage (ICH) is the most significant bleeding complication and occurs in 10%–20% of cases. Other locations of bleeding include the GI tract, vascular access sites, and pericardium (tamponade). Bleeding complications are best managed by titrating heparin to a lower ACT target of 180 seconds and aggressively maintaining a platelet count >100,000/

mm^3. ECMO is usually discontinued in response to confirmed ICH or uncontrollable bleeding.

b) Neurologic: During cannulation for VA ECMO, the RCC artery is ligated with only rare attempts to repair it after ECMO. Owing to collateral blood flow to the brain, acute neurologic sequelae directly related to this ligation are rare, although seizures have been reported in 10%–15% of patients. Interestingly, while VV ECMO avoids ligation of arteries for vascular access, seizures have occurred with similar frequency.

c) Other complications encountered include hemolysis, hyperbilirubinemia, renal insufficiency, cardiac arrhythmias, pulmonary hypertension, and sepsis.

C. Outcome and Follow-up.

As part of its charter, the Extracorporeal Life Support Organization (ELSO) maintains an international registry of all patients treated with ECMO. As of October 1990, the registry for neonatal ECMO had recorded 4,221 cases performed at 78 medical centers. Overall hospital survival of this population was 3,461 neonates (82%). By diagnosis, babies suffering MAS or PPHN had survival rates of 93% and 87%, respectively, while survival of patients with CDH or post cardiac surgery averaged 60%. Several reports of long-term follow-up describe approximately 75% of ECMO survivors as normal children.

SELECTED REFERENCES

MANAGEMENT OF THE PEDIATRIC SURGICAL PATIENT

Arnold WL: Parenteral nutrition, and fluid and electrolyte therapy. *Pediatr Clin North Am* 1990; 37:449.

Carter JM, Gerstmann DR, Clark RH, et al: High-frequency oscillatory ventilation and extracoporeal membrane oxygenation for the treatment of acute neonatal respiratory failure. *Pediatrics* 1990; 85:159.

Crone RK: Acute circulatory failure in children. *Pediatr Clin North Am* 1980; 27:525.

Perkin RM, Levin DL: Shock in the pediatric patient. Part I. *J Pediatr* 1982; 101:163.

EXTRACOPOREAL MEMBRANE OXYGENATION

Bartlett RH: Extracorporeal life support for cardiopulmonary failure. *Curr Probl Surg* 1990; 27:623–705.

Bartlett RH, Gazzaniga AB, Toomasian J, et al: Extracorporeal membrane oxygenation (ECMO) in neonatal respiratory failure: 100 cases. *Ann Surg* 1986; 204:236–245.

Klein MD, Shaheen KW, Wittlesey GC, et al: Extracorporeal membrane oxygenation for the circulatory support of children after repair of congenital heart disease. *J Thorac Cardiovasc Surg* 1990; 100:498–505.

O'Rourke PP, Crone RK, Vacanti JP, et al: Extracorporeal membrane oxygenation and conventional medical therapy in neonates with persistent pulmonary hypertension of the newborn: A prospective randomized study. *Pediatrics* 1989; 84:957–963.

Redmond CR, Graves ED, Falterman KW, et al: Extracorporeal membrane oxygenation for respiratory and cardiac failure in infants and children. *J Thorac Cardiovasc Surg* 1987; 93:199–204.

TRAUMA $\quad$ 19

I. INITIAL MANAGEMENT.

Patients arriving in the SICU from the ER or OR should be assumed to have unrecognized or inadequately managed problems. Late recognition of significant injuries is the rule rather than the exception in multiply-injured patients. Significant morbidity is associated with delay in diagnosis.

A. Initial Evaluation in the SICU.

1. **Initial evaluation** should proceed as in protocols followed in initial assessments in the ER.
2. The prime consideration is **thoroughness**.
3. **Airway management:**
   a. Goals of management are (1) to **secure** an adequate airway and (2) to **protect** the airway.
   b. **Assume cervical spine injury** until radiographic clearance is confirmed. Often, semirigid collars are maintained in the SICU until all views can be safely obtained.
   c. As a general principle, **hypothermic** patients should remain intubated.
4. **Ventilation and oxygenation:**
   a. Initial examination should include observation of chest expansion and confirmation of bilateral breath sounds.
   b. **ET tube** should be examined for a properly inflated cuff and the distance from the tip noted (usually 22–24 cm).
   c. Arterial blood gas measurement and CXR will provide additional data.
5. **Vascular access:**
   a. IV access should be identified by location, size, and current fluid type. IV location and patency should be confirmed. This step is essential should sudden decompensation occur.

      b. Arterial lines should be checked.

      c. Special lines such as central venous lines and Swan-Ganz catheters should be examined.

        1) Appropriate zero levels should be confirmed.

        2) Location of Swan-Ganz catheters should be ascertained and confirmed radiographically.

6. **Appropriate laboratory studies** should be obtained. In particular, a coagulation profile including fibrinogen level is useful in permitting rational treatment of bleeding diatheses.

7. **Fluid resuscitation:**

    a. Upon arrival in the SICU, many patients will not be fully resuscitated.

    b. Basic indices such as vital signs, assessment of peripheral perfusion, and UO can guide fluid management. Patients with multiple injuries and unclear fluid status should undergo early invasive monitoring (Swan-Ganz catheterization).

8. **Thorough physical examination:**

    a. A careful head-to-toe evaluation should be performed.

    b. Details of the accident should allow particular consideration of diagnoses associated with that mechanism of injury.

    c. Physical examination provides a baseline, maximizing the opportunity for diagnosing missed injuries and complications.

9. **An admission portable CXR** allows confirmation of central line, ET tube, NG tube, and chest tube placements. Careful attention should be directed to mediastinal and pulmonary structures.

10. **All previous studies should be reviewed** and the final reading by the radiologists noted.

11. The above information should allow decisions regarding further workup. Timing of further studies should be based on the stability of the patient for transport as well as the potential cost of delayed diagnosis.

II. THORACIC TRAUMA.

A. Simple and Complicated Pneumothorax.

1. Chest pain and shortness of breath are the most common symptoms.

2. **Physical findings** include decreased breath sounds and decreased chest wall motion. Patients on ventilators will demonstrate significantly higher airway pressures.

3. **CXR** demonstrates a hyperlucent area with absent lung markings. Small pneumothoraces may only be identified on expiratory films taken with the patient upright.

4. **Treatment** of a pneumothorax involves placement of a 28F or 32F chest tube.

5. **Complications:**

   a. **Incomplete reexpansion** of the lung following chest tube placement results in persistent air leaks and delay in resolution. Management involves higher suction pressures and sometimes placement of an additional chest tube into a residual space.

   b. **Large air leaks** should arouse suspicion of a tracheobronchial injury (see below).

   c. **Continuous air leaks** which do not vary with respiration can be associated with esophageal injury (see below).

B. Tension Pneumothorax.

1. Tension pneumothorax is an immediately life-threatening problem which in the SICU is most often seen as a complication of mechanical ventilation.

2. **A tension pneumothorax results** from a check-valve effect which allows accumulation of air under pressure within the pleural space, but does not allow egress of air. Positive intrapleural pressures of only 10–15 cm H_2O significantly impede venous return to the heart resulting in hemodynamic instability.

3. **The diagnosis is based on clinical findings.** Respiratory compromise and hypotension associated with decreased breath sounds and hyperresonance to percussion on the affected side identify a tension pneumothorax. The trachea may shift away from the affected side. Patients requiring mechanical ventilation will demonstrate elevated airway pressures.

4. **Treatment should be immediate** and precede radiographic confirmation. Decompression should be performed immediately. **A 14- or 16-gauge intracatheter inserted in the second or third intercostal space** in the midclavicular line is effective. A rush of air confirms the diagnosis. Placement of a standard chest tube should follow decompression.

C. **Pulmonary Contusion.**
   1. Pulmonary contusion is a direct injury to the lung associated with hemorrhage and subsequent edema.
   2. **Diagnosis** is based upon early (<4–6 hours) radiographic findings of pulmonary infiltrates and consolidation.
   3. **Mild contusions may be treated with:**
      a. Aggressive pulmonary toilet including chest physiotherapy and ET suctioning.
      b. Pain control of associated rib fractures.
      c. Avoidance of fluid overload.
   4. **Moderate to severe contusions require intubation** and mechanical ventilation based on standard criteria for intubation ($PaO_2 < 60$ mm Hg; $PaCO_2 > 55$ mm Hg; respiratory rate > 30).
      a. Treatment goals should be to maintain O_2 saturation >90% while maintaining $FIO_2 < 0.5$ to prevent O_2 toxicity.
      b. **PEEP** is effective in increasing functional residual capacity and in improving oxygenation. CO and pulmonary compliance measurements allow selection of optimal PEEP settings.
      c. **Fluid overload should be avoided.** Invasive hemodynamic monitoring including Swan-Ganz catheterization is indicated to allow optimal fluid management.
      d. **The Hct should be maintained >30 mL/dL** to optimize O_2 delivery.
   5. **Complications.**
      a. **Infection:**
         1) The injured lung is susceptible to bacterial colonization.
         2) Prophylactic antibiotics are not indicated.
         3) Frequent sputum cultures should be obtained.
         4) Antibiotic therapy is initiated for the treatment of documented pneumonia.
      b. **Barotrauma:** The most common manifestation is development of a pneumothorax.
   6. Patients with severe contusions are expected to have gradual improvement in ABGs and in clinical condition allowing ventilation weaning at 10–14 days. Failure to demonstrate improvement should arouse suspicion of superimposed pneumonia or PE.

D. Flail Chest.

1. Flail chest results when a segment of chest wall loses continuity with the remainder of the bony thorax.
2. The flail segment will demonstrate paradoxical respiratory movement. However, the primary pathophysiology results from injury to the underlying lung.
3. Therapy is essentially the treatment of the underlying lung injury, as discussed on p 735.

E. Hemothorax.

1. Patients treated for hemothorax will ideally arrive in the SICU with a large-bore chest tube.
2. **Indications for operation include**
   a. Initial output > 1,000 mL.
   b. Hourly output > 300 mL/hr.
   c. Total output > 2,000 mL.
3. An early clotted hemothorax not removed by chest tube should be managed by thoracotomy and evacuation of clot.
4. Delayed management may result in a fibrothorax with an entrapped lung or an empyema. Pleural decortication is required to treat an entrapped lung.

F. Tracheobronchial Injuries.

1. Only 30% of cases are diagnosed within the first 24 hours.
2. **Signs** include mediastinal or subcutaneous emphysema and presence of pneumothorax. A large air leak will often be present from chest tubes. Proximity of the path of a penetrating object should arouse suspicion.
3. **Diagnosis** is made by tracheobronchoscopy.
4. **Treatment** involves operative repair. The incision used is determined by the site of injury.
5. **Two clinical syndromes** are seen with delayed diagnosis:
   a. In patients with incomplete injuries, the bronchus will heal with a stricture.
      1) Atelectasis and recurrent infection will occur distally, and ultimately tissue destruction will occur.
      2) At this point, management involves pulmonary resection.

       b. In patients with circumferential lacerations, each end
         will heal over.
         1) The distal bronchial tree will fill with mucus and
            radiographic studies will demonstrate complete
            atelectasis.
         2) In this case, repair can be effected.

G. Myocardial Contusion.

1. This diagnosis should be considered in patients sustaining blunt trauma to the anterior chest.
2. **Diagnosis** may be based on ECG and cardiac isoenzyme determination. ECG findings include ST segment changes, PVCs, conduction system defects, atrial fibrillation.
3. **Echocardiography** will identify associated wall motion abnormalities and allow identification of a pericardial effusion.
4. **Management:**
   a. Monitoring for 48 hours.
   b. Measurement of cardiac isoenzymes q. 8 h. × 24 hours.
   c. Ventricular ectopy is treated with lidocaine.
5. **Complications:** Findings of a new postinjury murmur should be evaluated with an echocardiogram and possibly cardiac catheterization.

H. Aortic Transection.

1. The most common site of aortic transection is just distal to the left subclavian artery secondary to a deceleration injury.
2. A high index of suspicion based on the mechanism of injury is required. The most important sign on a CXR is a widened mediastinum, which should be evaluated with an aortogram. Additional CXR findings are (1) an apical cap, (2) fractures of the first and second ribs, (3) scapular fractures, (4) deviation of the esophagus (NG tube), (5) loss of the aortic knob, (6) depression of the left mainstem bronchus.
3. **Aortography** is the definitive test, and a low threshold for obtaining this study should be maintained.
4. **Therapy** involves left posterolateral thoracotomy with primary or graft repair.

5. **Complications:**
   a. Paraparesis or paraplegia occurs in ~5% of patients.
   b. ARF is usually reversible.
   c. Vigorous correction of coagulation abnormalities should be performed with correction of hypothermia. Continued bleeding suggests a mechanical source.

I. **Diaphragmatic Injury.**
   1. **Diaphragmatic rupture** usually occurs with significant blunt trauma. The tears are usually radical and most commonly on the left side.
   2. **Diagnosis** can be difficult in the early postinjury period. CXR findings include irregularity or elevation of the diaphragm, a loculated hydropneumothorax, or a subpulmonary hematoma.
      a. Contrast studies are utilized to confirm the diagnosis.
      b. The presence of an NG tube or abdominal viscera in the hemithorax on plain films will establish the diagnosis.
   3. The **stomach** is the most frequent organ involved in herniation, and gastric volvulus may result. Injuries to the liver and spleen are frequently associated.
   4. **Diaphragmatic tears** should be repaired in two layers with nonabsorbable suture. Repairs may be performed through an abdominal approach. Tears discovered at thoracotomy mandate celiotomy to evaluate associated abdominal injuries.
   5. **Late repairs** should be performed through a thoracotomy because of dense adhesions which are usually present.

J. **Esophageal Injuries.**
   1. This injury most commonly occurs with penetrating trauma, and should be suspected if the path of the object could have been in proximity to the esophagus.
   2. **Symptoms** include dysphagia and hematemesis.
   3. **Findings** include subcutaneous or mediastinal emphysema, fluid levels within the mediastinum, or pleural effusions.
      a. Chest tubes that exhibit air leaks which do not vary with respiration suggest an esophageal leak.
      b. Particulate matter in chest tube drainage should also lead to evaluation.
   4. **Esophagoscopy** can be used in patients unable to cooperate or in patients taken emergently to the OR for asso-

ciated injuries. A Gastrografin swallow will demonstrate a leak.

5. **Early treatment** involves primary repair with aggressive drainage with two or three large-bore chest tubes.

6. **Complex injuries and those recognized late** (>12 hours postinjury) may require diversion and drainage.

7. In patients undergoing repair, a Gastrografin swallow is obtained 5–7 days after repair. Oral feeding is resumed only after documentation of no extravasation. Adequate nutrition is an absolute priority after repair and can be obtained with TPN or with placement of an enteral tube into the small intestine.

III. ABDOMINAL TRAUMA.

A. One subset of patients will arrive in the SICU after blunt or occasionally penetrating abdominal trauma without having undergone laparotomy. A high index of suspicion for occult injuries is required. Repetitive and thorough physical examinations by the same examiners are required. Negative peritoneal lavage or CT scans do not absolutely exclude intraabdominal pathology.

B. A second group of patients will have undergone laparotomy. Meticulous attention must again be directed toward identification of occult injuries and toward early recognition of complications of injuries or the operative procedures. The SICU physician must have a thorough knowledge of pathologic conditions identified and therapeutic maneuvers performed during the laparotomy to assist in optimal care.

C. **Occult Injuries.**

1. Significant injuries may be missed during diagnostic workup or during laparotomy. Examples:

   a. **Unrecognized sources of bleeding:**

      1) Associated signs may include hemodynamic instability, falling Hct, peritoneal irritation, or increasing abdominal girth.

      2) A CT scan is a sensitive diagnostic test to evaluate intraabdominal sources in questionable cases.

   b. **Hollow viscus perforation:**

      1) Signs include peritoneal irritation, continued sepsis, and clinical deterioration.

      2) Both peritoneal lavage and a CT scan can miss this injury. In addition, intestinal perforation is a complication of peritoneal lavage.

2. Diagnosis can be based on serial physical examinations, repeat plain films, and supplemented by CT scanning.

D. Late Complications

1. **Intraabdominal abscess:**
   a. Most patients with abscesses will demonstrate **persistent fever,** often with a spiking character, as well as an elevated WBC count with a left shift.
   b. Ileus and abdominal distention are frequently present. In some cases, worsening hyperbilirubinemia or sepsis may occur. Multiorgan failure may follow with delay in diagnosis.
   c. **CT** is the diagnostic test of choice.
   d. **Management** of an abscess requires drainage. Options include:
      1) Percutaneous catheter drainage under CT control.
      2) Open surgical drainage.
2. The most common cause of **early postoperative bowel obstruction** is adhesions. Appropriate decompression will usually be successful.
3. **Stress gastritis** (see pp 457–459):
   a. Gastritis with associated upper GI bleeding is a frequent complication in the trauma patient.
   b. Prophylaxis with H_2 antagonists, antacids, or sucralfate should be utilized.

E. Splenic Trauma.

1. The spleen is the most frequently injured abdominal organ by blunt trauma.
2. **Symptoms** include LUQ pain and left shoulder pain (Kehr's sign).
3. **Findings** may include LUQ tenderness, tachycardia, and hypotension. A falling Hct and radiographic findings of left lower rib fractures, elevated left hemidiaphragm, and gastric displacement may be found.
4. Both delays in diagnosis and rupture of the spleen may occur.
5. In patients in the SICU who do not manifest a surgical abdomen, diagnosis can be established with a CT scan.
6. A current trend toward more conservative management of splenic injuries has been based upon the occurrence of postsplenectomy sepsis, particularly in children.
7. **Nonoperative management** has been used in patients who have (1) documented splenic injury or CT scan

which is thought to be isolated, (2) hemodynamic stability, (3) normal level of consciousness, and (4) absence of coagulopathy.

    a. This protocol has been used primarily in children with an 85% success rate.

    b. The success rate in adults is 60%, with most patients requiring surgery undergoing splenectomy.

    c. The protocol includes bed rest, NG suction, repetitive physical examinations, and Hct determinations.

8. **Operative management** includes both splenic salvage and splenectomy.

    a. **Splenic salvage** is appropriate in patients with (1) hemodynamic stability, (2) no major associated injuries, (3) limited splenic trauma (no avulsion or fragmentation injuries, injuries involving the hilum). Splenic salvage procedures should include full mobilization of the spleen.

    b. Drainage with a closed drainage system is used after splenectomy for trauma.

9. **Complications:**

    a. **Hemorrhage** is the most common complication following splenectomy. Coagulation abnormalities and hypothermia should be corrected. Continued evidence of blood loss mandates reexploration. Approximately 2%–3% of patients treated with splenorrhaphy will require splenectomy secondary to postoperative bleeding.

    b. **Subphrenic abscess** is treated by drainage

    c. **Pancreatitis** is managed with NG suction and hyperalimentation if required.

    d. **Postsplenectomy sepsis** is characterized by the abrupt onset of overwhelming sepsis with early death in patients with previous splenectomy

        1) The incidence is greatest in children.

        2) Polyvalent pneumococcal vaccine should be given to patients prior to discharge (protective against 80% of pneumococcal strains).

        3) Prophylactic penicillin should be given to children following splenectomy.

        4) Patients and families should be instructed about postsplenectomy sepsis.

F. **Hepatic Injury.**
   1. **Intraoperative management** of hepatic injury may include:
      a. Drainage (used in almost all cases).
      b. Direct suture ligation.
      c. Debridement.
      d. Hepatic resection.
      e. Hepatic artery ligation.
      f. Packing.
   2. **Postoperative management:**
      a. **Aggressive correction** of coagulation abnormalities which often necessitates transfusion with FFP.
      b. **Treatment of hypothermia.**
      c. **Prevention of hypoglycemia.** Standard practice is to administer D10 solutions following hepatic resection.
      d. **Prevention of hypoalbuminemia** by administration of albumin after liver resections.
   3. **Subcapsular hematomas** may be managed nonoperatively in stable patients with bed rest, serial physical examination and Hct determinations, and repeat CT scanning.
      a. One third of these patients require operation.
      b. Signs of rupture or abscess formation require immediate operative intervention.
      c. Enlargement of contained hematomas may be initially managed with arteriography and embolization, but may also require operative intervention.
   4. **Complications:**
      a. **Continued bleeding** despite correction of hypothermia and coagulation parameters should be treated with early reoperation.
      b. **Abscess** is common after hepatic trauma (10%–20%) secondary to retained bile, blood, and necrotic tissue. Prevention involves aggressive drainage at the original procedure.
         1) Clinical signs include fever, sepsis, persistent hyperbilirubinemia.
         2) Diagnosis is established by CT scan.
         3) Treatment is by percutaneous or open drainage.
      c. **Hyperbilirubinemia** is a common early finding related to multiple transfusions and transient hepatic dysfunction. Persistent elevation may be associated with infection.

d. **Hematobilia:**
1) Usually complicating subcapsular or central hematomas, may result from inadvisable closure of transcapsular lacerations.
2) **Clinical findings** include colicky abdominal pain and GI bleeding (usually melena) with a history of abdominal trauma.
3) **Diagnosis** is established by angiography.
4) **Embolization** is usually successful. Several operative strategies have been employed including resection, ligation of hepatic artery branches, and debridement.

G. Gastric Injury.
1. Gastric injuries most commonly occur with penetrating trauma. Diagnosis may be suspected with a bloody NG aspirate.
2. **Management:** Most gastric injuries can be repaired. External drainage is not warranted.
3. Postoperatively, NG suction should be maintained until peristalsis has returned.
4. **Complications:**
   a. **Significant bleeding** via the NG tube may originate from a suture line. Management involves reexploration for hemostasis.
   b. Subhepatic, subphrenic, or lesser sac **abscesses** are suspected in patients with persistent fever and elevated WBC counts. Treatment is drainage.

H. Duodenal Injury.
1. **Delays in diagnosis** of duodenal injuries are common.
   a. Retroperitoneal duodenal injuries may be missed at laparotomy unless meticulous care is given to inspection of the entire duodenum.
   b. Mortality rates of 25%–40% have been reported secondary to delay in diagnosis and severity of associated injuries.
2. **Clinical findings** are nonspecific but include fever, tachycardia, abdominal, back, or shoulder pain. Testicular pain is associated with retroperitoneal injuries.
3. **Plain films** may demonstrate free air, loss of the right psoas margin, air outlining the right kidney or right psoas muscle, or retroperitoneal gas bubbles.
4. **Gastrografin studies** will demonstrate duodenal leaks as well as intramural hematomas.

5. **CT scans** are very helpful in evaluation of pancreatic and duodenal injuries in unclear cases.
6. **Intramural hematoma:**
   a. Usually results from blunt trauma.
   b. Commonly causes partial small bowel obstruction with nausea, vomiting, and abdominal pain.
   c. UGI series is diagnostic, showing a coiled-spring appearance in the second and third portions of the duodenum.
   d. Nonoperative treatment is usually successful.
   e. The traditional surgical treatment is evacuation of the hematoma.
7. **Intraoperative management** depends on the location and severity of injury.
   a. The most important procedure is to establish effective drainage.
   b. Simple lacerations can be closed with transverse closure. Repairs can be buttressed with omental or jejunal patches.
   c. Resection may be required in more serious injuries.
   d. **Two useful techniques for severe injuries include:**
      1) **Duodenal diverticularization,** which involves antrectomy with Billroth II gastrojejunostomy and vagotomy, closure of the duodenal stump, repair of the duodenal laceration, decompression with a tube duodenostomy, T tube drainage of the common duct, and extensive drainage.
      2) **Pyloric exclusion:** repair of the duodenal laceration followed by closure of the pylorus with absorbable suture through a gastrotomy which is the site for a gastrojejunostomy.
   e. Tube duodenostomy may be helpful in difficult injuries. The tube may be removed after 2–4 weeks.
8. **Postoperative care:**
   a. Bowel rest with NG or gastrostomy tube decompression should be maintained 5–7 days.
   b. Water-soluble contrast studies can be obtained to evaluate the repair.
   c. Drains should be maintained until several days after an oral diet has been resumed.

9. **Complications.**
   a. **Duodenal fistula.**
      1) Initial management includes:
         a) Maintenance of gastric decompression.
         b) Sump drainage of the fistula.
         c) TPN.
      2) Fistulas that fail to close necessitate reoperation. Two surgical options include:
         a) Closure using a Roux-en-Y limb of jejunum.
         b) Disconnection of the duodenum with gastrojejunostomy.

I. Pancreatic Injury.

1. Following upper abdominal trauma, patients with pancreatic injuries often initially display only mild symptoms. The development of significant pain, tenderness with loss of bowel sounds, and peritoneal signs may be delayed. A common indication for exploration in these patients is associated IP injuries that require operation.
2. **Additional studies** which may be helpful include:
   a. **Serum amylase determinations.**
      1) Serum amylase levels are not reliable indicators of pancreatic trauma.
      2) Only 66% of patients with significant blunt pancreatic trauma have hyperamylasemia.
      3) Hyperamylasemia without other signs of injury should not lead to laparotomy. These patients deserve in-hospital observation and should undergo CT scanning.
   b. Retroperitoneal injuries may be missed by peritoneal lavage.
   c. **CT scan** is the best diagnostic study for pancreatic injury. Use of oral contrast is recommended since unopacified bowel loops in proximity to the pancreas are frequently the cause of false-positive results.
3. **Intraoperative management** is dictated by the extent of injury and is based on the location of the injury, involvement of the pancreatic duct, and associated injury to the duodenum and common bile duct.
   a. Isolated injuries not involving the duct should be treated with drainage with or without suturing of lacerations.

    b. Body or tail injuries including the duct can be treated with distal pancreatectomy.

    c. Isolated head and uncinate process injuries involving the duct should be treated by drainage.

4. **Complex injuries** involving the duodenum and pancreas are associated with a high mortality. Surgical options include:

    a. Duodenal diverticularization.

    b. Duodenal exclusion.

    c. Whipple procedure is a last resort. Mortality approaches 40%.

5. **Complications.**

    a. **Pancreatic fistulas** occur in approximately 10% of patients.

      1) These fistulas can usually be managed conservatively.

      2) Management of high-volume fistulas should include TPN.

      3) Somatostatin may be useful in shortening the time to closure.

    b. **Pancreatitis** occurs in up to 10% of cases.

      1) Management is conservative, including bowel rest. Provisions for adequate nutrition must be made.

      2) Recurrent pancreatitis should trigger evaluation for ductal stricture by ERCP.

    c. **Pancreatic pseudocysts.**

      1) **Clinical findings** include abdominal pain, nausea, abdominal mass, and a persistently elevated serum amylase.

      2) **Diagnostic tests** include ultrasound, CT, and ERCP.

      3) **Internal drainage** via cystogastrostomy or Roux-en-Y cystojejunostomy for mature pseudocysts is indicated. Clinical findings may include sepsis with associated pulmonary or renal insufficiency or progressive deterioration with fever and elevated WBC counts.

    d. **Pancreatic abcess.**

      1) Signs of sepsis evident.

      2) **CT scanning** is the diagnostic test of choice.

      3) Management necessitates **open drainage and sump drainage.**

e. **Hemorrhage:**
  1) Significant bleeding may occur secondary to erosion of retroperitoneal vessels.
  2) Immediate reexploration is necessary and is associated with a high mortality.

J. Small Bowel Injuries.
1. Most small bowel injuries are managed by repair or resection with reanastomosis.
2. **Complications.**
  a. Complications are unusual following these injuries.
  b. **Intraabdominal abscess or generalized peritonitis** may result from anastomotic breakdown.
    1) Signs include fever, abdominal pain and tenderness, and leukocytosis.
    2) Treatment is usually reexploration with resection and reanastomosis.
  c. **Enterocutaneous fistulas** also result from failure at a repair site or anastomosis.
    1) Most fistulas close with conservative management including TPN.
    2) High output fistulas often require resection with reanastomosis
  d. **Obstruction:**
    1) Early obstruction will frequently resolve with decompression.
    2) Criteria for operative intervention include fever, leukocytosis, tachycardia, or peritoneal signs as well as failure of conservative therapy.

K. Colon Injuries.
1. **Diagnosis:**
  a. The majority of colon injuries are caused by penetrating trauma. Injury to the colon is identified at laparotomy.
  b. Patients with colorectal injuries secondary to blunt trauma may require further evaluation.
    1) As stated previously, both peritoneal lavage and CT may miss hollow viscera injury. In-hospital observation is required despite negative studies.
    2) Particularly in the case of pelvic fractures, proctoscopy is required for evaluation of concomitant rectal injury.

2. **Management** is based on location and extent of injury as
   well as time to surgery.
   a. Primary repair is used in stable patients with minimal
      contamination and minimal delay.
   b. Repair and exteriorization:
      1) The repaired segment is returned to the peritoneal
         cavity in 10–14 days.
   c. Colostomy includes patients undergoing exterioriza-
      tion of the injury, repair with proximal colostomy, re-
      section with end colostomy. This strategy of diver-
      sion or exteriorization is used most commonly.
   d. **Rectal injuries** should be treated with proximal di-
      version. Drainage of the presacral space is impera-
      tive.
3. **Complications:** Intraabdominal abscess occurs in
   5%–15% of patients, and can usually be managed with
   percutaneous drainage.

BURNS 20

I. **INITIAL MANAGEMENT.**
A. **Stop the Burning Process.**
   1. Extinguish flames and remove all involved clothing.
   2. Flush chemical burns with copious amounts of water. The depth of injury is proportional to chemical concentration and duration of exposure.
B. **Standard ABCs of CPR.**
C. **Establish Venous Access.**
   1. Mandatory if cardiac arrhythmia is present, >30–45 minutes from a burn center, or significant blood loss has occurred.
   2. Insert 14- or 16-gauge IV catheter, through unburned skin if possible. Peripheral veins are almost always adequate.
D. **History: Underlying Medical Conditions, Current Medications, Allergies, Circumstances of Injury.**
E. **Physical Examination.**
   1. Examine for associated injuries.
   2. Monitor vital signs hourly.
   3. Obtain baseline body weight.
F. **Laboratory Evaluation.**
   1. ABG with carboxyhemoglobin level.
   2. RBC loss is proportional to extent of full-thickness burn injury. Hct should return to normal by 48–72 hours postburn.
   3. Electrolytes, BUN, creatinine.
   4. Urinalysis.
   5. Type and crossmatch.
G. **Tetanus Prophylaxis.**
   1. Tetanus toxoid 0.5 mL IM.
   2. If history of tetanus immunization unknown:
      a. Tetanus-immune globulin 250–500 units IM.
      b. Begin active immunization with tetanus toxoid.

H.   Estimate Extent of Burn.
1. "Rule of nines" for a rapid approximation of BSA burned (Fig 20–1).
2. The area of the patient's palm, which is ~1% BSA, is useful in estimating the % BSA burn.
3. Children have an increased percentage of surface area in the head and neck compared with an adult.

I.   Estimation of Burn Depth.
1. Partial thickness burn:
   a. Pink or mottled red color.
   b. Wet appearance.
   c. Covered with vesicles or bullae.
   d. Painful, often severely.
2. Full-thickness burns (all epithelial elements destroyed):
   a. Charred; may appear translucent.
   b. Dry appearance.
   c. May have thrombosed superficial veins.
   d. Insensate (nerve endings destroyed).
   e. Often requires excision.
   f. Always requires cutaneous autografting for wound closure.

II.   INDICATIONS FOR SICU OR BURN CENTER ADMISSION.
A.   Adults with ≥25% BSA burn.
B.   Children with ≥20% BSA burn.
C.   Full-thickness burns ≥10% of BSA.
D.   Burns of face, hands, feet, eyes, ears, or perineum (possible cosmetic or functional disability).
E.   High-voltage electric injury.
F.   Inhalation injury or associated trauma.
G.   Other medical conditions which increase medical risk (extremes of age, diabetes, cardiovascular disease).

III.   FLUID RESUSCITATION.
A.   IV hydration mandatory for all burns ≥15% BSA.
B.   Physiologic considerations: Blood volume decreases and edema forms most rapidly during the first 8 hours after thermal injury.
1. These processes decrease over the first postburn day.
2. Capillary permeability begins to return to normal on postburn day 2 and edema resorption begins.

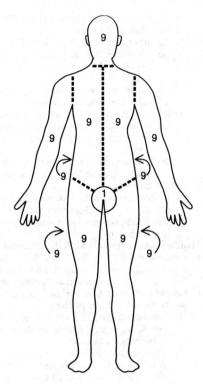

FIG 20-1.
"The rule of nines." Each of the above regions represents approximately 9% of BSA.

 3. Pulmonary edema, while uncommon during initial resuscitation, most often occurs during this resorptive phase (commonly 3–6 days postburn).
C. **IV Fluid Therapy.**
 1. **Duke method of initial resuscitation:**
 a. **Isotonic fluid** (150–160 mEq Na/L) for fluid resuscitation during the first 48 hours postburn.

1) Composition: Add ½ ampule of NaHCO$_3$ to each liter of lactated Ringer's.
2) Administration: Infuse 3 mL/kg/%BSA burn.
   a) Administer ½ of this calculated volume over the first 8 hours postburn (not postadmission).
   b) Administer the remaining ½ of calculated volume over the next 16 hours.
3) Reducing the rate of fluid administration:
   a) Attempt to decrease the infusion rate during the second 24 hours postburn after patient is stable.
   b) Reduce infusion rate by 25% q. 3 h., as tolerated, based on UO and vital signs.

b. **Colloid infusion:**
1) Reserve until capillary permeability returns to normal (i.e., second postburn day).
2) Infuse salt-poor albumin if serum albumin level is <2.5 gm/dL.

2. **Modified Brooke formula for initial resuscitation:**
a. **Lactated Ringer's** for fluid resuscitation during the first 24 hours. Infuse 2 mL/kg/%BSA burn in adults (3 mL/kg/%BSA in children) as described above.
b. **Colloid-containing fluid** for fluid resuscitation during the second 24 hours postburn.
1) Composition: Add 25 g albumin (one ampule) to 500 mL NS to yield a final concentration of 5 g/dL (physiologic concentration).
2) Administration: Estimate plasma volume deficit (based on BSA burn) and replace with the colloid-containing fluid over 24 hours.
   a) 30%–50% BSA burn: Infuse 0.3 mL/kg/% burn.
   b) 50%–70% BSA burn: Infuse 0.4 mL/kg/% burn.
   c) >70% BSA burn: Infuse 0.5 mL/kg/% burn.
3) An electrolyte-free water infusion, in addition to colloid, is utilized to maintain adequate UO.
   a) Administer IV D5W in the adult.
   b) In children, infuse D5 ¼ NS or D5 ½ NS (children tend to develop hyponatremia with D5W infusion).

3. **Estimate insensible fluid losses.** This is important after initial resuscitation (i.e., >48 hours postburn).

   a. Insensible water loss (mL/hr) = (25 + %BSA burn) × total BSA (m^2).

   b. Replace insensible losses with D5W.

   c. Inadequate free water replacement may lead to hypernatremia.

   d. Anticipate a decrease in evaporative losses when open wounds are grafted or covered with a biologic dressing.

4. **Blood replacement:** Transfuse PRBCs to maintain Hct at 30%–35%.

5. **In children,** in addition to calculated resuscitation volume, maintenance fluid may be required.

D. **Adequate fluid resuscitation must be clinically assessed.**

1. **Hourly UO** is the most readily available index of adequate volume resuscitation.

   a. Insert Foley catheter to record output hourly.

   b. Adequate UO is 30–50 mL/hr in an adult (1 mL/kg/hr in children <30 kg in weight).

      1) Low UO is usually prerenal oliguria. ARF is extremely uncommon in burn patients. Administer additional IV fluid as a fluid challenge and adjust maintenance and replacement fluid infusion based on the urine response.

      2) High UO (>75 mL/hr in the adult or >2 mL/kg/hr in the child) indicates overhydration, unless secondary to glucosuria, and necessitates decreasing fluid administration.

2. **The uses of PA (Swan-Ganz) catheterization are limited in the burn patient.** Indications include:

   a. Poor response to adequate volume resuscitation (inadequate UO, poor perfusion, etc.).

   b. Underlying cardiac disease.

   c. Extremes of age.

3. **Measure body weight on admission and every day.**

   a. The first 48 hours postburn: A weight gain of 10%–20% with adequate resuscitation should occur.

   b. After 48 hours: a 1%–2% weight loss occurs every day with return to preburn weight on postburn day 7–10.

4. **The Hct** is not an accurate indicator of adequacy of volume resuscitation.

IV. **CARDIOVASCULAR CONSIDERATIONS.**
A. **Vascular compromise** may occur in full-thickness encircling burns of the extremities because seared tissue will not expand as edema develops. This may lead to vascular insufficiency.
   1. **Signs and symptoms:**
      a. Progressive paresthesia and deep tissue pain.
      b. Cyanosis.
      c. Impaired capillary refill.
   2. **Doppler ultrasonic flow meter** is useful in evaluation because tissue edema may make palpation of pulses difficult. In the upper extremity, examine palmar arch pulses.
   3. **Prevention:**
      a. Elevation of the circumferentially burned limb above the level of the heart will reduce edema. A sling suspended from an IV pole may be used.
      b. Active exercise and muscular contraction for 2–3-minute periods q. 2 h. during the first 24–48 hours postburn may enhance venous return and reduce edema.
   4. **Escharotomy** may be indicated to release compressing eschar. It should be utilized for the following:
      a. Absence of pulsatile arterial flow.
      b. Progressive decrease in pulse on serial examination.
   5. **Technique of escharotomy:**
      a. **Bed side procedure,** performed sterilely.
      b. **No anesthesia necessary** (no sensation in areas of full-thickness burn).
      c. **Using scalpel or electrocautery,** make a mid-medial or midlateral incision, or both, through nonviable eschar (Fig 20–2).
         1) Make incisions only through full-thickness burns.
         2) Proceed from proximal to distal and always incise eschar across involved joints.
         3) Stay anterior to medial epicondyle of the upper extremity to avoid the ulnar nerve.
         4) Incise through the superficial fascia down to, but not through, underlying subcutaneous tissue. Cut eschar edges should separate.
      d. **Distal pulses should return within a few minutes.**
         1) Facilitate venous return by extremity elevation and exercise.

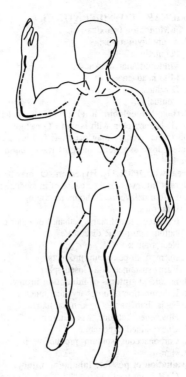

FIG 20-2.
Locations of properly placed escharotomy incisions.

 2) Failure of pulses to return may have several etiologies.
 a) Hypovolemia.
 b) Subfascial edema secondary to electrical or
 deep thermal burn, prolonged ischemia, or
 trauma. Fasciotomy may be needed.
 e. **A topical antimicrobial agent should be applied to
 all escharotomy** (and fasciotomy) **incisions** until
 fully healed (see pp 758, 759, and 764).

V. **PULMONARY CONSIDERATIONS.**
A. **Carbon Monoxide Intoxication.**
    1. **Signs and symptoms:**
        a. Palpitations.
        b. Mild muscular weakness.
        c. Mild headache.
        d. Dizziness.
        e. Confusion.
    2. **Carboxyhemoglobin level** should be determined by ABG. Hemoglobin with bound CO cannot transport O_2 and tissue hypoxia may occur. If CO level >40%, the patient may experience progressive collapse, coma, or death.
    3. **Treat with 100% O_2.** Hyperbaric O_2 may be beneficial.
B. **Inhalation injury** is rarely a cause of immediate hypoxia as onset is often delayed ≥24 hours postburn.
    1. **Risk factors.**
        a. Impaired mental status (ethanol or other drug intoxication, neurologic disease).
        b. Head trauma.
        c. Burns from petroleum products.
        d. Burns sustained in a closed space.
    2. **Signs and symptoms of inhalation injury.**
        a. Inflammation of oropharyngeal mucosa.
        b. Facial burns and singed nasal hair.
        c. Hoarseness, stridor, wheezing, rales.
        d. Unexplained hypoxemia.
        e. Carbonaceous sputum production is most specific sign.
    3. **Evaluation of possible inhalation injury:**
        a. CXR is insensitive.
        b. **Flexible fiberoptic bronchoscopy:**
            1) Perform when hemodynamically stable.
            2) Anesthetize nasal mucosa with topical agents.
            3) Administer 100% O_2 to patient for 3 minutes prior to examination.
            4) **Place an appropriately sized (no. 7 or 8) ET tube over scope prior to examination.** In the event intubation is necessary, the tube can easily be passed into the trachea over the scope.
            5) Signs of inhalation injury include mucosal erythema, edema, blisters, ulcers, hemorrhage, and carbon particles in major airways.

   c. ^{133}Xen perfusion lung scan: Delay in xenon clearance >90 seconds suggests significant inhalation injury.
   d. Follow ABG for evidence of hypoxia and carboxyhemoglobinemia.
4. **Treatment of inhalation injury:**
   a. Administer warm, humidified O_2.
   b. Pulmonary toilet: postural drainage, chest percussion, incentive spirometry, IPPB.
   c. Treat bronchospasm.
   d. Therapeutic bronchoscopy to clear debris.
   e. **Indications for intubation include:**
      1) Progressive hypoxia.
      2) Vocal cord edema threatening airway occlusion as assessed by bronchoscopy. Can usually extubate after several days of edema resorption, approximately postburn day 5.
   f. **Prophylactic steroids** are not beneficial and may increase the risk of infection.
   g. **Prophylactic antibiotics** are not beneficial and may lead to the emergence of resistant strains of bacteria.
   h. High-frequency positive pressure ventilation has reduced the incidence of pneumonia after inhalation injury in early clinical trials.
C. **Circumferential burns of the thorax may mechanically impair ventilation.**
   1. **Signs and symptoms:**
      a. Progressive use of accessory muscles of respiration.
      b. An increase in inspiratory pressures in mechanically ventilated patients is the most common indication for thoracic escharotomy.
      c. Tachypnea.
   2. **Thoracic escharotomy** (see also p 754–755).
      a. Incisions are made in anterior axillary lines bilaterally, extending from clavicle to costal margin (Fig 20–3).
      b. If full-thickness burn involves the anterior abdominal wall, connect the above mentioned escharotomies with a costal margin escharotomy.
D. **Unexpected respiratory depression.** If patient is accepted in transfer from another hospital, consider the possibility that IM or SC narcotics were given at the referring institution and have been systemically absorbed as resuscitation has increased tissue perfusion. Treat with IV naloxone.

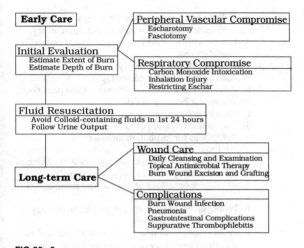

FIG 20–3.
Burn care algorithm.

VI.   WOUND CARE.

A.   Daily **examination** of wound until totally healed.

B.   Daily **gentle cleansing** with a non–alcohol-containing surgical detergent.

C.   **Gentle debridement** of nonviable tissue following cleansing.

   1. Continue to point of pain or bleeding. Administer IV analgesia as needed.
   2. Wash in shower or Hubbard tank but do not immerse.

D.   **Shave the wound** and an adjacent margin of approximately 1 in. Do not shave eyebrows!

E.   Allow wound to air-dry.

F.   **Apply a topical antimicrobial agent q. 12 h.**

   1. **Apply 11.1% mafenide acetate (Sulfamylon).**
      a. Leave wound open (do not apply dressing).
      b. Remove with shower for daily debridement.
      c. Advantages:
         1) Broadest spectrum of antimicrobial activity, especially against *Pseudomonas spp*.
         2) Penetrates eschar well.

      d. Disadvantages and side effects:
         1) Painful in areas of partial-thickness burn.
         2) Hyperchloremic metabolic acidosis due to carbonic anhydrase inhibition.

  2. **Apply 1% silver sulfadiazine (Silvadene).**
    a. Apply topically and leave wound open.
    b. Advantages:
      1) Nontoxic.
      2) Not painful.
    c. Disadvantages:
      1) Less effective penetration of eschar.
      2) Spectrum of antimicrobial activity narrower than mafenide.
      3) Neutropenia resolves with cessation of application.

  3. **Silver nitrate solution 0.5%.**
    a. Apply with multilayered dressings.
    b. Reserve for patients allergic to sulfonamides.
    c. Disadvantages:
      1) Dressings limit joint motion.
      2) Supplemental Na, K, and Ca may be needed.
      3) Poor eschar penetration.
      4) Stains environment.

G. Burn Wound Excision.
  1. **Indications:**
    a. Full-thickness burns.
    b. Patients requiring debridement of high-voltage electric injury.
  2. **Contraindications:**
    a. Hemodynamic instability. Burn excision is accompanied by large volume blood loss. Limit excision to 20% BSA or 2 hours' operative time.
    b. Pulmonary complications.
    c. Superficial partial-thickness injury.
  3. **Excision is performed after resuscitation is complete.**
  4. **Technique:**
    a. Adequate levels of systemic antibiotics prior to excision.
    b. Method:
      1) Tangential "shaving" method.
      2) Excision to fascia.

    c. Control of hemorrhage:
       1) Thrombin- or epinephrine-moistened gauze dressings.
       2) Tourniquet for excision on limb.
       3) IV or subeschar infiltration with vasopressin.
    d. May graft immediately or delay grafting.

H. Biologic Dressings.
  1. **Indications and uses:**
    a. Coverage of freshly excised wounds.
    b. Decreases bacterial proliferation and promotes granulation tissue formation.
    c. May be used to determine readiness of a site for grafting. If biologic dressing "takes" without suppuration, then it is highly likely that skin autografts will remain viable.
    d. Decreases pain of partial-thickness burns and maintains joint mobility.
    e. Decreases evaporative water loss.
  2. **Types of biologic dressings:**
    a. **Human cutaneous allografts** are dressing of choice. Donor must be minimal risk, documented HIV-seronegative.
    b. **Porcine xenografts:**
       1) Readily available.
       2) Less effective than allografts in decreasing bacterial proliferation.
    c. **Bilaminate synthetic dressing:**
       1) Use only when allo- or xenografts are not available.
       2) Ineffective in decreasing bacterial proliferation.
  3. **Technique:**
    a. Reapply new dressings q. 3–5 d.
    b. Remove and replace more frequently if suppuration occurs between wound and dressing.

I. Burn Wound Infection.
  1. **Signs of burn wound infection:**
    a. Intraeschar hemorrhage (black or dark hemorrhagic discoloration) is the most common sign but may be secondary to minor trauma.
    b. Conversion of a partial-thickness burn to full-thickness injury is pathognomonic.

    c. Erythema and edema at wound edges.

    d. Degeneration of granulation tissue.

    e. Marked subeschar suppuration.

    f. Premature or unexpected eschar separation.

    g. Hemorrhagic fat necrosis.

    h. Metastatic abscesses in unburned skin (ecthyma gangrenosum).

    i. Vesicular lesions on healing partial-thickness burns suggest viral infection.

2. **Diagnosis of burn wound infection:**

    a. Surface culture is unreliable.

    b. **Wound biopsy** is method of choice.

      1) Perform if signs of infection are present.

      2) Biopsy viable tissue subjacent or adjacent to burn wound.

      3) Excise a 500-mg lenticular portion of tissue.

      4) Divide this tissue sample in half.

        a) Send half of sample for culture and sensitivity. If $\geq 10^5$ organisms per gram of tissue, suggestive but not diagnostic of infection (possibility of surface colonization).

        b) Send half of sample for histologic examination. Place in 10% formalin for rapid processing, or examine by frozen section. Invasive infection is present if bacteria are detected in unburned tissue adjacent to wound.

3. **Treatment of documented bacterial wound infection:**

    a. **Change topical antimicrobial agent** to mafenide.

    b. **Administer systemic antibiotics** based on sensitivities of offending organisms.

    c. **Inject antibiotics** into infected wound below eschar.

      1) Especially useful in treatment of focal pseudomonal infections.

      2) Use prior to excision of infected wound to reduce bacteremia.

      3) Technique:

        a) One-half daily dose of semisynthetic penicillin (Piperacillin) in 150–1,000 mL NS q. 12 h.

        b) Inject beneath eschar using a no. 20 spinal needle to minimize number of injection sites.

    d. **Excise all infected tissue.**
      1) Adequate blood levels of antibiotics should be present prior to excision.
      2) Debride infected tissue. Amputation may be necessary.
      3) Cover immediately with a biologic dressing.
  4. **Nonbacterial burn wound infection.**
    a. *Candida* frequently colonizes but rarely causes invasive infection. May require systemic therapy with amphotericin B with or without 5-fluorocytosine if fungemia occurs.
    b. Treat HSV with systemic ara-A or acyclovir.

VII. COMPLICATIONS.
A. GI Complications.
  1. **Curling's ulcer:**
    a. May progress to hemorrhage or perforation and can be a life-threatening complication.
    b. Preventive therapy: Maintain gastric pH >5.
      1) H_2 blockers (cimetidine, ranitidine).
      2) Early feeding and antacids (30 mL q. 1–2 h. prn pH < 5).
  2. **Ileus** is almost always present in burns ≥20% BSA.
    a. Usually resolves spontaneously 2–3 days postinjury.
    b. Treat with NG suction, IV fluids.
  3. **Acalculous cholecystitis:**
    a. Usually causes RUQ pain and jaundice.
    b. Diagnosis is confirmed using abdominal ultrasound.
    c. Cholecystectomy is indicated if distended gallbladder is detected by ultrasonography.
  4. **Superior mesenteric artery syndrome:** usually occurs after significant weight loss.

B. Respiratory Complications.
Pneumonia is the most common infectious complication in burn patients. It is most commonly due to *Staphylococcus aureus* and gram-negative bacteria. Pneumonia due to hematogenous spread of organisms can occur with wound infection. This usually occurs late in the hospital course (>7 days postburn). Other sources include infected veins, soft tissue abscesses, perforated viscus.

C. Suppurative Thrombophlebitis.
  1. **Local signs** are present in less than half of patients with suppurative thrombophlebitis.

a. Maintain a high index of suspicion in a septic patient without an identifiable source of infection.

b. Every previously cannulated vein is a potential site for infection.

2. **Exploration of vein:**

a. Recovery of normal-appearing blood from the vein is a negative result.

b. Intraluminal pus confirms the diagnosis.

c. Excise veins which contain intraluminal clot.

1) Send one segment for histologic examination.

2) Send another segment for culture and sensitivity.

3. **Treatment:**

a. IV antibiotics.

b. Total surgical removal of infected vein.

4. **Prevention:** Change all IV catheters, including central lines, at least q. 72 h.

D. **Acute bacterial endocarditis.** Right heart involvement is most common, but all valves can be affected.

VIII. NUTRITION.

A. **Enteric tube feeding** is usually necessary initially. Diarrhea can be controlled by reducing the caloric density of feedings and with paragoric.

B. **Avoid TPN** if possible as there is a high risk of catheter-related sepsis.

C. **Caloric and protein requirements** based on %BSA burn and preburn weight. For patients with >40% total BSA burn:

1. 2,000–2,200 calories per total BSA (m^2) per day.

2. 12–18 g nitrogen per total BSA (m^2)/per day.

IX. SPECIAL CONSIDERATIONS.

A. **Electric Injury.**

1. **Arrhythmias** are common, especially asystole and ventricular fibrillation.

a. ACLS as needed.

b. Indications for continuous cardiac monitoring (≥48 hours):

1) Loss of consciousness.

2) Abnormal ECG.

2. **Associated skeletal fractures are common.**

a. Falls are often associated with the electric injury (e.g., falls from high-voltage towers).

b. Current-induced muscle contractions may cause vertebral fractures. Radiographs must exclude cervical spine injury.

3. **Vascular damage must be excluded.**
   a. Electric current may damage the intima producing thrombosis and hemorrhage.
   b. Arteriography may be useful to determine extent of tissue damage, and level for amputation.

4. **Renal damage** secondary to hemochromogens (hemoglobin and myoglobin) is common. May also occur with burn-associated crush injuries.
   a. **Prevention:**
      1) Increase infusion of IV fluids. Maintain UO of 1 mL/kg/hr until no hemochromogens are present in urine.
      2) If excretion of hemochromogens continues or there is risk of hypervolemia:
         a) Mannitol 25 g IV bolus, up to 300 g q. 24 h. prevents tubular deposition of pigment.
         b) IV NaHCO$_3$ to keep the urine pH >6.0. Alkalinization facilitates hemochromogen excretion.

5. **Neurologic damage includes spinal cord deficits.**
   a. Early-appearing deficits may be transient.
   b. Late-appearing deficits are generally permanent.

6. **Cataract formation** occurs days to months after head or neck electric injury.

7. **Wound care.**
   a. **Fasciotomy.**
      1) Indications:
         a) Cyanosis and impaired distal capillary refill.
         b) Hard stony muscle to palpation.
         c) Progressively diminishing or absent pulses by Doppler ultrasound.
         d) Compartment pressure by wick catheter of >30 mm Hg.
      2) Technique:
         a) Perform in OR.
         b) Incise fascia of each involved muscle compartment.
         c) If distal pulses do not return after compartment release, amputation may be indicated.

b. **Operative debridement:**
1) Delay until resuscitation is complete.
2) Debride all necrotic tissue; amputate if necessary.
3) Pack wound open.
4) Reexplore wound 24–72 hours later.
  a) Carry out further debridement, if necessary.
  b) If all necrotic tissue has been removed, close wound by skin approximation or by grafting.
c. Inspect wound daily with further debridement as necessary.

B. Chemical Burns.
1. **Initial treatment:**
  a. Remove all involved clothing.
  b. Flush with large amounts of water. Do not search for specific neutralizing agents. Chemicals burn continuously until washed off.
  c. IV fluid resuscitation: Extent and depth of chemical burn wound are often underestimated.
2. **Agents for which specific therapy is indicated:**
  a. **Hydrofluoric acid:**
    1) Prolonged irrigation with benzalkonium chloride or application of calcium gluconate gel.
    2) Local injection of 10% calcium gluconate into damaged tissue for treatment of severe pain.
    3) Treat hypocalcemia as necessary.
  b. **Phenol:**
    1) Initial water lavage.
    2) Wash with lipophilic solvent (polyethylene glycol, propylene glycol, glycerol) to remove residual phenol.
  c. **White phosphorus:**
    1) Irrigate wound with saline.
    2) Cover with moist gauze dressing to prevent ignition.
    3) 0.5%–1.0% copper sulfate wash followed by copious irrigation will turn retained particles blue-gray. This facilitates identification of particles, and impedes ignition.
  d. **Tar and bitumen burns:**
    1) Cool the hot material with cold water.
    2) Wound care:
      a) Do *not* remove material with petroleum-based solvent.

b) Cover with petrolatum-based ointment and dress daily.

3. **Treatment of chemical eye injury:**
    a. Continuous irrigation with water for at least 30 minutes.
    b. Topical antimicrobial agent.
    c. Cycloplegic eye drops to decrease synechia formation.
    d. Lubricant ointments without eye patches.
    e. Monitor intraocular pressure daily.
    f. Early consultation with ophthalmologist.

SELECTED REFERENCES

McManus WF, Pruitt BA Jr: Thermal injuries, in Mattox KL, Moore EV, Feliciano DV (eds): *Trauma*. Norwalk Conn, Appleton & Lange, 1988.

Moylan JA: Burn injury, in Moylan JA (ed): *Trauma Surgery*, ed 2. Philadelphia, JB Lippincott Co, 1991.

Pruitt BA Jr: The burn patient. I. Initial care. II. Later care and complications of thermal injury. *Curr Probl Surg* 1979; 16:

Pruitt BA Jr, Goodwin CW Jr: Thermal injuries, in Davis JH (ed): *Clinical Surgery*, vols 1, 2. St. Louis, CV Mosby Co, 1987.

Pruitt BA Jr, Goodwin CW Jr, Pruitt SK: Burns: Including cold, chemical and electrical injuries, in Sabiston DC Jr (ed): *Textbook of Surgery*, ed 14. Philadelphia, WB Saunders Co, 1991.

Waymack J, Pruitt BA Jr: Burn wound care. *Adv Surg* 1990; 23:261.

ANESTHETIC MANAGEMENT

21

I. INDUCTION AGENTS

A. Barbiturates.

1. Barbiturates such as thiopental and methohexital are the drugs most commonly used for induction. These drugs have several actions in the CNS such as depression of the reticular activating system, decreasing the release of excitatory neurotransmitters, and decreasing the dissociation rate of γ-aminobutyric acid (GABA).

2. CNS effects occur within 30 seconds and, although they have long T½ (hours), rapid awakening occurs because of rapid redistribution to tissues such as skeletal muscle and fat. Elimination depends almost entirely upon metabolism by liver and kidneys.

3. The typical induction dose of thiopental is 3–4 mg/kg and methohexital, 0.7–1.0 mg/kg (Table 21-1).

B. Etomidate.

1. Injection of etomidate produces an anesthetized state within 30 seconds and is followed by prompt awakening because of almost complete hydrolysis to inactive metabolites.

2. Etomidate produces less cardiovascular instability than do the barbiturates. There is less direct myocardial depression, and BP decreases are attenuated.

3. Although etomidate reduces cerebral blood flow, cerebral O_2 metabolism, and intracranial pressure, making it a useful drug for patients with an increased intracranial pressure or space-occupying lesion, it also activates seizure foci.

4. Etomidate supresses adrenocortical function for up to 8 hours following an induction dose.

TABLE 21–1.

Induction Agents

	Induction Dose (mg/kg)	Elimination Half-Life (hr)
Barbiturates		
Thiopental	3–4	
Methohexital	0.7–1.0	4
Etomidate	0.2–0.3	
Ketamine	1–3	3
Propofol	1.5–3.0	

    5. IV injection of etomidate is painful and causes involuntary skeletal muscle movements.

    6. The typical induction dose of etomidate is 0.2–0.3 mg/kg.

C. Ketamine.

    1. Ketamine produces a dissociative state of anesthesia in < 60 seconds following IV administration. It is less likely to produce apnea than the barbiturates. The eyes usually remain open with uncoordinated movements, and skeletal muscle tone is maintained (there may even be purposeful movements and phonation). There is, however, analgesia and amnesia.

    2. The sympathetic nervous system is activated causing an increase in HR and BP which makes it an ideal agent for hypovolemic patients. These effects may not be seen in chronically stressed patients who are catecholamine-depleted; in fact, the opposite may occur since ketamine is a direct myocardial depressant.

    3. Because of its sympathetic nervous system activation, ketamine should be used judiciously in patients with coronary artery disease or vascular aneurysms.

    4. **Ketamine is a potent cerebral vasodilator and is contraindicated in patients with an increased intracranial pressure or a space-occupying lesion.**

    5. Emergence delirium and hallucinations may occur in up to 30% of patients. Although benzodiazepines reduce this response, it is probably best to avoid this drug in patients with psychiatric disorders.

    6. Ketamine is very useful in the SICU for short painful procedures such as dressing changes or wound irrigation.

7. The typical induction dose is 1–3 mg/kg IV. Although its T½ is 3 hours, its redistribution to inactive tissues allows awakening in 10–15 minutes following a single IV dose.

8. There is an increase in oral secretions so pretreatment with an antisialagogue (glycopyrrolate 0.1–0.2 mg IV or IM or atropine 0.2 mg IV or IM) is recommended when intubation is not planned.

D. Propofol.

1. Propofol has recently been approved for use in the United States. Its pharmacologic profile is similar to that of thiopental with a rapid (< 30 seconds) onset of anesthesia followed by awakening in 4–6 minutes.

2. The circulatory and ventilatory depressant effects are similar to thiopental; however, there is much less residual sedation as well as less nausea and vomiting with propofol.

3. The typical induction dose is 1.5–3.0 mg/kg.

II. BENZODIAZEPINES.

A. Indications

Benzodiazepines are used routinely in the SICU setting for their anxiolytic and sedative properties, and are also frequently used as anticonvulsants, for amnesia, and for skeletal muscle relaxation. In higher doses they may be used for anesthesia induction, but their onset is not as rapid as other induction agents.

B. Mechanism of Action and Specific Agents.

1. The main mechanism of action of benzodiazepines is related to accumulation of the inhibitory neurotransmitter GABA. There are also specific benzodiazepine receptors on postsynaptic nerve endings in the CNS which enhance the inhibitory actions of GABA.

2. The most commonly used benzodiazepines are diazepam (Valium) and midazolam (Versed). The drugs are highly lipid-soluble in vivo which accounts for their rapid onset of action (2–3 minutes following IV dose). The action of both drugs is terminated by redistribution, and midazolam is rapidly metabolized by the liver (T½ 1–4 hours) into inactive metabolites. In contrast, diazepam has a much longer T½ (20–40 hours), and several of its metabolites are pharmacologically active (particularily des-

methyldiazepam), contributing to a prolonged effect of diazepam as compared with midazolam.

3. Sedation can be achieved with midazolam in doses of 0.02–0.08 mg/kg IV and with diazepam in doses of 0.03–0.10 mg/kg IV (Table 21-2).

C. **Complications.**

1. Cardiovascular effects of benzodiazepines are minimal when used by themselves.

2. Respiratory effects are also usually minimal when low doses are used; however, **profound respiratory depression may occur when these drugs are given in large doses, in combination with a narcotic, in patients with an abnormal ventilatory drive, or in chronically ill or elderly patients.** Their use, particularly in the SICU, should be carefully monitored.

3. **Withdrawal may be seen if benzodiazepines are abruptly discontinued after prolonged administration.**

4. Flumazenil is a specific benzodiazepine antagonist that also acts in the CNS and has almost no untoward side effects. Flumazenil has not been approved for use in the United States.

III. OPIOIDS.

A. **Effects of Opioids.**

1. Mechanism of action:

   a. Opioids are frequently utilized in the SICU, particularily for their analgesic and sedative properties. When used alone they do not reliably produce unconsciousness or anesthesia.

   b. The most commonly used opioids in the SICU are morphine, meperidine, fentanyl, and sufentanil. They all act as agonists at specific opioid receptors which are normally activated by endorphins.

TABLE 21–2.

Benzodiazepines

Drug	Induction Dose (mg/kg)	Sedative Dose (mg/kg)	Half-Life (hr)
Diazepam	0.3–0.4	0.03–0.10	20–40
Midazolam	0.15–0.35	0.02–0.08	1–4

c. Several different classes of receptors exist; mu receptors appear to play the greatest role in the brain, while delta and kappa receptors are dominant in the spinal cord.

d. Opioids are mainly metabolized in the liver and excreted through the kidneys. All have large volumes of distribution, and elimination $T\frac{1}{2}$ is largely determined by lipid solubility. The potency of these drugs varies widely, and analgesia is best achieved by incremental doses (Table 21–3).

2. Hemodynamic effects:

a. Cardiovascular effects of opioids are minimal in supine, normovolemic patients, but reductions in SVR caused by all narcotics may result in orthostatic hypotension. Venous pooling may exaggerate the hypotensive effects of hypovolemia.

b. Morphine and meperidine, but not fentanyl, can cause histamine release which can reduce SVR.

c. Stimulation of the central vagal nuclei by all opioids except meperidine causes bradycardia.

3. Complications:

a. Opioids cause a dose-dependent respiratory depression by decreasing the sensitivity of the CO_2 response. Minute ventilation is reduced mainly as a function of respiratory rate as TV may increase slightly. Decreased minute ventilation can also be caused by opioid-induced skeletal muscle rigidity.

b. These drugs stimulate smooth muscle which can cause urinary retention, constipation, and biliary colic.

TABLE 21–3.

Intravenous Opioids

Drug Life (hr)	Relative Potency	Analgesic Dose (mg/kg)	PCA (mg)*	Half-Life (hr)
Morphine	1	0.05–0.20	0.5–3.0	3–4
Meperidine	1/10	0.5–2.0	5–30	3–4
Fentanyl	100	0.001–0.002	0.01–0.08	4–7
Sufentanil	500		0.002–0.01	2–3
Alfentanil	20		0.05–0.30	1–2

*PCA = patient-controlled analgesia.

c. Direct stimulation of the chemoreceptor trigger zone causes nausea and vomiting.

d. **Withdrawal may be seen if opioids are abruptly stopped after prolonged administration.**

4. Regional administration: Subarachnoid, epidural, and caudal opioids in low doses have been used for postoperative analgesia (Table 21–4). They must be used cautiously, however, as delayed respiratory depression (6–24 hours) may occur as a consequence of their cephalad spread to the respiratory inhibitory centers near the fourth ventricle.

B. **Naloxone.**

1. Naloxone is used to reverse the receptor-mediated effects of the opioids.

2. Although the amount of naloxone needed is dependent on the total narcotic given, it should be carefully titrated in IV doses of ≤0.04 mg in adults.

3. The onset of action is 1–2 minutes following IV injection and may last for 30–60 minutes.

4. **Since many narcotics have a longer duration of action, all patients who require narcotic reversal warrant close observation. Abrupt reversal of analgesia and onset of postsurgical pain caused by overdosage may cause profound elevations in HR and BP. Acute pulmonary edema and ventricular arrhythmias may accompany this reaction.**

5. In patients with preexisting cardiac or pulmonary disease, ventilatory support until the undesirable narcotic effects are gone may be preferable to naloxone antagonism.

6. Naloxone may be used to reverse respiratory depression following epidural administration of narcotics.

IV. NEUROMUSCULAR BLOCKING AGENTS.

A. Neuromuscular blocking agents (relaxants) are commonly used in the SICU. These drugs interrupt the action of acetylcholine (Ach). They are used to facilitate tracheal intubation, provide optimal surgical conditions, decrease O_2 metabolism in critically ill patients (where increased O_2 consumption by muscle contraction is detrimental), and facilitate mechanical ventilation. **They do not provide anesthetic or analgesic effects and must be used in conjunction with other agents (opioids, benzodiazepines). Also, me-**

TABLE 21-4.
Neuroaxial Opioids

Drug	Epidural			Subarachnoid		
	Dose (mg)	Duration (hr)	Onset (min)	Dose (mg)	Duration (hr)	Onset (min)
Morphine	4–5	12–24	20	0.5–1.0	18–48	10
Meperidine	100	4–20	5	10–30	?–48	5
Fentanyl	0.1	2–4	5	0.025	3–6	5

chanical ventilation must be instituted when these drugs are used secondary to paralysis of the respiratory muscles.

B. **Mechanism of Action and Specific Agents.**

1. Mechanism of action:

   Neuromuscular blocking agents structurally resemble ACh. Succinylcholine is actually two molecules of ACh linked by methyl groups, and while nondepolarizing muscle relaxants are bulky molecules, they also contain portions similar to ACh. All contain at least one positively charged quaternary ammonium group which is important for its attraction to the negatively charged cholinergic receptor.

2. Depolarizing neuromuscular blocking agents:

   a. The only clinically used depolarizing neuromuscular blocker is succinylcholine, which mimics the action of ACh and depolarizes the postjunctional membrane.

   b. Metabolism of succinylcholine occurs via hydrolysis by plasma cholinesterase. Because this enzyme is not present at the neuromuscular junction, succinylcholine must diffuse into the ECF in order for its action to be terminated.

   c. *Sustained depolarization caused by succinylcholine causes ion channels to remain open producing an elevation in serum potassium of approximately 0.5 mEq/L. Therefore, succinylcholine should not be used in patients in whom this rise in potassium would be detrimental such as those with ARF or with diseases which produce abnormal numbers or function of the neuromuscular junction (e.g., burns or spinal cord injuries).*

   d. Patients with atypical plasma cholinesterase will have a prolonged neuromuscular block following succinylcholine administration.

3. Nondepolarizing neuromuscular blocking agents:

   a. Commonly used nondepolarizing neuromuscular blocking agents can be divided into long-acting (pancuronium) and intermediate-acting (vecuronium and atracurium) agents.

   b. These drugs compete with ACh for binding sites on the postjunctional receptor, depolarization does not occur, and muscle paralysis ensues. They are highly ionized at physiologic pH and do not cross the blood-brain barrier, placenta, or other lipid membranes.

c. Their actions are mainly terminated by redistribution and they are subsequently metabolized by the liver (pancuronium, vecuronium), kidneys (pancuronium), or Hofmann elimination (atracurium).

d. Commonly used doses and duration are given in Table 21–5.

4. Reversal of neuromuscular blockade.

a. Antagonism of nondepolarizing neuromuscular blockade is achieved by administration of anticholinesterases such as neostigmine 0.05–0.07 mg/kg IV and edrophonium 0.5–1.0 mg/kg IV (see Table 21–5).

b. These agents inhibit the action of acetylcholinesterase leading to an increase in ACh which competes with the neuromuscular blockers for receptor sites at the neuromuscular junction.

c. These drugs also increase the amount of ACh at the cholinergic muscarinic receptors which causes peripheral effects such as bradycardia and salivation, which may be attenuated by the coadministration of atropine 0.2–0.4 mg IV or IM or glycopyrrolate 0.1–0.2 mg IV or IM.

I. LOCAL ANESTHETICS.
A. Mechanism of Action.

1. Local anesthetics (LAs) (Tables 21–6 and 21–7) produce nerve impulse conduction blockade by acting at specific receptor sites in the nerve membrane which prevent increases in sodium permeability caused by an action potential.

2. The sites of action are receptors located on the inner portion of the sodium channel; therefore, the uncharged LA must diffuse through the cell membrane before binding to the receptor in the ionized form, explaining why LAs are ineffective with local tissue acidosis, as caused by infections.

B. Specific Agents.

1. LAs are comprised of an aromatic portion (lipophilic) connected to a tertiary amine portion (hydrophilic) through either an ester or an amide bond. The differences between these two classes form the basis for their differences in metabolism and adverse effects.

TABLE 21–5.
Neuromuscular Blocking Agents

Type	Dose (mg/kg)	Onset (min)	Infusion (µg/kg/min)	Duration (min)	Metabolism
Depolarizing					
Succinylcholine	0.6–2.0	0.5–1.0		5–10	Plasma cholinesterase
Nondepolarizing					
Pancuronium	0.04–0.1	3–5		60–100	80% renal
Vecuronium	0.1	3–5	1	25–40	80% hepatic
Atracurium	0.3–0.5	3–5	6–8	25–40	Hofmann elimination
Anticholinesterases					
Neostigmine	0.3–0.6	5–7		55–75	
Edrophonium	0.5–1.0	1		40–65	

TABLE 21-6.
Local Anesthetics

	Relative Potency	Onset	Maximum Recommended Dose (mg)		Toxic Plasma Concentration (μg/kg)	Concentration (%)	Infiltration Duration (hr)	
			Plain	With Epinephrine			Plain	With Epinephrine
Esters								
Procaine	1	Slow	400	600		0.5–1.0	0.25–0.5	0.5–1.0
Chloroprocaine	4	Rapid	800	1000		0.5–1.0	0.25–0.5	0.5–1.0
Tetracaine	16	Slow	100	200				
Amides								
Lidocaine	1	Rapid	300	500	5	0.5–1.0	0.5–2.0	1–4.0
Bupivacaine	4	Slow	175	225	1.5	0.5–1.0	2–4	4–8.0
Etidocaine	4	Slow	300	400	2			

TABLE 21–7.
Neuroaxial Local Anesthetics

	Epidural			Subarachnoid		
Drug	Concentration	Duration (hr)	Dose (mL)	Concentration	Duration (hr)	Dose (mg)
Procaine				5% in 5% glucose	0.5–1.0	120
Chloroprocaine	2%–3%	0.5–1.0	40 (2%)			
Tetracaine				5% in 5% glucose	1.5–2.0	12
Tetracaine with epinephrine				5% in 5% glucose	3–5	12
Lidocaine	1%–2%	0.75–1.5	50 (1%)	5% in 7.5% glucose	0.5–1.0	60
Bupivacaine	0.25%–0.50%	2–4	45 (0.5%)	0.75% in 8.25% glucose	1.5–2.0	9

2. Metabolism of ester LAs is hydrolysis by cholinesterase; therefore, the plasma $T^{1}/_{2}$ is very short. However one of the metabolites, para-aminobenzoic acid, is an allergen in some patients.

3. Amide LAs undergo initial dealkylation followed by hydrolysis in the liver, and the elimination half-lives are 2–3 hours. Patients with liver disease are more susceptible to toxic reactions with amide LAs.

4. Different LAs have different potencies (within classes), rapidity of onset, and duration. Addition of epinephrine (1:200,000) produces local vasoconstriction which slows systemic absorption and thus prolongs the anesthetic effect.

C. **Toxicity of Local Anesthetic Agents.**

1. Toxicity of LAs is directly related to an elevated plasma concentration which is usually due to accidental intravascular injection but which may result from systemic absorption from the injection site. CNS and cardiovascular toxic reactions are the most pronounced.

2. Early CNS changes include restlessness, dizziness, vertigo, circumoral numbness, and slurred speech. With additional LAs given or continued absorption, generalized seizures occur and may be followed by profound CNS depression, apnea, cardiovascular collapse, and death.

   a. Treatment of CNS toxicity is to stop the drug, hyperventilate with 100% O_2, and treat seizures with incremental doses of diazepam 0.1 mg/kg IV or thiopental 0.5–2.0 mg/kg IV.

   b. If this is ineffective, neuromuscular blockade and ET intubation are indicated.

3. In low doses, LAs such as lidocaine are used to treat arrhythmias by decreasing the automaticity of ectopic pacemaker foci and increasing the fibrillatory threshold of ventricular myocardium. In high doses, however, hypotension occurs owing to the relaxation of arteriolar smooth muscle. Moreover, normal cardiac automaticity and conduction is impaired causing a wide QRS complex and a prolonged PR interval. Treatment of hypotension centers on fluid administration, vasoconstrictors, and inotropic agents.

4. **Bupivacaine is especially cardiotoxic** and its intravascular injection may result in profound hypotension, intract-

able ventricular arrhythmias, and complete heart block.

    a. Cardiac arrhythmias caused by bupivacaine are especially difficult to treat because of extensive tissue binding.

    b. **Prolonged CPR is indicated in this setting since the toxic effects will subside as the drug redistributes.**

VI. REGIONAL ANESTHESIA.

A. Spinal Anesthesia.

  1. Regional anesthetic techniques have become increasingly popular for a wide variety of clinical situations ranging from sole anesthetic for a certain procedure, as an adjunct to a general anesthetic, or as a mechanism for providing postoperative analgesia.

  2. Subarachnoid (spinal) anesthesia is one of the simplest regional techniques used. The most commonly used drugs are lidocaine (30–60-minute duration), tetracaine (90–120-minute duration), and bupivacaine (90–120-minute duration). The duration of tetracaine can be increased two- or threefold by the addition of epinephrine 0.2 mg (see Table 21–7).

  3. Postoperative analgesia can be provided by the addition of morphine 0.6–1.0 mg or fentanyl 0.05–0.10 mg. Intrathecal narcotics are especially useful in attenuating upper abdominal and thoracotomy incisional pain and decreasing the respiratory compromise secondary to splinting which usually accompanies these incisions.

  4. **The possibility of opioid-induced delayed respiratory depression must be appreciated. It can be reversed with naloxone.**

B. Epidural Anesthesia.

  1. Local anesthetics (Table 21–7):

    a. The LA is placed in the epidural space, typically in the lumbar region, by a single injection or through a catheter placed for repeated injections. The site of action are the spinal nerve roots. Doses necessary to produce anesthesia are larger, and the potential for toxic reactions exists.

    b. Chlorprocaine and bupivacaine are most commonly used.

    c. The initial dose of LA can be estimated by giving 1.0 mL of LA solution per spinal segment to be anesthetized plus 0.1 mL of solution for every 2 in. above 5 ft in patient height. This dose should be reduced by approximately 50% in the elderly and 25% in pregnant patients.

   d. Additional "top up" doses should be given in anticipation of a waning block and should be approximately 50% of the initial dose. Alternatively, an infusion can be used to maintain a constant level.

2. Narcotics:

   a. Similar to subarachnoid blocks, opioids can be given in the epidural space for postoperative analgesia (see Table 21–4).

   b. Morphine 4–5 mg can provide postoperative analgesia for 12–24 hours, while fentanyl 0.10 mg can persist for 2–4 hours.

   c. Neuroaxial opioids, while providing excellent analgesia and more normal pulmonary mechanics following upper abdominal and thoracotomy incisions, have the **potential to produce delayed respiratory depression** which should be treated with naloxone.

   d. **In patients requiring heparin anticoagulation there is a risk of epidural hematoma following epidural anesthesia.**

C. **Nerve Blocks.**

1. Peripheral nerve blocks can also be used for intraoperative anesthesia and postoperative analgesia.

2. Brachial plexus blocks are widely used for procedures on the upper extremity. In addition to providing surgical anesthesia, the sympathetic block is useful in increasing blood flow to the extremity which is very important following some vascular surgical procedures such as digit reimplantation.

3. Intercostal blocks are another commonly used peripheral nerve block.

   a. They are usually performed with the patient in the lateral or supine position to facilitate access to the nerve approximately 8–10 cm from the posterior midline.

   b. The neurovascular bundle is located in the inferior groove of the rib, and the nerve can be blocked with 5 mL of an LA solution.

   c. Multiple segments can be blocked to provide postoperative thoracotomy analgesia.

4. Other peripheral nerve blocks such as ankle blocks and femoral-sciatic nerve blocks are less common but are useful in selected situations.

III. ACUTE PAIN MANAGEMENT.

One of the most common, most frustrating, and most important problems in the SICU is the treatment of acute postoperative pain and chronic pain in selected patients. There are many different chemical mediators of pain (e.g., substance P, serotonin, prostaglandins, cholecystokinin) and many different pain receptors and pathways that lead to the clinical perception of pain. Many pain syndromes can be treated effectively by drugs.

A. Narcotics.

The mainstay in the treatment of acute postoperative pain has been systemic (IV, IM) narcotics. Mixed agonist-antagonist drugs such as butorphanol have also been used and are favored by some because of their apparent attenuation of respiratory depression.

B. Epidural Anesthesia.

1. More recently, epidural and subarachnoid narcotics have been used to treat acute pain. Kappa and delta opioid receptors are present in the spinal cord and can block afferent pain transmission. Theoretically, neuroaxial opioids would provide analgesia while avoiding respiratory depression and preserving pulmonary function. However, delayed respiratory depression, pruritus, nausea and vomiting, and urinary retention can occur with this route of delivery.

2. While epidural narcotics are most commonly employed because of the ease of repeat dosing and lack of dural puncture, single-dose subarachnoid narcotics are used in conjunction with local anesthetics to provide both surgical anesthesia and postoperative analgesia.

3. With epidural narcotics at therapeutic doses, morphine (which is water-soluble) is more likely to cause respiratory depression than is fentanyl (which is more lipid-soluble and thus less diffusion to the CSF occurs).

C. Patient-Controlled Analgesia.

1. A newer route of narcotic delivery which has rapidly gained widespread acceptance and popularity is patient-controlled analgesia (PCA). Since individual variations in

pharmacokinetics and pharmacodynamics make it difficult to predict the amount of narcotic needed to produce
analgesia, the patient is allowed to titrate the narcotic to
his own end point.

2. PCA is provided by an initial dose (which may be repeated) prescribed by a physician, and the patient is allowed to give himself subsequent bolus doses after a pre-
set "lockout" interval between doses. Newer PCA pumps
also allow a continuous background narcotic infusion to
be given in addition to bolus dosing.

3. Although not yet fully evaluated, many studies have reported a greater degree of patient analgesia, lower total
dose of narcotic used (compared with intermittent IV bolus dosing), a higher activity level, and a decreased
length of hospital stay.

SELECTED REFERENCES

Barash PG, Cullen BF, Stoelting RK (eds): *Clinical Anesthesia.*
Philadelphia, JB Lippincott Co, 1989.

Fireston LL, Lebowitz PW, Cook CE (eds): *Clinical Anesthesia
Procedures of the Massachusetts General Hospital,* ed 3. Boston, Little, Brown & Co, 1988.

Stoelting RK, Dierdorf SF: *Anesthesia and Co-Existing Disease.*
New York, Churchill Livingstone Inc, 1983.

Stoelting RK, Miller RD: *Basics of Anesthesia,* ed 2. New York,
Churchill Livingstone Inc, 1989.

PROCEDURES 22

I. CENTRAL VENOUS CATHETERIZATION.
A. Indications.
1. Access to the central venous circulation is frequently required for administration of fluids, vasoactive drugs, drugs that irritate veins, and TPN.
2. To obtain vascular access when peripheral access is poor.
3. Hemodialysis.
4. Plasmapheresis.
5. Access to the central venous compartment and right heart for physiologic monitoring.

B. General Approach.
1. Central venous cannulation is performed as a sterile procedure, requiring adequate preparation, including the following supplies: 18-gauge needle and guidewire (several centimeters longer than the catheter to be placed); catheter (single-, double-, or triple-lumen) or 8F introducer-sheath combination; povidone-iodine solution; cap, mask, sterile gloves, sterile towels; lidocaine (1% solution without epinephrine).
2. Prior to placement, obtain a CXR for comparison with subsequent films.
3. For internal jugular vein and subclavian vein cannulation, the patient should be supine, in the Trendelenburg position (15 degrees), so as to distend the veins and to reduce the incidence of air embolism. Turn the patient's head away from the desired side of cannulation.
4. Don cap, mask, and sterile gloves; prepare the skin with povidone-iodine solution; drape the field with sterile towels. Determine the length for catheter placement (catheter tip in the SVC) by measuring from the point of insertion to the angle of Louis (Fig 22–1).

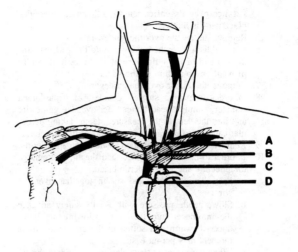

FIG 22–1.
Superficial anatomic landmarks used to determine the depth of central venous catheters. *(A)* Sternoclavicular joint—subclavian vein. *(B)* Manubrium—brachiocephalic vein. *(C)* Angle of Louis—SVC. *(D)* 5 cm inferior to Angle of Louis—RA. (From: Intravenous techniques, in *Textbook of Advanced Cardiac Life Support*. Dallas, American Heart Association, 1987, p 148. Used by permission.)

C. **Seldinger Technique.**
   The Seldinger (guidewire) technique is preferable to the catheter-over-needle technique and may be used for central venous as well as arterial access.
   1. Infiltrate the desired area with lidocaine.
   2. Puncture the skin with the 18-gauge needle mounted on a 10-mL syringe, maintaining constant negative pressure; advance slowly until blood appears.
   3. Upon entering the vein, disengage the syringe and cover the needle with a sterile gloved finger in order to minimize bleeding and to prevent air embolism.
   4. Insert the wire through the needle and advance slowly into the vein. **The wire must pass with minimal re**

        sistance over its entire length, otherwise improper placement is likely.

5. Remove the needle over the guidewire.
6. Pass a dilator over the guidewire into the vein, **retaining control of the guidewire at all times in order to prevent embolization of the wire.**
7. Remove the dilator over the guidewire.
8. In order to pass a single-, double-, or triple-lumen catheter, simply thread the catheter over the guidewire and into the vein to the measured depth, taking particular care not to contaminate any part of the catheter.
9. Remove the wire through the catheter and cap all ports.
10. In order to insert an introducer and sheath, first enlarge the puncture site with a sterile blade.
    a. Pass the introducer and sheath together over the wire.
    b. Slow, gentle pressure will usually safely advance the introducer into the vein. Allowing the introducer to warm and soften in the circulation for a moment may permit easier passage.
    c. When certain of correct placement, remove the introducer and wire through the sheath, and immediately cap the sheath with its previously flushed connector.
11. Aspirate all ports of the catheter or sheath to ascertain intraluminal placement. Each lumen should then be flushed with saline solution.
12. Secure the catheter to the skin with a suture. Dress the venipuncture site with povidone-iodine ointment, sterile gauze, and clear polyurethane.
13. Verify the location of the catheter with a CXR immediately after placement. Catheters should descend toward the heart, and the tip should be found in the SVC or at the cavoatrial junction. The film should also be inspected for the presence of pneumothorax.

D.   **Internal Jugular Vein Cannulation.**

1. **Anatomy:**
   a. As the internal jugular vein emerges at the base of the skull, it enters the carotid sheath posterior to the internal carotid artery, and continues posterior and lateral to the common carotid artery, until it crosses anterior to the common carotid artery near its termination.

    b. The internal jugular vein is medial to the sternoclei-
       domastoid muscle superiorly, crossing deep to it
       and emerging at the triangle between the sternal and
       clavicular heads of the sternocleidomastoid, and
       continuing behind the clavicular head, where it
       joins the subclavian vein (Fig 22–2).
2. **Central approach:**
    a. Identify the triangle formed by the sternal and cla-
       vicular heads of the sternocleidomastoid muscle
       (Fig 22–3).
    b. Palpate the adjacent carotid artery pulse and retract
       the carotid medially with gentle digital pressure.
    c. Insert the needle at the apex of the triangle of the
       sternocleidomastoid, directing the needle inferiorly
       and laterally along the medial aspect of the clavicu-
       lar head, toward the ipsilateral nipple.

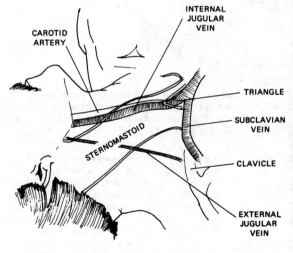

FIG 22–2.
Anatomy of the internal jugular vein. (From: Intravenous techniques, in
Textbook of Advanced Cardiac Life Support. Dallas, American Heart Asso-
ciation, 1987, p 147. Used by permission.)

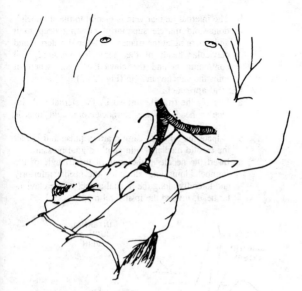

FIG 22–3.
Anatomic landmarks for cannulation of the internal jugular vein using the central approach. (From Kaye W: Intravenous techniques, in *Textbook of Advanced Cardiac Life Support*. Dallas, American Heart Association, 1987, p 150. Used by permission.)

      d. If the vein is not entered on the first pass (3–4 cm), maintain negative pressure in the syringe while slowly withdrawing the needle. (In difficult cases, a 22-gauge "seeker" needle may be useful in locating the jugular vein prior to inserting the 18-gauge needle.) If venous blood is encountered, remove the syringe and follow the Seldinger technique.

      e. If venous blood is not encountered, reassess the landmarks and make a second pass.

      f. **If arterial blood is encountered, immediately remove the needle and maintain pressure over the artery for 10 minutes before resuming.**

      g. **If air is aspirated, the procedure should be terminated and a CXR obtained to rule out pneumothorax prior to further attempts at cannulation.**

  3. **Posterior approach:**

      a. Identify the lateral border of the sternocleidomastoid muscle and introduce the needle deep to it, 5 cm superior to the clavicle, and just superior to the junction of the sternocleidomastoid and the external jugular vein (Fig 22–4).

      b. Direct the needle inferiorly and anteriorly toward the suprasternal notch.

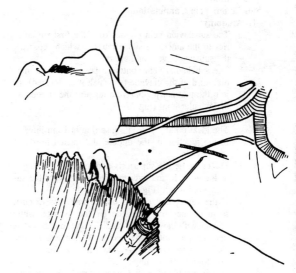

FIG 22–4.
Anatomic landmarks for cannulation of the internal jugular vein using the posterior approach. (From Kaye W: Intravenous techniques, in *Textbook of Advanced Cardiac Life Support*. Dallas, American Heart Association, Dallas, 1987, p 150. Used by permission.)

      c. If the vein is not entered on the first pass (5 cm), maintain negative pressure in the syringe while slowly withdrawing the needle. If venous blood is encountered, remove the syringe and follow the Seldinger technique as described above.

      d. If venous blood is not encountered, reassess the landmarks and make a second pass.

      e. **If arterial blood is encountered, immediately remove the needle and maintain pressure over the artery for 10 minutes before resuming.**

      f. **If air is aspirated, the procedure should be terminated and a CXR obtained to rule out pneumothorax prior to further attempts at cannulation.**

E.   **Subclavian Vein Cannulation.**

    1. **Anatomy:**

      a. The subclavian vein crosses over the first rib anterior to the anterior scalene muscle, which separates the subclavian vein and artery.

      b. The subclavian vein continues posterior to the medial third of the clavicle (to which it is attached), to join the internal jugular vein deep to the sternocostoclavicular joint (Fig 22–5).

    2. **Infraclavicular approach:**

      a. The ideal point for needle insertion is 1 cm inferior to the junction of the middle and medial thirds of the clavicle.

      b. Direct the needle superiorly and medially, just deep to the clavicle and over the first rib, toward the suprasternal notch (Fig 22–6).

      c. If the vein is not entered on the first pass (5 cm), maintain negative pressure in the syringe while slowly withdrawing the needle. If venous blood is encountered, rotate the needle 90 degrees, so that the bevel faces inferiorly. Then remove the syringe and follow the Seldinger technique.

      d. If venous blood is not encountered, reassess the landmarks and make a second pass.

      e. **If arterial blood is encountered, remove the needle immediately. Owing to the anatomy, arterial compression for hemostasis is not possible. Thus, the patient must be observed closely for signs of**

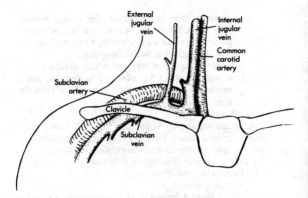

FIG 22–5.
Anatomy of the subclavian vein. (From Sladen A: *Invasive Monitoring and Its Complications in the Intensive Care Unit.* St Louis, CV Mosby Co, 1990, p 102. Used by permission.)

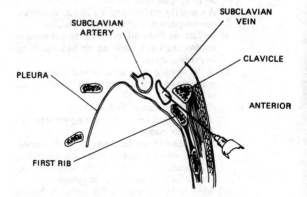

FIG 22–6.
Sagittal section through the medial third of the clavicle. (From Kaye W: Intravenous techniques, in *Textbook of Advanced Cardiac Life Support.* Dallas, American Heart Association, 1987, p 148. Used by permission.)

hemodynamic compromise, indicating hemorrhage. A CXR should be obtained to evaluate for
possible hemothorax. Usually, hemostasis occurs
and the patient is not endangered.

f. If air is aspirated, the procedure should be terminated and a CXR obtained to rule out pneumothorax prior to further attempts at cannulation.

F. **Complications.**

Life-threatening complications may develop during insertion of central venous catheters. The overall complication
rate for internal jugular vein cannulation is 5%–20%, and
for subclavian vein cannulation, 6%–10%.

1. **Venous air embolism.**

a. Pathophysiology:

1) **During insertion of the catheter, air embolism may occur any time the catheter is not
occluded.**

2) If the patient inspires during catheter placement, negative intrathoracic pressure may cause
air to be drawn into the site.

3) A 4 mm Hg gradient across a 20-gauge catheter
permits air to flow at a rate of 90 mL/sec.

4) **As little as 5–10 mL of air in the pulmonary
outflow tract can cause an air lock resulting
in cardiac arrest.**

5) In the absence of an atrial or ventricular septal
defect no cerebral or coronary air embolism can
occur.

b. Prevention of venous air embolism:

1) **Air embolism can occur during catheter insertion or removal.**

2) The patient should be supine or in the Trendelenburg position during catheter manipulation.

3) The needle or catheter should always be occluded with a finger, wire, or syringe.

4) Modern introducers for PA catheters have a
valve designed to prevent air embolism; however, malfunction has been reported, especially
after removal of the PA catheter.

c. Management of venous air embolism:

1) Air may be noted entering the catheter or there
may be a sudden cardiac arrest.

2) Place the patient in the Trendelenburg positon (if not already done) turned to the left lateral decubitus position to trap the air in the right ventricular apex (Fig 22–7).
3) The catheter should be aspirated to attempt to return the air.
4) A precordial thump may dislodge air trapped in the outflow tract.
5) If the patient is stable, a cross-table CXR is obtained to determine the amount of air in the

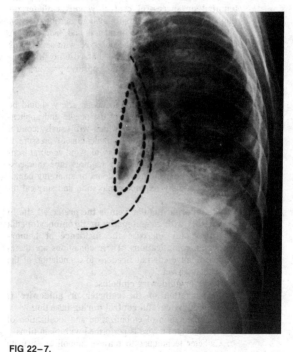

FIG 22–7.
Left lateral decubitus CXR showing air trapped in the right ventricular apex. (Courtesy of Dr. John Grant.)

RV. The patient is maintained in this position until the air is dissolved into the blood, as documented by repeat films.

6) If the patient is hemodynamically unstable or cardiac arrest ensues, a thoracotomy should be performed for open cardiac massage to force air from the pulmonary outflow tract. Needle aspiration of the RV apex may aid in recovery of the air.

2. **Pneumothorax:**
   A CXR must always be obtained following attempted or successful central venous catheterization. If hypotension occurs following insertion, tension pneumothorax must be considered and managed. A small pneumothorax may be observed with serial films but must be treated with tube thoracostomy if symptomatic, or if the patient requires positive pressure ventilation.

3. **Arterial puncture:**
   a. Puncture of carotid or subclavian artery should be managed by withdrawal of the needle and application of digital pressure, which will usually control the hemorrhage. Careful application of pressure is required on the carotid artery to avoid cerebral ischemia. Hemothorax usually requires tube thoracostomy. An expanding hematoma or enlarging hemothorax usually requires exploration and surgical repair.

   b. **The internal jugular vein is the preferred site in patients with coagulopathy or thrombocytopenia which may increase the incidence of hemorrhagic complications.** These conditions are therefore relative contraindications to cannulation of the subclavian vein.

4. **Catheter or guidewire embolus:**
   a. **Embolization of the catheter or guidewire is avoided by careful control during insertion.**
   b. Documentation of embolization and localization of the catheter or wire is performed with plain films.
   c. Catheter techniques to retrieve emboli are usually performed in the vascular radiology suite.
   d. Operative extrication is rarely required.

5. Other complications of central venous cannulation include hematoma formation, hemomediastinum, brachial plexus injury, tracheal laceration, subclavian and jugular vein thrombosis, and sepsis.

G. **Special Considerations.**

1. Success rates for internal jugular vein cannulation range from 60%–95%; for subclavian vein cannulation, 85%–90%.

2. **If an unsuccessful attempt at central venous catheterization is made, obtain a CXR prior to attempting to cannulate the contralateral site, in order to avoid undetected bilateral pneumothorax.**

3. Central venous catheters should be changed over a wire (if the site is not infected) or replaced every 3–5 days, to minimize infectious and thromboembolic complications. In cases of suspected catheter-borne infections, nonessential catheters should be removed and the tip submitted under sterile condition for culture. Evaluation of line sepsis is discussed in Chapter 17 (p. 670).

4. The subclavian vein is the preferred site for long-term central venous access, providing greater patient comfort and facilitating catheter care.

5. Retrograde passage of the catheter into the internal jugular vein after attempted cannulation of the subclavian vein may occur. Manual compression of the internal jugular vein or rotation of the patient's head toward the side of cannulation while passing the guidewire may prevent this complication. When retrograde passage occurs, the catheter must be removed and cannulation attempted once again.

II. **PULMONARY ARTERY CATHETERIZATION.**
A. **Indications.**

1. Continuous hemodynamic monitoring, in an unstable or potentially unstable patient, utilizing CVP, PA systolic and diastolic pressures, PCWP, and CO (see Chapter 2).

2. To guide fluid management in complicated patients

3. Sampling of mixed venous (pulmonary arterial) blood for O_2 saturation.

4. Access to the RV for cardiac pacing.

B.   General Approach.

1. PA catheterization is performed as a sterile procedure, requiring the following equipment: supplies for catheter sheath placement including sterile gowns and sterile drapes; PA catheter (7F); transducer, oscilloscope, monitor (all calibrated); and cardiac defibrillator, lidocaine, and atropine (at bedside).

2. Patient preparation:

    a. The patient should be monitored continuously with ECG and should have a functioning IV catheter in place for treatment of dysrhythmias.

    b. Sterile preparation should be performed as previously described, including cap, mask, sterile gown, sterile gloves, sterile drapes, and skin preparation.

C.   Technique.

1. Cannulate the internal jugular vein or the subclavian vein, using the Seldinger technique, and insert the catheter sheath.

2. After securing the sheath, ensure that the PA catheter has been properly flushed and that the balloon is functional.

3. Thread the catheter through its sterile protective sleeve.

4. With the balloon deflated, insert the catheter through the sheath to a depth of 20 cm, at which point the tip will be beyond the end of the sheath.

5. Inflate the balloon and advance the catheter slowly, while inspecting the ECG for dysrhythmias and the pressure tracing for the succession of characteristic waveforms (Fig 22–8).

6. Once the proper position has been reached (pulmonary capillary wedge), the balloon should be deflated. At this point, the tracing should return to that of the PA.

7. After the catheter has been successfully positioned, draw the protective sleeve over it and secure the connector.

8. Verification of catheter position:

    a. The disappearance of the characteristic PA waveform when the balloon is inflated and its prompt return when the balloon is deflated is mandatory.

    b. The O_2 saturation of blood samples drawn with balloon inflated should be greater than that of systemic arterial blood.

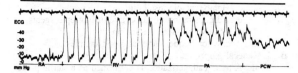

FIG 22–8.
Succession of pressure waveforms observed during the advancement of the PA catheter, through the right atrium *(RA)*, right ventricle *(RV)*, pulmonary artery *(PA)*, and to the pulmonary capillary wedge *(PCW)* position. (From: Intravenous techniques, in: *Textbook of Advanced Cardiac Life Support.* Dallas, American Heart Association, 1987, p 173. Used by permission.)

      c. Obtain a CXR to ascertain that the tip of the catheter is in a main branch of the PA. If the tip is peripherally positioned (>5 cm from the mediastinum) the catheter should be repositioned to prevent PA rupture. The film should also be inspected for the presence of pneumothorax.

D.   **Complications.**

Complications associated with the PA catheter include cardiac dysrhythmias (PVCs, ventricular tachycardia, ventricular fibrillation, RBBB), pulmonary hemorrhage, PA rupture, pulmonary infarction, catheter entanglement or knotting, cardiac perforation, valvular damage, endocarditis, and sepsis.

E.   **Special Considerations.**

The presence of LBBB prior to placement is a relative contraindication to the use of a PA catheter, as its passage may result in complete heart block. Fluoroscopic guidance may facilitate the passage of the catheter into the PA in difficult cases. Placement of a temporary pacing wire or use of a pacing PA catheter may be necessary.

III.   **ARTERIAL CATHETERIZATION.**

A.   **Indications.**

    1. Continuous monitoring of arterial pressure (see Chapter 2).

    2. Any condition in which the factors influencing cardiac function may change rapidly.

      a. Hypertensive crisis.

      b. Shock.

        c. Hemodynamic instability.

        d. Administration of vasoactive or inotropic agents.

        e. Positive pressure ventilation.

    3. Access for frequent arterial blood samples.

B.   **General Approach.**

    1. Arterial catheterization is performed as a sterile procedure, requiring the following supplies: appropriately sized catheter-over-needle; flexible guidewire; povidone-iodine solution; cap, mask, sterile gloves, sterile towels; lidocaine (1% solution without epinephrine); pressure tubing, transducer, and monitor.

    2. Although the catheter-over-needle technique is acceptable, particularly for the radial artery, the Seldinger technique is preferred for femoral and axillary arterial cannulation. An introducer needle may be used, or the guidewire may be passed through the catheter, prior to advancing the catheter entirely into the artery.

C.   **Radial Artery Catheterization.**

    1. Equipment: 20-gauge (2-in.) catheter-over-needle; arm board, roll of gauze; other supplies, as listed above.

    2. Assess collateral circulation by performing the Allen test.

        a. Occlude the radial and ulnar arteries digitally until blanching of the hand is noted.

        b. Release the ulnar artery (maintaining occlusion of the radial artery) and observe the hand for blushing.

        c. Ulnar collateral circulation is considered inadequate if >5 seconds elapse before blushing of the hand occurs, in which case another site should be selected.

    3. Insertion technique:

        a. Support the patient's hand in dorsiflexion with a roll of gauze under the wrist. Secure the palm and lower arm to the board. Use sterile precautions, as previously described.

        b. Palpate the radial artery just proximal to the head of the radius. Insert the 20-gauge needle-catheter at a 30-degree angle to the skin with the bevel down.

        c. Advance the catheter and needle until blood appears at the hub of the needle. Maintain the position of the needle and advance the catheter into the artery.

d. If arterial blood is not encountered, reassess the landmarks and make a second pass. If arterial blood is encountered but the catheter cannot be passed, immediately remove the needle and maintain pressure over the artery for 10 minutes before resuming.

e. **If the artery cannot be cannulated in three attempts, discontinue the procedure and choose another site.**

f. Once the catheter has been successfully passed, remove the needle and attach the hub of the catheter to the pressure tubing.

g. Secure the catheter to the skin with suture or tape. Apply povidone-iodine to the puncture site and cover with a sterile dressing.

D. Femoral Artery Catheterization.

1. Equipment: 16- or 18-gauge (4-in.) catheter-over-needle; razor, surgical soap; other supplies, as listed above.

2. The femoral artery is found at the midpoint of a line between the anterior superior iliac spine and the symphysis pubis. Medial to the femoral artery is the femoral vein; lateral to the femoral artery is the femoral nerve.

3. Scrub and shave the groin area and prepare the skin with povidone-iodine solution. Use sterile precautions, as previously described. Infiltrate the skin with lidocaine.

4. Insertion technique:

a. Palpate the femoral pulse.

b. Enter the skin at a 45-degree angle, with the catheter-over-needle or the needle alone (Seldinger technique). **If the Seldinger technique is chosen, the wire must pass without any resistance, indicating that it is in the lumen, and that it has not dissected.**

c. If the artery is not entered on the first pass (3–4 cm), maintain negative pressure in the syringe while slowly withdrawing the needle. If arterial blood is encountered, remove the syringe and follow the Seldinger technique.

d If arterial blood is not encountered, reassess the landmarks and make a second pass. If arterial blood is encountered but the guidewire cannot be passed, immediately remove the needle and maintain pressure over the artery for 10 minutes before resuming.

e. **If the artery cannot be cannulated in three attempts, discontinue the procedure and choose another site.**

f. Once the catheter has been successfully passed, remove the needle or wire and attach the hub of the catheter to the pressure tubing.

g. Secure the catheter to the skin with a suture. Dress the site with povidone-iodine ointment, sterile gauze, and clear polyurethane.

E. **Dorsalis Pedis Artery Catheterization.**

1. Equipment: 20-gauge (2-in.) catheter-over-needle; other supplies, as listed above.

2. Anatomy:

   a. The dorsalis pedis artery, the extension of the anterior tibial artery, is found on the dorsum of the foot, parallel and lateral to the extensor hallucis longus.

   b. In 12% of the population, the dorsalis pedis artery is absent. Demonstrate the presence of collateral flow by assessing the flow in the posterior tibial artery, by palpation, or using a Doppler flowmeter.

3. Sterile conditions are maintained, as previously described. Infiltrate the skin with lidocaine.

4. Insertion technique:

   a. Palpate the dorsalis pedis artery.

   b. Insert the 20-gauge needle-catheter at a 30-degree angle to the skin with the bevel down. Advance the catheter and needle until blood appears at the hub of the needle. Maintain the position of the needle and advance the catheter into the artery.

   c. If arterial blood is not encountered, reassess the landmarks and make a second pass. If arterial blood is encountered but the catheter cannot be passed, immediately remove the needle and maintain pressure over the artery for 10 minutes before resuming.

   d. **If the artery cannot be cannulated in three attempts, discontinue the procedure and choose another site.**

   e. Once the catheter has been successfully passed, remove the needle and attach the hub of the catheter to the pressure tubing.

f. Secure the catheter to the skin with suture or tape. Apply povidone-iodine to the puncture site and cover with a sterile dressing.

F. Axillary Artery Catheterization.

1. Equipment: 18-gauge (6-in.) catheter-over-needle; razor and surgical soap; other supplies, as listed above.
2. Anatomy:
   a. The axillary artery is the continuation of the subclavian artery, entering the axilla at the lateral border of the first rib; at the teres major muscle, it becomes the brachial artery.
   b. The axillary sheath contains the axillary artery, axillary vein, and brachial plexus (Fig 22–9).
   c. Interruption of flow in the axillary artery will not lead to ischemia in the arm because of extensive

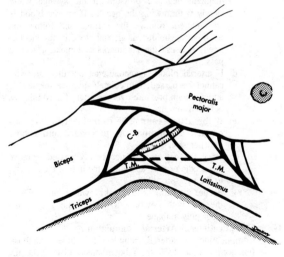

FIG 22–9.
Anatomic landmarks for cannulation of the axillary artery. *C-B.* =coracobrachialis muscle, *T.M.* = teres major muscle. (From Sladen A: *Invasive Monitoring and Its Complications in the Intensive Care Unit.* St Louis, CV Mosby Co, 1990, p 187. Used by permission.)

collateral flow from the thyrocervical trunk and the subscapular artery.

d. The arm should be hyperabducted, externally rotated, and immobilized.

3. Shave the axilla and prepare the skin with povidone-iodine solution. Sterile conditions are maintained as previously described. Infiltrate the skin with lidocaine.

4. Insertion technique:

   a. Palpate the axillary artery.

   b. Enter the skin as high as possible in the axilla, with the catheter-over-needle or needle alone (Seldinger technique). **If the Seldinger technique is chosen, the wire must pass without any resistance, indicating that it is in the lumen, and that it has not dissected.**

   c. If the artery is not entered on the first pass (5 cm), maintain negative pressure in the syringe while slowly withdrawing the needle. If arterial blood is encountered, remove the syringe and follow the Seldinger technique. If arterial blood is not encountered, reassess the landmarks and make a second pass.

   d. If arterial blood is encountered but the guidewire cannot be passed, immediately remove the needle and maintain pressure over the artery for 10 minutes before resuming.

   e. **If the artery cannot be cannulated in three attempts, discontinue the procedure and choose another site.**

   f. Once the catheter is successfully passed, remove the needle or wire and attach the hub of the catheter to the pressure tubing.

   g. Secure the catheter to the skin with a suture. Dress the site with povidone-iodine, sterile gauze, and clear polyurethane.

G. Complications of Arterial Cannulation.

Complications of arterial cannulation include thrombosis (temporary, 10%–15%) thromboembolism, distal ischemia, hemorrhage, hematoma, infection, arteriovenous fistula, and neurologic complications (brachial plexus).

H. Special Considerations.
1. Arterial catheters should be changed over a wire (if the site is not infected) or replaced every 3–5 days to minimize infectious and ischemic complications.
2. Catheters should be immediately removed when signs of distal ischemia appear.
3. Risk factors for ischemic complications include female sex; low CO state; use of vasoconstricting agents; multiple failed attempts to cannulate; peripheral vascular disease; and prolonged duration of cannulation.
4. **Brachial artery cannulation is not recommended, owing to the inadequate collateral circulation and the unacceptably high incidence of complications.**

IV. ENDOTRACHEAL INTUBATION.
A. Indications for Endotracheal Intubation (see Chapter 7).
1. Inability to ventilate an unconscious patient with conventional methods.
2. To protect the airway in an unresponsive patient.
3. Respiratory insufficiency.
4. Cardiopulmonary arrest.
5. To hyperventilate a patient with elevated ICP.
B. General Approach.
1. ET intubation may be performed electively, as in a patient with progressive respiratory insufficiency, or emergently, as for cardiopulmonary arrest. In either case, ET tube placement must be performed promptly yet carefully, and requires the following equipment: laryngoscope; ET tubes of various sizes; malleable stylet; rigid pharyngeal suction apparatus and flexible tracheal suction catheter; bag-valve-mask ventilation unit; and an oxygen source.
2. The ideal position for direct visualization of the glottic opening requires alignment of three axes: mouth, pharynx, and trachea. Extend the head and flex the neck to obtain this alignment, known as the "sniffing position" (Fig 22–10).
C. Technique for Orotracheal Intubation.
1. Prior to attempting ET intubation, hyperventilate the patient with 100% O_2 via face mask. The patient may be monitored with a transcutaneous O_2 sensor if indicated.

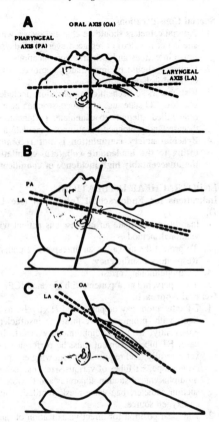

FIG 22–10.
Proper head position is important for successful orotracheal intubation. **A,** oral (OA), pharyngeal (PA), and laryngeal (LA) axes must be aligned for direct laryngoscopy. **B,** elevate head 10 cm above shoulders with folded towel to align PA and LA. **C,** extend atlanto-occipital joint to achieve straightest possible line from incisors to glottis. (From Stone DJ, Gal TJ: Airway management, in Miller RD (ed): *Anesthesia,* ed 3. New York, Churchill-Livingstone, 1990, p 1271. Used with permission.)

2. Suction the oropharynx. Dentures and any foreign material should be removed.
3. Standing at the head of the patient, hold the laryngoscope in the left hand and open the patient's mouth with the right hand.
4. Insert the blade of the laryngoscope in the right side of the mouth, displace the tongue to the left, and advance the blade in the midline to the base of the tongue. **Care must be taken to avoid injury to the upper lip and teeth.**
   a. If using a curved blade, the tip is advanced into the vallecula, exposing the glottic opening.
   b. If using a straight blade, the tip is inserted under the epiglottis directly.
5. At this point, the epiglottis, arytenoid cartilage, vocal cords, and glottic opening should be visualized clearly (Fig 22–11).
6. The upper airway and trachea may be anesthetized with lidocaine 4% aerosolized solution (5 mL).

ANATOMY

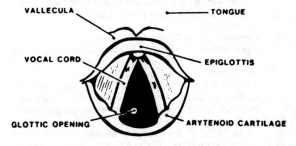

FIG 22–11.
Anatomic structures visualized during direct laryngoscopy for orotracheal intubation. (From Adjuncts for airway control, ventilation, and supplemental oxygen, in *Textbook of Advanced Cardiac Life Support*. Dallas, American Heart Association, 1987, p 32. Used by permission.)

7. The ET tube is placed under direct vision through the vocal cords, advancing the cuff 2 cm past the vocal cords into the trachea.

8. **If after 30 seconds intubation has not been achieved, ventilate the patient once again with 100% O_2 via face mask prior to further attempts at intubation.**

9. Once intubation is successful, inflate the cuff and ventilate the patient with 100% O_2 manually, auscultating the axillae bilaterally. If breath sounds are clear and equal, the tube may be secured to the patient's face and mechanical ventilation initiated.

10. If gurgling sounds are present, indicating esophageal intubation, the tube is immediately removed and the patient is ventilated via face mask prior to another attempt.

11. If breath sounds are observed to be greater on the right, indicating right mainstem bronchus intubation, the cuff is deflated, the tube withdrawn slightly, and the cuff then reinflated. If auscultation then reveals equal breath sounds bilaterally, the tube may be secured.

12. After the initiation of mechanical ventilation, a CXR should be obtained to verify correct positioning of the tip of the ET tube. In addition, an arterial blood sample should be obtained to verify adequate oxygenation and ventilation.

D. **Complications of Orotracheal Intubation.**

Complications of orotracheal intubation, which occur more frequently in the emergent setting, include oropharyngeal and dental trauma, tracheal laceration or rupture, vocal cord injury, avulsion of the arytenoid cartilage, esophageal perforation, vomiting and aspiration, intubation of the right mainstem bronchus, and intubation of the pyriform sinus.

E. **Special Considerations.**

1. A "difficult" airway may be encountered, characterized by laryngeal edema, upper airway trauma, trachea not in the midline, tumor obstructing the airway, and limited range of motion at the cervical or temporomandibular joints. **Cricothyroidotomy may be necessary in life-threatening situations.**

2. **Assume that all patients have a full stomach and take precautions against aspiration during intuba-**

tion: maintain the patient's protective reflexes by
withholding heavy sedation; instruct an assistant to
apply cricoid pressure during the procedure.

3. **For patients with a suspected or known spinal injury, orotracheal intubation is contraindicated.
Blind nasotracheal intubation may be attempted for
airway control; otherwise, cricothyroidotomy is recommended.**

4. A malleable stylet may facilitate intubation in some patients.

V. EMERGENT CRICOTHYROIDOTOMY.
A. Indications for Emergent Cricothyroidotomy.

1. Immediate airway management after trauma to the oropharynx that precludes direct visualization of the glottic opening

2. Immediate airway management after unsuccessful ET intubation

3. Upper airway obstruction.

B. General Approach.

1. **Although the technical details are critical, the success of emergent cricothyroidotomy depends on
sound judgment concerning the timing of the procedure. Anticipation that this approach to airway
management may be necessary contributes to its
success.**

2. For the most expedient placement, the following equipment is required:
   a. Knife blade and handle.
   b. Povidone-iodine or other antiseptic solution.
   c. Tracheostomy tube, pediatric ET tube, or 14-gauge catheter-over-needle.
   d. Bag-valve ventilation unit and oxygen source.

3. The patient must be supine with the head extended.
The standard precautions for sterility should be attempted, but the emergent nature of this procedure usually does not permit complete surgical preparation. If
possible, the area should be prepared with povidone-iodine solution.

C. Technique for Cricothyroidotomy.

1. Palpate the cricothyroid membrane between the thyroid
and cricoid cartilages (Fig 22–12).

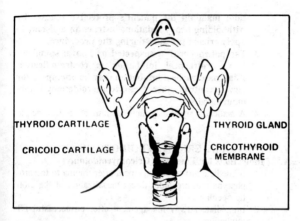

FIG 22–12.
Anatomic landmarks for locating the cricothyroid membrane. (From Adjuncts for airway control, ventilation, and supplemental oxygen, in *Textbook of Advanced Cardiac Life Support*. Dallas, American Heart Association, 1987, p 33. Used by permission.)

2. A vertical skin incision is made and the cricothyroid membrane incised horizontally.
3. Insert the knife handle through the cricothyroidotomy and rotate 90 degrees.
4. Pass an ET or tracheostomy tube through the opening, inflate the cuff, and begin ventilation with the bag-valve unit and 100% O_2.
5. Alternatively, one may puncture the cricothyroid membrane with a catheter-over-needle and remove the needle. The hub of the catheter is then mounted with the barrel of a 12-mL syringe, which serves as a connector for ventilation.

D. Complications.
Complications of emergent cricothyroidotomy include hemorrhage; perforation of the esophagus; and inability to cannulate the trachea.

E. **Special Considerations.**
1. **Assume that all trauma patients requiring cricothyroidotomy have a cervical spine injury and take all necessary precautions to protect the spinal cord.**
2. **Cricothyroidotomy is the procedure of choice when emergent surgical airway access is necessary.**
3. Cricothyroidotomy is associated with a lower complication rate than emergent tracheostomy. Furthermore, cricothyroidotomy is performed more easily and rapidly.
4. Following cricothyroidotomy in an emergent setting, airway control may be converted electively to a standard tracheostomy.

VI. **THORACENTESIS.**
A. **Indications for Thoracentesis.**
1. To obtain a sample of pleural fluid for diagnosis (see Chapter 7).
2. Drainage of a restricting pleural effusion to relieve respiratory compromise.
B. **General Approach.**
1. Thoracentesis is performed as a sterile procedure, requiring the following equipment: 18-gauge catheter-over-needle, stopcock, 20-mL syringe; extension tubing and collecting vessel; povidone-iodine solution and sterile drapes; lidocaine (1% solution without epinephrine).
2. If possible, the patient is placed in the sitting position, with the arms supported on a bedside table (Fig 22–13). Alternatively, the patient may be supine, with the head of the bed elevated to 90 degrees.
3. The fluid level is located by percussion. Thoracentesis is performed two interspaces below the percussed fluid level, but not lower than the eighth intercostal space.
4. Prepare the skin with povidone-iodine solution and drape the field.
C. **Technique for Thoracentesis.**
1. Infiltrate the skin with lidocaine, using a 25-gauge needle. Anesthetize the deeper tissues with a 20-gauge needle, including the periosteum of the rib below the chosen intercostal space.

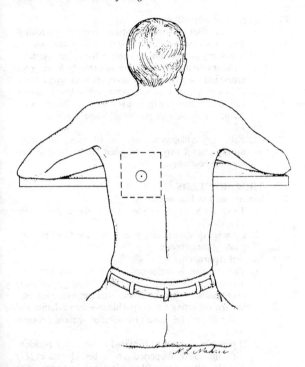

FIG 22–13.
Ideal position for thoracentesis. (From Yeston NS, Niehoff JM: Important procedures in the intensive care unit, in Civetta JM, Taylor RW, Kirby RR (eds): *Critical Care*. Philadelphia, JB Lippincott Co, 1988, p 244. Used by permission.

2. **While aspirating the syringe to avoid intravascular injection of lidocaine, enter the pleural cavity over the superior aspect of the rib,** thus avoiding the intercostal neurovascular bundle. Lidocaine should be administered through the pleura, and subsequent aspiration should confirm the presence of pleural fluid.

3. Remove the needle and reenter the pleural space with the catheter-over-needle attached to a syringe. Remove the needle, covering the hub of the catheter to prevent pneumothorax.

4. Mount the stopcock and the 20-mL syringe to the catheter. For diagnostic purposes, fluid may be aspirated directly. For drainage of a large effusion, the extension tubing is connected to the stopcock, so that the pleural fluid can be withdrawn into the syringe and ejected through the tubing into a collecting container. Upon completion of the procedure, a small sterile dressing is placed.

5. Obtain a CXR in order to document the removal of the pleural fluid. In addition, the film should be inspected for the presence of pneumothorax.

D. Evaluation of Pleural Effusions.
The pleural fluid should be collected under sterile conditions and a specimen sent for laboratory evaluation.

1. Total and differential cell count.
2. Gram's stain and bacterial culture.
3. Fungal and mycobacterial cultures.
4. Cytology.
5. Protein.
6. Glucose.
7. Amylase.
8. LDH.
9. pH.

E. Complications.
Complications of thoracentesis include pneumothorax, hemothorax, and puncture of the lung, liver, or spleen.

VII. TUBE THORACOSTOMY.
A. Indications.

1. Pneumothorax (>20% in magnitude or associated with positive pressure ventilation) (see Chapter 7).
2. Hemothorax, hydrothorax, or chylothorax.
3. Prophylaxis for high-risk patients (rib fractures, penetrating thoracic trauma) prior to positive pressure ventilation.
4. Empyema.

B. General Approach.

1. Tube thoracostomy is performed as a sterile procedure, and requires the following equipment: thoracostomy

tube (24F–28F for pneumothorax; 28F–36F for hemothorax); povidone-iodine solution; cap, mask, and sterile gown, gloves, towels and drapes; lidocaine (1% solution without epinephrine); sterile instruments (knife, scissors, Kelly clamp); and collection-suction apparatus.

2. The patient is placed in the supine position.

3. The preferred site for tube thoracostomy is the fifth intercostal space, in the anterior axillary line, although an alternative site may be indicated if there is loculated pneumothorax or effusion.

4. Prepare the skin with povidone-iodine solution. Don cap, mask, sterile gown, and sterile gloves. Create a sterile field with towels and drapes.

C. **Technique of Chest Tube Insertion.**

1. Measure the chest tube from the desired insertion site to the apex, and mark the chest tube with a suture.

2. Infiltrate the skin with lidocaine, using a 25-gauge needle. Anesthetize the deeper tissues using a 20-gauge needle, including the periosteum of the ribs above and below the chosen intercostal space.

3. While aspirating the syringe to avoid intravascular injection of lidocaine, enter the pleural cavity over the superior aspect of the rib, thus avoiding the intercostal neurovascular bundle. Lidocaine should be administered through the pleura, and subsequent aspiration should confirm the presence of pleural air or fluid.

4. Remove the needle and incise the skin one interspace below the desired site of insertion.

5. Create a subcutaneous tunnel with blunt dissection using the Kelly clamp (Fig 22–14).

6. Enter the pleural space with the tip of the clamp, just over the superior margin of the rib; open the clamp, spreading the pleura.

7. With a gloved finger, confirm penetration into the chest by palpating the lung, sweeping away pleural adhesions, if present (see Fig 22–14).

8. Grasp the tip of the thoracostomy tube with the Kelly clamp, and insert both into the pleural space. Direct the tube posteriorly and superiorly for drainage of hemothorax or hydrothorax, or anteriorly for pneumothorax (Fig 22–15).

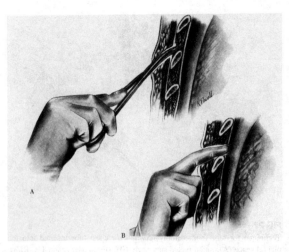

FIG 22–14.
Technique for tube thoracostomy: creation of a subcutaneous tunnel **(A)**, and digital penetration into the pleural space **(B)**. (From Marsicano TH, Rippe JM: Chest tube insertion and care, in Rippe JM, Irwin RS, Albert JS, et al (eds): *Intensive Care Medicine*. Boston, Little, Brown & Co, 1985, p 65. Used by permission.)

   9. Ensure that the last hole in the tube is within the thoracic cavity. Secure the tube to the chest wall with a suture. Cover the wound with a sterile dressing, consisting of petrolatum-soaked gauze and sponges.
   10. Inspect the collecting system for an adequate water seal and measure the amount of drainage. Inspect and secure all connections.
   11. Obtain a CXR to assess the position of the catheter and the evacuation of air or fluid from the thoracic cavity.
D. **Complications of Tube Thoracostomy.**
   1. Hemorrhage.
   2. Laceration of the lung.
   3. Infection.
   4. Cardiac injury.

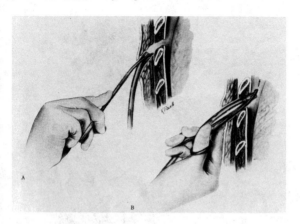

FIG 22–15.
Technique for tube thoracostomy *(continued):* chest tube inserted into the pleural space **(A),** and directed superiorly **(B).** (From Marsicano TH, Rippe JM: Chest tube insertion and care, in Rippe JM, Irwin RS, Alpert JS, Dalen JE (eds): *Intensive Care Medicine.* Boston, Little, Brown & Co, 1985, p 66. Used by permission.)

     5. Subcutaneous placement.
     6. Reexpansion pulmonary edema.
     7. Intraperitoneal placement of tube.
E.   **Special Considerations.**
     Trocar tube thoracostomy is associated with a high complication rate and therefore is not recommended.

VIII. PERICARDIOCENTESIS.
A.   **Indications for Pericardiocentesis.**
     1. For relief of cardiac tamponade emergently, in patients with respiratory distress or progressive hypotension (see Chapter 5).
     2. To obtain fluid for diagnostic study.
B.   **General Approach.**
     1. Pericardiocentesis is performed as a sterile procedure, with complete monitoring available, and requires the following supplies: 16-gauge (4-in.) needle, short-bev-

eled; 50-mL syringe; sterile alligator connector (for ECG V lead); povidone-iodine solution; cap, mask, and sterile gown, gloves, towels, and drapes; and lidocaine (1% solution without epinephrine).

2. If the indication for pericardiocentesis is cardiac tamponade, the IV infusion of volume will improve cardiac performance until the pericardium can be drained. If the patient is hypotensive and unresponsive to volume infusion, isoproterenol may be administered, in order to increase stroke volume and lower SVR.

3. The patient is placed in the supine position. Continuous ECG is mandatory.

4. Prepare the skin with povidone-iodine solution. Don cap, mask, sterile gown, and sterile gloves. Create a sterile field with towels and drapes.

C. **Technique of Pericardiocentesis (Subxiphoid Approach).**

1. The ECG V lead is connected to the needle with the sterile alligator clip. ST segment elevation during the procedure indicates ventricular contact with the needle, and PR segment elevation suggests atrial contact (Fig 22–16).

2. Infiltrate the skin and subcutaneous tissue to the left of the xiphoid process with lidocaine.

3. Insert the needle 1 cm to the left of the xiphoid, at a 30-degree angle to the frontal plane, continuously aspirating the syringe. Advance the needle while observing the ECG (Fig 22–16).

4. If grossly bloody fluid is obtained, it is assessed for coagulation. Clotting suggests intracardiac penetration, whereas pericardial blood has been defibrinated and should not coagulate.

5. If successfully entered, the pericardium should be completely drained; this may require the placement of a catheter, either through the needle, or using a guidewire.

D. **Complications of Pericardiocentesis.**

1. Cardiac dysrhythmias.

2. Cardiac puncture.

3. Myocardial laceration.

4. Coronary artery laceration.

5. Air embolism to a cardiac chamber or coronary artery.

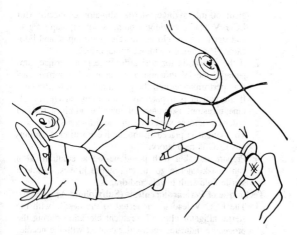

FIG 22–16.
Subxiphoid approach for pericardiocentesis. (From Invasive therapeutic techniques, in *Textbook of Advanced Cardiac Life Support*. Dallas, American Heart Association, 1981, p 193. Used by permission.)

      6. Pneumothorax.
      7. Hemorrhage.
E. **Special Considerations.**
      1. The pericardial sac normally contains only 50 mL of fluid; in the acute setting, it can accommodate an additional 100 mL before cardiac tamponade results (see Chapter 5).
      2. Pericardiocentesis to remove bloody fluid after trauma is a temporary maneuver, and should be followed by thoracotomy (see Chapter 19).

IX. **INSERTION OF THE INTRAAORTIC BALLOON PUMP**
A. **Methods of Insertion (see Chapter 6).**
      1. The most common method for IABP insertion is percutaneously via the femoral artery (Fig 22–17).

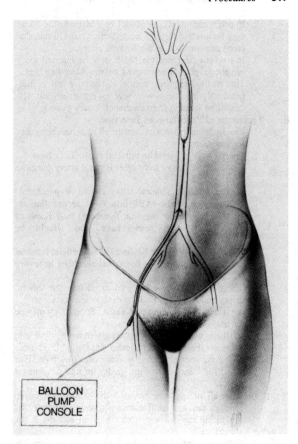

FIG 22–17.
Percutaneous insertion of an IABP. Note position of the tip of balloon distal to the origin of the left subclavian artery. (From Reetsma K, Bregman D, Colten S, et al: Mechanical circulatory support—advance in intra aortic balloon pumping, in Shoemaker WC, Ayres S, Grenvik A, et al: *Textbook of Critical Care*. Philadelphia, WB Saunders Co, 1989, p 423. Used by permission.)

2. If percutaneous access cannot be obtained, the IABP
   may be inserted through a prosthetic graft (10 mm Dacron) anastomosed to the femoral artery.
3. In exceptional cases the IABP may be inserted via a
   prosthetic graft anastomosed to the ascending aorta.
   This method requires median sternotomy and is indicated only in patients with severe vascular disease who
   cannot be weaned from cardiopulmonary bypass.

B. Technique of Percutaneous Insertion.

1. The IABP insertion kits contain all materials necessary
   for insertion.
2. The groin is prepared and draped in sterile fashion.
3. Using the Seldinger technique, femoral artery puncture
   is performed.
   a. The common femoral artery should be punctured.
   b. **Insertion of the IABP into the external iliac ar-
      tery (above the inguinal ligament) may result in
      retroperitoneal hemorrhage and should be
      avoided.**
   c. **Insertion of the IABP into the superficial femoral
      artery may occlude the vessel resulting in severe
      limb ischemia.**
4. The flexible guidewire is introduced into the femoral
   artery and advanced into the descending aorta.
   a. If the wire does not pass easily, fluoroscopy may be
      useful.
   b. If the wire cannot be passed it will be impossible to
      insert the IABP, and another site should be chosen.
5. Using the arterial dilator, an introducer sheath (9.5F or
   10.5F) is inserted over the guidewire into the femoral
   artery.
6. After all air has been aspirated, the balloon is removed
   from its package and the insertion length estimated by
   measuring the distance from the groin incision to the
   sternal angle.
7. Following removal of the arterial dilator from the
   sheath (the sheath must be compressed between two
   fingers to prevent hemorrhage), the balloon is passed
   over the guidewire to the predetermined length.
8. The guidewire is removed and a stopcock and pressure
   tubing attached for measurement of MAP. **The lumen**

    must be carefully aspirated prior to flushing to prevent air emboli.

   9. A separate tubing is attached to the balloon lumen for inflation and deflation.

  10. The IABP is secured to the thigh with several heavy sutures.

  11. A CXR must be obtained to confirm postioning of the IABP distal to the origin of the left subclavian artery (Fig 22–17).

C. **Removal of the IABP.**

   1. When the balloon was inserted via a femoral sheath the deflated balloon is withdrawn until the hub of the balloon engages the sheath (Fig 22–18,A).

   2. The sheath and balloon are then removed simultaneously with coincident pressure applied to the distal superficial femoral artery (Fig 22–18,B). This maneuver allows any intravascular thrombus to exit via the arteriotomy site which is flushed for several seconds with antegrade arterial blood flow and avoids a distal shower of emboli.

   3. Direct pressure is then applied to the insertion site (the arteriotomy is generally 1–2 cm proximal to the skin site and pressure should be applied at this point) (Fig 22–18,C).

   4. The pedal pulses are assessed frequently, and the amount of pressure applied should be slightly less than that which ablates the palpable or Doppler audible pulse.

   5. Local pressure is applied for an initial period of 30 minutes, followed by a second period of 30 minutes if bleeding persists.

     a. If bleeding persists beyond 1 hour, suture repair of the arteriotomy generally is necessary.

     b. If bleeding stops with pressure, a sandbag is applied, and the patient is maintained supine with the leg straight for 12 hours. The pulses are assessed frequently.

X. **PARACENTESIS.**

A. **Indications for Paracentesis.**

   1. Diagnosis of unexplained ascites.

   2. Suspicion of spontaneous bacterial peritonitis.

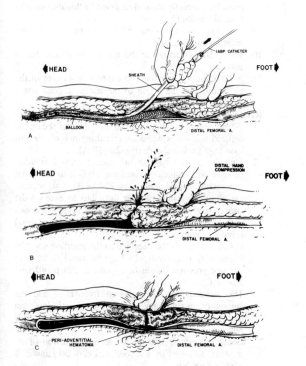

FIG 22–18.
Removal of the IABP. **A,** the deflated balloon is withdrawn to the sheath. **B,** the sheath and balloon are removed while pressure is held on the distal femoral artery to prevent emboli. The insertion site is allowed to bleed to wash out any thrombus. **C,** direct pressure is applied to the insertion site while distal pulses are assessed. (From Reemtsma K, Bregman D, Colten S, et al: Mechanical circulatory support—advance in intra aortic balloon pumping, in Shoemaker WC, Ayres S, Grenvik A, et al : *Textbook of Critical Care*. Philadelphia, WB Saunders Co, 1989, p 423. Used by permission.

3. Relief of severe ascites causing respiratory compromise.

B. General Approach.

1. Paracentesis is performed as a sterile procedure, and requires the following equipment: 20-gauge catheter-over-needle, stopcock, 50-mL syringe; extension tubing and collecting vessel; povidone-iodine solution; sterile gloves and drapes; and lidocaine (1% solution without epinephrine).

2. Place the patient in the supine position. Confirm the presence of fluid by percussion. The preferred site for paracentesis is lateral to the rectus abdominis muscle in the lower abdomen (Fig 22–19).

3. Prepare the skin with povidone-iodine solution and drape the field.

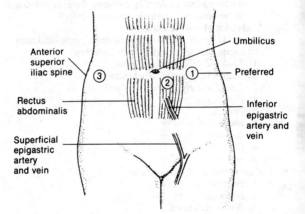

FIG 22–19.
Anatomic landmarks for paracentesis. *(1)* Preferred location lateral to rectus sheath. *(2)* Periumbilical. *(3)* Adjacent to anterior iliac spine. (From Yeston NS, Niehoff: Important procedures in the intensive care unit, in Civetta JM, Taylor RW, Kirby RR (eds): *Critical Care*. Philadelphia, JB Lippincott Co, 1988, p 252. Used by permission.)

C. **Technique for Paracentesis.**
1. Infiltrate the skin with lidocaine, using a 25-gauge needle. Anesthetize the deeper tissues with the 20-gauge needle, making the needle track discontinuous using the z-track technique.
2. While aspirating the syringe, advance the needle through the fascia and into the peritoneum, until ascitic fluid returns; remove the needle.
3. Insert the catheter-over-needle in the same manner; when ascitic fluid is again encountered, advance the catheter and remove the needle. Attach a three-way stopcock and the 50-mL syringe.
4. For diagnostic purposes, fluid may be aspirated directly. For drainage of massive ascites, the extension tubing is connected to the stopcock, so that the fluid can be withdrawn into the syringe and ejected through the tubing into a collecting container. Upon completion of the procedure, a sterile dressing is placed.

D. **Evaluation of Ascitic Fluid.**
The ascitic fluid should be collected under sterile conditions and a specimen sent for laboratory evaluation.
1. Total and differential cell count.
2. Gram's stain and bacterial culture.
3. Fungal and mycobacterial cultures.
4. Cytology.
5. Protein.
6. Glucose.
7. Amylase.
8. LDH.
9. pH.

E. **Complications of Paracentesis.**
1. Hemorrhage.
2. Infection.
3. Bowel perforation.
4. Bladder perforation.
5. Persistent ascitic leak.
6. Hypotension (secondary to withdrawal of excessive volume).

XI. PERITONEAL DIALYSIS: INSERTION OF THE TENCKHOFF CATHETER.

A. **Indications for Peritoneal Dialysis.**
   1. Temporary management of acute renal insufficiency.
   2. Long-term management of end-stage renal disease with continuous ambulatory peritoneal dialysis.

B. **The Tenckhoff Catheter.**
   The Tenckhoff catheter is a flexible silicone rubber tube with an inner diameter of 2.6 mm and an outer diameter of 5 mm, comprised of three segments: intraperitoneal segment (11–15 cm), intramural segment (5–7 cm), and external segment. The intraperitoneal segment has multiple 0.5-mm perforations. The intramural segment includes one or two Dacron cuffs.

C. **General Approach.**
   1. The bedside insertion of the peritoneal dialysis (Tenckhoff) catheter is performed as a sterile procedure and requires the following equipment: Tenckhoff catheter and obturator; detachable trocar and obturator; priming trocar or priming catheter; Faller guide; povidone-iodine solution; cap, mask, and sterile gown, gloves, towels, and drapes; lidocaine (1% solution without epinephrine); sterile instruments (knife, scissors, clamps, forceps); and peritoneal dialysis fluid and administration tubing.
   2. Contraindications to the insertion of a peritoneal dialysis catheter at the bedside include extreme obesity and previous abdominal surgery.
   3. Ascertain that the patient's bladder and rectum have been emptied. An NG tube should be placed to suction to empty the stomach.
   4. Place the patient in the supine position. The preferred site for placement is in the midline, inferior to the umbilicus.
   5. Prepare the skin with povidone-iodine solution. Don cap, mask, sterile gown, and sterile gloves, and create a sterile field with towels and drapes.

D. **Technique for Insertion of a Tenckhoff Catheter.**
   1. Infiltrate the skin and subcutaneous tissue with lidocaine. Make a 3 cm midline incision, 2 cm inferior to the umbilicus. Using blunt dissection, identify the linea alba and provide upward traction with a suture or a

clamp. Enter the peritoneum with a catheter-over-needle or trocar. Connect the priming catheter or trocar to the administration tubing and instill approximately 2 L of dialysis solution.

2. Lubricate the Tenckhoff catheter, its obturator, and the Dacron cuffs with sterile saline; insert the obturator into the Tenckhoff catheter. Remove the priming catheter or trocar and insert the detachable trocar and obturator. After correct positioning within the peritoneum, remove the obturator from the trocar.

3. Insert the Tenckhoff catheter and its obturator through the trocar, into the peritoneum, directing the catheter deeply into the pelvis. Remove the trocar over the catheter, after which it may be detached. Remove the obturator from the catheter, and position the inner Dacron cuff to rest at the fascial level. Test the catheter for patency. Secure the catheter to the fascia.

4. Create an exit site lateral and inferior to the entrance with a stab wound, so that the subcutaneous cuff is 2 cm below the skin; this site should be just large enough for the catheter. Create a subcutaneous tunnel with the Faller guide, and carefully pull the end of the catheter through the tunnel; insert the titanium connector. Suture the insertion wound and apply sterile dressings.

5. Attempt to direct the obturator and catheter into the pelvis. After correct positioning within the peritoneum, remove the obturator from the catheter.

6. Position the inner Dacron cuff to rest at the fascial level. Test the catheter for patency.

7. Instill 1 L of dialysis fluid into the abdomen. Allow it to drain.

8. Create an exit site lateral and inferior to the entrance with a stab wound, so that the subcutaneous cuff is 2 cm below the skin; this site should be just large enough for the catheter.

9. Create a subcutaneous tunnel with the Faller guide, and carefully pull the end of the catheter through the tunnel; insert the titanium connector.

10. Suture the insertion wound and apply sterile dressings.

E. **Complications of Tenckhoff Catheter Insertion.**

1. Bleeding from the abdominal wall, recognized as bloody effluent, occurs in 30% of cases.

2. Dialysis solution leak (15%–35%).
3. Inadequate drainage.
4. Extraperitoneal extravasation.
5. Intestinal perforation.
6. Peritonitis.

F. **Special Considerations.**

1. Other types of peritoneal dialysis catheters, such as any of the rigid dialysis catheters, may be placed at the bedside; however, the Tenckhoff catheter appears to be the safest and the most widely used.
2. The most common cause of early catheter failure is omental entanglement, due to placement anteriorly in the peritoneum, rather than deeper in the pelvis.

XII. SENGSTAKEN-BLAKEMORE TUBE.

A. **Indications for Placement of the Sengstaken-Blakemore Tube.**

1. To compress endoscopically proven variceal hemorrhage by tamponade of the gastroesophageal junction or lower esophagus.
2. The Sengstaken-Blakemore tube is usually inserted after other methods such as vasopressin or sclerotherapy have failed to control variceal bleeding.

B. **General Approach.**

1. **Adequate fluid resuscitation should take precedence over attempts to treat upper GI bleeding and is accomplished with two large-bore IV catheters in the forearm.**
2. After adequate fluid resuscitation is achieved, the placement of a Sengstaken-Blakemore tube may be performed in conjunction with other therapeutic modalities in the management of variceal hemorrhage, such as the administration of vasopressin (0.2–0.4 units/min IV) or in the event of bleeding following endoscopic sclerotherapy.
3. The placement of a Sengstaken-Blakemore tube should be performed with continuous ECG monitoring, with supplemental oxygen available, and requires the following equipment: Sengstaken-Blakemore tube, suction apparatus, 50-mL syringe, pressure manometer, NG tube (10F–12F), Ewald tube, lubrication, and supplies for ET intubation.

C.   **Technique for Insertion.**
1. Place the patient in the left lateral decubitus position.
2. Empty the stomach by passing a large orogastric or Ewald tube.
3. Test the balloons of the Sengstaken-Blakemore tube carefully prior to insertion; lubricate the tube well.
4. Pass the tube nasally to the 50-cm mark.
5. Fill the gastric balloon with 250–500 mL air or a dilute radiocontrast solution. Clamp the tube (Fig. 22–20).
6. Using gentle traction, withdraw the tube until resistance is encountered at the gastroesophageal junction.

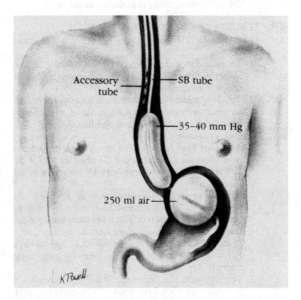

FIG 22–20.
Proper insertion of the Sengstaken-Blakemore (SB) tube. (From Eastwood GL: Variceal bleeding, in Rippe JM, Irwin RS, Alpert JS, et al (eds): *Intensive Care Medicine.* Boston, Little, Brown & Co, 1985, p 737. Used by permission.)

Secure the tube to the patient's face under minimal traction. A football helmet with face mask is useful to anchor the tube.

7. Irrigate the distal tube with saline. In the absence of continued bleeding, the esophageal tube is left deflated. If bleeding has not ceased, the esophageal balloon should be inflated to 40 mm Hg.

8. Pass the NG tube through the contralateral nostril until resistance is sensed at the level of the esophageal balloon. **The blind esophageal segment should be aspirated continuously to prevent regurgitation and aspiration of esophageal secretions.**

9. Obtain a CXR to confirm correct positioning.

10. Some tubes (Minnesota tube) have an additional esophageal lumen. so that an NG tube is unnecessary.

D. Management.

1. The esophageal tube may remain deflated in the absence of bleeding, but should be inflated to 40 mm Hg if bleeding ensues in the first 24 hours after placement.

2. The balloon(s) of the Sengstaken-Blakemore tube remain inflated for 24 hours, at which time they are deflated if no further bleeding has occurred.

3. **The esophageal balloon should be deflated transiently every 4–6 hours to prevent mucosal ischemia.**

4. The tube may be removed after a second 24-hour period without bleeding.

E. Complications.

1. Esophageal rupture secondary to malposition of the gastric balloon.

2. Aspiration of blood, gastric secretion, or saliva.

3. Refractory variceal hemorrhage.

F. Special Considerations.

Consider ET intubation for airway protection in all cases of altered consciousness, respiratory compromise, aspiration, shock, or complex medical problems.

XIII. LUMBAR PUNCTURE.

A. Patient in lateral knee-chest position at edge of bed, or sitting on edge of bed, flexed over bedside table (cannot measure pressure accurately this way).

B. Palpate superior iliac crest; spinous process at this level is usually L4. Puncture may be performed at L3–4, L4–5, or L5-S1.

C. Prepare the skin with povidone-iodine and drape as sterile field, but do not mask key landmarks.

D. Anesthetize the skin with 1% lidocaine, raising a small wheal in midline of chosen interspace with a 27-gauge needle. Change to a 22-gauge 1.5-in. needle for anesthetizing the deeper tissue, including lumbodorsal fascia.

E. Insert a 20-gauge spinal needle with bevel parallel to longitudinal axis of spine (to minimize dural opening) in midline, aiming slightly cephalad.

F. With dural penetration, a distinct "give" may be felt.

G. Remove the stylet slowly and confirm flow of CSF.

H. If no CSF (or bone) is encountered, withdraw needle completely and reassess landmarks prior to repeated attempt.

I. When CSF flow has been obtained, have patient lie on side and straighten legs and attach manometer to measure pressure.

J. Collect CSF for cell count and differential, glucose, protein, Gram's stain, culture and sensitivity, as well as cytology, TB, and fungal cultures as indicated (Table 22–1).

K. Replace stylet, remove needle, and apply sterile dressing.

L. The patient should remain flat in bed for 6 hours to minimize CSF leak.

XIV. INTRACRANIAL PRESSURE MONITORING.

Because of the potentially devastating effects of infection, sterility in insertion and maintenance of these systems is critical. During the time that these devices are in use, patients should be given prophylactic antistaphylococcal antibiotics, e.g., vancomycin 500 mg IV q.6h.

A. Ventriculostomy is usually performed on the right (nondominant) side (see Fig 22–21).

1. The patient should be supine, with the head slightly elevated and immobilized (sandbags, tape, etc.).

2. Shave area about coronal suture from 1 cm beyond midline to at least 8 cm lateral, from 3 cm posterior to coronal suture to 3 cm anterior to coronal suture.

3. Wearing mask and sterile gloves, prepare shaved area with povidone-iodine and drape as sterile field, taking

TABLE 22–1.
Spinal Fluid Laboratory Values*

	Appearance	RBC	WBC	Glucose	Protein
Normal	Clear	0	0 PMNs, 0–5 lymphocytes	50–80 (mg/dL)	20–50 (mg/dL)
Subarachnoid hemorrhage	Bloody, xanthochromic	>100	2/1,000 RBCs	WNL	Increased (1 mg/1,000 RBCs)
Viral meningitis	Occasionally xanthochromic	Few	Increased, mainly mononuclear cells	WNL	Slightly increased
Bacterial meningitis	Cloudy	Few	Increased, mainly PMNs	Decreased	Increased

*WNL = Within normal limits.

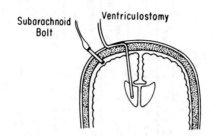

FIG 22–21.
Coronal view of the brain demonstrating ICP monitoring techniques. (From Fuchs HE: Neurosurgical intensive care, in Lyerly HK (ed): *The Handbook of Surgical Intensive Care,* ed 2. Chicago, Year Book Medical Publishers, Inc, 1988.)

care to allow nasal bridge and external auditory canal to be palpated through drapes.

4. Change gloves and inject 1% lidocaine with epinephrine to raise a wheal 1 cm anterior to the coronal suture, 3 cm from midline, and another approximately 5 cm lateral to this site (this is for the catheter exit site).

5. Using a no. 15 blade, make a 5-mm stab wound in each of these locations.

6. Insert a curved hemostat into the lateral incision and create a subcutaneous tunnel to the medial incision. Be sure that the tips of the hemostat can be opened within the medial incision.

7. Using a twist drill, drill a hole at the medial point in the coronal plane, aiming toward the medial canthus of the ipsilateral eye. As the drill reaches the inner table of the skull, it will "catch." Slowly rotate the drill in the same direction while pulling back, to prevent plunging, and then withdraw the drill, continuing to rotate it. (This method removes bone chips along with the drill.)

8. The dura is penetrated using a spinal needle and the dural opening enlarged with progressively larger ventricular needles.

9. Measure 6 cm on the ventricular catheter, place thumb at this point, and advance catheter (with stylet in place)

through twist drill hole in the same direction as in (9.). By 4–5 cm, the frontal horn should be entered (with a slight give). The stylet is pulled back and the catheter advanced 1 cm. Free flow of CSF should be noted as the stylet is removed. If no fluid is obtained by 6 cm, the catheter should be withdrawn, landmarks re-checked, and the catheter reinserted (three attempts maximum).

10. Once CSF is obtained, the catheter should be occluded with manual pressure and the distal end inserted into the hemostat tips in the medial incision and carefully pulled through the subcutaneous tunnel to the lateral incision.

11. Spontaneous flow of CSF is confirmed, the medial incision is closed with a single monofilament suture (taking care not to pierce the catheter), and the exit wound closed around the catheter with one monofilament suture (securing the catheter in place as the suture is tied).

12. The drainage and monitoring tubing system is then attached to the catheter and a good waveform tracing is confirmed on the monitor.

13. Sterile dressings are applied. (*Note:* In patients with head trauma, intracranial shifts may occur which alter the position of the ventricular system. For this reason, after an initial attempt at catheterization using the above landmarks, in an emergency situation, without a CT scan to document the position of the ventricular system, a second attempt should be directed at the ipsilateral lateral canthus and a third attempt at the contralateral medial canthus.)

B. **Subarachnoid Bolt.**
   1. Shave and prepare the head as above for ventriculostomy.
   2. Make a 3-cm incision over the frontal region, preferably the nondominant side.
   3. Make a 0.5-cm twist drill hole.
   4. Open dura with a cruciate incision.
   5. Measure depth of the hole in the bone.
   6. Insert hollow, metal, self-threading plug into hole so that bottom of plug is even with bottom of hole.

7. Flush system with saline to remove blood and ensure adequate communication with subarachnoid space. (Pulsations should be visible in fluid within the plug.)
8. Connect a stopcock and pressure tubing to plug.
9. Close skin incision and apply a sterile dressing.
   (*Note:* This method of ICP monitoring does not allow drainage of CSF.)

XV. ASPIRATION OF VENTRICULOPERITONEAL SHUNT.

To obtain fluid from the reservoir of a ventriculoperitoneal or ventriculoatrial shunt:

1. Plain skull film to document hardware, presence of reservoir which may be tapped to obtain fluid, location and connections of intracranial catheter(s).
2. Palpate reservoir to be tapped.
3. Shave 4-cm area around reservoir.
4. Prepare area with multiple layers of povidone-iodine and drape as sterile field.
5. Insert a 23-gauge butterfly catheter into center of reservoir. There should be free flow of CSF. If no CSF, attempt to reposition needle.
6. Once flow is established, attach manometer to read pressure.
7. Collect CSF for desired studies. (*Note:* Avoid aspiration of CSF with syringe as this may draw choroid plexus into ventricular catheter and cause hemorrhage or catheter occlusion.)
8. Withdraw needle, apply sterile dressing.

SELECTED REFERENCES

Berk JL, Sampliner JE (eds): *Handbook of Critical Care*. Boston, Little, Brown & Co, 1990.

Civetta JM (ed): *Intensive Care Therapeutics*. New York, Appleton-Century-Crofts, 1980.

Civetta JM, Taylor RW, Kirby RR (eds): *Critical Care*. Philadelphia, JB Lippincott Co., 1988.

Daldec DL, Krome RL: Thoracostomy. *Emerg Med Clin North Am* 1986; 4:441.

Dauphinee K: Orotracheal intubation. *Emerg Med Clin North Am* 1988; 6:699.

Kaye W: Intravenous techniques, in *Textbook of Advanced Cardiac Life Support*. Dallas, American Heart Association, 1987, pp 141–153.

Nolph KD (ed): *Peritoneal Dialysis*. Dordecht, Netherlands, Kluwer Academic, 1989.

Putterman C: Central venous catheterization. *Acute Care* 1986; 12:219.

Sladen A: *Invasive Monitoring and Its Complications in the Intensive Care Unit*. St Louis, CV Mosby Co, 1990.

Taylor RW, Civetta JM, Kirby RR (eds): *Techniques and Procedures in Critical Care*. Philadelphia, JB Lippincott Co, 1990.

Walls RM: Cricothyroidotomy. *Emerg Med Clin North Am* 1988; 6:725.

MEDICATIONS **23**

Drug*	Use	Form	Dose
Acebutolol (Sectral)	Antihypertensive; β-antagonist	**Cap:** 200, 400 mg	200–600 mg PO BID
Acetaminophen (Tylenol)	Antipyretic	**Cap:** 325 mg; **Elixir:** 160 mg/5 mL; **Supp:** 125, 325, 650 mg	650 mg PO/PR q.3–4h.
Acetaminophen with codeine (Tylenol #3 or #4)	Analgesic	**Tab #3:** 300 mg acetaminophen/30 mg codeine; **Tab #4:** 300 mg acetaminophen/60 mg codeine; **Elix:** 120 mg acetaminophen/12 mg codeine	1–2 PO q.3–4h. prn; 15 mL PO q.3–4h. prn
Acetaminophen with oxycodone (Percocet)	Analgesic	**Tab:** 325 mg acetaminophen/5 mg oxycodone	1–2 PO q.3–4h. prn
Acetazolamide (Diamox)	Diuretic; carbonic andydrase inhibitor; HCO$_3$ excretion	**Inj:** 500 mg; **Tab:** 125, 250 mg; **Sustained release:** 500 mg	250–375 mg PO q.d.; 250–500 mg IV q.8h × 3
Acyclovir (Zovirax)	Antiviral	**Inj:** 500 mg/10 mL; **Cap:** 200 mg	5–10 mg/kg IV q.8h.
Adenosine (Adenocard)	Antiarrhythmic	**Inj:** 6mg/2 mL	6 mg bolus, then 12 mg bolus if needed
Albuterol (Proventil, Ventolin)	Bronchodilator; β-agonist	**Inhaler:** 90 µg/dose; **Tab** 2, 4 mg; **Solution:** 0.4 mg/mL	1–2 puffs q.4–6h.; 2–4 mg PO t.i.d.-q.i.d.
Allopurinol (Zyloprim)	Inhibitor of uric acid synthetase	**Tab:** 100, 300 mg	200–600 mg PO q.d.

*Trade name given in parentheses.

(Continued.)

835

Drug*	Use	Form	Dose
Amiloride (Midamor)	Potassium sparing diuretic	**Tab:** 5 mg	1–4 PO q.d.
Aminocarproic acid (Amicar)	Coagulant	**Inj:** 250 mg/mL **Tab:** 500 mg; **Solution:** 250 mg/mL	**Load:** 4 g; **Infusion:** 1 g/h × 4
Aminophylline	Bronchodilator	**Inj:** 25 mg/mL	See theophylline
Amiodarone (Cordarone)	Antiarrythmic	**Tab:** 200 mg	**Load**—1,600 mg PO/day **Maintenance:** 400 mg q. day
Amitriptyline (Elavil)	Antidepressant	**Inj:** 10 mg/mL; **Tab:** 10, 25, 50, 75, 100, 150 mg	25–50 mg PO t.i.d.; 20–30 mg IM q.i.d.
Amphotericin B (Fungizone)	Antifungal	**Inj:** 5 mg/10 mL	**Systemic:** 0.3–1 mg/kg/day; **Bladder irrigation:** 50 mg/L D5W
Amrinone (Inocor)	Inotrope	**Inj:** 5 mg/mL (20 mL)	**Load:** 0.75 mg/kg; **Infusion:** 5–10 µg/kg/min; (see Chapter 5)
Aspirin (ASA)	Analgesic; antipyretic; antiinflammatory; antiplatelet activity	**Cap:** 325 mg; **Enteric coated:** 325 mg; **Supp:** 125, 325, 650 mg; **Tab:** 325 mg	650 mg PO/PR q.3–4h. prn
Atenolol (Tenormin)	Antihypertensive; β-antagonist	**Tab:** 50, 100 mg	50–100 mg PO q.d.
Atracurium (Tracrium)	Nondepolarizing neuromuscular blocking agent	**Inj:** 10 mg/mL	0.3–0.5 mg/kg IV (see Chapter 21)

Atropine	Anticholinergic	**Inj:** 0.05, 0.1, 0.3, 0.4, 0.5, 0.8, 1 mg/mL	0.5 mg IV (see Chapter 5)
Azathioprine (Imuran)	Immunosuppressive	**Inj:** 5 mg/ml; **Tab:** 50 mg	(See Chapter 16)
Beclomethasone (Vanceril)	Antiasthmatic; corticosteroid	**Inhaler:** 42 µg/dose	2 puffs q.3–4 h.
Bumetanide (Bumex)	Diuretic	**Inj:** 0.25 mg/mL; **Tab:** 0.5, 1 mg	0.5–2 mg/day PO; 0.5–1 mg IV q4h up to 10 mg/day
Bretylium tosylate (Bretylol)	Antiarrhythmic	**Inj:** 50 mg/mL (10 mL)	**Load:** 5–10 mg/kg/ **Infusion:** 1–2 mg/min (see Chapter 5)
Brompton's mix	Analgesic	**Solution:** 1 mg morphine/mL, 0.67 mg cocaine/mL of alcohol cherry syrup	5–10 mL PO q.3–4 h. prn
Calcifediol (Calderol)	Vitamin D supplement in CRF	**Cap:** 20, 50 µg	20–100 µg PO q.d.
Calcium chloride	Calcium supplement	**Inj:** 100 mg/mL (10 mL); 13.6 mEq (272 mg) Ca/g of CaCl₂	**For CPR:** 0.5–1.0 g IV; **For Ca:** 0.5–1.0 g IV q1–3d
Calcium gluconate	Calcium supplement	**Inj:** 100 mg/mL (10 mL); 4.5 mEq (90 mg) Ca/g of Ca gluconate (Neo-calglucon) 155 mg Ca/5 mL	**For Ca:** 0.5–2.0 g IV; 15–30 mL PO t.i.d. (Neo-calglucon)
Captopril (Capoten)	Antihypertensive; ACE inhibitor	**Tab:** 12.5, 25, 50, 100 mg	25–150 mg PO t.i.d.

*Trade name given in parentheses.

(Continued.)

Drug*	Use	Form	Dose
Chlorpromazine (Thorazine)	Antipsychotic; tranquilizer; antihypertensive	**Inj:** 25 mg/mL; **Supp:** 25,100 mg; **Tab:** 10, 25, 50, 100 mg	10–25 mg PO/IM t.i.d.; 1 mg IV prn BP
Cimetidine (Tagament)	Antiulcer; H_2 antagonist	**Inj:** 150 mg/mL; **Tab:** 200, 300, 400, 800 mg; **Liq:** 300 mg/5 mg	300 mg PO/IV q.6h; 37.5 mg/hr
Codeine	Narcotic; analgesic; antitussive	**Inj:** 15, 30, 60 mg/mL; **Tab:** 15, 30, 60 mg	30–60 mg PO/IM q.3–4h. prn
Clonidine (Catapress)	Antihypertensive	**Tab:** 0.1, 0.2, 0.3 mg; **Transdermal patch:** 3.5 cm^2, 7 cm^2, 10.5 cm^2	0.1–0.8 mg PO q.8–12h.; **Topical:** q.7d.
Cyclosporine (Sandimmune)	Immunosuppressive	(see Chapter 16)	
Dantrolene (Dantrium)	Malignant hyperthermia therapy	**Inj:** 0.32 mg/mL; **Cap:** 25, 50, 100 mg	2.5 mg/kg IV q.6h. (see Chapter 17)
Darvocet-N-100	Analgesic	**Tab:** 100 mg propoxyphene/650 mg acetaminophen	1–2 PO q.3–4h. prn
Deferoxamine (Desferal)	Iron intoxication	**Inj:** 500 mg/2 mL	1 g IV followed by 500 mg IV q.4–12h.
Desmopressin acetate (DDAVP)	DI; bleeding	**Inj:** 4 μg/mL	**DI:** 1 μg–2μg IV q.12.; **Bleeding:** 0.3 μg/kg IV

Dexamethasone (Decadron)	Corticosteroid	**Inj:** 4, 10, 20, 24 mg/mL; **Tab:** 0.25, 0.5, 0.75, 1, 1.5, 2, 4, 6 mg; **Elixir:** 0.5 mg/mL	10 mg IV q.6h. (see Chapter 13)
Diazepam (Valium)	Antianxiety; tranquilizer	**Inj:** 5 mg/mL; **Tab:** 2, 5, 10 mg	5–10 mg PO/IM q.4h. prn; 2.5 mg IV q15–20 min prn (see Chapter 21)
Diazoxide (Hyperstat)	Antihypertensive	**Inj:** 15 mg/mL (20 mL)	1–3 mg/kg IV (see Chapter 9)
Digoxin (Lanoxin)	Inotrope	**Inj:** 0.1, 0.25 mg/mL; **Elixir:** 0.05 mg/mL; **Tab:** 0.125, 0.25, 0.5 mg	**Load:** 12–15 µg/kg/24 hr; **Maintenance:** 0.125–0.5 mg q.d. (see Chapter 5)
Dihydrotachysterol (Hytakerol)	Vitamin D analogue	**Cap:** 0.125 mg; **Solution:** 0.25 mg/mL	**Load:** 0.8–2.4 mg PO q.d.; **Maintenance:** 0.2–1.0 mg PO q.d.
Diltiazem (Cardizem)	Antianginal; calcium channel blocker	**Tab:** 30, 60, 90, 120 mg	30–90 mg PO q.i.d.
Diphenhydramine (Benadryl)	Antihistamine	**Inj:** 10, 50 mg/mL; **Cap:** 25, 50 mg; **Elixir:** 2.5 mg/5mL	25–50 mg PO/IM q.3–4h. prn
Diphenoxylate (Lomotil)	Antidiarreal	**Tab, Solution:** 2.5 mg diphenoxylate 0.025 mg atropine per tab or 5 mL	1–2 tab PO 4 × day prn

*Trade name given in parentheses.

(Continued.)

Drug*	Use	Form	Dose
Dipyridamole (Persantine)	Anti-platelet aggregation	Tab 25, 50, 75 mg	50–75 mg PO t.i.d.
Disopyramide (Norpace)	Antiarrhythmic	**Cap**: 100, 150 mg; **Controlled release**: 100, 150 mg	100–200 mg PO q.6–8h.; 200–400 mg PO q.12h.
Dobutamine (Dobutrex)	Inotrope	**Inj**: 50 mg/mL (5 mL)	2.0–20.0 μg/kg/min (see Chapter 5)
Docusate sodium (Colace)	Stool softener	**Cap**: 50, 100, 250 mg; **Tab**: 50, 100 mg; **Syrup**: 60 mg, Liq 10 mg/ml	100 mg PO b.i.d.–t.i.d.
Dopamine (Inotropin)	Inotrope	**Inj**: 40, 80 160 mg/mL (15 mL)	1.0–20.0 μg/kg/min (see Chapter 5)
Edrophonium (Tensilon)	Cholinergic; curare antagonist	**Inj**: 10 mg/mL	10 mg IV to convert PAT to NSR (1 mg test dose); 0.5–1.0 mg/kg IV (see Chapter 21)
Enalapril (Vasotec)	ACE inhibitor	**Inj**: 1.25 mg/mL; **Tab**: 5, 10, 20 mg	10–40 mg PO q.d.; 1.25–5.0 mg IV q.6h.
Encainide (Enkaid)	Antiarrhythmic	**Tab**: 25, 35, 50 mg	25–50 mg PO t.i.d.
Epinephrine (Adrenalin)	Inotrope; pressor; bronchodilator	**Inj**: 1 mg/mL (1:1000); **Inj**: 0.1 mg/mL (1:10,000)	0.01–0.15 μg/kg/min (see Chapter 5)
Esmolol (Brevibloc)	β-antagonist	**Inj**: 250 mg/mL (10 mL)	**Load**: 500 μg/kg/min; **Infusion**: 50–200 μg/kg/min

Ethacrynic acid (Edecrin)	Diuretic	**Inj:** 50 mg/vial; **Tab:** 25, 50 mg	25–100 mg PO q.d.; 0.5–1.0 mg/kg/IV
Etomidate (Amidate)	Induction agent	**Inj:** 1 mg/mL	0.2–0.3 mg/kg IV (see Chapter 21)
Famotidine (Pepcid)	H₂-antagonist	**Inj:** 10 mg/mL; **Tab:** 20, 40 mg	20 mg PO/IV q.12h.
Fentanyl (Sublimaze)	Analgesic	**Inj:** 0.05 mg/mL	0.001–0.002 mg/kg IV (see Chapter 21)
Flecainide (Tambocor)	Antiarrhythmic	**Tab:** 100 mg	100–200 mg PO b.i.d.
Flucytosine (Ancobon)	Antifungal	**Cap:** 250, 500 mg	12.5–37.5 mg/kg PO q.6h.
Fluconazole (Diflucan)	Antifungal	**Inj:** 2 mg/mL; **Tab:** 50, 100, 200 mg	200–400 mg PO/IV q.d. × 1, then 100–200 mg PO IV q.d.
Flurazepam (Dalmane)	Hypnotic	**Cap:** 15, 30 mg	15–30 mg PO q.h.s. prn
Furosemide (Lasix)	Diuretic	**Inj:** 10 mg/mL; **Tab:** 20, 40, 80 mg; **Solution:** 10 mg/mL	20–80 mg PO q.d.; 20–40 mg IV (see Chapter 9)
Ganciclovir (Cytovene)	Antiviral	**Inj:** 500 mg	5 mg/kg IV q.8h.
Glucagon	Hypoglycemia treatment	**Inj:** 1 unit/ 1 mL	0.5–1 units IV/IM

*Trade name given in parentheses.

(Continued.)

Drug*	Use	Form	Dose
Glycopyrrolate (Roginul)	Anticholinergic	**Inj:** 0.2 mg/mL; **Tab:** 1, 2 mg	**To reverse neuromuscular blocking agent;** 0.2 mg IV for each 1 mg Neostigmine
Guanethidine (Ismelin)	Antihypertensive	**Tab:** 10, 25 mg	10–25 mg PO q.d.
Haloperidol (Haldol)	Antipsychotic	**Inj:** 5 mg/mL; **Solution:** 2 mg/mL; **Tab:** 0.5, 1, 2, 5, 10, 20 mg	2–5 mg PO/IM q.$\frac{1}{2}$–1h prn (see Chapter 13)
Hydralazine (Apresoline)	Antihypertensive; vasodilator	**Inj:** 20 mg/mL; **Tab:** 10, 25, 50, 100 mg	10–40 mg PO q.i.d.; 10–40 mg; IM q.1–2h. prn; 10–20 mg IV prn (see Chapter 9)
Hydrochlorothiazide (Hydrodiuril)	Diuretic (thiazide)	**Tab:** 25, 50, 100 mg; **Solution:** 10, 100 mg/mL	25–100 mg PO q.d.
Hydrocortisone (Solu-Cortef)	Corticosteroid	**Inj:** 100, 250, 500, 1,000 mg/vial	100 mg IV q.8h. (see Chapter 14)
Hydromorphone (Dilaudid)	Analgesic	**Inj:** 1, 2, 3, 4 mg/10 mL; **Tab:** 2, 3, 4 mg; **Supp:** 3 mg	2–4 PO/IM q.4–6h. prn; 3 mg PR q.6–8h.
Hydroxyzine (Atarax, Vistaril)	Antianxiety	**Inj:** 25, 50 mg/mL; **Syrup:** 2 mg/mL; **Tab:** 10, 25, 50, 100 mg	25–100 mg PO/IM q.i.d.

Imipramine (Tofranil)	Antidepressant	**Inj:** 12.5 mL; **Cap:** 75, 100, 125, 150 mg; **Tab:** 10, 25, 50 mg	25–50 mg PO/IM q.i.d.
Indomethacin (Indocin)	Anti-inflammatory	**Cap:** 25, 50 mg; **Supp:** 50 mg; **Susp:** 25 mg/5 mL	25–50 mg PO/PR b.i.d.–t.i.d.
Isoproterenol (Isuprel)	β-agonist	**Inj:** 0.2 mg/mL (5 mL)	0.01–0.10 µg/kg/min (see Chapters 1–3)
Ketamine (Ketalap)	Induction agent	**Inj:** 10 mg/mL	1–3 mg/kg IV (see Chapter 21)
Ketoconazole (Nizoral)	Antifungal	**Tab:** 200 mg; **Susp:** 100 mg/5 mL	200–400 mg PO q.d.
Labetalol (Trandate)	Antihypertensive	**Inj:** 5 mg/mL; **Tab:** 100, 200, 300 mg	100–400 mg PO b.i.d.; **Load:** 20 mg; **Infusion:** 0.5–2.0 mg/min
Lactulose (Cephulac)	Hepatic encephalopathy	**Syrup:** 67%	15–50 mL PO t.i.d.; 300 mL in 700 mL NS PR q.4–6h.
Levarterenol/Norepinephrine (Levophed)	Hypotension; vasopressor	**Inj:** 1 mg/mL (4 mL)	0.01–0.20 µg/kg/min (see Chapters 3–5)
Loperamide (Imodium)	Antidiarrheal	**Cap:** 2 mg; **Liq:** 1 mg/5 mL	**Load:** 4 mg; 2 mg after each stool up to 16 mg/day
Mannitol	Osmotic diuretic	**Inj:** 5%, 10%, 15%, 20%, 25%	12.5–25 mg IV prn

*Trade name given in parentheses.

(Continued.)

Drug*	Use	Form	Dose
Meperidine (Demerol)	Analgesic	**Inj:** 25, 50, 100 mg; **Elixir:** 50 mg/5 mL; **Tab:** 50 mg	0.5–2.0 mg/kg IV q.2–3h.; 50–75 mg PO/IM q.3–4h. (see Chapter 21)
Methohexital (Brevital)	Induction agent	**Inj:** 10 mg/mL	0.7–1.0 mg/kg IV (see Chapter 21)
Methyldopa (Aldomet)	Antihypertensive	**Inj:** 50 mg/mL; **Tab:** 125, 250, 500 mg; **Susp:** 250 mg/mL	250–500 mg PO b.i.d.–t.i.d.; 250–500 mg IV q.6–8h.
Methylprednisone (Solu-Medrol)	Corticosteroid	**Inj:** 40, 125, 500, 1,000, 2,000 mg/vial; **Tab:** 2, 4, 8, 16, 24, 32 mg	(See Chapters 14 and 16)
Metoclopramide (Reglan)	Gastric motility	**Inj:** 5 mg/mL; **Tab:** 10 mg; **Syrup:** 1 mg/mL	10 mg PO/IV q.6h.
Metolazone (Zaroxolyn)	Diuretic	**Tab:** 2.5, 5, 10 mg	5–20 mg PO q.d.
Metoprolol (Lopressor)	Antihypertensive	**Inj:** 1 mg/mL; **Tab:** 50, 100 mg	50–200 mg PO b.i.d.; 5 mg IV prn
Mexiletine (Mexitil)	Antiarrhythmia	**Tab:** 150, 200, 250 mg	200–400 mg PO q.8h.
Midazolam (Versed)	Antianxiety	**Inj:** 1, 5 mg/mL	0.15–0.35 mg/kg IV (see Chapter 21)
Monoctanoin (Moctanin)	Dissolve gallstones	**Solution:** 120 mL/bottle	3–5 mL/hr in perfusion into bile duct

Morphine	Analgesic	**Inj:** 1 mg/mL	0.05–0.20 mg/kg IV q.1h.; 8–10 mg IM q.3–4h. (see Chapter 21)
Nadolol (Corgard)	Antihypertensive; β-antagonist	**Tab:** 20, 40, 80, 120, 160 mg	40–80 mg PO q.d.
Naloxone (Narcan)	Narcotic antagonist	**Inj:** 0.02, 0.4, 1.0 mg/mL	0.3 mg IV prn
Neostigmine	Anticholinesterase	1:1,000 1 mg/1 mL 1:2,000 0.5 mg/1 mL	0.3–0.6 mg/kg IV (see Chapter 21)
Nifedipine (Procardia)	Calcium channel blocker	**Cap:** 10, 20 mg	10–20 mg PO t.i.d.
Nitroglycerin	Vasodilator	**Inj:** 0.5, 0.8, 5, 10 mg/mL; **Tab:** 0.15, 0.3, 0.4, 0.6 mg; **Ointment:** 2% (1 in. = 15 mg)	0.3–0.6 mg sublingually; 1–4 in. topically q.4–8h.; 0.1–2.0 µg/kg/min (see Chapter 5)
Nitroprusside (Nipride)	Antihypertensive; vasodilator	**Inj:** 10 mg/mL (5 mL)	1–10 µg/kg/min (see Chapters 5 and 9)
Octreotide acetate (Sandostatin)	Somatostatin analog	**Inj:** 0.05 mg, 0.1 mg, 0.5 mg	50–100 µg SQ q.8–12h.
OKT3	Immunosuppressive		(See Chapter 16)
Omeprazole (Prilosec)	Proton pump inhibitor	**Cap:** 20 mg	20 mg PO q.d.
Oxazepam (Serax)	Antianxiety; tranquilizer	**Cap:** 10, 15, 30 mg; **Tab:** 15 mg	10–30 mg PO t.i.d.–q.i.d.

*Trade name given in parentheses.

(Continued.)

Drug*	Use	Form	Dose
Oxycodone (Percodan)	Analgesic	**Tab:** 325 mg ASA/0.38 oxycodone terephthalate/4.5 mg oxycodone HCl	1–2 PO q.4h. prn
Pancreatin	Pancreatic enzyme replacement	**Tab:** (Pancreatin, 325 mg; lipase, 650 U; protease, 8,125 U; amylase, 8,125 U)	1–3 tab PO with meals
Pancrelipase (Cotazym, Viokinase)	Pancreatic enzyme replacement	**Cotazym Cap:** Lipase, 8,000 U; protease, 30,000 U; amylase, 30,000 U; calcium carbonate, 25 mg; **Viokinase Tab:** lipase, 8,000 U; protease, 30,000 U; amylase 30,000 U	1–3 tab PO before meals
Pancuronium bromide (Pavulon)	Nondepolarizing neuromuscular blocking agent	**Inj:** 1, 2 mg/mL	**Load:** 0.04–0.1 mg/kg IV; then 0.01 mg/kg IV increments
Paregoric (Donnagel)	Antidiarrheal	**Liq:** 2 mg/5 mL (0.04% MSO$_4$)	5–10 mL PO q.i.d. prn
Phenobarbital	Anticonvulsant	**Inj:** 30, 60, 130 mg/mL; **Tab:** 8, 16, 32, 65, 100 mg; **Elixir:** 4 mg/mL	1–5 mg/kg/day PO/IV
Phenylephrine (Neosynephrine)	Vasopressor	**Inj:** 10 mg/mL (1 mL)	0.6–5.0 µg/kg/min (see Chapter 5)

Phenoxybenzamine (Dibenzyline)	Alphadrenergic blocker	Tab: 10 mg	10 – 40 mg PO q.8 – 12h. (see Chapter 14)
Phentolamine	α-antagonist	Inj: 5 mg/mL	5 mg IM/IV prn
Phenytoin (Dilantin)	Anticonvulsant; antiarrhythmic	Inj: 50 mg/mL; Cap: 30, 100 mg; Suspension: 30, 125 mg/5 mL	100–300 mg PO t.i.d.; Load: 10–15 mg/kg/IV; Maintenance: 4 – 5 mg/kg/day
Prazosin (Minipress)	Antihypertensive	Cap: 1, 2, 5 mg	5 mg PO t.i.d.
Prednisone	Corticosteroid	Tab: 1, 2.5, 5, 20 50 mg Solution: 5 mg/5 mL	(See Chapters 14 and 16)
Procainamide (Pronestyl)	Antiarrhythmic	Inj: 100, 500 mg/mL; Cap: 250, 375, 500 mg; Sustained release: 250, 500, 750, 1,000 mg	Load: 750–1,000 mg; Infusion: 3 mg/kg/hr; Maintenance: PO 250–500 mg q.4h. or 500–1,000 mg q.6h. (see Chapter 5)
Prochlorperazine (Compazine)	Antiemetic	Inj: 5 mg/mL; Tab: 5, 10, 25 mg; Supp: 2.5, 5, 25 mg	10 mg PO/IM q.4–6h. prn; 25 mg PR b.i.d. prn
Promethazine (Phenergan)	Antiemetic	Inj: 25, 50 mg/mL; Tab: 12.5, 25, 50 mg; Supp: 12.5, 25, 50 mg	12.5–25 mg PO/IM; q4–6h prn; 25 mg PR t.i.d.–q.i.d. prn
Propofol (Diprivan)	Induction agent	Inj: 10 mg/mL	1.5 – 3.0 mg/kg IV (see Chapter 21)

Trade name given in parentheses.

(Continued.)

Drug*	Use	Form	Dose
Propranolol (Inderal)	Antiarrhythmic; β-antagonist; antihypertensive	**Inj:** 1 mg/mL; **Tab:** 10, 20, 40, 60, 80, 90 mg; **Sustained release cap:** 60, 80, 120, 160 mg	IV 1 mg q20min up to total of 0.15 mg/kg; PO 10–60 mg q.6h. (see Chapters 5 and 9)
Propylthiouracil	Antithyroid	**Tab:** 50 mg	(see Chapter 14)
Protamine sulfate	Heparin antagonist	**Inj:** 10 mg/mL	1 mg to reverse 90 U bovine heparin, 100 U porcine heparin (Ca²⁺), 115 U porcine heparin (Na⁺)
Quinidine sulfate (Quinidex)	Antiarrhythmic	**Inj:** 200 mg/mL; **Tab:** 100, 200, 300 mg; **Sustained release:** 300 mg	200–300 mg PO/IM t.i.d.–q.i.d. (see Chapter 5)
Ranitidine (Zantac)	H₂ antiulcer antagonist	**Inj:** 25 mg/mL; **Tab:** 150, 300 mg	150 mg PO q.12h.; 50 mg IV q.8h.
Sodium bicarbonate	Alkalinizing agent	**Amp:** 50 mEq/50 mL	(See Chapter 4)
Spironolactone (Aldactone)	Diuretic; anti-aldosterone	**Tab:** 25, 50, 100 mg	25–200 mg PO q.d.
Succinylcholine	Depolarizing neuromuscular blocking agent	**Inj:** 20 mg/mL	0.6–2.0 mg/kg IV (see Chapter 21)
Sucralfate (Carafate)	Antiulcer; cytoprotective	**Tab:** 1 g; **Solution:** 1 g/10 mL	1 g PO/via NG tube q.4h.

Sufentanil (Sufenta)	Analgesic	(see Chapter 21)
Terbutaline (Brethine)	Bronchodilator; β-agonist	**Inhaler:** 200 μg/dose; **Inj:** 1 mg/mL; **Tab:** 2.5, 5 mg	1–2 puffs q.4–6h.; 0.25–0.5 mg SC q.4h.; 5 mg PO q.6h.
Theophylline	Bronchodilator	**Inj** (aminophylline): 25 mg/mL; **Solution:** 80, 150 mg/15 mL; **Tab:** 100, 200, 300, 400 mg	**Load:** 6 mg/kg IV; **Infusion:** 0.6–0.9 mg/kg/hr; 5–8 mg/kg PO q.6–8h.
Thiopental	Induction agent		3–4 mg/kg IV (see Chapter 21)
Thioridazine (Mellaril)	Antipsychotic	**Tab:** 10, 15, 25, 50, 100, 150, 200 mg; **Susp:** 25, 100 mg/5 mL	50–250 mg PO t.i.d.
Thyroxine (Synthroid)	Hypothyroidism	**Inj:** 200, 500 μg/vial; **Tab:** 20, 50, 75, 100, 125, 150, 175, 200, 300 mg	100–200 μg/day; 200–500 μg IV for myxedema coma
Timolol (Blocadren)	Antihypertensive; β-antagonist	**Tab:** 5, 10, 20 mg	10–20 mg PO b.i.d.
Tocainide (Tonocard)	Antiarrhythmic	**Tab:** 400, 600 mg	400–800 mg PO q.8h.
Tolazamide (Tolinase)	Oral hypoglycemic	**Tab:** 100, 250, 500 mg	100–500 mg PO q.d.–b.i.d.
Triazolam (Halcion)	Hypnotic	**Tab:** 0.125, 0.25, 0.5 mg	0.125–0.5 mg PO q.h.s.
Trimethaphan (Arfonad)	Antihypertensive	**Inj:** 10 mg/mL (10mL)	3–4 mg/min (see Chapters 5 and 9)

*Trade names given in parentheses.

(Continued.)

Drug*	Use	Form	Dose
Vasopressin (Pitressin)	GI bleeding; diabetes insipidus	**Inj:** 20 units/mL; **Susp:** 5 units/mL	(For GI bleeding see Chapter 11; for DI see Chapter 14)
Verapamil (Isoptin)	Antiarrhythmic; calcium channel blocker	**Inj:** 5 mg/2 mL; **Tab:** 80, 120 mg; **Sustained release:** 240 mg	**Load:** 0.75–0.150 µg/kg; **Infusion:** 5 µg/kg/min; 40–80 mg PO q.6h. (see Chapter 5)
Vecuronium (Norcuron)	Nondepolarizing neuromuscular blocking agent	**Inj:** 1 – 2 mg/mL	0.1 mg/kg IV (see Chapter 21)
Warfarin (Coumadin)	Oral anticoagulant	**Tab:** 2, 2.5, 5, 7.5, 10 mg	5–15 mg q.d. (monitor prothrombin time)
Xylocaine (Lidocaine)	Antiarrhythmic	**Inj:** 40, 100, 200 mg/ml	**Load:** 1 mg/kg then 0.5 mg/kg in 5 min; **Infusion:** 1–4 mg/min

*Trade name given in parentheses.

BODY SURFACE NOMOGRAMS **A**

NOMOGRAM FOR THE DETERMINATION OF BODY SURFACE AREA OF CHILDREN AND ADULTS*

*From Way LW (ed): *Current Surgical Diagnosis and Treatment*, ed 7. Los Altos, Calif, Lange Medical Publications, 1985, p 1188. Used by permission.

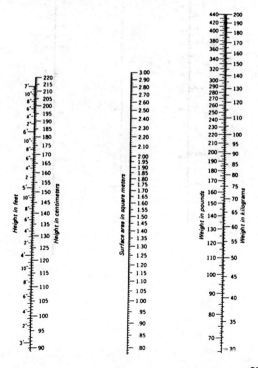

NOMOGRAM FOR THE DETERMINATION OF BODY SURFACE AREA OF CHILDREN*

*From Way LW (ed): *Current Surgical Diagnosis and Treatment*, ed 7. Los Altos, Calif, Lange Medical Publications, 1985, p 1188. Used by permission.

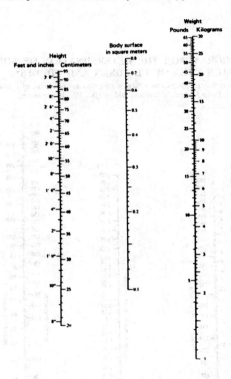

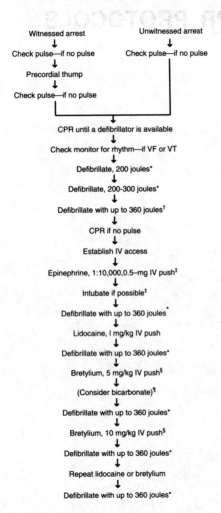

Witnessed arrest
↓
Check pulse—if no pulse
↓
Precordial thump
↓
Check pulse—if no pulse

Unwitnessed arrest
↓
Check pulse—if no pulse

↓

CPR until a defibrillator is available
↓
Check monitor for rhythm—if VF or VT
↓
Defibrillate, 200 joules*
↓
Defibrillate, 200-300 joules*
↓
Defibrillate with up to 360 joules†
↓
CPR if no pulse
↓
Establish IV access
↓
Epinephrine, 1:10,000, 0.5–mg IV push‡
↓
Intubate if possible‡
↓
Defibrillate with up to 360 joules*
↓
Lidocaine, I mg/kg IV push
↓
Defibrillate with up to 360 joules*
↓
Bretylium, 5 mg/kg IV push§
↓
(Consider bicarbonate)¶
↓
Defibrillate with up to 360 joules*
↓
Bretylium, 10 mg/kg IV push§
↓
Defibrillate with up to 360 joules*
↓
Repeat lidocaine or bretylium
↓
Defibrillate with up to 360 joules*

FIG B–1 (facing page).

Ventricular fibrillation (and pulseless ventricular tachycardia). This sequence was developed to assist in teaching how to treat a broad range of patients with ventricular fibrillation (VF) or pulseless ventricular tachycardia (VT). Some patients may require care not specified herein. This algorithm should not be construed as prohibiting such flexibility. Flow of algorithm presumes that VF is continuing. CPR indicates cardiopulmonary resuscitation. (Note: pulseless VT should be treated identically to VF.

*Check pulse and rhythm after each shock. If VF recurs after transiently converting (rather than persists without ever converting), use whatever energy level has previously been successful for defibrillation.

†Epinephrine should be repeated every five minutes.

‡Intubation is preferable. If it can be accomplished simultaneously with other techniques, then the earlier the better. However, defibrillation and epinephrine are more important initially if the patient can be ventilated without intubation.

§Some may prefer repeated doses of lidocaine, which may be given in 0.5-mg/kg boluses every eight minutes to a total dose of 3 mg/kg.

¶Value of sodium bicarbonate is questionable during cardiac arrest, and it is not recommended for routine cardiac arrest sequence. Consideration of its use in a dose of 1 mEq/kg is appropriate at this point. Half of original dose may be repeated every ten minutes if it is used. (From Albarran-Sotelo R, Atkins JM, Bloom RS, et al: *Textbook of Advanced Cardiac Life Support,* ed 2. Chicago, American Heart Association, 1987, p. 238. Used with permission.)

If rhythm is unclear and possibly ventricular
fibrillation, defibrillate as for VF.   If asystole is present*
↓
Continue CPR
↓
Establish IV access
↓
Epinephrine, 1:10,000, 0.5–mg IV push†
↓
Intubate when possible‡
↓
Atropine, l.0 mg IV push (repeated in 5 min)
↓
(Consider bicarbonate)§
↓
Consider pacing

FIG B–2.

Asystole (cardiac standstill). This sequence was developed to assist in teaching how to treat a broad range of patients with asystole. Some patients may require care not specified herein. This algorithm should not be construed to prohibit such flexibility. Flow of algorithm presumes asystole is continuing. VF indicates ventricular fibrillation; IV, intravenous.

*Asystole should be confirmed in two leads.

†Epinephrine should be repeated every five minutes.

‡Intubation is preferable; if it can be accomplished simultaneously with other techniques, then the earlier the better. However, cardiopulmonary resuscitation (CPR) and use of epinephrine are more important initially if patient can be ventilated without intubation. (Endotracheal epinephrine may be used.)

§Value of sodium bicarbonate is questionable during cardiac arrest, and it is not recommended for the routine cardiac arrest sequence. Consideration of its use in a dose of 1 mEq/kg is appropriate at this point. Half of original dose may be repeated every ten minutes if it is used. (From Albarran-Sotelo R, Atkins JM, Bloom RS, et al: *Textbook of Advanced Cardiac Life Support,* ed 2. Chicago, American Heart Association, 1987, p. 239. Used with permission.)

Continue CPR
↓
Establish IV access
↓
Epinephrine, 1:10,000, 0.5–mg IV push*
↓
Intubate when possible†
↓
(Consider bicarbonate)‡
↓
Consider hypovolemia,
cardiac tamponade,
tension pneumothorax,
hypoxemia,
acidosis,
pulmonary embolism

FIG B–3.
Electromechanical dissociation. This sequence was developed to assist in teaching how to treat a broad range of patients with electromechanical dissociation. Some patients may require care not specified herein. This algorithm should not be construed to prohibit such flexibility. Flow of algorithm presumes that electromechanical dissociation is continuing. CPR indicates cardiopulmonary resuscitation; IV, intravenous.

*Epinephrine should be repeated every five minutes.

†Intubation is preferable. If it can be accomplished simultaneously with other techniques, then the earlier the better. However, epinephrine is more important initially if the patient can be ventilated without intubation.

‡Value of sodium bicarbonate is questionable during cardiac arrest, and it is not recommended for routine cardiac arrest sequence. Consideration of its use in a dose of 1 mEq/kg is appropriate at this point. Half of original dose may be repeated every ten minutes if it is used. (From Albarran-Sotelo R, Atkins JM, Bloom RS, et al: *Textbook of Advanced Cardiac Life Support,* ed 2. Chicago, American Heart Association, 1987, p. 240. Used with permission.)

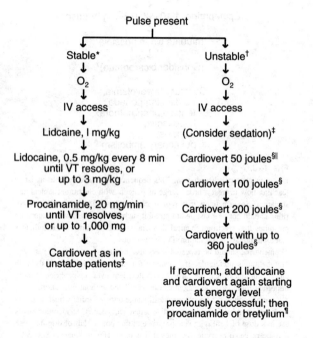

Pulse present

Stable* | Unstable†

Stable*:
- O₂
- IV access
- Lidcaine, I mg/kg
- Lidocaine, 0.5 mg/kg every 8 min until VT resolves, or up to 3 mg/kg
- Procainamide, 20 mg/min until VT resolves, or up to 1,000 mg
- Cardiovert as in unstabe patients‡

Unstable†:
- O₂
- IV access
- (Consider sedation)‡
- Cardiovert 50 joules§‖
- Cardiovert 100 joules§
- Cardiovert 200 joules§
- Cardiovert with up to 360 joules§
- If recurrent, add lidocaine and cardiovert again starting at energy level previously successful; then procainamide or bretylium¶

FIG B–4 (facing page).

Sustained ventricular tachycardia (VT). This sequence was developed to assist in teaching how to treat a broad range of patients with sustained VT. Some patients may require care not specified herein. This algorithm should not be construed as prohibiting such flexibility. Flow of algorithm presumes that VT is continuing. VF indicates ventricular fibrillation.

*If patient becomes unstable (see footnote b for definition) at any time, move to "Unstable" arm of algorithm.

†Unstable indicates symptoms (e.g., chest pain or dyspnea), hypotension (systolic blood pressure <90 mmHg), congestive heart failure, ischemia, or infarction.

‡Sedation should be considered for all patients, including those defined in footnote b as unstable, except those who are hemodynamically unstable (e.g., hypotensive, in pulmonary edema, or unconscious).

§If hypotension, pulmonary edema, or unconsciousness is present, unsynchronized cardioversion should be done to avoid delay associated with synchronization.

‖In the absence of hypotension, pulmonary edema, or unconsciousness, a precordial thump may be employed prior to cardioversion.

¶Once VT has resolved, begin intravenous (IV) infusion of antiarrhythmic agent that has aided resolution of VT. If hypotension, pulmonary edema, or unconsciousness is present, use lidocaine if cardioversion alone is unsuccessful, followed by bretylium. In all other patients, recommended order of therapy is lidocaine, procainamide, and then bretylium. (From Albarran-Sotelo R, Atkins JM, Bloom RS, et al: *Textbook of Advanced Cardiac Life Support,* ed 2. Chicago, American Heart Association, 1987, p. 241. Used with permission.)

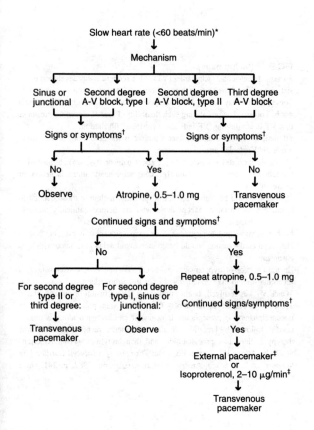

FIG B−5 (facing page).

Bradycardia. This sequence was developed to assist in teaching how to treat a broad range of patients with bradycardia. Some patients may require care not specified herein. This algorithm should not be construed to prohibit such flexibility. AV indicates atrioventricular.

*A solitary chest thump or cough may stimulate cardiac electrical activity and result in improved cardiac output and may be used at this point.

†Hypotension (blood pressure <90 mmHg), premature ventricular contractions, altered mental status or symptoms (e.g., chest pain or dyspnea), ischemia, or infarction.

‡Temporizing therapy. (From Albarran-Sotelo R, Atkins JM, Bloom RS, et al: *Textbook of Advanced Cardiac Life Support,* ed 2. Chicago, American Heart Association, 1987, p. 242. Used with permission.)

INDEX